PROGRESS IN BRAIN RESEARCH

VOLUME 115

BRAIN FUNCTION IN HOT ENVIRONMENT

PROGRESS IN BRAIN RESEARCH

VOLUME 115

BRAIN FUNCTION IN HOT ENVIRONMENT

EDITED BY

H.S. SHARMA AND J. WESTMAN

*Laboratory of Neuroanatomy, Department of Anatomy, Uppsala University Biomedical Centre,
S-751 23 Uppsala, Sweden*

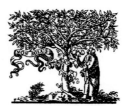

ELSEVIER

AMSTERDAM – LAUSANNE – NEW YORK – OXFORD – SHANNON – SINGAPORE – TOKYO

1998

ISBN 0-444-82377-8 (volume)
ISBN 0-444-80104-9 (series)

1001463408

Published by:
Elsevier Science B.V.
P.O. Box 211
1000 AE Amsterdam
The Netherlands

Library of Congress Cataloging in Publication Data
A catalog record from the Library of Congress has been applied for.

∞ The paper used in this publication meets the requirements of ANSI/NISO Z39.48-1992 (Permanence of Paper).

Printed in The Netherlands.

List of Contributors

P. Alm, Department of Pathology, University Hospital, Lund University, S-221 85 Lund, Sweden

C.M. Blatteis, Department of Physiology and Biophysics, University of Tennessee, Memphis, TN 38163, USA

J.A. Boulant, Department of Physiology, College of Medicine, Ohio State University, Columbus, OH 43210, USA

E. Bongcam-Rudloff, Department of Zoological Cell Biology, The Wenner-Gren Institute, University of Stockholm, S-712 34 Stockholm, Sweden

D.D. Breimer, Division of Pharmacology, Leiden/Amsterdam Center for Drug Research, Leiden University, Sylvius Laboratories, P.O. Box 9503, 2300 RA Leiden, The Netherlands

C. Cao, Department of Neuroscience, Osaka Bioscience Institute, Suita, Osaka 565, Japan

J. Cervós-Navarro, Institute of Neuropathology, Free University Berlin, Klinikum Steglitz, Hindenburgerdamm 30, D-12203 Berlin, Germany

X.-M. Chen, Department of Physiology, Osaka University Faculty of Medicine, Yamadaoka 2-2, Suita, Osaka 565, Japan

C.A. Conn, Lovelace Respiratory Research Institute, P.O. Box 5890, Albuquerque, NM 87185, USA, email: cconn@lrri.org

A.G. De Boer, Division of Pharmacology, Leiden/Amsterdam Center for Drug Research, Leiden University, Sylvius Laboratories, P.O. Box 9503, 2300 RA Leiden, The Netherlands

V. Fraifeld, Department of Clinical Pharmacology, Faculty of Health Sciences, Ben-Gurion University of the Negev, P.O. Box 653, Beer-Sheva 84105, Israel

T. Hori, Department of Physiology, Kyushu University Faculty of Medicine, Fukuoka 812-82, Japan, email: thori@physiol.med.kyushu-u.ac.jp

T. Hosono, Department of Physiology, Osaka University Faculty of Medicine, Yamadaoka 2-2, Suita, Osaka 565, Japan

M.C.C.M. Hulshof, Department of Radiotherapy, Academic Medical Center, University of Amsterdam, P.O. Box 22700, 1100 DE Amsterdam, The Netherlands

M. Iriki, Vice-President, Yamanashi Medical University, Tamaho, Nakakoma, Yamanashi 409-38, Japan

T. Itoh, Department of Physiology, Kyoto Prefectural University of Medicine, Kamigyo-ku, Kyoto 602, Japan

K. Kanosue, Department of Physiology, School of Allied Health Sciences, Osaka University Faculty of Medicine, Yamadaoka 1-7, Suita, 565 Osaka, Japan, email: kanosue@sahs. med.osaka-u.ac.jp

J. Kaplanski, Department of Clinical Pharmacology, Faculty of Health Sciences, Ben-Gurion University of the Negev, P.O. Box 653, Beer-Sheva 84105, Israel

T. Katafuchi, Department of Physiology, Kyushu University Faculty of Medicine, Fukuoka 812-82, Japan

M.J. Kluger, Lovelace Respiratory Research Institute, P.O. Box 5890, Albuquerque, NM 87185, USA, email: mkluger@lrri.org

W. Kozak, Lovelace Respiratory Research Institute, P.O. Box 5890, Albuquerque, NM 87185, USA, email: wkozak@lrri.org

L.R. Leon, Lovelace Respiratory Research Institute, P.O. Box 5890, Albuquerque, NM 87185, USA, email: lleon@lrri.org

P. Lomax, School of Medicine, University of California, Los Angeles, CA 90024, USA or corresponding address: 25 Avenue du Soleil d'Or, 06230 Villefranche-sur-Mer, France

C.D.P. Lynch, Department of Neurology, University of Otago, Dunedin Hospital, P.O. Box 913, Dunedin, New Zealand

K. Matsumura, Department of Neuroscience, Osaka Bioscience Institute, Suita, Osaka 565, Japan

A.S. Milton, Department of Pharmacology, University of Cambridge, Tennis Court Road, Cambridge CB2, 1QJ, UK

T. Morimoto, Department of Physiology, Kyoto Prefectural University of Medicine, Kamigyo-ku, Kyoto 602, Japan, email: morimoto@phys.kpu-m.ac.jp

F. Nyberg, Department of Pharmaceutical Biosciences, Division of Biological Research on Drug Dependence, Biomedical Centre, Uppsala University, S-751 23 Uppsala, Sweden

U. Pehl, Max-Planck-Institute for Physiological and Clinical Research, W.G. Kerckhoff-Institute, Parkstrasse 1, D-61231 Bad Nauheim, Germany

F.-K. Pierau, Max-Planck-Institute for Physiological and Clinical Research, W.G. Kerckhoff-Institute, Parkstrasse 1, D-61231 Bad Nauheim, Germany, email: fpierau@kerckhoff.mpg.de

M. Pollock, Department of Neurology, Department of Medicine, University of Otago Medical School, P.O. Box 913, Dunedin, New Zealand, email: jan.kettink@stonebow.otago.ac.nz

W. Riedel, Max-Planck-Institute, W.G. Kerckhoff-Institute, Parkstrasse 1, D-61231 Bad Nauheim, Germany

A.A. Romanovsky, Director, Thermoregulation Laboratory, Legacy Holladay Park Medical Center, Portland, OR 97208-3950, USA, email: aromanov@lhs.org

J. Roth, Physiologisches Institut, Klinikum der Justus-Liebig-Universität Giessen, Aulweg 129, 35392 Giessen, Germany, email: eugen.zeisberger@physiologie.med.uni-giessen.de

T. Saigusa, Yamanashi Medical University, Tamaho, Nakakoma, Yamanashi 409-38, Japan

H. Sann, Max-Planck-Institute for Physiological and Clinical Research, W.G. Kerckhoff-Institute, Parkstrasse 1, D-61231 Bad Nauheim, Germany

H.A. Schmid, Max-Planck-Institute for Physiological and Clinical Research, W.G. Kerckhoff-Institute, Parkstrasse 1, D-61231 Bad Nauheim, Germany, email: hschmid@kerckhoff.mpg.de

E. Schönbaum, Department of Medical Pharmacology, LACDR, Leiden State University, Leiden, The Netherlands

H.S. Sharma, Department of Anatomy, Laboratory of Neuroanatomy, Biomedical Centre, P.O. Box 571, S-751 23 Uppsala, Sweden, email: Sharma@anatomi.uu.se

R.R. Shivers, Department of Zoology, University of Western Ontario, London, Ont. N6A 5B7, Canada, email: rshrivers@julian.uwo.ca

E. Simon, Max-Planck-Institute, W.G. Kerckhoff-Institute, Parkstrasse 1, D-61231 Bad Nauheim, Germany

P. Sminia, Department of Radiotherapy, Academic Medical Center, University of Amsterdam, P.O. Box 22700, 1100 DE Amsterdam, The Netherlands, email: p.sminia@amc.uva.nl

D. Soszynski, Department of Physiology, University School of Medical Science, 24 Karlowicza Street, PL-85-092 Bydgoszcz, Poland, email: darek@aci.amb.bydgoszcz.pl

A. Takamata, Department of Physiology, Kyoto Prefectural University of Medicine, Kamigyo-ku, Kyoto 602, Japan

Yasuyoshi Watanabe, Department of Neuroscience, Osaka Bioscience Institute, Suita, Osaka 565, Japan

Yumiko Watanabe, Subfemtomole Biorecognition Project, Research Development Corporation, Osaka, Japan

J. Westman, Uppsala Experimental CNS Injury Group, Department of Anatomy, Laboratory of Neuroanatomy, Biomedical Centre, P.O. Box 571, Uppsala University, S-751 23 Uppsala, Sweden

J.A. Wijsman, Department of Zoology, University of Western Ontario, London, Ont. N6A 5B7, Canada

K.S. Yakimova, Max-Planck-Institute for Physiological and Clinical Research, W.G. Kerckhoff-Institute, Parkstrasse 1, D-61231 Bad Nauheim, Germany

E. Zeisberger, Physiologisches Institut, Klinikum der Justus-Liebig-Universität Giessen, Aulweg 129, 35392 Giessen, Germany, email: eugen.zeisberger@physiologie.med.uni-giessen.de

Y.-H. Zhang, Department of Physiology, Osaka University Faculty of Medicine, Yamadaoka 2-2, Suita, Osaka 565, Japan

Preface

The new challenge of global warming on the biological system has recently received wide attention in scientific literature. However, the influence of heat as a physiological or pathological stimulus on the structure and function of the nervous system is largely ignored.

Hyperthermia is a common problem frequently encountered in everyday life due to fever associated with bacterial or viral infections. The major cause of hyperthermia is associated with heat stress and heat-related illness due to exposure at high environmental temperature particularly during hot summer seasons in many parts of the globe. The other common cause of hyperthermia is due to radiotherapy of tumours in combination with whole body heating and/or ionizing radiation. This therapy poses a great danger to normal tissue while making an attempt to kill the tumour cell by local heat treatment.

To our knowledge, this is the first book which deals with the influence of brain function in hot environment in great detail ranging from molecular biology to behavioural neurosciences. This book is a refereed collection of 24 chapters written by several eminent scientists from different disciplines engaged in basic and applied research in the CNS from various parts of the world.

The book is divided into five sections. Section I deals in five chapters, with basic aspects of thermoregulation. Thermal pathways in the CNS are still a matter of considerable research and are usually described with touch and pressure sensation. Recent research on thermal sensitive and insensitive neurones in the CNS provides a new role of temperature sensitive neurons in the mechanism of thermoregulation. The current thinking on temperature sensitive neurons in hypothalamus is summarised in Chapter 1 (Boulant). In Chapter 2 (Hori and Katafuchi), a critical overview of new knowledge and the cell biology of thermosensitive neurones is presented. Chapter 3 (Simon et al.) deals with thermosensitive neurons in the spinal cord based on both in vivo and in vitro findings in relation to hypothalamic neuronal thermosensitivity. However, apart from thermosensitive neurons in the CNS, body temperature is regulated by multiple thermoregulatory effectors distributed throughout the body and controlled by 'neuronal networks'. Chapter 4 (Kanosue et al.) reviews the current concepts of neuronal network controlling thermoregulatory effectors and provides some new emerging concepts in this field. There is recent evidence that the distribution of temperature sensitive and insensitive neurons is influenced by long-term adaptation in ambient temperature showing plasticity of the hypothalamic neuronal network. In Chapter 5 (Pierau et al.), current concepts of neuronal plasticity among hypothalamic temperature sensitive neurons is reviewed and new experimental evidence is presented.

In Section II, the pharmacology of thermoregulation is covered in seven chapters. Research on the pharmacology of thermoregulation in the last 25 years suggests the involvement of several neurochemicals in the basic mechanisms of thermoregulation.

However, this subject is expanding rapidly and the new role of many other factors influencing neuronal communication, signal transduction and immune system in influencing thermoregulation is emerging. Nitric oxide (NO) is one such recently discovered free radical gaseous molecule which is capable of influencing neuronal communication and signal transduction mechanisms in the CNS (Dawson and Snyder, 1994). Chapter 6 (Schmid et al.) presents some new evidence regarding the involvement of NO in temperature regulation in the light of recent experimental findings. In the CNS, however, a large number of neurochemicals such as opioids, prostaglandins and biogenic amines are involved in the mechanisms of neurotransmission and thermoregulation. The opioid peptides are often co-localised with many other neurotransmitters in the CNS and are now known to be involved in various physiological and pathological processes (Hökfelt et al., 1987). Recently, their role in influencing thermoregulation has also emerged. Chapter 7 (Romanovsky and Blatteis) reviews the current concepts of opioids in hyperthermia and provides new evidence indicating that opioid antagonists can be useful in treatment of several hyperthermic states in clinical conditions in the near future. The other most important mediator of fever is prostaglandin (Dey et al., 1974). However the detailed mechanisms of prostaglandin-induced fever is still unclear. Chapter 8 (Milton) updates this knowledge and describes the new concepts in this challenging subject. Further evidence regarding the involvement of prostaglandins in fever is presented in Chapter 9 (Fraifeld and Kaplanski) which describes the influence of age and species on brain eicosanoids production in fever based on new experimental evidence. The concept of biogenic amines in fever is still valid and some new research has been done in the recent past. Chapter 10 (Zeisberger) reviews the current state of knowledge regarding involvement of biogenic amines in temperature regulation and provides some new evidence. In view of the emerging role of immunomodulators and their interaction with the neuroendocrine system in temperature regulation, Chapter 11 (Roth) provides some new evidence in this rapidly advancing field and describes the immunological and neuroendocrine modulation of fever in stress. Recently, some data suggest that the influence of drugs can be modified in the biological system in hot environments. Thus it is very important to understand the basic mechanisms of altered drug metabolism in the CNS during hyperthermic states. Chapter 12 (Lomax and Schönbaum) provides new data which suggest that the drug metabolism is somehow influenced in hyperthermic states. On the basis of this new information, one may speculate that the drug metabolism is altered in hyperthermia. However, this is entirely a new subject which requires further investigation.

Section III is devoted to new molecular aspects of brain function in hyperthermic states and is represented by four chapters. The molecular mechanisms involved or affected during hyperthermia in the CNS are not well known. Heat shock proteins (HSP), as the name implies, are the most sensitive markers of cellular stress caused by hyperthermia. However, the functional significance of HSP expression in the CNS during hyperthermic states is not well characterised. Thus, it is not yet certain whether the upregulation of HSP in various disease conditions may represent a sign of cellular stress or whether this induction has something to do with neuroprotection. Chapter 13 (Westman and Sharma) describes the current concepts of HSP expression in the CNS and its functional significance in hyperthermia in view of the new experimental findings. Interestingly, nerve cells in the CNS are the main focus of current research activity in the field of hyperthermia or thermoregulation. Although glial cells outnumber neurons and are known to participate actively in CNS homeostasis, their role in thermoregulation is still unknown. Chapter 14 (Cervós-Navarro et al.) reviews the current concepts of glia cells in modulating brain function and provides new experimental evidence which supports the idea that glial cells are one of the most sensitive indicators in the CNS during hyperthermia-induced brain damage. The detailed molecular mechanisms of brain dysfunction caused by various neurotransmitter and neuromodulator substances are still unclear. With the discovery of new molecular markers of brain function, the involvement of various neurotransmitters and their receptors in the CNS can now be well characterised. Using these new techniques, Chapter 15 (Matsumura et al.) describes the involvement of prostaglandin biosynthesis and their receptor sites in the CNS during normal and hyperthermic states. In general, during any disease or experimental condition, no single chemical compound is responsible for all the pathological disturbances seen in the CNS. Thus, it appears that many more neurochemicals/factors are contributing simultaneously to such disease processes. The recently identified gaseous molecules NO and CO (carbon monoxide) thus seem to participate in the brain pathology caused by trauma and ischemia. However, their role in hyperthermia-induced brain dysfunction is not yet known. Chapter 16 (Sharma et al.) reviews the current concepts of NO and CO in brain function and provides new experimental data which support the idea that these molecules are actively engaged in the brain pathology of heat stress.

The pathophysiological aspects of hyperthermia-induced cellular alteration are described in Section IV which contains five chapters. One of the common causes of brain pathology in heat stress is due to local heat treatment of tumour cells in the CNS. However this procedure also induces damage in normal brain cells resulting in many other neurological or behavioural symptoms (Britt et al., 1983). Thus, further research is required in this important area in order to improve the techniques for routine clinical use. Chapter 17 (Sminia and Hulshof) reviews the present status of new knowledge in this field and provides some new ideas in this exciting subject.

The pathological aspect of hyperthermia and heat-related illnesses in humans has been known since Biblical times (Judith 8: 2–3). Sporadic reports in the literature often deal with heat-induced death in the human population. Scientific reports on this subject date back to 1743 when 11 000 people died in China during hot weather conditions in July. Another incidence of heat death was recorded in 1841 in Liverpool, when 33 British soldiers died in one day due to hot weather in a ship sailing from Muscat to Bushier. Similarly, during 1873 in the 'Black Hole of Calcutta', 123 out of 186 British prisoners died in one night (Wakefield and Hall, 1929). This heat-induced death is still prominent in many parts of the World. Thus, in the Netherlands, about 1000 deaths due to hot weather in 1996 occurred in nursing homes in Rotterdam (*The Lancet* 1997, 349: 1297–1298). About 700 people died in 1995 due to hot weather conditions in Chicago during summer months. In many heat deaths, the CNS damage is largely ignored because most emphasis is placed on cardiovascular and renal damage as the principal cause of death. In one classical study of 125 fatal cases, Malamud et al. (1946) described the histopathology of brain in some detail using routine histological techniques available at that time. This indicates that the brain is an important organ susceptible to heat-induced damage. However, even 50 years after this report, new studies on the probable cause of brain damage in heat stress are not available and the mechanisms responsible for brain injury in heat stress still remain uncertain. It appears that breakdown of the blood–brain barrier (BBB) permeability in heat stress (Sharma and Dey, 1987) contributes to the mechanism of vasogenic edema formation and cell changes in the brain. Chapter 18 (Sharma et al.) reviews the current concepts of edema formation and provides new experimental evidence indicating a prominent role of BBB in edema formation and structural damage in the CNS using newly available morphological techniques in an experimental model of heat stress. Further evidence in this line is provided in Chapter 19 (Shivers and Wijsman) which confirms that hyperthermia in anaesthetised mice can lead to an increase in the permeability of the BBB to the protein tracer, horseradish peroxidase, visualised at the ultrastructural level. The other way of understanding the role of BBB in hyperthermia is to test the ability of several endogenous compounds known to be involved in fever and to study their influence on the breakdown of BBB permeability. Chapter 20 (De Boer and Breimer) provides new experimental evidence that cytokines, an endogenous molecule influencing fever and thermoregulation, can indeed increase the BBB transport of many substances. However, CNS is not the only organ vulnerable to heat-induced damage. Recent reports suggest that hyperthermia can also induce profound damage to the peripheral nervous system (PNS). Like CNS, the PNS is also equipped with the blood–nerve barrier (BNB) similar to the BBB and changes of permeability is mediated by several neurochemical mediators (Olsson, 1990). In Chapter 21 (Lynch and Pollock) this aspect is reviewed briefly and new ideas on thermal nerve injury are presented.

Section V is based on the clinical aspects of hyperthermia and contains three chapters. In recent years the clinical significance of hyperthermia and thermoregulation has attracted great attention. With the identification of the various endogenous antipyretics or cryogens, current interest in endogenous compounds involved in the mechanisms of fever and antipyresis has increased tremendously among clinicians. Chapter 22 (Kluger et al.) reviews the concept of fever and antipyresis in the light of current research in this rapidly advancing field. Nowadays, the sympathetic nervous system is regarded as one of the most important mediators between central temperature control and peripheral heat production mechanisms. Chapter 23 (Iriki and Saigusa) reviews the current knowledge regarding involvement of sympathetic efferents in fever in the light of new data. In view of the recent clinical significance attached to body fluid homeostasis in temperature regulation as well as in many diseases processes, Chapter 24 (Morimoto et al.) reviews the present concepts in the field and provides new information on body fluid homeostasis in hot environments.

We hope that the new aspects of brain function in hot environment compiled in this volume will provide an up-to-date ready reference which may serve as a strong scientific stimulus to many workers in this emerging field of neuroscience to explore the subject with novel ideas and/or experimental and clinical approaches in future.

Hari Shanker Sharma and Jan Westman

References

Britt, R.H., Lyons, B.E., Pounds, D.W. and Prionas, S.D. (1983) Feasibility of ultrasound hyperthermia in the treatment of malignant brain tumours. *Med. Instrum.*, 17: 172–177.

Dawson, T.M. and Snyder, S.H. (1994) Gases as biological messengers: nitric oxide and carbon monoxide in the brain. *J. Neurosci.*, 14: 5147–5159.

Dey, P.K., Feldberg, W., Gupta, K.P., Milton, A.S. and Wendlandt, S. (1974) Further studies on the role of prostaglandins in fever. *J. Physiol. (Lond.)*, 241: 639–646.

Hökfelt, T., Johansson, O., Holets, V., Meister, B. and Melander, T. (1987) Distribution of neuropeptides with special reference to their coexistence with classical neurotransmitters. In: H.Y. Meltzer (Ed.), *Psychopharmacology: The Third Generation of Progress*, Raven Press, New York, pp. 401–416.

Malamud, N., Haymaker, M.W. and Custer, R.P. (1946) Heat stroke. A clinico-pathologic study of 125 cases. *Milit. Surg.*, 99: 397–449.

Olsson, Y. (1990) Microenvironment of the peripheral nervous system under normal and pathological conditions. *Crit. Rev. Neurobiol.*, 5: 265–311.

Sharma, H.S. and Dey, P.K. (1987) Influence of long-term acute heat exposure on regional blood–brain barrier permeability, cerebral blood flow and 5-HT level in conscious normotensive young rats. *Brain Res.*, 424: 153–162.

Wakefield, E.G. and Hall, W.W. (1929) Heat injuries: A preparatory study for experimental heat stroke. *J. Am. Med. Assoc.*, 89: 92–95.

Contents

SECTION I

Basic aspects

H.S. Sharma and J. Westman (Eds.)
Progress in Brain Research, Vol 115

CHAPTER 1

Cellular mechanisms of temperature sensitivity in hypothalamic neurons

J.A. Boulant

Department of Physiology, College of Medicine, The Ohio State University, Columbus, OH 43210, USA

In warm and cool environments, neural structures in the septum and rostral hypothalamus are important in the regulation of body temperature. This is especially true of the preoptic region and anterior hypothalamus (PO/AH). In thermode-implanted animals, local changes in PO/AH temperature evoke a variety of thermoregulatory responses that are appropriate both for the species and for the environmental conditions (Boulant, 1980, 1996). PO/AH warming, for example, can produce an increase in skin blood flow, along with an increase in evaporative heat loss due to panting or sweating. In addition to physiological responses, PO/AH warming can also evoke behavioral responses, such as moving to a cooler environment or postural changes that facilitate heat loss. PO/AH cooling, on the other hand, elicits skin vasoconstriction, along with behavioral heat retention responses to conserve body heat. PO/AH cooling also produces heat production responses that increase metabolic rate. Besides shivering, these heat production responses include non-shivering thermogenesis initiated by metabolic endocrines and sympathetic activation of brown adipose tissue.

All of these thermoregulatory responses are controlled by certain PO/AH neurons, many of which are sensitive to changes in temperature. Both *in vivo* and *in vitro* electrophysiological studies classify the majority of PO/AH neurons as temperature insensitive (Boulant and Dean,

1986). As illustrated in Fig. 1A, temperature insensitive neurons show little or no change in their firing rates when hypothalamic temperature is changed. When neuronal firing rate (impulses/s) is plotted as a function of temperature, the thermal coefficient or slope (impulses/s/°C) is the criterion for thermosensitivity. Temperature insensitive neurons can be divided into two subcategories (Boulant, 1996). As shown in Fig. 1A, low-slope temperature insensitive neurons show almost no change in their firing rate, even when temperature is changed several degrees. These neurons have thermal coefficients of 0.2 impulses/s/°C or less. Other neurons are classified as moderate slope temperature insensitive and show only slight increases in their firing rates during warming. Moderate-slope temperature insensitive neurons have thermal coefficients greater than 0.2 but less than 0.8 impulses/s/°C.

In contrast to the temperature insensitive neurons, about 30% of PO/AH neurons are considered to be warm sensitive (Boulant and Dean, 1986). As shown in Fig. 1B, these neurons dramatically increase their firing rates during hypothalamic warming or decrease their firing rates during hypothalamic cooling. Warm sensitive neurons have thermal coefficients of 0.8 impulses/s/°C or more. Also, there is a very small population of PO/AH cold sensitive neurons whose firing rates increase during hypothalamic cooling or decrease during hypothalamic warming.

4

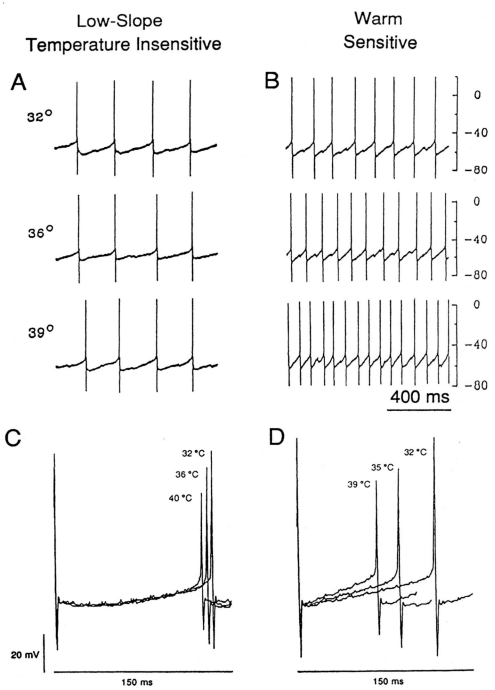

Low-Slope
Temperature Insensitive

Warm
Sensitive

Fig. 1. Effect of temperature on the firing rate, interspike interval, and depolarizing prepotential of two types of PO/AH neurons: temperature insensitive neurons (A and C) and warm sensitive neurons (B and D). A and B show one-second records at three different temperatures; and C and D show superimposed records of individual action potentials and subsequent depolarizing prepotential and action potential. Both types of neurons display depolarizing prepotentials, and action potentials occur when the prepotentials reach threshold. In warm sensitive neurons, warming increases the prepotential's rate of depolarization which shortens the interspike interval and increases the firing rate. In both types of neurons, warming decreases the amplitudes of the action potentials [adapted from Griffin, Kaple, Chow and Boulant (Griffin and Boulant, 1995) reprinted with kind permission of The Physiological Society, London, UK].

These neurons may not be intrinsically thermosensitive, but rather, they appear to be synaptically inhibited by nearby warm sensitive neurons (Boulant, 1980, 1996).

In addition to sensing changes in their own core temperature, many of the thermosensitive neurons in the PO/AH receive synaptic input from pathways relaying afferent information about skin and spinal cord temperature (Boulant and Hardy, 1974). Accordingly, these PO/AH thermosensitive neurons integrate peripheral and central thermal information, allowing them to evoke thermoregulatory responses that are appropriate for different environmental conditions. This chapter summarizes recent electrophysiological studies in rat hypothalamic slices addressing the cellular mechanisms that determine differences between warm sensitive and temperature insensitive neurons.

Cellular mechanisms of neuronal thermosensitivity are best studied *in vitro*. Whole-cell recordings in hypothalamic tissue slices permit the intracellular activity of neurons to be examined free from anesthesia and without afferent input. Previous *in vitro* studies have shown that hypothalamic slices contain the same proportions of neuronal types as found *in vivo*; and, of the spontaneously firing PO/AH neurons, more than 60% are temperature insensitive, about 30% are warm sensitive, and less than 10% are cold-sensitive (Boulant and Hardy, 1974; Kelso et al., 1982; Boulant and Dean, 1986; Dean and Boulant, 1989a). Some studies have also perfused the tissue slices with media that block all synaptic activity (Hori et al., 1980; Kelso and Boulant, 1982; Dean and Boulant, 1989b); and these synaptic blockade studies indicate that most PO/AH warm sensitive neurons have inherent, cellular mechanisms that determine their thermosensitivity. Subsequent studies with intracellular recordings have explored the mechanisms for this inherent thermosensitivity (Griffin and Boulant, 1995; Griffin et al., 1996).

One of the more controversial issues regarding neuronal thermosensitivity is the role of resting membrane potential. Early studies of invertebrate neurons (Gorman and Marmor, 1970; Carpenter, 1981) and recent studies of mammalian hypothalamic neurons (Nakashima et al., 1989; Kiyohara et al., 1990; Kobayashi and Takahashi, 1993) suggest that thermally-induced changes in membrane potential are the primary mechanisms for neuronal warm-sensitivity and cold-sensitivity. These studies imply, for example, that some neurons depolarize during warming and hyperpolarize during cooling, thus producing the warm-induced increases in firing rate and cold-induced decreases in firing rate that are observed in warm sensitive neurons. Unfortunately, this hypothesis is not supported by recent intracellular studies using sharp-tip (Curras et al., 1991) or whole-cell recordings (Griffin and Boulant, 1995; Griffin et al., 1996) in rat hypothalamic slices. Fig. 1B shows the action potentials and membrane potential of a warm sensitive neuron recorded with a whole-cell patch microelectrode. In this neuron, warming caused the firing rate to increase, but there was no change in the underlying resting membrane potential.

This finding raises an important question: why did other intracellular studies suggest that membrane potential is the basis of neuronal thermosensitivity? Answers to this question come from a recent study (Griffin and Boulant, 1995) that identified certain conditions in previous studies that produce erroneous thermally-induced changes in membrane potential. These errors occur: (1) when holding current is injected in a recorded neuron and (2) when the ground electrode is exposed to temperature changes.

1. Because temperature changes the input resistance of all neurons, if a holding current is applied, the resulting 'holding potential' will change with temperature. The diagram in Fig. 2 shows that injected negative current produces concomitant hyperpolarization of the membrane; and a neuron's input resistance is represented by the slope of this current-voltage plot (i.e. $R = V/I$). All neurons show similar thermal changes in their input resistance; resistance increases during cooling and decreases during warming (Curras et al., 1991; Griffin and Boulant, 1995; Boulant, 1996). In the example in Fig. 2, warming from 36°C to

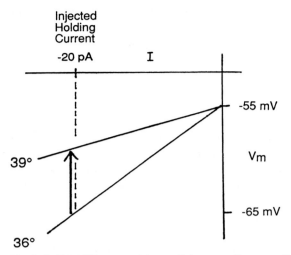

Fig. 2. In PO/AH neuronal intracellular recordings, negative current injections (I) produce comparable hyperpolarizations in the membrane potential (V_m). Input resistance is determined by the slope of this current-voltage plot, and all neurons display decreased resistance (or slope) during warming. These plots converge near resting membrane potential (e.g. -55 mV); and when no holding current is injected, temperature has minimal effects on V_m. This is not the case, however, when a holding current is applied. At 36°C, a negative holding current may be injected to produce hyperpolarization of V_m; however, because resistance decreases during warming, there is a relative depolarization (indicated by the upward arrow) when temperature changes from 36°C to 39°C [adapted from Griffin, Kaple, Chow and Boulant (Griffin and Boulant, 1995), reprinted with kind permission of The Physiological Society, London, UK].

39°C decreases the resistance (slope), but it causes no change in the -55 mV resting membrane potential (i.e. when there is no injected current). On the other hand, if a -20 pA holding current is applied, the neuron becomes hyperpolarized, and the measured membrane potential may be -65 mV at 36°C. If this 'current injected' neuron is then warmed to 39°C, there is an apparent depolaraization (indicated by the upward arrow) simply because of the decreased input resistance. It is likely that some previous studies have erroneously identified this as a mechanism for warm-sensitivity.

2. Tip potentials are recorded with all micro-

electrodes. These recorded potentials are affected by temperature in high resistance electrodes, particularly if the grounding electrode is not isolated from the temperature changes (Purves, 1981). These temperature effects are minimal if whole-cell electrodes are used and the ground electrode is maintained at a constant temperature. However, temperature can cause substantial changes in the recorded tip potential if high resistance, sharp-tip microelectrodes are used and the temperature of the ground electrode is allowed to change (Griffin and Boulant, 1995). Since these conditions existed in earlier studies, they are another likely source of error in the conclusions of these studies.

If neuronal thermosensitivity is not due to changes in resting potential, it is likely that the basis of this sensitivity rests in the effect of temperature on transient potentials that determine the interspike interval between successive action potentials. As indicated in Fig. 1, an important transient potential is the depolarizing prepotential that precedes each spontaneous action potential. This prepotential occurs in both temperature insensitive neurons (Fig. 1A,C) and warm sensitive neurons (Fig. 1B,D); however, there are differences between these two types of neurons in the conductances that determine the prepotentials. Warming increases the rate of depolarization in warm sensitive neurons (Fig. 1D) but not in temperature insensitive neurons (Fig. 1B) (Curras et al., 1991; Griffin et al., 1996).

The effect of temperature on the prepotential's depolarization determines whether or not the interspike interval (and thus, the firing rate) will change. For a warm sensitive neuron at three different temperatures, Fig. 1D shows the superimposed action potentials and subsequent depolarizing prepotentials that lead to the next action potentials. In this neuron, warming increased the prepotential's rate of depolarization; and this shortened the interspike interval between action potentials, leading to an increased firing rate. In contrast, Fig. 1C shows that temperature has no effect on the rate of depolarization in prepotentials of a low-slope temperature insensitive neuron; and accordingly, interspike intervals and firing rate remain constant when the neuron is warmed or cooled.

Although depolarizing prepotentials occur in both warm sensitive neurons and temperature insensitive neurons, a recent study (Griffin et al., 1996) suggests that there are neuronal differences in the ionic conductances underlying these prepotentials. The prepotentials may be due to increased depolarizing conductances (e.g. inward Na^+ or Ca^{2+}), or they may be due to decreasing hyperpolarizing conductances (e.g. inactivation of outward K^+ (Pahapill and Schlichter, 1990; Hille, 1992). In one intracellular study (Griffin et al., 1996), brief -50 pA current injections were given at different times during the interspike interval. Since $V = IR$, measured voltage drops show the relative changes in resistance at different times during this brief interval. In the temperature insensitive neurons, resistance remained constant during the interspike interval. Resistance is the inverse of conductance. Since the net ionic conductance (i.e. resistance^{-1}) did not change, this indicates that the prepotential of temperature insensitive neurons may be due to a constant conductance or to a combination of both increasing depolarizing conductances and decreasing hyperpolarizing conductances. In warm sensitive neurons, however, resistance increased (and conductance decreased) as the prepotential depolarized, suggesting that much of the prepotential is due to a decrease in hyperpolarizing (K^+) current, rather than an increase in depolarizing (Na^+ and Ca^{2+}) currents. Therefore, the prepotentials of warm sensitive neurons are more dependent on inactivation of outward K^+ conductances, while the prepotentials of temperature insensitive neurons appear to depend on a more balanced combination of inward and outward conductances.

These intracellular studies reveal cellular mechanisms of neuronal thermosensitivity, which are important to our understanding the hypothalamic control of body temperature during both short-term and long-term heat exposures. Any conditions that change temperature's effect on the ionic conductances or on the depolarizing prepotential have the capacity to drastically alter the ability of PO/AH neurons to respond to central and peripheral temperature. A variety of conditions present the opportunity for intracellular messengers to alter conductances underlying the prepotential. These conditions include both short-term events associated with synaptic activity, as well as long-term events associated with circadian rhythm and adaption to heat and exercise. The influence of these events on intracellular mediators determines the temperature sensitivity of PO/AH neurons; and this, in turn, determines the ability of the hypothalamus to evoke thermoregulatory responses that are appropriate for different thermal environments.

Acknowledgements

Most of the research described in this chapter was supported by NIH grant NS14644. J.A. Boulant is the Hitchcock Professor of Environmental Physiology.

References

Boulant, J.A. (1980) Hypothalamic control of thermoregulation: neurophysiological basis. In: P.J. Morgane and J. Panksepp (Eds.), *Handbook of the Hypothalamus: Behavioral Studies of the Hypothalamus*, Vol. 3, part A, Dekker, New York, pp. 1–82.

Boulant, J.A. (1996) Hypothalamic neurons regulating body temperature. In: M.J. Fregly and C.M. Blatteis (Eds.), *APS Handbook of Physiology*, section 4 *Environmental Physiology*, Oxford University Press, New York, pp. 105–126.

Boulant, J.A. and Dean, J.B. (1986) Temperature receptors in the central nervous system. *Annu. Rev. Physiol.*, 48: 639–654.

Boulant, J.A. and Hardy, J.D. (1974) The effect of spinal and skin temperatures on the firing rate and local thermosensitivity of preoptic neurons. *J. Physiol. (Lond.)*, 216: 1371–1374.

Carpenter, D.O. (1981) Ionic and metabolic bases of neuronal thermosensitivity. *Fed. Proc.*, 40: 2808–2813.

Curras, M.C., Kelso, S.R. and Boulant, J.A. (1991) Intracellular analysis of inherent and synaptic activity in hypothalamic thermosensitive neurones in the rat. *J. Physiol. (Lond.)*, 440: 257–271.

8

Dean, J.B. and Boulant, J.A. (1989a) *In vitro* localization of thermosensitive neurons in the rat diencephalon. *Am. J. Physiol.*, 257: R57–R64.

Dean, J.B. and Boulant, J.A. (1989b) Effects of synaptic blockade on thermosensitive neurons in rat diencephalon *in vitro*. *Am. J. Physiol.*, 257: R65–R73.

Gorman, A.L.F. and Marmor, M.F. (1970) Temperature dependence of the sodium potassium permeability ratio of a molluscan neurone. *J. Physiol. (Lond.)*, 210: 919–931.

Griffin, J.D. and Boulant, J.A. (1995) Temperature effects on membrane potential and input resistance in rat hypothalamic neurones. *J. Physiol. (Lond.)*, 488: 407–418.

Griffin, J.D., Kaple, M.L., Chow, A.R. and Boulant, J.A. (1996) Cellular mechanisms for neuronal thermosensitivity in the rat hypothalamus. *J. Physiol. (Lond.)*, 492: 231–242.

Hille, B. (1992) *Ionic Channels of Excitable Membranes*, Sinauer Assoc. Inc., Sunderland, MA, pp. 116–121.

Hori, T., Nakashima, T., Kiyohara, T., Shibata, M. and Hori, N. (1980) Effect of calcium removal on thermosensitivity of preoptic neurons in hypothalamic slices. *Neurosci. Lett.*, 20: 171–175.

Kelso, S.R. and Boulant, J.A. (1982) Effect of synaptic blockade on thermosensitive neurons in hypothalamic tissue slices. *Am. J. Physiol.*, 243: R480–R490.

Kelso, S.R., Perlmutter, M.N. and Boulant, J.A. (1982) Thermosensitive single-unit activity of *in vitro* hypothalamic slices. *Am. J. Physiol.*, 242: R77–R84.

Kiyohara, T., Hirata, M., Hori, T. and Akaike, N. (1990) Hypothalamic warm-sensitive neurons possess a tetrodotoxin-sensitive channel with a high Q_{10}. *Neurosci. Res.*, 8: 48–53.

Kobayashi, S. and Takahashi, T. (1993) Whole-cell properties of temperature-sensitive neurons in rat hypothalamic slices. *Proc. R. Soc. Lond.*, 251: 89–94.

Nakashima, T., Hori, T. and Kiyohara, T. (1989) Intracellular recording analysis of septal thermosensitive neurons in the rat. In: J.B. Mercer (Ed.), *Thermal Physiology — 1989*, Excerpta Medica, Amsterdam, pp. 69–72.

Pahapill, P.A. and Schlichter, L.C. (1990) Modulation of potassium channels in human T lymphocytes: effect of temperature. *J. Physiol. (Lond.)*, 422: 103–126.

Purves, R.D. (1981) *Microelectrode Methods For Intracellular Recording and Iontophoresis*, Academic Press, New York, pp. 51–54.

H.S. Sharma and J. Westman (Eds.)
Progress in Brain Research, Vol 115
© 1998 Elsevier Science BV. All rights reserved.

CHAPTER 2

Cell biology and the functions of thermosensitive neurons in the brain

Tetsuro Hori* and Toshihiko Katafuchi

Department of Physiology, Kyushu University Faculty of Medicine, Fukuoka 812-82, Japan

Introduction

Our modern conception of the central control of thermoregulation has developed mainly based on the research results of thermosensitive neurons in the brain and the whole body thermoregulatory responses (for reviews, see Boulant, 1980; Nakayama, 1985: Simon et al., 1986; Hori, 1991). Major contributions have been made towards the understanding of: (1) the properties and functions of thermosensitive neurons and (2) the autonomic and behavioral thermoregulatory responses during thermal, neural and chemical stimulation. These findings have shown a good correlation between the activity of the thermosensitive neurons and thermoregulatory responses. The thermosensitive neurons have been recorded in the rostral hypothalamus, the lower brainstem and the spinal cord of ectothermic as well as endothermic vertebrates. In parallel with the existence of such thermosensitive neurons, the thermal stimulation of these localized regions has been found to produce adaptive thermoregulatory responses.

Thermosensitive neurons which alter the firing rate in response to small changes in the local temperature were first discovered in the preoptic and anterior hypothalamus (POA) of anesthetized cats by Nakayama et al. (1961). In 1980, our in vitro studies utilizing brain tissue slices revealed the existence of thermosensitive neurons which have an inherent thermosensitivity in the POA (Hori et al., 1980a,b). Furthermore, thermosensitive neurons have also been widely found in such extraPOA tissue as the ventromedial hypothalamus (Hori et al., 1988a), midbrain (Nakayama and Hardy, 1969; Hori and Harada, 1976a,b), the medulla oblongata (Inoue and Murakami, 1976) and the spinal cord (Simon and Iriki, 1971). These POA and extraPOA thermosensitive neurons respond not only to local temperatures but also to temperatures in remote sites where the thermosensitive neurons are found. The high degree of convergence of thermal information from local and remote sites on thermosensitive neurons, and the sparsity of such convergence on thermally insensitive neurons, suggests that thermosensitive neurons in one site of CNS are connected to the thermosensitive neurons in the other sites, thus forming a neural network of thermosensitive neurons which is hierarchically organized in the CNS (for reviews, see Satinoff 1978; Boulant 1980; Hori, 1984).

Furthermore, studies from different laboratories have revealed that some thermosensitive neurons in the POA respond to changes in the parameters of non-thermal homeostatic functions such as blood pressure, local and peripheral os-

---

*Corresponding author. Tel: +81 92 6426085; fax: +81 92 6426093; e-mail: thori@physiol.med.kyushu-u.ac.jp

molality, sex steroids, glucose and emotional stimuli. Such multimodal responsiveness of the POA neurons indicate that POA thermosensitive neurons may thus be involved in the coordination of thermoregulation and non-thermal homeostatic functions controlled in the hypothalamus (Silva and Boulant, 1984, 1986; Nakashima et al., 1985b; Hori et al., 1986a; Koga et al., 1987a,b).

The goal of this review is to elucidate: (1) the thermal transduction mechanisms of central thermosensitive neurons, (2) their specific key roles in central thermoregulation, and (3) the responsiveness of POA thermosensitive neurons to non-thermal signals as a basis of the interactions between thermoregulation and the non-thermal homeostatic functions.

Thermal transduction mechanisms of central thermosensitive neurons

As discussed earlier (Hori and Shinohara, 1979), there are two methods for characterizing neuronal thermosensitivity, i.e. the thermal coefficient (the slope of thermal-response curve) and the Q_{10}. While the thermal coefficient designation is not suitable for a comparison of the thermosensitivity of neurons, which have quite different basal rates of discharge, the Q_{10} expression does tend to favor neurons that have a low spontaneous firing rate. Since the extracellular recording technique which is conventionally employed to explore the central thermosensitive neurons depends largely on the spontaneous discharges, the neurons which are either silent or fire at a very low rate (e.g. < 1 impulse/s) have often been neglected. Although such limitations exist, the thermosensitive neurons have generally been defined as neurons which respond to local temperatures in the range between 35 and 41°C with Q_{10} over 2 and/or thermal coefficients of greater than 0.8 imp./s/°C (warm-sensitive neurons) and with Q_{10} of less than 0.5 and/or thermal coefficients of smaller than −0.6 imp./s/°C (cold-sensitive neurons) (Boulant and Dean, 1986; Nakashima et al., 1987; Hori, 1991). In a wide species of homeotherms (Hori and Shinohara,

1979; Boulant, 1980; Hori et al., 1980a,b; Hori et al., 1986a; Nakashima et al., 1987; Kiyohara et al., 1990) and poikilotherms (Cabanac et al., 1967; Nelson and Prosser, 1981) that have been studied both in vivo and *in vitro*, it has been shown that the proportions of warm-sensitive and cold-sensitive among the POA neurons are about 20–30% and 5–10%, respectively.

Since the first demonstration of thermosensitive neurons in the cat POA (Nakayama et al., 1961), the issue as to whether thermosensitive neurons are actually endowed with a direct thermosensitivity or whether neuronal thermosensitivity merely derives from the temperature dependency of synaptic transmission has remained unresolved. With the advent of *in vitro* brain slice studies, we first demonstrated the existence of warm-sensitive neurons and cold-sensitive neurons in the rat POA demonstrating an inherent thermosensitivity which was preserved during synaptic blockade (Hori et al., 1980a,b). Subsequent brain slices studies revealed the existence of such 'primary' thermosensitive neurons in the duck POA (Nakashima et al., 1987) and rat extra POA tissue such as the ventromedial hypothalamus (Hori et al., 1988a), the organum vasculosum lamina terminalis (Matsuda et al., 1992), the septum (Nakashima et al., 1989a), the suprachiasmatic nucleus (Derambure and Boulant, 1994), the red nucleus (Asami et al., 1988a), the medulla oblongata (Kobayashi and Murakami, 1982) and the dorsal motor nucleus of the vagus (Muratani et al., 1991).

To elucidate the temperature transduction mechanisms, the membrane properties of thermosensitive neurons in the central nervous system have been examined using current- and voltage clamp techniques (Carpenter, 1981; Nakashima et al., 1989a; Curras et al., 1991; Muratani et al., 1991; Kobayashi and Takahashi, 1993; Griffin and Boulant, 1995). Although controversy still remains concerning the ionic mechanisms of the thermosensitivity, the most common finding on temperature-sensitive neurons is that the input resistance of the neurons increases during cooling and decreases during warming. Since these changes in the input resistance were pre-served in a free or low Ca^{2+}–high Mg^{2+} solution, they were not mediated by synaptic transmission (Nakashima et al., 1989a; Muratani et al., 1991; Kobayashi and Takahashi, 1993).

In Aplysia neurons, it has been suggested that the ratio of Na^+ conductance (gNa^+) to K^+ conductance (gK^+) is important in determining the temperature sensitivity of neurons. When Q_{10} of gNa^+ is higher than gK^+, the neuron tends to depolarize with an increasing temperature (Carpenter, 1981). Similar mechanisms have also been suggested in the rat POA (Kobayashi and Takahashi, 1993) and DMV (Muratani et al., 1991) neurons. It has been reported that (1) the warming-induced inward current or depolariza-tion was accompanied by a decrease in the input resistance and (2) that the average equilibrium potential of the responses was more positive than the resting potential. In the case of POA neurons, Cl^- ions may also be involved since the equilib-rium potential of warm-sensitive neurons was shifted by changing the external concentration of not only Na^+ and K^+ but also Cl^- (Kobayashi and Takahashi, 1993). On the other hand, other studies showed that the membrane potentials of warm-sensitive neurons in the POA (Griffin and Boulant, 1995) and septum (Nakashima et al., 1989a) were not affected, or only slightly if at all, by warming in spite of an increase in input resis-tance, thus indicating that the equilibrium poten-tial of the responses was very near the resting membrane potential. Since the extracellular con-centration of K^+ in the these two experiments (6.24 mM) was higher than that (5 and 3 mM) in the former studies (Muratani et al., 1991; Kobayashi and Takahashi, 1993), it is thus possi-ble that the resting membrane potential is more depolarized (according to the Nernst equation, the difference would be more than 5–7 mV). If the equilibrium potential determined by gNa^+/gK^+ is not markedly affected by the extra-cellular concentration of K^+, the driving force to the equilibrium potential may become smaller in these experiments (Griffin and Boulant, 1995; Nakashima et al., 1989a). The decrease in the

input resistance induced by warming was also observed in the temperature-insensitive neurons in the hippocampus (Thompson et al., 1985) and in the POA demonstrating a low- or moderate-slope thermal coefficient (Griffin and Boulant, 1995). Therefore, it is possible that the change in the input resistance during warming may be a general feature of the CNS neurons while the temperature transduction mechanisms in the warm-sensitive neurons are characterized by the positive shift of the equilibrium potential of the responses by warming, which may be determined by the ratio of gNa^+ to gK^+.

By the use of single neurons dissociated from the rat POA, we recorded the membrane current responses to changes in the cellular temperature over a range from 32 to 40°C (Kiyohara et al., 1990). The K^+ and Ca^{2+} currents were both, respectively eliminated by replacing K^+ with Cs^+ and by the intracellular perfusion of F^-. About three quarters of the neurons exhibited a linear increase in a non-inactivating inward current with Q_{10} of about 2 during warming over the entire range of cellular temperatures examined (Fig. 1C,D). On the other hand, the inward current responses of the remaining one quarter of the neurons demonstrated high Q_{10} (< 4.0) charac-teristics in the hyperthermic range (35–40°C) and low Q_{10} (about 2) characteristics in the hy-pothermic range (32–35°C) (Fig. 1A,B,D). Based on the thermosensitivity, the population and the shape of the thermal response characteristics, it is suggested that the former type of neurons are thermally insensitive neurons while the latter type neurons are warm-sensitive neurons. The non-lin-ear thermal response characteristics of the latter type of neurons coincide with the shape of the temperature vs. the firing rate response curves (more thermosensitive in the hyperthermic range and less thermosensitive in the hypothermic range) of the warm-sensitive neurons found in POA tissues *in vitro* (Hori et al., 1980a,b).

Tetrodotoxin (TTX) reversibly eliminated the inward current response with a high Q_{10} in the hyperthermic range, but no similar finding was observed in the current response with a low Q_{10}

12

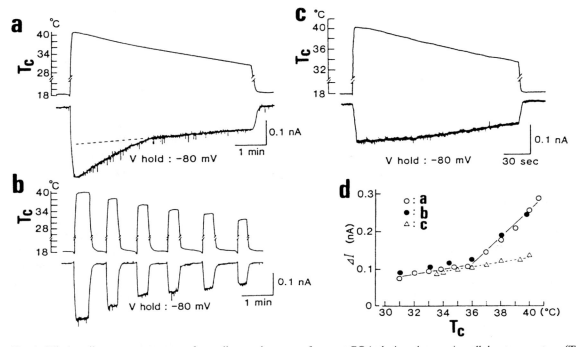

Fig. 1. Whole-cell current responses of two dispersed neurons from rat POA during changes in cellular temperature (Tc). In the experiments shown in Figs. 1 and 2, K^+ and Ca^{2+} currents were eliminated, respectively by replacing K^+ with Cs^+ and by intracellular perfusion of F^-. The holding potential (Vhold) was -80 mV. (a) and (b) Changes in the current of a warm-sensitive neuron during continuous (a) and step (b) changes in Tc. (c) Changes in the current of a thermally-insensitive neuron during continuous changes in Tc. (d) Thermal response curves of these two neurons showing changes in the currents (I) from the values at Tc of 18°C as a function of Tc. Data were taken from a, b and c (reprinted from Neuroscience Research, 8, Kiyohara et al., Hypothalamic warm-sensitive neurons possess a tetrodotoxin-sensitive sodium channel with a high Q_{10}, 48–53, 1990, with kind permission from Elsevier Science Ireland, Shannon).

in the hypothermic range (Fig. 2A). TTX demonstrated no change in the current response to temperature in the thermally insensitive neurons with a low Q_{10} (Fig. 2C). These results thus indicate that the warm-sensitive neurons possess a non-inactivating, TTX-sensitive Na^+ channel (Gilly and Armstrong, 1984) with a high Q_{10}. These findings closely correlate with our findings that warm-sensitive neurons in the septum (Nakashima et al., 1989a) and the DMV (Muratani et al., 1991) decreased the input resistance to warming in a TTX-sensitive way.

It is also possible that temperature affects other ion channels, such as the Ca^{2+}-activated K^+ and hyperpolarization-activated cation ('pace-maker')

channels, which can modulate the firing rate of the action potentials, even if these channels do not markedly affect the membrane potential. For example, it was reported that a slow depolarizing potential preceding an action potential increased its rate of rise with an elevation of the temperature in the POA warm-sensitive neurons, although the ionic mechanism was not examined (Curras et al., 1991). Sah and McLachlan (1991) found that in the guinea pig DMV neurons, an apamin-insensitive Ca^{2+}-activated K^+ current, which contributed to an afterhyperpolarization and was activated by the Ca^{2+}-induced Ca^{2+} release through the ryanodine receptors, was highly temperature-sensitive. Both the rising phase and

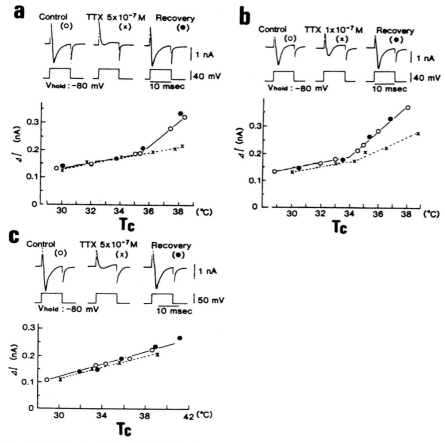

Fig. 2. Effects of tetrodotoxin (TTX) on the current responses of two POA warm-sensitive neurons (a and b) and a thermally-insensitive neuron (c) to Tc. In each panel, the upper trace shows the Na$^+$ current response generated by potential step from a holding potential of -80 mV (second trace) before (left) and during (middle) addition of TTX and after (right) removal of TTX, and the bottom graph shows the thermal response curve of each neuron with (cross) and without (open and filled circles) exposure to TTX (reprinted from Neuroscience Research, 8, Kiyohara et al., Hypothalamic warm-sensitive neurons possess a tetrodotoxin-sensitive sodium channel with a high Q_{10}, 48–53, 1990, with kind permission from Elsevier Science Ireland, Shannon).

the decay of this current were markedly accelerated by warming with the average Q_{10} of 4.6 and 2.9, respectively. It is thus possible to consider that the shortening of the time course of the Ca^{2+}-activated K^+ current during warming thereby results in an increase in the firing rate.

Some experiments on the Aplysia neurons (Carpenter, 1981) and the rat peripheral thermoreceptors (Pierau et al., 1975) have suggested that an electrogenic Na^+–K^+ pump might underlie the thermal transduction process of cold-sensi-

tive neurons and peripheral cold receptors. An inhibition of the pump, which may be induced by cooling, has been confirmed to produce the depolarization and increase in neuronal excitability. Cold-sensitive neurons in the rat DMV also showed membrane depolarization by cooling (Muratani et al., 1991). In these neurons the input resistance increased during cooling and decreased during warming, in the same manner as that observed in warm-sensitive neurons (see above). The reversal potential of the cooling-in-

14

duced depolarization was close to the K^+ equilibrium potential and the depolarization was partially sensitive to tetraethylammonium chloride (TEA). Although the input resistance was shown to either decrease (Schlue, 1991) or increase (McCarren and Alger, 1987) during depolarization by pump inhibitors, the above findings could not be explained solely by the temperature dependency of the electrogenic pump activity. It is thus suggested that the cooling-induced depolarization in cold-sensitive neurons may be mainly caused by a decrease in the membrane K^+ conductance. This conclusion closely correlates with the finding that ouabain does not affect the thermosensitivity of cold-sensitive and warm-sensitive neurons in the POA of rat brain slices (Curras and Boulant, 1989). It has been reported that the K^+ channels of Aplysia ganglion cells are activated by warming, thus resulting in hyperpolarization with an increase in membrane conductance (Tamazawa et al., 1991). These K^+ channels were suggested to be regulated by GTP-binding protein, since the current was depressed by an intracellular injection of GDPβS, a blocking analogue of GDP. There is no doubt that further studies are needed to elucidate the thermal transduction mechanisms of mammalian cold-sensitive neurons.

Activity of central thermosensitive neurons related to thermoregulation

It has not yet been fully determined as to whether all the thermosensitive neurons in the brain are involved in thermoregulation, or whether thermally insensitive neurons do have any roles in thermoregulation. However, it has been generally believed that the thermosensitive neurons in the hypothalamus, lower brainstem and spinal cord do play specific key roles in thermoregulation by functioning as a core temperature detector on the one hand and by integrating the thermal signals from different parts of body on the other. This view is based largely on the strikingly good correlation observed between the activity of thermosensitive neurons and the whole body thermoregulatory responses during changes in the thermal, neural and chemical inputs.

The thermally induced changes in the activity of thermosensitive neurons and thermoregulatory responses

While the local warming and cooling of POA, medulla oblongata and spinal cord induce heat-defense thermoregulatory responses and cold-defense ones, respectively, electrophysiological studies have demonstrated that thermosensitive neurons are recorded abundantly in these thermoreactive regions. Most of these thermosensitive neurons also respond to the temperatures of remote sites where thermosensitive neurons or thermoreceptors are found, and thus show the convergence of thermal signals from different sites of body (Simon, 1972; Boulant and Hardy, 1974; Hori and Harada, 1976a; Asami et al., 1988a,b). When the effects of different combinations of POA and skin temperatures were studied on the thermoregulatory effector responses and the discharge responses of POA thermosensitive neurons, both responses displayed the 'multiplicative' integration of thermal information from the two sites (Boulant, 1980). The pattern of integration of thermal information in the warm-sensitive neurons and the cold-sensitive neurons was similar to that of the heat-defense responses and cold-defense responses, respectively.

In order to see whether the POA thermosensitive neurons actually alter the activity during ongoing thermoregulation, we analyzed the activity of POA neurons of conscious monkeys during bar press behavior to lower the ambient temperature when exposed to warm air (Hori et al., 1987). While almost all the thermosensitive neurons (43 of 46) altered their activity during this cooling behavior, only 45% (29 of 64) of the thermally insensitive neurons responded ($P < 0.05$), thus suggesting that POA thermosensitive neurons are more closely involved in the thermoregulatory cooling behavior. The frequently observed responses included sustained increases or decreases in activity during the bar press period (the bar press-related response) and the cooling period (the cooling phase-related response) (Fig. 3I). The bar press-related response was largely dependent on the strength of motivation of the monkeys to seek cool air. The cooling phase-related response was not a simple sensory response to skin cooling, but it occurs only when the cooling air has a 'rewarding' value for the animal. Moreover, when

the deep body temperature was higher, this response continued longer until the skin was cooled down to lower levels (Fig. 3II). This could be correlated with the hedonic response in man: the subjects feel a lower skin temperature to be more pleasant when the deep body temperature is higher (Cabanac, 1969). The bar press-related response and the cooling phase-related response both appear to be somehow involved in the drive

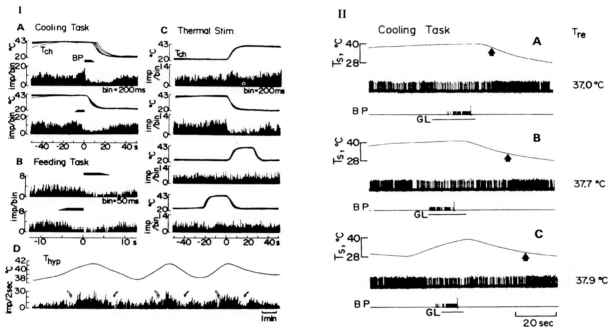

Fig. 3. **I.** Bar press-related and cooling phase-related responses of a warm-sensitive neuron during bar press cooling behavior, bar press feeding behavior and ambient temperature stimulation. (A) Peri-event histograms of neuronal activity during cooling behavior with time zero at the moment of the first bar press (BP) (upper) and at the last BP (lower) of task. (B) Peri-event histograms of neuronal activity during feeding behavior with time zero at the moment of the first BP (upper) and the last BP (lower) of task. (C) Peri-event histograms of neuronal activity during ambient thermal stimulation with two different time courses. Ambient temperature was raised and then lowered by experimenter, with a similar time course (upper two panels) as it was during cooling behaviors in A and more quickly (lower two panels). In each histogram, time zero indicates the time of switching the valve from cool-neutral air to warm air (first and third panels) and from warm to cool-neutral air (second and fourth panels). (D) Neuronal responses to changes in hypothalamic temperature (Thyp). Arrows indicate transient decreases of firing rate in the early parts of rising and falling phases of Thyp, in addition to the static increase and decrease in firing rate to a rise and a fall of Thyp. **II.** Bar press-related and cooling phase-related responses of a POA neuron at different rectal temperature (Tre). From the top to the bottom of records in each trial, skin temperature (Ts) at the back, neuronal spikes, bar press (BP) and time of cue (green) lamp (GL) on which the monkey was allowed to press the bar to cool the air. Arrows indicate the time when the neuronal activities returned to their original levels. When the rectal temperature was higher, the bar press-related responses appeared at lower Ts and the cooling phase-related responses continued longer until the skin was cooled down to lower levels [reprinted from Brain Research Bulletin 18: 48–53 (1990), Hori et al., with kind permission of Elsevier Science, Inc., New York, USA].

and reward mechanisms of thermoregulatory cooling behavior. The dynamic responses of the POA thermosensitive neurons thus observed imply that they participate in the phasic information processing which is necessary for the performance of thermoregulatory behavior.

Birzis and Hemingway (for review, see Hemingway, 1963) proposed an 'efferent shivering pathway' in the cat which descends from the hypothalamus via the midbrain reticular formation (Rf) dorsolateral to the red nucleus and then the dorsolateral side of the pons and medulla to the lateral columns of the spinal cord, the regions which correspond roughly to the reticulospinal (RfS) tract. Electrical lesion and stimulation of these areas, respectively, inhibits and enhances shivering in the cold. Our single neuron studies on the thermal responsiveness of neurons in these brainstem area of rats revealed a high degree of convergence of 'cold' signals from both local and remote (hypothalamus and skin) sites on the RfS neurons, which were identified by antidromic responses to stimulation of the RfS tract in the spinal cord (Asami et al., 1988a,b). Microinjections of procaine and glutamate into these areas decreased and increased the cold-induced shivering without any correlated changes in the cardiovascular and respiratory parameters as well as the pilomotor activity. Localized neuronal death induced by the injection of kainic acid into the same sites abolished shivering in a cold environment. In contrast, RfS and non-RfS neurons in the ventromedial part of brainstem Rf tended to show the convergence of 'warm' signals and neither localized anesthetization nor neuronal excitation in these areas affected the EMG activity. The congruency between the neuronal responses and the shivering observed in these studies therefore implies that cold-sensitive RfS neurons in the dorsolateral part of the rat brainstem are involved in the control of shivering.

Neurally-induced changes in the activity of POA thermosensitive neurons and thermoregulatory responses

The congruency between the activity of POA thermosensitive neurons and the thermoregulatory responses has been observed during the 'reversible ablation' of the prefrontal cortex induced by cortical spreading depression (CSD). In rats, in which an electrical lesion was induced unilaterally in the POA, a single CSD, which was produced in the frontal cortex contralaterally, but not ipsilaterally to the POA lesion, enhanced the cold-defense responses (skin-warming behavior and autonomic heat production) and inhibited the heat-defense response (skin-cooling behavior) (Shibata et al., 1983a,b, 1985). Upon the entrance of CSD into the ipsilateral prefrontal cortex, the increases and decreases of the firing rate were observed in the cold-sensitive and warm-sensitive neurons of the ipsilateral POA, respectively (Shibata et al., 1984). These neuronal responses during ipsilateral CSD also correlated to the changes in the thermoregulatory responses in terms of the direction of changes and the time courses. The majority of thermally-insensitive neurons, however, was not affected by CSD. Furthermore, the electrical stimulation of the prefrontal cortex inhibited 68.7% of cold-sensitive neurons and excited 35% of warm-sensitive neurons in the ipsilateral POA (Hori et al., 1984). The results clearly indicate a tonic facilitatory and inhibitory influence of the prefrontal cortex on the warm-sensitive and cold-sensitive neurons of ipsilateral POA, respectively.

The inhibition of the activity in a majority (69.8%) of both warm-sensitive and cold-sensitive neurons in the POA after the electrical stimulation of the ventral subiculum of the hippocampus in the anesthetized rat (Hori et al., 1982c) may also explain the poikilothermic effect of the same stimulus in the conscious rat (Osaka et al., 1984).

The chemically-induced changes in the activity of POA thermosensitive neurons and thermoregulatory responses

It has been demonstrated that the direction of changes in the firing rate of POA thermosensitive neurons which are induced by the local application of various endogenous and exogenous substances may explain the basis of changes in the whole body thermoregulatory responses after the injection of these chemicals into the POA. The local application of endotoxin (Nakashima et al., 1985a), cytokines (Hori et al., 1988c; Nakashima et al., 1988, 1989b, 1991), TRH (Saltzman and Beckman, 1981; Hori et al., 1988d), noradrenaline (Hori and Nakayama, 1973; Hori et al., 1982a) and dopamine (Scott and Boulant, 1984) has been demonstrated to decrease the activity in 60–95% of POA warm-sensitive neurons and excite a similar population of cold-sensitive neurons. An intraPOA injection of these chemicals may thus decrease the heat-defense responses and increase the cold-defense responses thereby producing hyperthermia. In contrast, hypothermia-producing substances (serotonin, histamine, angiotensin II and III, morphine and capsaicin) which facilitate and inhibit the heat-defense and cold-defense responses, respectively, excite and inhibit the activity of POA warm-sensitive and cold-sensitive neurons, respectively (Hori and Nakayama, 1973; Baldino et al., 1980; Kiyohara et al., 1984a; Hori et al., 1988b, Shibata et al., 1988b; Tsai et al., 1989). On the other hand, 60–80% of thermally-insensitive neurons were unaffected by these hyperthermic and hypothermic agents. Poikilo-thermia-producing peptides (bombesin and neurotensin), which inhibit the heat-defense and cold-defense responses, respectively, decreased the firing rate in 50–70% of the POA neurons, regardless of the type of their thermosensitivity (Hori et al., 1986b).

The multiple thermostats system with a 'warm signal' network and a 'cold signal' network

The modern concepts of central thermoregulation that have emerged from various studies of the brain have generally been expressed as a multiple thermostats model, which consists of multiple integrators with almost separate and independent sets of thermosensors and effectors (Roberts and Mooney, 1974; Simon, 1974; Satinoff, 1978; Hori, 1984; Simon et al., 1986). There is ample evidence indicating that different types of autonomic and behavioral thermoregulation can be dissociated

from one another by thermal stimuli given to different sites in the body and by lesioning of the CNS (for reviews, see Hori, 1984). Furthermore, the presumed independent controller networks can be collectively grouped into at least two sets of thermoregulatory signal processing systems in the CNS, i.e. a 'warm signal' network and a 'cold signal' network. The high degree of convergence of thermal information from local and remote sites on thermosensitive neurons, without hardly any such convergence on thermally-insensitive neurons, thus implies the existence of synaptic networks of thermosensitive neurons in the CNS. A majority of such warm-sensitive and cold-sensitive neurons respond to thermal stimulation of remote sites with positive and negative thermal coefficients, respectively (Simon, 1972; Boulant and Hardy, 1974; Hori and Harada, 1976a; Inoue and Murakami, 1976; Asami et al., 1988a,b). These observations may thus offer a basis for the view of the 'warm signal' network and the 'cold signal' network which increase the activity, respectively, to a rise and a fall in body temperature. One of the strongest pieces of evidence for this view is the finding that the capsaicin-desensitized animals have an impaired function of heat-defense thermoregulation with an almost completely intact cold-defense thermoregulation (for reviews, see Hori, 1984).

Even though the medulla oblongata and the spinal cord, which contain thermosensitive neurons, exhibit the thermoregulatory capacity (Lipton, 1973; Simon, 1974), the disconnection of the upper brain produces progressively less powerful and higher threshold thermoregulatory responses. Thus, a hypothesis has been put forward that the multiple thermostats system is hierarchically organized and the hypothalamus may 'serve to coordinate and adjust the activity of thermoregulatory systems located at several lower levels of the neuraxis' (Satinoff, 1978). Thermosensitive neurons in the POA, on the abundant neural and humoral inputs as well as by the neural descending connections from the POA thermosensitive neurons to the lower brain (Nutik, 1973; Murakami and Sakata, 1978; Hori et al., 1982a,b; Ishikawa et al., 1984; Asami et al., 1988a,b), may selectively induce the effector responses, which are most appropriate to changes in the internal and external environments, among a variety of repertoires of autonomic and behavioral thermoregulatory responses.

The multimodal responsiveness of hypothalamic neurons and interactions among regulatory systems

Studies in different laboratories have revealed that 40–70% of POA thermosensitive neurons *in vivo* and *in vitro* respond to divergent types of non-thermal homeostatic signals, such as osmolality (Silva and Boulant, 1984; Nakashima et al., 1985b; Koga et al., 1987a), glucose (Silva and Boulant, 1984), blood pressure (Koga et al., 1987b), sex steroids (Silva and Boulant, 1986), noxious stimuli (Kanosue et al., 1984), carbon dioxide (Tamaki et al., 1986) and non-thermal emotional events (Hori et al., 1986a). There is also a higher incidence of such non-thermal responsiveness among thermosensitive neurons than among thermally insensitive neurons in the POA. Furthermore, the activity of some hypothalamic neurons, which are presumed to control osmoregulation or feeding, has been shown to be affected by body temperature (Yamamoto et al., 1981; Nakayama and Imai-Matsumura, 1984; Matsumura et al., 1985; Hori et al., 1988a). Such overlapping of sensitivity to thermal and non-thermal homeostatic parameters may explain many of the interactions observed between thermoregulation and the non-thermal homeostatic functions. As discussed previously (Hori, 1984, 1991), these interactions are inevitable because the thermoregulatory system has no specific effectors organs of its own and 'borrows' them from other regulation systems. Homeothermic animals generate body heat mainly in skeletal muscles and brown adipose tissues which are shared with the control systems of motor functions and the diet balance, respectively. They dissipate body heat by cutaneous vasomotion and evaporation which are related to the cardiovascular and osmoregulatory systems, respectively. In some circumstances,

competition may thus occur between the thermal and non-thermal drives. Various strategies in thermoregulation have been used in the animal to overcome such a situation where these drives are competing against each other (Johnson and Hales, 1984).

One example of such strategies is the decreased evaporative heat loss under hypohydrated conditions, which at first protects osmoregulation at the expense of thermoregulation. However, when the body temperature subsequently rises over about 40°C, the animals begin to dissipate heat by evaporative means thereby defending the body from further overheating. In a hot environment with water shortage, this whole sequence of responses provides a longer survival time than the reversed sequence manifesting two regulatory responses (Schmidt-Nielsen et al., 1957) and the POA thermosensitive neurons having osmosensitivity may be involved in this phenomenon. Our *in vitro* studies have demonstrated that about 60% of the thermosensitive neurons and 12% of the thermally-insensitive neurons in the examined POA tissue slices have an inherent sensitivity to changes in local osmolality of less than 15 mOsm/kg changes (estimated threshold, less than 5 mOsm/kg) (Nakashima et al., 1985b) (Fig. 4). Furthermore, a similar population of thermosensitive neurons and thermally-insensitive neurons in the POA of anesthetized rats was affected by changes in the hepatoportal osmolality of less than 10 mOsm/kg (Koga et al., 1987a). The type of responses of POA neurons to both local and peripheral osmolality was predominantly such that the firing rate was reduced by hyperosmotic stimuli, regardless of the type of thermosensitivity, while the thermal coefficient was barely affected. The decreased activity of POA thermosensitive neurons in hyperosmotic conditions may thus explain, at least in part, the inhibition of evaporative and non-evaporative heat loss and the decreased heat production in dehydrated animals (Baker and Doris, 1982).

Hypothermia after acute blood loss has been regarded as an adaptive response which enables the organism to adapt to hypoxic conditions by

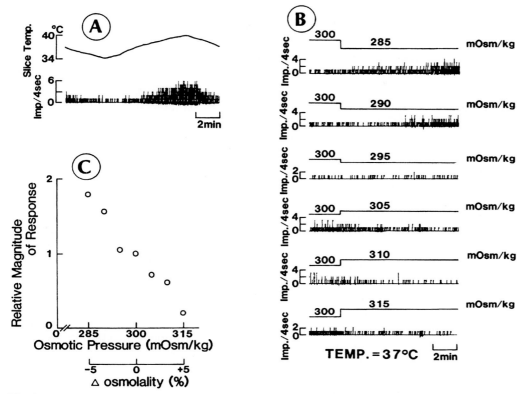

Fig. 4. Firing rate responses of a POA warm-sensitive neuron to changes in local temperature (a) and in local osmolality (b, c). In c, the relative magnitude of each response at steady state was plotted taking the firing rate in 300 mOsm/kg medium as 1 [reprinted from *Pflueger Archiv* 405: 112–117 (1985), Nakashima et al., with kind permission of Springer-Verlag, Berlin/Heidelberg, Germany].

decreasing the cellular metabolism at a lower temperature. This is supported by the finding that keeping the hemorrhagic rats at a lower body temperature by extracorporeal cooling prolonged their survival time, while, on the other hand, keeping them at normothermia by warming shortened it (Tanaka et al., 1983). While this hypothermic response is taken to be the result of reduced heat production due to the lower oxygen supply, it is considered to involve a centrally-mediated component. We found a high incidence of baro/volume receptor inputs to POA thermosensitive neurons (60%) and thermally insensitive neurons (28.4%) (Koga et al., 1987b). Hypotension by 15 mmHg or less increased and decreased the firing rate of about half of the

warm-sensitive neurons and cold-sensitive neurons, respectively. While this finding suggests the involvement of POA thermosensitive neurons in cardiovascular functions, it may explain, at least in part, the hypothermia observed during acute bleeding (Tanaka et al., 1983).

Non-thermal emotional and behavioral stimuli also affect the activity of POA thermosensitive neurons in alert monkeys when they see and receive rewards (food) or aversive objects (an air puffer, a toy snake) (Hori et al., 1986a). One type of neuronal response was dependent upon the degree of perturbation such as a positive or negative emotional state aroused by stimuli which were presented to the animals. Another type of response appeared to reflect some internal drive state to obtain the rewarding objects which varied depending on the degree of hunger. These types of non-thermal responsiveness were found more frequently among thermosensitive neurons (45 of 52 or 86.5%) than among thermally insensitive neurons (51 of 91 or 56.0%). These neuronal responses seem to explain the modulation of thermoregulatory responses by non-thermal events, which was exemplified by a transient decrease and increase in the rate of sweating on general body surface during mental arithmetic and administration of pain or noise stimulus, respectively (Ogawa, 1975).

Such overlapping of the responsiveness to thermal and non-thermal stimuli has been documented as well among the hypothalamic neurons which are considered to be primarily involved in osmoregulation and food intake. About 70% of the neurosecretory cells in the supraoptic nucleus alter the activity in response to changes in the POA temperature (Matsumura et al., 1985). This neuronal response may mediate the increase in vasopressin release during heat exposure, which may be understood as a feedforward response to conserve body water before the manifestation of evaporative heat loss responses in a hot environment. Similarly, about 39% of the neurons in the ventromedial hypothalamus, a satiety center for feeding control, demonstrate inherent thermosensitivity (Hori et al., 1988a). While glucoreceptor neurons in the ventromedial hypothalamus, which inhibit feeding, increase their activity with a rise in the POA temperature (Nakayama and Imai-Matsumura, 1984), the glucosensitive neurons in the lateral hypothalamus, which facilitate feeding, increase the activity with a decrease in the POA temperature. These neuronal responses may offer an explanation for the increase and decrease in food intake during hypothermia and hyperthermia, respectively, which are also considered to be adaptive responses. It thus appears that the modifications of thermoregulation by non-thermal signals should not be regarded as an undesirable disturbance of thermoregulation. Rather, the interactions may be understood as a part of the adaptive responses of the organism as a whole.

The POA thermosensitive neurons demonstrating responsiveness to non-thermal homeostatic parameters, together with their abundant mutual connections with divergent areas of brain including the limbic system and the association cortices (Hori et al., 1982a–c; Kiyohara et al., 1984b; Shibata et al., 1988a), may thus be involved in the coordination of thermal and non-thermal homeostatic functions controlled in the hypothalamus.

Acknowledgements

This work was supported in part by Grants-in-Aid to T. Hori (No. 09557006 and No. 08877017) from the Ministry of Education, Science and Culture, Japan. We also express our sincere thanks, particularly, to our collaborators Drs K. Kiyohara, T. Nakashima, M. Shibata, H. Koga, T. Osaka, A. Asami, T. Asami and H. Muratani for their valuable contributions, without which this review could not have been completed.

References

Asami, A., Asami, T., Hori, T., Kiyohara, T. and Nakashima, T. (1988a) Thermally induced activities of the mesencephalic reticulospinal and rubrospinal neurons in the rat. *Brain Res. Bull.*, 20: 387–398.

Asami, T., Hori, T., Kiyohara, T. and Nakashima, T. (1988b) Convergence of thermal signals on the reticulospinal neurons in the midbrain, pons and medulla oblongata. *Brain Res. Bull.*, 20: 581–596.

Baker, M.A. and Doris, P.A. (1982) Effect of dehydration on hypothalamic control of evaporation in the cat. *J. Physiol. (Lond.)*, 322: 457–468.

Baldino, F., Jr., Beckman, A.L. and Adler, M.W. (1980) Actions of iontophoretically applied morphine on hypothalamic thermosensitive units. *Brain Res.*, 196: 199–208.

Boulant, J.A. and Hardy, J.D. (1974) The effect of spinal and skin temperatures on the firing rate and thermosensitivity of preoptic neurones. *J. Physiol. (Lond.)*, 240: 639–660.

Boulant, J.A. (1980) Hypothalamic control of thermoregulation. neurophysiological basis. In: P.J. Morgane and J. Panksepp (Eds.), *Handbook of the Hypothalamus*, Vol. 3, Part A, Dekker, New York, pp. 1–82.

Boulant, J.A. and Dean, J.B. (1986) Temperature receptors in the central nervous system. *Annu. Rev. Physiol.*, 48: 639–654.

Cabanac, M. (1969) Plasir ou deplasir de la sensation thermique et homeothermie. *Physiol. Behav.,* 4: 359–364.

Cabanac, M., Hammel, H.T. and Hardy, J.D. (1967) Tiligua scincoides: temperature sensitive units in lizard brain. *Science,* 158: 1050–1051.

Carpenter, D.O. (1981) Ionic and metabolic bases of neuronal thermosensitivity. *Fed. Proc.,* 40: 2808–2813.

Curras, M.C. and Boulant, J.A. (1989) Effects of ouabain on neuronal thermosensitivity in hypothalamic tissue slices. *Am. J. Physiol.,* 257: R21–R28.

Curras, M.C., Kelso, S.R. and Boulant, J.A. (1991) Intracellular analysis of inherent and synaptic activity in hypothalamic thermosensitive neurones in the rat. *J. Physiol. (Lond.)* 440: 257–271.

Derambure, P.S. and Boulant, J.A. (1994) Circadian thermosensitive characteristics of suprachiasmatic neurons in vitro. *Am. J. Physiol.,* 266: R1876–R1884.

Gilly, W.F. and Armstrong, C.M. (1984) Threshold channels a novel type of sodium channel in squid giant axon. *Nature,* 309: 448–450.

Griffin, J.D. and Boulant, J.A. (1995) Temperature effects on membrane potential and input resistance in rat hypothalamic neurones. *J. Physiol.,* 488: 407–418.

Hemingway, A. (1963) Shivering. *Physiol. Rev,* 43: 397–422.

Hori, T. (1984) Capsaicin and central control of thermoregulation. *Pharmacol. Ther.,* 206: 389–416.

Hori, T. (1991) An update on thermosensitive neurons in the brain: from cellular biology to thermal and non-thermal homeostatic functions. *Jpn. J. Physiol.,* 41: 1–22.

Hori, T. and Nakayama, T. (1973) Effects of biogenic amines on central thermoresponsive neurones in the rabbit. *J. Physiol. (Lond.),* 232: 71–85.

Hori, T. and Harada, Y. (1976a) Midbrain neuronal responses to local and spinal cord temperatures. *Am. J. Physiol.,* 231: 1573–1578.

Hori, T. and Harada, Y. (1976b) Responses of midbrain raphe neurons to local temperature. *Pflug. Arch.,* 364: 205–207.

Hori, T. and Shinohara, K. (1979) Hypothalamic thermoresponsive neurones in the newborn rat. *J. Physiol. (Lond.),* 294: 541–560.

Hori, T., Kiyohara, T., Nakashima, T. and Shibata, M. (1982a) Responses of preoptic thermosensitive neurons to medial fore-brain bundle stimulation. *Brain Res. Bull.,* 8: 667–675.

Hori, T., Kiyohara, T., Osaka, T., Shibata, M. and Nakashima, T. (1982b) Responses of preoptic thermosensitive neurons to mediobasal hypothalamic stimulation. *Brain Res. Bull.,* 8: 677–683.

Hori, T., Kiyohara, T., Shibata, M. and Nakashima, T. (1984) Involvement of prefrontal cortex in the central control of thermoregulation. In: J.R.S. Hales (Ed.), *Thermal Physiology,* Raven Press, New York, pp. 71–74.

Hori, T., Kiyohara, T., Shibata, M., Oomura, Y., Nishino, H., Aou, S and Fujita, I. (1986a) Responsiveness of monkey preoptic thermosensitive neurons to non-thermal emotional stimuli. *Brain Res. Bull.,* 17: 75–82.

Hori, T., Kiyohara, T., Oomura, Y., Nishino, H., Aou, S. and Fujita, I. (1987) Activity of thermosensitive neurons of monkey preoptic hypothalamus during thermoregulatory operant behavior. *Brain Res. Bull.,* 18: 649–655.

Hori, T., Kuriyama, K. and Nakashima, T. (1988a) Thermal responsiveness of neurons in the ventromedial hypothalamus. *J. Physiol. Soc. Jpn.,* 50: 619.

Hori, T., Nakashima, T., Hori, N. and Kiyohara, T. (1980a) Thermosensitive neurons in hypothalamic tissue slices *in vitro. Brain Res.,* 186: 203–207.

Hori, T., Nakashima, T., Kiyohara, T., Shibata, M. and Hori, N. (1980b) Effect of calcium removal on thermosensitivity of preoptic neurons in hypothalamic slices. *Neurosci. Lett.,* 20: 171–175.

Hori, T., Osaka, T., Kiyohara, T., Shibata, M. and Nakashima, T. (1982c) Hippocampal input to preoptic thermosensitive neurons in the rat. *Neurosci. Lett.,* 32: 155–158.

Hori, T., Shibata, M., Kiyohara, T., Nakashima, T. and Asami, A. (1988b) Responses of anterior hypothalamic-preoptic thermo-sensitive neurons to locally applied capsaicin. *Neuropharmacology,* 27: 135–142.

Hori, T., Shibata, M., Nakashima, T., Yamasaki, M., Asami, A., Asami, T. and Koga, H. (1988c) Effects of interleukin-1 and arachidonate on the preoptic and anterior hypothalamic neurons. *Brain Res. Bull.,* 20: 75–82.

Hori, T., Yamasaki, M., Asami, T., Koga, H. and Kiyohara, T. (1988d) Responses of anterior hypothalamic-preoptic thermosensitive neurons to TRH and Cyclo (His-Pro). *Neuropharmacology,* 27: 895–901.

Hori, T., Yamasaki, M., Kiyohara, T. and Shibata, M. (1986b) Responses of preoptic thermosensitive neurons to poikilothermia-inducing peptides–bombesin and neurotensin. *Pflug. Arch.,* 407: 558–560.

Inoue, S. and Murakami, N. (1976) Unit responses in the medulla oblongata of rabbit to changes in local and cutaneous temperature. *J. Physiol. (Lond.),* 259: 339–356.

Ishikawa, Y., Nakayama, T., Kanosue, K. and Matsumura, K. (1984) Responses of medial medullary neurons to preoptic and scrotal thermal stimulation and to preoptic microinjection of capsaicin. *J. Therm. Biol.,* 9: 47–50.

Johnson, K.G. and Hales, J.R.S. (1984) An introductory analysis of competition between thermoregulation and other homeostaic systems. In: J.R.S. Hales (Ed.), *Thermal Physiology,* Raven Press, New York, pp. 295–298.

Kanosue, K., Nakayama, T., Ishikawa, Y. and Imai-Matsumura, K. (1984) Responses of hypothalamic and thalamic neurons to noxious and scrotal thermal stimulations in rats. *J. Therm. Biol.,* 9: 11–13.

Kiyohara, T., Hirata, M., Hori, T. and Akaike, N. (1990) Hypothalamic warm-sensitive neurons possess a tetrodotoxin-sensitive sodium channel with a high Q_{10}. *Neurosci. Res.,* 8: 48–53.

Kiyohara, T., Hori, T., Shibata, M. and Nakashima, T. (1984a) Effects of angiotensin II on preoptic thermosensitive neurones in the rat. In: J.R.S. Hales (Ed.), *Thermal Physiology*, Raven Press, New York, pp. 141–144.

Kiyohara, T., Hori, T., Shibata, M., Nakashima, T. and Osaka, T. (1984b) Neural inputs to preoptic thermosensitive neurons-histological and electrophysiological mapping of central connections. *J. Therm. Biol.*, 9: 21–26.

Kobayashi, S. and Murakami, N. (1982) Thermosensitive neurons in slice preparations of rat medulla oblongata. *Brain Res. Bull.*, 8: 721–726.

Kobayashi, S. and Takahashi, T. (1993) Whole-cell properties of temperature-sensitive neurons in rat hypothalamic slices. *Proc. R. Soc. Lond. B.*, 251: 89–94.

Koga, H., Hori, T., Inoue, T., Kiyohara, T. and Nakashima, T. (1987a) Convergence of hepatoportal osmotic and cardiovascular signals on preoptic thermosensitive neurons. *Brain Res. Bull.*, 19: 109–113.

Koga, H., Hori, T., Kiyohara, T. and Nakashima, T. (1987b) Responses of preoptic thermosensitive neurons to changes in blood pressure. *Brain Res. Bull.*, 18: 749–755.

Lipton, J.M. (1973) Thermosensitivity of medulla oblongata in control of body temperature. *Am. J. Physiol.*, 224: 890–897.

Matsuda, T., Hori, T. and Nakashima, T. (1992) Thermal and PGE2 sensitivity of the organum vasculosum lamina terminalis region and preoptic area in rat brain slices. *J. Physiol. (Lond.)*, 454: 197–212.

Matsumura, K., Nakayama, T. and Tamaki, Y. (1985) Effects of preoptic and hypothalamic thermal stimulation on electrical activity of neurosecretory cells in the supraoptic nucleus. *Brain Res.*, 346: 327–332.

McCarren, M. and Alger, B.E. (1987) Sodium-potassium pump inhibitors increase neuronal excitability in the rat hippocampal slice: role of a Ca^{2+}-dependent conductance. *J. Neurophysiol.*, 57: 496–509.

Murakami, N. and Sakata, Y. (1978) Influences of thermal stimulation in various thermosensitive structures on the activity of the medullary thermo-responsive neurones of rabbits. In: Y. Houdas and J.D. Guieu (Eds.), *New Trends in Thermal Physiology*, Masson, Paris, pp. 94–97.

Muratani, H., Katafuchi, T., Hori, T. and Kosaka, T. (1991) Extracellular and intracellular recordings from thermosensitive neurons in the rat dorsal motor nucleus of the vagus. *Soc. Neurosci. Abstr.*, 834.

Nakashima, T., Hori, T. and Kiyohara, T. (1989a) Intracellular recording analysis of septal thermosensitive neurons in the rat. In: J.B. Mercer (Ed.), *Thermal Physiology 1989*, Elsevier, Amsterdam, pp. 69–72.

Nakashima, T., Hori, T., Kiyohara, T. and Shibata, M. (1985a) Effects of endotoxin and sodium salicylate on the preoptic thermosensitive neurons in tissue slices. *Brain Res. Bull.*, 15: 459–463.

Nakashima, T., Hori, T., Kiyohara, T. and Shibata, M. (1985b) Osmosensitivity of preoptic thermosensitive neurons in hypothalamic slices *in vitro*. *Pflug. Arch.*, 405: 112–117.

Nakashima, T., Hori, T., Kuriyama, K. and Matsuda, T. (1988) Effects of interferon-α on the activity of preoptic thermosensitive neurons in tissue slices. *Brain Res.*, 454: 361–367.

Nakashima, T., Hori, T., Mori, T., Kuriyama, K. and Mizuno, K. (1989b) Recombinant human interleukin-1β alters the activity of preoptic thermosensitive neurons *in vitro*. *Brain Res. Bull.*, 23: 209–213.

Nakashima, T., Kiyohara, T. and Hori, T. (1991) Tumor necrosis factor-β specifically inhibits the activity of preoptic warm-sensitive neurons in tissue slices. *Neurosci. Lett.*, 128: 97–100.

Nakashima, T., Pierau, F.K., Simon, E. and Hori, T. (1987) Comparison between hypothalamic thermoresponsive neurons from duck and rat slices. *Pflug. Arch.*, 409: 236–243.

Nakayama, T. (1985) Thermosensitive neurons in the brain. Jpn. J. Physiol., 35: 375–389.

Nakayama, T. and Hardy, J.D. (1969) Unit responses in the rabbit's brain stem to changes in brain and cutaneous temperature. *J. Appl. Physiol.*, 27: 848–857.

Nakayama, T. and Imai-Matsumura, K. (1984) Response of glucose-responsive ventromedial hypothalamic neurons to scrotal and preoptic thermal stimulation in rats. *Neurosci. Lett.*, 45: 129–134.

Nakayama, T., Eisenman, J.S. and Hardy, J.D. (1961) Single unit activity of anterior hypothalamus during local heating. *Science*, 134: 560–561.

Nelson, D.O. and Prosser, C.L. (1981) Intracellular recordings from thermosensitive preoptic neurons. *Science*, 213: 787–789.

Nutik, St.L. (1973) Posterior hypothalamic neurons responsive to preoptic region thermal stimulation. *J. Neurophysiol.*, 36: 238–249.

Ogawa, T. (1975) Thermal influence on palmar sweating and mental influence on generalized sweating in man. *Jpn. J. Physiol.*, 25: 525–536.

Osaka, T., Hori, T., Kiyohara, T., Shibata, M. and Nakashima, T. (1984) Changes in body temperature and thermosensitivity of preoptic and septal neurons during hippocampal stimulation. *Brain Res. Bull.*, 13: 93–98.

Pierau, F.K., Torrey, P. and Carpenter, D.O. (1975) Effect of ouabain and potassium free solution on mammalian thermosensitive afferents *in vitro*. *Pflug. Arch.*, 359: 349–356.

Roberts, W.W. and Mooney, R.D. (1974) Brain areas controlling thermoregulatory grooming, prone extension, locomotion, and tail vasodilatation in rats. *J. Comp. Physiol. Psychol.*, 86: 470–480.

Sah, P. and McLachlan, E.M. (1991) Ca^{2+}-activated K^+ currents underlying the afterhyperpolarization in guinea pig vagal neurons: a role for Ca^{2+}-activated Ca^{2+} release. *Neuron*, 7: 257–264.

Saltzman, S.K. and Beckman, A. (1981) Effects of thyrotropin releasing hormone on hypothalamic thermosensitive neurons of the rat. *Brain Res. Bull.,* 7: 325–332.

Satinoff, E. (1978) Neural organization and evolution of thermal regulation in mammals. *Science,* 201: 16–22.

Schlue, W.R. (1991) Effects of ouabain on intracellular ion activities of sensory neurons of the leech central nervous system. *J. Neurophysiol.,* 65: 736–746.

Schmidt-Nielsen, K., Schmidt-Nielsen, B., Jearum, S.A. and Houpt, T.R. (1957) Body temperature of camel and its relation to water economy. *Am. J. Physiol.,* 188: 103–112.

Scott, I.M. and Boulant, J.A. (1984) Dopamine effects on thermosensitive neurons in hypothalamic tissue slices. *Brain Res.,* 306: 157–163.

Shibata, M., Hori, T., Kiyohara, T. and Nakashima, T. (1983a) Facilitation of thermoregulatory heating behavior by single cortical spreading depression in the rat. *Physiol. Behav.,* 31: 651–656.

Shibata, M., Hori, T., Kiyohara, T., Nakashima, T. and Osaka, T. (1983b) Impairment of thermoregulatory cooling behavior by single cortical spreading depression in the rat. *Physiol. Behav.,* 30: 599–605.

Shibata, M., Hori, T., Kiyohara, T. and Nakashima, T. (1984) Activity of hypothalamic thermosensitive neurons during cortical spreading depression in the rat. *Brain Res.,* 308: 255–262.

Shibata, M., Hori, T., Kiyohara, T. and Nakashima, T. (1988a) Convergence of skin and hypothalamic temperature signals on the sulcal prefrontal cortex in the rat. *Brain Res.,* 443: 37–46.

Shibata, M., Hori, T., Kiyohara, T., Nakashima, T. and Asami, T. (1988b) Responses of anterior hypothalamic-preoptic thermo-sensitive neurons to substance P and capsaicin. *Neuropharmacology,* 27: 143–148.

Shibata, M., Hori, T. and Nagasaka, T. (1985) Effects of single cortical spreading depression on the metabolic heat production in the rat. *Physiol. Behav.,* 343: 563–567.

Silva, N.L. and Boulant, J.A. (1984) Effects of osmotic pressure, glucose, and temperature on neurons in preoptic tissue slices. *Am. J. Physiol.,* 247: R335–R345.

Silva, N.L. and Boulant, J.A. (1986) Effects of testosterone, estradiol, and temperature on neurons in preoptic tissue slices. *Am. J. Physiol.,* 250: R625–R632.

Simon, E. (1972) Temperature signals from skin and spinal cord converging on spinothalamic neurons. *Pflug. Arch.,* 337: 323–332.

Simon, E. (1974) Temperature regulation: The spinal cord as a site of extrahypothalamic thermoregulatory functions. *Rev. Physiol. Biochem. Pharmacol.,* 71: 1–76.

Simon, E. and Iriki, M. (1971) Sensory transmission of spinal heat and cold sensitivity in ascending spinal neurons. *Pflug. Arch.,* 328: 103–120.

Simon, E., Pierau, F.K. and Taylor, D.C.M. (1986) Central and peripheral thermal control of effectors in homeothermic temperature regulation. *Physiol. Rev.,* 66: 253–300.

Tamaki, Y., Nakayama, T. and Matsumura, K. (1986) Effects of carbon dioxide inhalation on preoptic thermosensitive neurons. *Pflug. Arch.,* 407: 8–13.

Tamazawa, Y., Matsumoto, M., Kudo, A. and Sasaki, K. (1991) Potassium ion channels operated by receptor stimulation can be activated simply by raising temperature. *Jpn. J. Physiol.,* 41: 117–127.

Tanaka, J., Sato, T., Berezesky, I.K., Jones, R.T., Trump, B.F. and Cowley, R.A. (1983) Effect of hypothermia on survival time and ECG in rats with acute blood loss. *Adv. Shock Res.,* 9: 219–232.

Thompson, S.M., Masukawa, L.M. and Prince, D.A. (1985) Temperature dependence of intrinsic membrane properties and synaptic potentials in hippocampal CA1 neurones *in vitro. J. Neurosci.,* 5: 817–824.

Tsai, L.L., Matsumura, K., Nakayama, T., Itowi, N., Yamatodani, A. and Wada, H. (1989) Effects of histamine on thermosensitive neurons in rat preoptic slice preparations. *Neurosci. Lett.,* 102: 297–302.

Yamamoto, K., Nakayama, T. and Ishikawa, Y. (1981) Response of the lateral hypothalamic neurons to preoptic thermal stimulation in rats. *Neurosci. Lett.,* 22: 257–262.

H.S. Sharma and J. Westman (Eds.)
Progress in Brain Research, Vol 115

CHAPTER 3

Spinal neuronal thermosensitivity *in vivo* and *in vitro* in relation to hypothalamic neuronal thermosensitivity

Eckhart Simon*, Herbert A. Schmid and Ulrich Pehl

Max-Planck-Institute for Physiological and Clinical Research, William G. Kerckhoff-Institute, Parkstrasse 1, D-61231 Bad Nauheim, Germany

Introduction

Interest in the thermosensitivity of central nervous neurons derives, in the first place, from their presumed role as deep-body temperature sensors in temperature regulation. This function was primarily attributed to central nervous elements by the observation of adequate thermoregulatory responses to local thermal stimulations within the central nervous system. In this way the preoptic and anterior hypothalamic (POAH) region was identified first as a site of origin of deep-body thermosensory inputs and, in connection with its thermointegrative functions, provided the experimental basis for the concept of hypothalamic temperature regulation (Hammel, 1968). The discovery of thermoreceptive elements in the spinal cord was pivotal for the establishment of the currently accepted multiple-input, multiple-level concept of thermoregulation (Simon, 1974; Satinoff, 1978; Jessen, 1990).

The present report is concerned with spinal neuronal thermosensitivity evaluated previously *in vivo* and more recently *in vitro*. As in reviews on hypothalamic neuronal thermosensitivity

(Boulant, 1980; Boulant and Dean, 1986), a brief introductory report will illustrate the function of spinal deep-body temperature sensors in temperature regulation. Unlike the hypothalamus, the spinal cord offered the advantage of a distinct topography of afferent and efferent systems which was of particular importance as a guide in the early *in vivo* analysis of neuronal thermosensitivity. Because most of the properties of thermosensitive neurons in the POAH region were disclosed in recent years by recording from brain slices (Hori, 1991; Boulant, 1994) we established a spinal cord slice preparation (Pehl et al., 1994a) to directly compare the local thermosensitivity of spinal cord neurons with properties reported for hypothalamic neurons.

Thermo-physiological evaluation of spinal cord thermosensitivity

Evidence for the thermosensory function of the spinal cord was provided by experiments in mammals in which thermal stimulation within the vertebral canal elicited shivering, vasoconstriction and behavioral cold defence in response to local cooling, and skin vasodilatation, thermal panting, sweating and behavioral heat defence in response to local warming (Simon et al., 1963, 1965; Simon,

---

* Corresponding author.

1974). Stimulation of panting by warming within the vertebral canal was found to persist after dorsal and ventral root transections and, thus, indicated that the spinal cord itself was most likely the site of deep-body temperature perception (Jessen and Simon-Oppermann, 1976). The spinal thermosensory function exists in both mammals and birds, and probably also in lower vertebrates, and is distributed over many segments from the cervico-thoracic to the thoracolumbar spinal cord (Simon, 1974).

The afferent transmission of spinal temperature signals to supraspinal levels was amply documented by the efficiency of spinal thermal stimulations to influence panting in dogs (Jessen, 1967), pigeons (Rautenberg, 1969), rats (Lin et al., 1972) and other mammals and birds (Simon, 1974; Simon et al., 1986) and to elicit behavioral thermoregulatory activities in pigeons (Rautenberg, 1969; Schmidt, 1978), dogs (Cormarèche-Leydier and Cabanac, 1973), pigs (Carlisle and Ingram, 1973) and poikilotherms (Cabanac and Jeddi, 1971). Common integration of hypothalamic and spinal thermal stimuli was concluded from their ability to mutually cancel or potentiate each other in the control of thermoregulatory activity (Jessen et al., 1968; Jessen and Simon, 1971). As a neurophysiological correlate, changes in activity of hypothalamic neurons in response to spinal thermal stimulations were observed (Guieu and Hardy, 1970; Wünnenberg and Hardy, 1972; Boulant and Hardy, 1974), and the underlying temperature-dependent neuronal activity in ascending fibre tracts was demonstrated at the pontine-medullary (Wünnenberg and Brück, 1968a, 1970) and spinal level (Simon and Iriki, 1970). The present report concentrates on the properties of spinal thermosensitive neurons for which an afferent function can be inferred from their location within the spinal cord.

A particular aspect of spinal thermoregulatory functions was disclosed by the observation that spinal thermal stimuli may be converted into adequate thermoregulatory responses in spinalized animals (Kosaka et al., 1967; Walther et al., 1971) suggesting the existence of vestigial thermointe-grative mechanisms at the segmental spinal level. Indeed, an increase in excitability of motoneurons with decreasing local temperature was detected (Klussmann and Pierau, 1972) and is considered as a component in the activation of shivering by spinal cord cooling (Kleinebeckel and Klussmann, 1990). The underlying temperature-dependent changes of membrane conductance provided a general model for neuronal thermosensitivity and were reviewed elsewhere (Pierau et al., 1976).

Spinal neuronal thermosensitivity in vivo

The search for ascending spinal thermosensitive neurons was guided by the deficits in thermoregulatory efficiency of spinal thermal stimulation after partial spinal transections in guinea pigs (Wünnenberg and Brück, 1968b) and rabbits (Kosaka et al., 1969b) which excluded the dorsal columns as a pathway. The studies showed that important fractions of spinal thermosensory signals were conducted ventrally in medial-to-lateral fiber tracts known to originate in mammals from cells in the spinal dorsal horn. Corresponding studies in an avian species, the pigeon, pointed to a more lateral location of the pathway for the thermosensory signals ascending in the spinal cord (Necker, 1975).

Experimental approach to single unit recording

In cats, experimental conditions were established which ensured that temperature-dependent discharge rates of recorded neurons could be unequivocally classified as afferent: (1) extracellular recordings were made from neuraxons, mostly at the level of the 3rd to 4th cervical segment, rostral to the thermally stimulated part of the spinal cord; (2) the stimulation thermode, which consisted of a water-perfused, U-shaped polyethylene tube located in the peridural space, was placed along the spinal cord from the lumbosacral to the upper thoracic/lower cervical segments to stimulate a section of the spinal cord as large as possible, but was kept distant sufficiently from the site of recording to avoid any local temperature changes (Simon and Iriki, 1971b); (3) in several series of experiments the spinal cord was transected rostral to the site of recording to eliminate descending neuronal activity. An approach similar to that established for the cat was also pursued in a study on pigeons in which ascending spinal cold thermosensitivity was analyzed (Necker, 1975). For both cats and pigeons as representatives of the two homeothermic classes of vertebrates, the existence of a minority of ascending neuraxons excited by warming or by cooling the spinal cord could be demonstrated among a majority of neuraxons not affected by spinal thermal stimulation. Because of the very time consuming search for stable recordings from the rather fine neuraxons of the anterior and lateral tracts, it was not possible to quantify the relationship between thermoinsensitive and thermosensitive neurons.

The only possible way to apply thermal stimulations to the spinal cord *in vivo* without causing damage was the use of thin flexible tubes placed in the peridural space alongside the spinal cord. With this method, temperature gradients across the spinal cord could not be avoided. Further, by recording from a thermosensitive neuraxon, the site of origin of the temperature signal could not be identified. Because of these limitations, quantitative figures could only be estimated for the relationships between the discharge rates and the temperatures monitored within the vertebral canal, either close to or distant from the stimulation thermode.

Location of spinal thermosensitive neuraxons

In the cat, both cold and warm sensitive neuraxons were found in the ventrolateral to lateral parts of the spinal fiber tract systems which serve afferent functions according to ample anatomical evidence (Simon and Iriki, 1971b). In the pigeon, the thermosensitive ascending fibers occupied a more dorsal and medial position in the lateral funiculus in agreement with the evidence for afferent temperature signal conduction obtained in transection experiments (Necker, 1975). In both

mammals and birds, the ascending spinal thermosensitive neurons apparently run in the so-called protopathic afferent pathway transmitting temperature and pain signals from the periphery.

Relationship between warm and cold sensitivity

In recordings at the medullary level from spinothalamic tract neurons in guinea pigs, only warm sensitive neurons were described (Wünnenberg and Brück, 1970). In the cat (Simon and Iriki, 1970) and in the pigeon (Necker, 1975) recordings at the cervical spinal level from antero-lateral and lateral tracts demonstrated the presence of neurons activated by either heating or cooling of the spinal cord distal to the recording site. Thermosensitive neuraxons activated by spinal cord warming were more frequent than those activated by cooling. In a sample of 25 thermosensitive neurons recorded in spinalized cats, 18 were warm sensitive and seven cold sensitive (Simon and Iriki, 1970). In a sample of 53 thermosensitive neurons recorded in non-spinalized cats, 40 were warm sensitive and 13 cold sensitive (Hackmann and Simon, 1975). Among 49 thermosensitive neurons recorded in spinalized pigeons, 35 were warm sensitive and 14 cold sensitive (Necker, 1975). Thus, the observations in a mammal and a bird agreed in demonstrating a relationship of about 3:1 between warm and cold sensitive ascending spinal neuraxons.

Temperature-response characteristics

In the cat as well as in the pigeon, the temperature range within which neuraxons exhibited cold or warm sensitivity, encompassed the natural variations of body core temperature. As a rule, both cold and warm sensitive neurons were spontaneously active. Evaluation of static and dynamic response components followed the criteria established for skin cold and warm receptors (Hensel, 1970). The average static response curves of spinal warm and cold sensitive neurons intersected at a spinal canal temperature of about 37°C in the cat (Simon and Iriki, 1971b) and of about 37.5°C in the pigeon (Necker, 1975). At the point of intersection the average discharge rates were approximately 7 Imp./s in the cat, but distinctly higher, approximately 20 Imp./s, in the pigeon.

Static temperature-response relationships

In a sample of 20 warm sensitive units recorded in cats, average static activity increased in a linear to exponential fashion when vertebral canal temperature was raised above 35°C, the slope being steepest in the range of 38–40°C, and tended to level off around 41–43°C at an average discharge rate of 21 Imp./s. Below 35°C, average activity was between 5 and 6 Imp./s and did not change significantly with decreasing temperature (Simon and Iriki, 1971b). In the same study, a sample of 20 cold sensitive spinal neuraxons exhibited an average minimum activity of approximately 4 Imp./s, when vertebral canal temperature was around 40°C. The rise in discharge rate with falling vertebral canal temperature was not rectilinear, the slope being steepest in the range of 37–34°C, and a broad maximum of about 15.5 Imp./s was attained in the range of 28–32°C. Above 40°C, part of the cold sensitive neurons became silent, one neuron responded to intense heating with a re-increase in discharge rate.

For warm sensitive ascending spinal neuraxons in cats an average static temperature coefficient of +3.9 to +6.1 Imp./s/°C was estimated for the temperature range between 38 and 41°C. For the cold sensitive neuraxons, the average temperature coefficient estimated for the temperature range of 35 to 32°C was between −2.2 and −4.4 Imp./s/°C (Simon and Iriki, 1971b). In a smaller sample of thermosensitive neuraxons recorded in the cat, average temperature coefficients of +3.73 Imp./s/°C for warm sensitive units and of −1.33 Imp./s/°C for cold sensitive units were determined by regression analysis (Simon and Iriki, 1971a). In non-spinalized cats, the static temperature-response relationships of warm and cold sensitive neuraxons were not different from those in spinalized cats (Hackmann and Simon, 1975).

In the pigeon, the static temperature-response

characteristics of both cold and warm sensitive neurons were approximately linear in the range of normal core temperature variations. The average temperature coefficients, +4.2 Imp./s/°C for warm sensitive neurons and −2.3 Imp./s/°C for cold sensitive neurons, were very similar to those in the cat (Necker, 1975).

In cats and pigeons, spinal cold and warm sensitive neurons exhibited a considerable overlap of the temperature ranges in which the static temperature dependence of their discharge rates was near its maximum. Thus, both systems could contribute to deep-body temperature monitoring in a rather large range around its normal level. For the cat, the striking similarity of the 'working range' of the spinal cold and warm sensitive neurons with that of the skin warm and cold receptors (Hensel, 1973) suggested similar functions in body temperature regulation (Fig. 1).

Dynamic temperature-response relationships

Both cold and warm receptors of the skin are characterized, apart from their static thermosensitivity, by transient, enhanced activation (overshoot) of the discharge rate, depending on the rate at which stimulus intensity increases, and transient, enhanced inhibition (undershoot), depending on the rate at which stimulus intensity decreases (Hensel, 1981). This kind of dynamic temperature sensitivity has, so far, not been reported in studies on hypothalamic thermosensitive neurons, neither *in vivo* nor *in vitro* (Boulant et al., 1989; Hori, 1991). Spinal thermosensitive neurons recorded *in vivo* seem to occupy an intermediate position. In the guinea pig, 17 among 20 warm sensitive units recorded at the medullary level exhibited a dynamic response component when cervical spinal cord temperature was increased (Wünnenberg and Brück, 1970). Dynamic responses were observed in nine out of 20 warm sensitive and in six out of 20 cold sensitive ascending spinal neurons recorded in spinalized cats (Simon and Iriki, 1971b). The combined static and dynamic responses of several spinal neurons (Figs. 2 and 3) resembled those of skin cold and warm receptors (Simon and Iriki, 1970, 1971a). Neurons

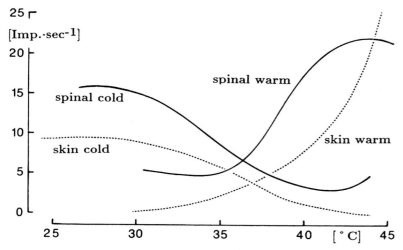

Fig. 1. Average static discharges of warm and cold sensitive units originating in nasal skin (stippled lines) and spinal cord (solid lines) of cats as a function of temperature [from Hensel (1973) (modified), reprinted with kind permission of the American Physiological Society, Belthesda, MD, USA].

with purely dynamic responses to spinal thermal stimulation were not observed *in vivo*. Whether the only partial expression of dynamic response components in spinal thermosensitive neurons reflected different modes of thermoresponsiveness or varying degrees of signal integration could not be experimentally decided in the *in vivo* studies. However, the absence of the dynamic components in the responses of hypothalamic neurons to thermal stimulation of the spinal cord (Guieu and Hardy, 1970; Wünnenberg and Hardy, 1972; Boulant and Hardy, 1974) suggests that only the static response is transmitted as relevant information to the central controller of body temperature.

Synaptic inputs to spinal thermosensitive neurons

Since ascending spinal thermosensitive neuraxons are running in the protopathic sensory tracts they originate most likely from cell somata in the superficial laminae of the dorsal horn, which also receive inputs from peripheral sensory fibers. In recordings made in spinalized cats, non-thermal modulation of discharge rate was occasionally observed, for instance, in correlation with respiratory movements. Especially, however, thermal sti-

mulation of large areas of the skin often affected the discharge rate (Simon and Iriki, 1971b; Simon, 1972). The most consistent observation was activation by skin cooling of neurons that were also activated by spinal cord cooling, but intense skin heating above 40°C also activated these neurons. Spinal warm sensitive neurons were more weakly and less consistently influenced by changes of skin temperature. Thus, convergence of cutaneous and spinal thermosensory inputs deviated from a simple additive interaction of cold signals and, respectively, warm signals of cutaneous and spinal origin (Simon, 1972).

Moreover, convergence of temperature signals from the skin and from the spinal cord on the ascending neurons in the anterolateral tract could be observed only in spinalized animals. While the expression of spinal cold and warm sensitivity was not altered in non-spinalized cats, the effects of peripheral thermal stimulations were greatly diminished (Hackmann and Simon, 1975). This suggests that signal transmission of thermosensory inputs from the skin to the ascending neurons transmitting spinal cold and warm sensitivity is under strong, descending inhibitory control. This degree of inhibition seems to be qualitatively different from the descending control of signal

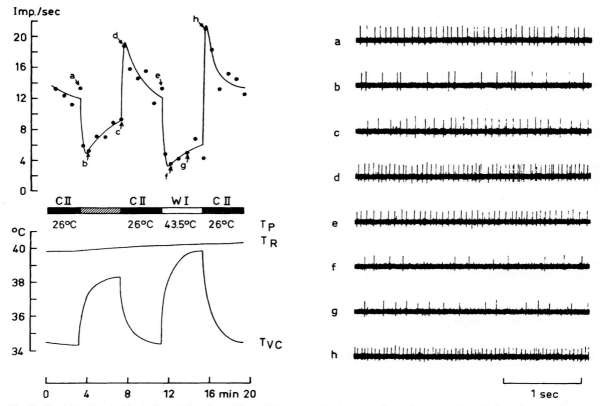

Fig. 2. Combined static/dynamic activity of a cold sensitive neuron in the anterolateral tract of the spinal cord responding to spinal cord temperature changes. Left: Upper diagram, discharge rate; lower diagram, temperature in the vertebral canal (T_{VC}) and rectal temperature (T_R); middle bar: perfusion of the peridurally located thermode with cool (black) or warm (white) water or no perfusion (hatched) with temperature of the perfusion fluid (T_P). Right: recordings of single unit activity at the points of the response curve indicated by the letters [from Simon and Iriki (1970), reprinted with kind permission of Birkhäuser Verlag AG, Basel, Switzerland).

transmission from cutaneous thermoreceptors to dorsal horn neurons in general (Pierau et al., 1980), since under comparable experimental conditions, signals from skin thermoreceptors undoubtedly reach supraspinal levels, as amply documented by the influence of skin temperature on thermoregulatory activities of non-spinalized, conscious as well as anesthetized animals. Therefore, the pathways by which spinal temperature signals are afferently transmitted, do not seem to be essential for the supraspinal transmission of skin temperature signals. Convergence of cutaneous and spinal temperature signals at the segmental level, as observed in spinalized animals,

probably reflected the vestigial thermointegrative functions of the spinal cord which were disclosed by the persistence of elementary thermoregulatory reactions after spinal cord transection (Simon, 1974).

Spinal neuronal thermosensitivity in vitro

The recent analysis of hypothalamic thermosensitivity has been carried out mainly by recording from single neurons in tissue slices. For this reason, the method was adapted to the spinal cord to characterize spinal thermosensitive neurons according to criteria applied also to hypothalamic neurons. So far, only the extracellular recording technique has been applied in the in vitro analysis of spinal cord thermosensitivity.

Experimental approach to single unit recording

Details of spinal cord slice preparation have been described elsewhere (Pehl et al., 1994a). The tissue slices, about 500 μm thick, were incubated and superfused with a medium (pH 7.4, 290 mosmol/kg) of the following composition (in mmol): NaCl, 124; KCl, 5; NaH_2PO_4, 1.2; $MgSO_4$, 1.3; $CaCl_2$, 1.2; $NaHCO_3$, 26; glucose 10, equilibrated with 95% O_2 and 5% CO_2. By lowering $[Ca^{2+}]$ to 0.3 mmol and elevating $[Mg^{2+}]$ to 9.0 mmol to block synaptic transmission, synaptic and inherent temperature dependence of neuronal activity could be separated. In addition, agents from which support in the characterization of neurons was expected were temporarily added to the perfusion fluid. Especially, however, the incubation chamber for the slice was specifically designed for the close control of slice temperature in a range between 33 and 41°C, with 37°C as maintenance temperature, and could be changed: (1) sinusoidally in a cycle of 7 min; (2) in a ramp-like manner at 0.02°C/s; and (3) in steps with a maximum rate of 0.4°C/s to separate static from dynamic response components. Neurons were extracellularly recorded with glass-coated platinum-iridium microelectrodes of about 2 μm tip diameter. Computerized evaluation of the single unit

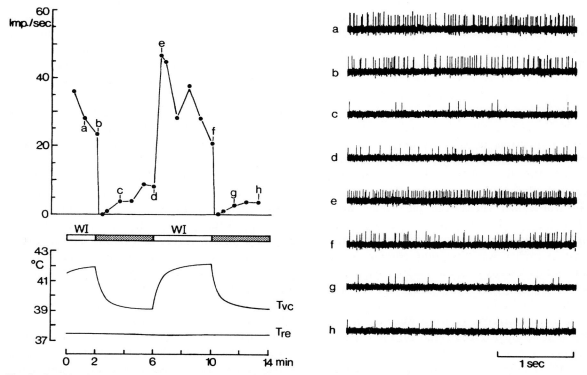

Fig. 3. Combined static/dynamic activity of a warm sensitive neuron in the anterolateral tract of the spinal cord responding to spinal cord temperature changes. Left: Upper diagram, discharge rate; lower diagram, temperature in the vertebral canal (T_{vc}) and rectal temperature (Tre); middle bar, perfusion of the peridurally located thermode with warm water of 41.5°C (WI, white) or no perfusion (hatched). Right: recordings of single unit activity at the points of the response curve indicated by the letters [from Simon and Iriki (1971a), reprinted with kind permission of Publications Elsevier, Paris, France].

activity was based on a bin width of 10 s to determine discharge rates.

The evaluation of temperature effects on unit discharge had to take into account some uncertainty about the temperature coefficient of the static temperature response as an indicator to discriminate between thermosensitive and insensitive neurons, ± 0.6 Imp./s/°C (Schmid and Pierau, 1993) or $+0.8$ Imp./s/°C for warm and -0.6 Imp./s/°C for cold sensitive units (Boulant, 1994) being conventionally taken as the limiting figures. Arguments derived from recordings in slice preparations, however, do not seem pertinent for the choice between one or the other convention, considering that minor variations in $[Ca^{2+}]$ in the superfusion media of different laboratories may modify the temperature coefficient (Schmid and Pierau, 1993). As expected, the tentative classification of spinal neurons according to either coefficient did not disclose relevant differences apart from minor changes in the relationship between warm sensitive and insensitive neurons.

Location of thermosensitive spinal cord neurons

As in the *in vivo* studies, the analysis of thermosensitive neurons in slice preparations from the spinal cord took advantage of the topography of the spinal cord which provided clues for the afferent or efferent function of an investigated cell. In transversal slices, the electrodes were placed under visual control observing the well-known histological landmarks. Longitudinal slices were cut in such a way that they contained the neurons of interest. Most studies were carried out by probing dorsal horn neurons between the surface of the spinal cord and the central canal. At all levels thermosensitive neurons were found. So far, the analysis has concentrated on the superficial laminae I and II of Rexed as part of the sensory afferent system, and on the lamina X surrounding the central canal as a region analogous to the periventricular neuropil of the hypothalamus. Ventral horn neurons were excluded from the analysis because of their efferent func-

tion, although their thermosensitivity had previously been demonstrated (Klussmann and Pierau, 1972; Pierau et al., 1976).

Relation between warm and cold sensitivity

In the *in vivo* studies on ascending spinal neuraxons about 75% of the thermosensitive neurons were warm sensitive and 25% cold sensitive. In this respect, the result obtained *in vitro* on slice preparations was distinctly different in that neuronal cold sensitivity was a rare observation. Table 1 summarizes the fractions of thermoinsensitive, warm sensitive and cold sensitive neurons recorded in extended studies on transversal slices. The percentages of warm and cold sensitive neurons were 45.9 and 1.6% in laminae I + II and 58.6 and 4.3% in lamina X. Basal discharge rates of both warm-sensitive and insensitive neurons were significantly higher in the sample of lamina X neurons compared to laminae I + II. For the small numbers of cold-sensitive neurons in each sample, the statistical comparison did not reveal a difference in the basal discharge rates.

In a small sample of 22 neurons recorded in an exploratory study on longitudinal slices containing dorsal horn neurons, 7 were insensitive and 15 warm sensitive but no cold sensitive neuron was observed (Pehl et al., 1994a). Compared with the laminae I + II neurons recorded in transversal slices, the average basal discharge rate of the warm-sensitive neurons in the longitudinal slices (13.5 ± 3.3 Imp./s) was significantly higher, suggesting a higher degree of synaptic interaction.

The scarcity or absence of cold sensitivity in each of the recording samples suggests that the more frequent appearance of this modality in the ascending tract neurons is the result of signal integration, reflecting synaptic inhibition of a spontaneously active neuron by a warm sensitive neuron. The neuronal interconnections existing within a transversal tissue slice were apparently not sufficient to generate an appreciable fraction of cold sensitive neurons. Further, the absence of cold sensitive neurons in longitudinal slice preparations containing the dorsal horn neurons of

TABLE 1

Fractions of thermosensitive and insensitive neurons recorded in transversal tissue slices from lumbar spinal cord of rats and frequency of dynamic response components

	No. of neurons	Discharge rate at 37°C (Imp./s/)	Temperature coefficient (Imp./s/°C)	Phasic response component (%)
Laminae I + II	183			
Warm sensitive	84	5.5 ± 0.4^a	1.6 ± 0.1	73^c
Cold sensitive	3	8.8 ± 5.5	-2.3 ± 0.6	0
Insensitive	96	3.0 ± 0.2^b	0.3 ± 0.03	59^d
Lamina X	116			
Warm sensitive	68	15.3 ± 1.0^a	1.8 ± 0.1	9^c
Cold sensitive	5	4.1 ± 2.7	-1.1 ± 0.2	40
Insensitive	43	6.2 ± 0.7^b	0.3 ± 0.04	3^d

Means ± standard errors; significant differences between laminae I + II and lamina X were found for: basal discharge rates of warm sensitive ([a]) and insensitive ([b]) neurons ($2P < 0.05$; t-test) and for the frequencies of occurrence of phasic components in the responses to thermal stimulations of warm sensitive ([c]) and insensitive ([d]) neurons ($2P < 0.001$, chi-square test); (Pehl et al., 1997).

several segments also seemed to exclude a longitudinal, trans-segmental organization of the presumed neuronal network generating the cold signal. At the current state of analysis it seems unlikely that a population of cold sensitive neurons with projections to the anterolateral ascending tracts might have been overlooked in the slice recordings.

Temperature-response characteristics

The temperature coefficient of a neuronal response was determined by linear regression analysis of the static relationship between discharge rate and slice temperature. Different from most studies on hypothalamic neurons, the starting points of the linear regressions were not determined by visual inspection but, instead, with a piecewise regression procedure to discriminate between monophasic and biphasic temperature-response relationships (Vieth, 1989). For monophasic responses the temperature coefficient was determined by the slope of the entire regression and for biphasic responses by the slope of the regression describing the steeper part of the response curve (Pehl et al., 1994a). According to this coefficient a neuron was characterized as insensitive, warm sensitive ($\geq +0.6$ Imp./s/°C) or cold sensitive (≤ -0.6 Imp./s/°C).

Dynamic components in the response of a neuron, depending on the rate of change of slice temperature, were usually obvious from the effects of stepwise temperature changes. As a limiting figure, a temporary rise in activity by 30% or more above the static response level was chosen.

Static temperature-response relationships

As summarized in Table 1, the temperature coefficients of insensitive, warm sensitive and cold sensitive neurons recorded in transversal slices did not differ between laminae I + II and lamina X neurons. They also did not differ from the corresponding coefficients of 1.5 ± 2.2 and 0.2 ± 0.03 Imp./s/°C obtained for the warm sensitive and insensitive neurons, respectively, in the longitudinal slices. Fig. 4 presents the activity of a

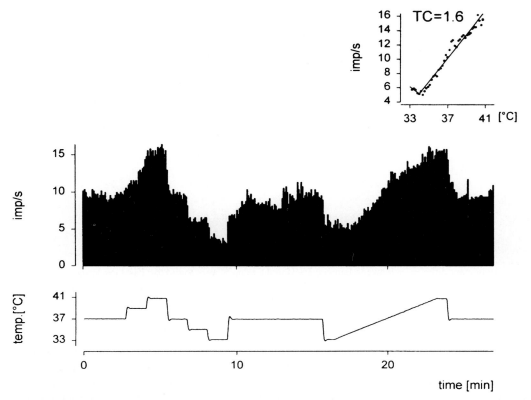

Fig. 4. Continuous rate meter recording (imp/s, upper trace) of a neuron in lamina X of a transversal lumbar spinal cord tissue slice. Slice temperature (temp., lower trace) was changed in a step-like and ramp-like fashion between 33 and 41°C. The neuron is warm sensitive and displays purely static thermosensitivity. The inset shows the result of piecewise linear regression analysis which disclosed a nearly monotonous relationship between temperature and static discharge rate in response to the ramp-like temperature change (TC, temperature coefficient). Pehl, unpublished data.

neuron recorded in lamina X which exhibits only static thermosensitivity. Fig. 5 presents a neuron from lamina II in which static warm sensitivity is combined with a dynamic response component.

Dynamic temperature-response relationships

As summarized in Table 1, a majority of warm sensitive neurons exhibited combined static/dynamic responses in laminae I + II, which differed significantly, in this respect, from neurons of lamina X, where purely static warm sensitivity was prevailing. Dynamic warm sensitivity was characterized by the transient overshoot of discharge rate after stepwise temperature increases.

In addition, 20% of the warm sensitive neurons of laminae I + II transiently exhibited a more pronounced suppression of discharge rate after stepwise decreases of stimulation temperature. This combination of dynamic over- and undershoots of discharge rate closely resembled the characteristics of many peripheral warm receptors (Hensel, 1981).

From the small number of cold sensitive neurons no conclusions about possible topographical differences in the distribution of dynamically responsive neurons could be drawn. None of the three cold sensitive neurons recorded in laminae I + II was dynamically responsive. Among the five cold sensitive neurons of lamina X, two were

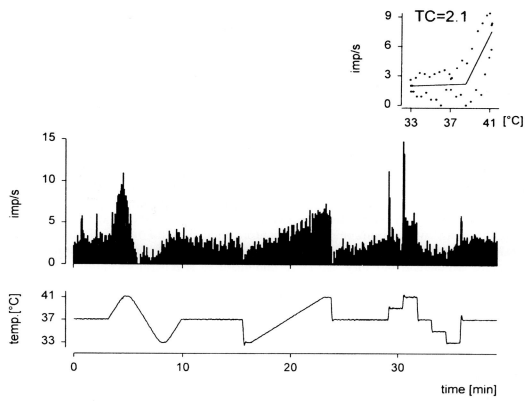

Fig. 5. Continuous rate meter recording (imp/s, upper trace) of a neuron in lamina II of a transversal spinal cord tissue slice. Slice temperature (temp., lower trace) was changed in a sinusoidal, ramp-like and step-like fashion between 33 and 41°C. The neuron is warm sensitive and displays static thermosensitivity as well as a dynamic response component which is visible when temperature is altered in steps. The inset shows the result of piecewise linear regression analysis which disclosed a thermoinsensitive and a warm sensitive range of the relationship between temperature and static discharge in the response to the sinusoidal temperature change with a switch point at about 38.5°C (TC, temperature coefficient of the warm sensitive range) [from Schmid et al. (1994), reprinted with kind permission of Birkhäuser Verlag AG, Basel, Switzerland].

dynamically sensitive, however, only one neuron responded adequately with a temporary overshoot of activity to rapid cooling, whereas the other neuron exhibited an inadequate transient activation in response to rapid warming.

A surprising observation was the frequent occurrence of dynamic response components among the thermo-insensitive neurons of laminae I + II, which typically consisted in a very transient activation by stepwise increases in slice temperature. Dynamic thermoresponsiveness alone cannot be relevant in monitoring deep-body temperature. However, its appearance in both warm sensitive

and insensitive neurons suggests that the underlying membrane properties may be common to the superficial dorsal horn neurons which, irrespective of their static thermosensitivity, serve as relay stations for peripheral sensory inputs.

Synaptic inputs of thermosensitive neurons

Neurons analyzed for thermosensitivity at the spinal segmental level generally have to be considered as interneurons involved in the integration of signals at the spinal level, as well as in the afferent conduction of primary or segmentally processed sensory information to supraspinal levels. Neurons of laminae I + II are relay stations in the temperature and pain pathway from the periphery and give rise to ascending anterolateral tract axons (Perl, 1990). Neurons of lamina X were shown to receive mixed sensory inputs from visceral and somatic afferents, and supraspinal projections were also documented (Honda, 1985). Especially in rat lumbar spinal segments, neurons which are clustered dorsally adjacent to the central canal (Hancock and Peveto, 1979) may be preganglionic sympathetic neurons with efferent axons running towards the intermedio-lateral columns (Anderson et al., 1989). As amply discussed for the hypothalamus, interneurons may exhibit thermosensitivity, because synaptic transmission is temperature dependent, but may as well possess inherent thermosensitivity independent of the synaptic input.

Synaptic vs. inherent thermosensitivity

The temperature sensitivity of 25 spontaneously active spinal cord neurons (13 warm sensitive, one cold sensitive and 11 temperature insensitive units) could be studied in the control incubation fluid as well as when the $[Ca^{2+}]$ had been lowered to 0.3 mmol and $[Mg^{2+}]$ had been elevated to 9.0 mmol in order to block synaptic transmission. Only 10 out of the 25 neurons remained spontaneously active during superfusion with the blocking solution for 35 or more min. However, nine of the 13 warm sensitive neurons retained their responsiveness to warming and remained warm sensitive, the temperature coefficient being increased in four neurons and slightly reduced in five neurons. Out of seven warm sensitive neurons recorded in laminae I + II, five retained their sensitivity in the low Ca^{2+}/high Mg^{2+} medium as illustrated by the example of Fig. 6. All five neurons exhibiting dynamic responsiveness retained this property during synaptic blockade. The one cold sensitive neuron investigated lost its temperature sensitivity in the blocking solution. Among the 11 thermoinsensitive neurons, synaptic blockade altered the temperature coefficient of only one neuron to a degree (from 0.5 to 1.0

Imp./s/°C) that made it warm sensitive. Taken together the results showed that the majority of the warm sensitive neurons were intrinsically thermosensitive, independent of their synaptic input.

Responsiveness to putative transmitters

With special respect to the possible function of thermosensitive neurons as interneurons in the temperature and pain pathway, an exploratory study was carried out on 21 neurons (10 warm sensitive and 11 insensitive units) in which the slices were temporarily exposed to substance P as a neuropeptide released in the dorsal horn by peripheral thermal and nociceptive afferents and to glutamate as a general excitatory transmitter (Schmid et al., 1994). The only notable observation was the absence of any influence of substance P on each of six warm sensitive neurons in laminae I + II, suggesting that peripheral warm receptors may not directly innervate these neurons. However, this impression has, so far, not been confirmed statistically on a larger sample.

Some degree of functional separation of neurons in laminae I + II from those in lamina X has recently been disclosed by the effects of nitric oxide (NO) at the lumbar spinal level (Pehl et al., 1994b). Staining for NADPH diaphorase, an enzyme involved in NO-formation, clearly indicated the presence of reactive fibres and cell bodies in the superficial laminae of the dorsal horn as well as in lamina X lateral and dorsal to the central canal (Fig. 7). As NO donors, sodium nitroprusside (SNP; Sigma, Deisenhofen; Schwarz, Monheim, Germany), *S*-nitroso-*N*-acetyl-D,L- penicillamine (SNAP; Alexis, Grünberg, Germany) or 3-morpholinosydnonimine (SIN-1; a generous gift from Cassella, Frankfurt, Germany) were applied to the incubation medium. Among the warm sensitive neurons of lamina X more than 90% were excited and only 3% inhibited by NO, while among the warm sensitive neurons of laminae I + II, 34% were excited and 44% inhibited (see accompanying article of Schmid et al.). Inhibitors of NO synthesis produced adequate effects indicating that endogenously produced NO was effective in

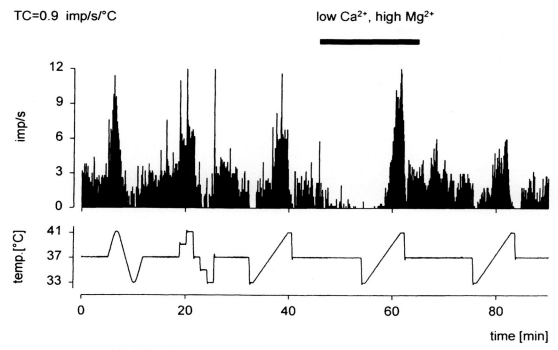

TC=0.9 imp/s/°C

low Ca²⁺, high Mg²⁺

Fig. 6. Continuous rate meter recording (imp/s, upper trace) of a neuron in lamina II of a transversal lumbar spinal cord tissue slice. Slice temperature (temp., lower trace) was changed in a sinusoidal, step-like, and ramp-like fashion between 33 and 41°C. The neuron is warm sensitive, displaying static and dynamic thermosensitivity. The middle ramp response was recorded during slice superfusion (bar) with a medium low in Ca^{2+} and high in Mg^{2+} to block synaptic transmission and shows that warm sensitivity was retained despite a decrease in spontaneous activity [from Pehl et al. (1994a), reprinted with kind permission of John Libbey Eurotext, Paris, France].

the same manner as exogenously applied NO. For both effects cellular mediation by cGMP could be confirmed by demonstrating parallel effects of NO donors and the membrane-permeable cGMP analogue 8Br-cGMP (Pehl and Schmid, 1997). The data suggest that the neurons of lamina X belong to a system that is functionally different from that represented by at least a majority of the neurons of laminae I + II. The well-known involvement of neurons of the superficial dorsal horn layers in the transduction of temperature signals suggests the hypothesis that thermosensitivity inherent to laminae I + II neurons most likely generates the specific spinal thermosensory signals which could be traced *in vivo* in ascending antero-lateral tract neurons. Whether their different susceptibilities to NO reflect a functional difference within this population, remains to be clarified.

Spinal in relation to hypothalamic neuronal thermosensitivity

Because of the powerful thermosensory function of the *hypothalamus* in mammals, especially of the preoptic and anterior hypothalamic (POAH) area, neuronal thermosensitivity has been most frequently analyzed in this region, starting with the discovery of hypothalamic warm sensitive neurons (Nakayama et al., 1961). In the earlier *in vivo* studies the rostrally located areas of maximum thermosensitivity, as disclosed by their role in temperature regulation, were chosen first as recording sites, but subsequently more caudal parts were also probed with the intention to obtain information from the comparison of areas of prevailing thermointegrative functions with those dominant in thermoreception. With the introduc-

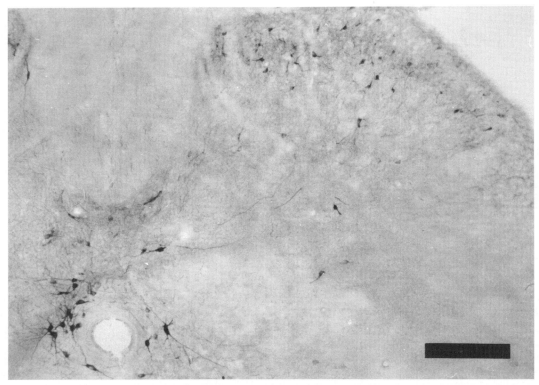

Fig. 7. Transversal section through the lumbar spinal cord of a rat in which neurons and fibers exhibit dark staining by NADPH diaphorase histochemistry. Concentrations of stained material indicating nitrergic innervation are found in the superficial dorsal horn layers and in lamina X near the central canal (bar: 200 μm).

tion of the *in vitro* technique using superfused tissue slice preparations, interest was again focused on the thermoreceptive function of hypothalamic neurons, making use of changes in composition of the incubation medium to study synaptic interactions.

In the analysis of *spinal cord* thermosensitivity, the early *in vivo* studies proceeded in the first place from the topography of the spinal cord which allowed study of neurons with confirmed, efferent or afferent functions (Simon, 1974). The recently started *in vitro* studies on spinal cord tissue slices, while also taking advantage of the structural clues offered by the spinal cord, have otherwise pursued the approaches prescribed by the *in vitro* analysis of hypothalamic neuronal thermosensitivity, including the conventional tem-

perature coefficients to discriminate between thermosensitive and insensitive neurons.

The problem of thermosensory specificity

In attempts to associate neuronal thermosensitivity with thermosensory functions, a general problem has arisen from the observation that thermosensitive neurons are not restricted to areas of the central nervous system with proven thermosensory functions. This was revealed first by *in vivo* studies on cortical neurons (Barker and Carpenter, 1970). Recently, the classification of neurons as thermosensitive or insensitive was shown to be affected *in vitro* by changes in extracellular Ca^{2+} concentration and by neuropeptides known to be present in hypothalamic neurons

(Schmid and Pierau, 1993; Schmid et al., 1993). For these reasons, discrimination between sensory and non-sensory neuronal thermoresponsiveness has remained a key issue in studies on the hypothalamus as well as on the lower brain stem and the spinal cord and cannot be solved by classifying neurons according to their temperature coefficients.

For the *hypothalamus*, *in vivo* studies revealed a continuous distribution of thermosensitive neurons, partly with different proportions of warm and cold sensitive neurons, which extended from its preoptic to its posterior portions and further into the midbrain and medulla (Boulant and Dean, 1986) without reflecting the different contributions of these brain stem sites to the thermosensory input in temperature regulation. Recent in vitro recordings from tissue slices of the rat diencephalon demonstrated similar thermosensitivities within the POAH region and within rostral brain stem regions outside of this classical thermosensory area (Dean and Boulant, 1989; Derambure and Boulant, 1994). Moreover, the distributions of thermosensitive neurons in the hypothalamus of the duck evaluated *in vivo* (Simon et al., 1977; Lin and Simon, 1982) were very similar to those in the mammalian hypothalamus, and *in vitro* studies revealed no differences between the temperature-response relationships of POAH neurons in the rat and duck (Nakashima et al., 1987), although the thermosensory function of the POAH region is strongly expressed in mammals but only weakly in birds (Simon et al., 1986).

As previously emphasized, the thermosensory function of *spinal cord* neurons is amply documented by thermophysiological data obtained in mammals, birds and lower vertebrates (Simon et al., 1986). At the supraspinal level, electrophysiological evidence for the afferent conduction of spinal temperature signals was provided by the responses of the cortical electroencephalogram to both spinal cord heating and cooling (Kosaka et al., 1969a) and by changes in neuronal activity evoked by spinal thermal stimulation at the anterior and posterior hypothalamic levels (Guieu and Hardy, 1970; Wünnenberg and Hardy, 1972; Boulant and Hardy, 1974), where neurons often displayed the same type of thermosensitivity in response to local and spinal thermal stimulations. At the spinal level, neuronal thermosensitivity is a property of many neurons including those with efferent functions (Simon, 1974), however, the anatomical organization of the spinal cord provides unequivocal evidence that the afferent thermosensory contribution of the spinal cord to thermoregulation can only be provided by the two populations of ascending, cold and warm sensitive neuraxons.

Primary thermodetectors vs. thermosensory interneurons

For the *hypothalamus* the early *in vivo* recordings from the POAH region suggested the hypothesis that neurons with linear-to-exponential relationships between discharge rate and temperature and little sensitivity to a variety of non-thermal stimulations might represent primary thermodetectors, whereas neurons which exhibited non-linear, biphasic temperature-response characteristics and were sensitive to remote, thermal and non-thermal stimuli were considered as interneurons (Hardy, 1972, 1973). However, for theoretical reasons bell-shaped response curves were also postulated for hypothalamic thermosensors (Bligh, 1972). Especially in later in vitro studies, the shape of the temperature response curve was no longer considered as a property to discriminate between thermosensors and interneurons taking into account that interneurons could also function as temperature signal generators.

For the *spinal cord*, the *in vivo* recordings on ascending anterolateral tract neuraxons showed that both cold and warm sensitive units frequently displayed responsiveness to inputs from the periphery and thereby revealed their function as interneurons. The function of interneurons has also to be attributed to those thermosensitive units which have, so far, been studied *in vitro* on spinal slice preparations, considering their location in the laminae of the dorsal horn. As for the hypothalamus, no convincing evidence seems to exist for the spinal cord that specific temperature signals are generated by primary sensory neurons without synaptic input; however, at present, this possibility cannot be definitely excluded.

Neuronal thermosensitivity as an inherent or synaptic property

For the *hypothalamus*, numerous *in vivo* studies of the POAH region unanimously reported proportions of warm sensitive, cold sensitive and thermally insensitive neurons in the order of 20–40%, 10–30%, and 40–70%, respectively (Boulant and Dean, 1986). It was earlier suggested that inherent thermosensitivity might be restricted to warm sensitive neurons, whereas cold sensitive neurons rather would be represented by insensitive interneurons receiving an inhibitory input from a warm sensitive cell (Hammel, 1968). Subsequent *in vitro* studies on hypothalamic tissue slices, in which at least a considerable fraction of neuronal interconnections is interrupted, supported this idea by showing that the occurrence of cold sensitive neurons relative to the warm sensitive ones was clearly diminished (Boulant and Dean, 1986; Hori, 1991). In addition the question of intrinsic vs. synaptic thermosensitivity of hypothalamic neurons was assessed *in vitro* by exposing slices to a medium low in Ca^{2+} and high in Mg^{2+} in order to block synaptic transmission. Generally, warm sensitivity was frequently retained after synaptic blockade. The disappearance of cold sensitivity supported the idea of an inherent warm sensitivity and a synaptically induced cold sensitivity (Kelso and Boulant, 1982), however, the persistence of cold sensitivity was also sometimes observed (Hori et al., 1980; Dean and Boulant, 1992).

For the *spinal cord*, studies *in vivo* revealed a relationship of about 1:3 between cold and warm sensitive neurons, but in the *in vitro* studies cold sensitive neurons were extremely scarce, less than 1:10 in relation to warm sensitive neurons. As for the hypothalamus, this difference suggests that cold sensitivity is secondary to synaptic intercon-

nections which were severed by the slice preparation. Experiments using slice superfusion with a low Ca^{2+}/high Mg^{2+} medium to block synaptic input confirmed that the majority of warm sensitive neurons retained their sensitivity, while the scarcity of cold sensitive neurons precluded a statistically relevant analysis. However, considering the *in vivo* and *in vitro* observations together, the data favor the hypothesis of an inherent warm sensitivity and a synaptically produced cold sensitivity also for the spinal cord.

Putative mechanisms of temperature responsiveness

Studies on tissue slices from the *hypothalamus* were recently carried out to elucidate the mechanisms responsible for the transduction of temperature changes into changes of neuronal activity. Particular properties like large temperature coefficients of sodium channels (Kiyohara et al., 1990), temperature dependent, non-synaptic depolarizing prepotentials (Curras et al., 1991), differential temperature effects on membrane conductances for different ions (Kobayashi and Takahashi, 1993), and temperature dependence of membrane potential and input resistance (Griffin and Boulant, 1995) are being discussed as indicators for the specificity of central nervous thermosensors. In addition, plasticity of neuronal temperature dependence has been analyzed as a property of potential thermosensory relevance (Pierau et al., 1994). Different from the responses of warm sensitive neurons which mostly follow local temperature changes with little delay, a delayed activation by local temperature changes, mostly of inherently cold sensitive neurons, was recently reported (Dean and Boulant, 1992), suggesting a basic difference between intrinsic warm and cold responsiveness.

In the *spinal cord*, cellular mechanisms of thermosensitivity have, so far, not been investigated in afferent neurons. However, because of the established thermosensitivity of spinal motoneurons their membrane properties were analyzed. Apart from the possible role of motoneuron cold sensitivity as a component in the activation of shivering (Klussmann and Pierau, 1972), this property was further investigated as a model for thermosensitivity in general (Klussmann, 1964; Pierau et al., 1969, 1976). From these studies, the hypothesis was put forward that neuronal thermoresponsiveness results from differential temperature coefficients of passive ionic conductance and electrogenic sodium transport, and was considered in the analysis of the mechanisms of temperature transduction in peripheral thermoreceptors (Pierau et al., 1974, 1975; Braun et al., 1980; Hensel, 1981; Braun et al., 1990). The relevance of this model for spinal afferent thermosensitivity remains to be tested.

Pharmacological analysis of synaptic control

In attempts to characterize the *hypothalamus* as a site of temperature signal generation as well as signal integration, the responsiveness of hypothalamic neurons to a variety of humoral factors, biogenic amines, neuropeptides, transmitters, pyrogens and cytokines was compared with the thermoregulatory effects elicited by the same agents *in vivo* (Boulant and Silva, 1987; Hori et al., 1987; Myers and Lee, 1989; Hori, 1991). Inasmuch as these agents affected the discharge rates of thermosensitive neurons the results were used either to interpret the roles of these mediators in body temperature control or, vice versa, to explain effects of hypothalamic temperature on non-thermoregulatory homeostatic control. The neurophysiological studies had been initiated by the observation of hypothermic effects of noradrenaline (NA) and hyperthermic effects of 5-hydroxytryptamine (5-HT) in cats (Feldberg and Myers, 1965). While subsequent thermophysiological studies confirmed these findings in dogs and monkeys, hyperthermic responses to NA and hypothermic responses to 5-HT were observed in rabbits, sheep, rats, guinea pigs and pigeons and were found to depend, in part, on the state of thermally induced thermoregulatory activities (Bligh, 1973; Hissa, 1988; Brück and Zeisberger, 1990). Early microiontophoresis studies in cats and rats revealed little responsiveness of highly

thermosensitive hypothalamic neurons to acetylcholine (ACh), 5-HT and NA, but presented evidence for opposing actions of NA on warm and cold sensitive interneurons, while 5-HT rarely affected neuronal activity and ACh excited a minority of warm sensitive neurons (Beckman and Eisenman, 1970). The role of dopamine (DA) was also considered in a later study (Scott and Boulant, 1984). The observation that NA and 5-HT affected warm and cold-sensitive neurons in the POAH region differently (Hori and Nakayama, 1973) was subsequently confirmed, although sometimes only as a statistically unproven tendency (Hellon, 1975). In further studies consistent as well as inconsistent relationships between thermosensitivity and responsiveness to biogenic amines were demonstrated (Jell, 1973; Murakami, 1973; Sato and Simon, 1988), and the opposing actions of NA and 5-HT on thermosensitive units were found to be differently organized at different levels of the brain stem (Watanabe et al., 1986). According to more recent reviews (Myers and Lee, 1989; Brück and Zeisberger, 1990), the roles of biogenic amines as transmitters of brain stem systems modulating thermoregulatory (and probably also non-thermoregulatory) mechanisms appear firmly established, irrespective of obvious species differences. The systematic analysis of hormones and pyrogens in addition to the biogenic amines revealed, at least as a general tendency, that compounds inducing hyperthermic responses reduced the activity of warm sensitive and enhanced the activity of cold sensitive neurons, whereas compounds inducing hypothermia had opposite effects on hypothalamic thermosensitive neurons (Hori, 1991).

The role of the *spinal cord* in temperature regulation was not systematically analyzed with the pharmacological approach, considering that its thermointegrative function is only vestigial (Simon, 1974). As briefly reported, testing spinal cord neurons in slice preparations with a neuropeptide and an excitatory transmitter has, so far, not provided evidence for a relationship between the observed responses and the topographical distribution of thermosensitive neurons (Schmid et al., 1994).

Hypothalamic integration of local, spinal and peripheral temperature signals

Unlike the *spinal cord*, the cytoarchitecture of the POAH region provides little information to apply afferent, integrative or efferent functions to single hypothalamic neurons. Various neuronal models of hypothalamic temperature regulation were devised with the intention to reconcile the observed properties of hypothalamic neurons with the function of the hypothalamus as the center of temperature regulation, where locally generated signals as well as signals transmitted from extrahypothalamic thermosensory structures are transformed into signals controlling the thermoregulatory effectors (Hammel, 1968; Myers and Yaksh, 1969; Bligh et al., 1971; Hardy, 1972; Bligh, 1972, 1973; Jell, 1974; Myers, 1975; Boulant, 1980; Lin, 1984; Boulant et al., 1989; Brück and Hinckel, 1982, 1990). Several models incorporated the spinal cord as a site of extrahypothalamic temperature signal generation. A model taking into account the vestigial thermointegrative functions of the spinal cord was devised with the intention to put forward the hypothesis of the multi-level organization of central nervous control in temperature regulation (Simon, 1974).

Neuronal networks of different complexity were derived from the presumed function of linearly and non-linearly temperature-dependent hypothalamic neurons as thermosensory neurons and interneurons, respectively (Hammel, 1968; Hardy, 1972). For thermosensory neurons, the assumption of a bell-shaped temperature-response relationship was also introduced for theoretical reasons (Bligh, 1972). While these models were helpful in explaining the interaction of hypothalamic temperature with extrahypothalamic, spinal and cutaneous thermal inputs in the control of body temperature, they remained unproven at the neuronal level (Bligh, 1973) and seem to have had little predictive value for the

analysis of the topographical distribution of thermosensitive neurons with the *in vitro* approach.

Unlike mammals, the thermosensory function of the *hypothalamus* is little developed in birds, and inadequate thermoregulatory effects may be elicited especially by hypothalamic cooling. Proceeding from this observation, attempts were made to discriminate conceptually between non-sensory, synaptic temperature-dependence of neurons as a general property of integrative hypothalamic networks and a sensory temperature-dependence providing input signals for thermoregulatory control (Simon, 1981). Indeed, the existence of a non-sensory temperature-dependence expressing itself as a positive temperature coefficient of the gain at which an input signal was transduced into an effector response was suggested by several studies. Lowering the temperature in the posterior hypothalamus with its mainly thermointegrative function reduced the thermoregulatory efficiency of anterior hypothalamic cooling in the goat (Puschmann and Jessen, 1978). Cold defence of birds in response to peripheral cooling was attenuated by hypothalamic cooling (Simon-Oppermann et al., 1978). The more recent demonstrations of positive temperature coefficients of hypothalamic osmotic control of antidiuretic hormone release in a bird (Simon and Nolte, 1990) and a mammal (Keil et al., 1994) suggest that non-sensory temperature-dependence is a general property of integrative networks underlying thermal as well as non-thermal hypothalamic control functions, and there is no reason to assume that this property should not exist at other levels of the central nervous system.

For the hypothalamus it is assumed that neurons with thermosensory functions are concentrated more in the POAH region, while the posterior hypothalamus mainly serves integrative and efferent functions (Bligh, 1973; Hardy, 1973). This conclusion was drawn from thermoregulatory deficits observed after hypothalamic lesioning, from the distribution of different types of hypothalamic thermosensitive neurons in the rostro-caudal direction, and from the degrees of convergence of local and remote temperature signals at the different hypothalamic levels. The hypothesis is in line with thermophysiological studies in conscious animals (Jessen, 1976; Puschmann and Jessen, 1978). However, at the neuronal level, thermointegrative functions, as indicated by the convergence of local and remote thermal stimuli in single neurons, reside in the preoptic as well as the posterior hypothalamus (Guieu and Hardy, 1970; Wünnenberg and Hardy, 1972; Boulant and Hardy, 1974). Consequently, the differences in the presentation of thermosensory, thermointegrative, and effector functions at the two hypothalamic levels can be only considered as quantitative ones. Thus, spatial separation of thermosensory and thermointegrative neurons is not distinct enough to derive criteria for these functions from the comparison of anterior and posterior hypothalamic thermosensitive neurons.

The incorporation of monoaminergic pathways and synapses into neuronal models of temperature regulation represents a further attempt to classify hypothalamic thermosensitive neurons. As the consequence of deviating thermoregulatory effects of the amines in different experimental animals, differently organized models were put forward (Bligh, 1972; Myers, 1975; Brück and Hinckel, 1982, 1990; Lin, 1984).

With the *in vitro* approach, the topographical distribution of thermosensitive diencephalic neurons was recently analyzed in horizontal tissue slices. In a comparison of several nuclei within as well as outside of the classical thermosensory POAH region, a relationship of about 35/5/60 between warm-, cold-, and thermo-insensitive neurons, respectively, was found in most hypothalamic regions, apart from a majority of warm sensitive neurons in the septum and in the lateral hypothalamus, suggesting the involvement of neurons with similar temperature-response characteristics in thermoregulatory as well as non-thermoregulatory control systems (Dean and Boulant, 1989). Neuronal responses to differential, local and remote thermal stimulations applied in a similar slice preparation seemed to underline the interneuron character of the thermosensitive neu-

rons and suggested their organization in a bi-directional rostro-caudal network, with some evidence for lateral dendritic projections toward the medial forebrain bundle (Dean et al., 1992).

Summary

In the spinal cord, temperature signals are generated which serve as specific inputs in the central nervous control of body temperature. Because of the spatially distinct organization of afferent and efferent neuronal systems at the spinal level, the afferent pathway for temperature signal transmission could be identified *in vivo* in the ascending, anterior and lateral tracts with a relationship of about 75:25% between warm and cold sensitive neuraxons. Analysis of spinal neuronal thermosensitivity *in vitro* on spinal cord tissue slices has been concerned, so far, with the superficial laminae of the dorsal horn as the site of origin of ascending nerve fibers conveying mostly temperature and pain signals, and with lamina X as a site of origin of afferent as well as efferent neurons. A relationship of about 95:5% between warm and cold sensitive neurons was found at the segmental level, indicating that warm sensitivity is the prevailing, primary property of spinal neurons, whereas cold sensitivity seems to be mainly generated by synaptic interaction as a secondary modality. Dynamic responses to temperature changes were frequently displayed in vitro at the spinal segmental level in lamina I + II but not in lamina X, even by neurons whose static activity was little influenced by local temperature. Dynamic thermosensitivity was found less frequently in ascending tract neuraxons and was not observed in hypothalamic neurons receiving temperature signal inputs from the spinal cord, and thus, does not seem to be relevant for the thermosensory function of spinal cord neurons, unlike peripheral warm and cold receptors. A majority of spinal warm sensitive neurons displayed both static and dynamic warm sensitivity as an inherent property after synaptic blockade. In the further analysis of spinal cord thermosensitivity, the *in vitro* approach permits application of the same electrophysiological and neuropharmacological methods as were established for the analysis of hypothalamic thermosensitivity. In addition, the topography of the spinal cord will provide additional structural and possibly histochemical information to characterize the functions of neurons independently of their thermal properties.

Acknowledgement

The studies carried out on spinal cord tissue slices were supported by the Deutsche Forschungsgemeinschaft: grant Si 230/8-1.

References

Anderson, C.R., McLachlan, E.M. and Srb-Christie, O. (1989) Distribution of sympathetic preganglionic neurons and monoaminergic nerve terminals in the spinal cord of rats. *J. Comp. Neurol.*, 283: 269–284.

Barker, J.L. and Carpenter, D.O. (1970) Thermosensitivity of neurons in the sensorimotor cortex of the cat. *Science*, 169: 597–598.

Beckman, A.L. and Eisenman, J.S. (1970) Microelectrophoresis of biogenic amines on hypothalamic thermosensitive cells. *Science*, 170: 334–336.

Bligh, J. (1972) Neuronal models of mammalian temperature regulation. In: J. Bligh and R.E. Moore (Eds.), *Essays on Temperature Regulation*, North-Holland, Amsterdam, pp. 105–120.

Bligh, J. (1973) *Temperature Regulation in Mammals and other Vertebrates*, North-Holland/Elsevier, Amsterdam, 436 pp.

Bligh, J., Cottle, W.H. and Maskrey, M. (1971) Influence of ambient temperature on the thermoregulatory responses to 5-hydroxytryptamine, noradrenaline, and acetylcholine injected into the lateral cerebral ventricles of sheep, goats and rabbits. *J. Physiol. (Lond.)*, 212: 377–392.

Boulant, J.A. (1980) Hypothalamic control of temperature regulation. In: P.J. Morgane and J. Panksepp (Eds.), *Handbook of the Hypothalamus*, Dekker, New York, Vol. 3, Part A, pp. 1–82.

Boulant, J.A. (1994) Cellular and synaptic mechanisms of thermosensitivity in hypothalamic neurons. In: E. Zeisberger, E. Schönbaum and P. Lomax (Eds.), *Thermal Balance in Health and Disease, Advances in Pharmacological Sciences*, Birkhäuser, Basel, pp. 19–29.

Boulant, J.A. and Dean, J.B. (1986) Temperature receptors in the central nervous system. *Annu. Rev. Physiol.*, 48: 639–654.

Boulant, J.A. and Hardy, J.D. (1974) The effect of spinal and skin temperatures on the firing rate and thermosensitivity of preoptic neurones. *J. Physiol. (Lond.)*, 240: 639–660.

Boulant, J.A. and Silva, N.L. (1987) Interactions of reproductive steroids, osmotic pressure, and glucose on thermosensitive neurons in preoptic tissue slices. *Can. J. Physiol. Pharmacol.*, 65: 1267–1273.

Boulant, J.A., Curras, M.C. and Dean, J.B. (1989) Neurophysiological aspects of thermoregulation. In: L.C.H. Wang (Ed.), *Advances in Comparative and Environmental Physiology*, Springer, Berlin, pp. 117–160.

Braun, H.A., Bade, H. and Hensel, H. (1980) Static and dynamic discharge patterns of bursting cold fibers related to hypothetical receptor mechanisms. *Pflüg. Arch.*, 386: 1–9.

Braun, H.A., Schäfer, K. and Wissing, H. (1990) Theories and models of temperature transduction. In: J. Bligh and K. Voigt (Eds.), *Thermoreception and Temperature Regulation*, Springer, Berlin, pp. 19–29.

Brück, K. and Hinckel, P. (1982) Thermoafferent systems and their adaptive modifications. *Pharmacol. Ther.*, 17: 357–381.

Brück, K. and Hinckel, P. (1990) Thermoafferent networks and their adaptive modifications. In: E. Schönbaum and P. Lomax (Eds.), *Thermoregulation: Physiology and Biochemistry*, Pergamon, Oxford, pp. 129–152.

Brück, K. and Zeisberger, E. (1990) Adaptive changes in thermoregulation and their neurophysiological basis. In: E. Schönbaum and P. Lomax (Eds.), *Thermoregulation: Physiology and Biochemistry*, Pergamon, Oxford, pp. 255–307.

Cabanac, M. and Jeddi, E. (1971) Thermopreferendum et thermoregulation comportementale chez trois poikilothermes. *Physiol. Behav.*, 7: 375–380.

Carlisle, H.J. and Ingram, D.L. (1973) The effects of heating and cooling the spinal cord and hypothalamus on thermoregulatory behavior in the pig. *J. Physiol. (Lond.)*, 231: 353–364.

Cormarèche-Leydier, M. and Cabanac, M. (1973) Influence de stimulations thermiques de la moelle épinière sur le comportement thermorégulateur du chien. *Pflüg. Arch.*, 341: 313–324.

Curras, M.C., Kelso, S.R. and Boulant, J.A. (1991) Intracellular analysis of inherent and synaptic activity in hypothalamic thermosensitive neurones in the rat. *J. Physiol. (Lond.)*, 440: 257–271.

Dean, J.B. and Boulant, J.A. (1989) *In vitro* localization of thermosensitive neurons in the rat diencephalon. *Am. J. Physiol.*, 257: R57–R64.

Dean, J.B. and Boulant, J.A. (1992) Delayed firing rate responses to temperature in diencephalic slices. *Am. J. Physiol.*, 263: R679–R684.

Dean, J.B., Kaple, M.L. and Boulant, J.A. (1992) Regional interactions between thermosensitive neurons in diencephalic slices. *Am. J. Physiol.*, 263: R670–R678.

Derambure, P.S. and Boulant, J.A. (1994) Circadian thermosensitive characteristics of suprachiasmatic neurons in vitro. *Am. J. Physiol.*, 266: R1876–R1884.

Feldberg, W. and Myers, R.D. (1965) Changes in temperature produced by microinjections of amines into the anterior hypothalamus of cats. *J. Physiol. (Lond.)*, 177: 239–245.

Griffin, J.D. and Boulant, J.A. (1995) Temperature effects on membrane potential and input resistance in rat hypothalamic neurones. *J. Physiol. (Lond.)*, 488: 407–418.

Guieu, J.D. and Hardy, J.D. (1970) Effects of heating and cooling of the spinal cord on preoptic unit activity. *J. Appl. Physiol.*, 29: 675–683.

Hackmann, E. and Simon, E. (1975) Single unit activity in spinal anterolateral tracts influenced by cold stimulation of the spinal cord and skin. In: L. Jansky (Ed.), *Depressed Metabolism and Cold*, Charles University, Prague, pp. 197–201.

Hammel, H.T. (1968) Regulation of internal body temperature. *Annu. Rev. Physiol.*, 30: 641–710.

Hancock, M.B. and Peveto, C.A. (1979) A preganglionic autonomic nucleus in the dorsal gray commissure of the lumbar spinal cord of the rat. *J. Comp. Neurol.*, 183: 65–72.

Hardy, J.D. (1972) Peripheral inputs to the central regulator for body temperature. In: S. Ito, K. Ogata and H. Yoshimura (Eds.), *Advances in Climatic Physiology*, Igaku Shoin, Tokyo, pp. 3–21.

Hardy, J.D. (1973) Posterior hypothalamus and the regulation of body temperature. *Fed. Proc.*, 32: 1564–1571.

Hellon, R.F. (1975) Monoamines, pyrogens and cations: their actions on central control of body temperature. *Pharmacol. Rev.*, 26: 289–321.

Hensel, H. (1970) Temperature receptors in the skin. In: J.D. Hardy, A.Ph. Gagge and J.A.J. Stolwijk (Eds.), *Physiological and Behavioral Temperature Regulation*, Thomas, Springfield, IL, pp. 442–453.

Hensel, H. (1973) Neural processes in thermoregulation. *Physiol. Rev.*, 53: 948–1017.

Hensel, H. (1981) *Thermoreception and Temperature Regulation*, Academic Press, London, 321 pp.

Hissa, R. (1988) Controlling mechanisms in avian temperature regulation: a review. *Acta Physiol. Scand.*, 132 (Suppl. 567): 1–148.

Honda, C.N. (1985) Visceral and somatic afferent convergence onto neurons near the central canal in the sacral spinal cord of the rat. *J. Neurophysiol.*, 53: 1059–1078.

Hori, T. (1991) An update of thermosensitive neurons in the brain: from cellular biology to thermal and non-thermal homeostatic functions. *Jpn. J. Physiol.*, 41: 1–22.

Hori, T. and Nakayama, T. (1973) Effects of biogenic amines on central thermoresponsive neurones in the rabbit. *J. Physiol. (Lond.)*, 232: 71–85.

Hori, T., Nakashima, T., Kiyohara, T., Shibata, M. and Hori, N. (1980) Effect of calcium removal on thermosensitivity of preoptic neurons in hypothalamic slices. *Neurosci. Lett.*, 20: 171–175.

Hori, T., Kiyohara, T., Nakashima, T., Shibata, M. and Koga, H. (1987) Multimodal responses of preoptic and anterior hypothalamic neurons to thermal and non-thermal homeostatic parameters. *Can. J. Physiol. Pharmacol.*, 65: 1290–1298.

Jell, R.M. (1973) Responses of hypothalamic neurones to local temperature and to acetylcholine, noradrenaline and 5-hydroxytryptamine. *Brain Res.*, 55: 123–134.

Jell, R.M. (1974) Responses of rostral hypothalamic neurones to peripheral temperature and to amines. *J. Physiol. (Lond.)*, 240: 295–307.

Jessen, C. (1967) Auslösung von Hecheln durch isolierte Wärmung des Rückenmarks am wachen Hund. *Pflüg. Arch.*, 297: 53–70.

Jessen, C. (1976) Two-dimensional determination of thermosensitive sites within the goat's hypothalamus. *J. Appl. Physiol.*, 40: 514–520.

Jessen, C. (1990) Thermal afferents in the control of body temperature. In: E. Schönbaum and P. Lomax (Eds.), *Thermoregulation: Physiology and Biochemistry*, Pergamon, Oxford, pp. 153–183.

Jessen, C. and Simon, E. (1971) Spinal cord and hypothalamus as core sensors of temperature in the conscious dog. III. Identity of functions. *Pflüg. Arch.*, 324: 217–226.

Jessen, C. and Simon-Oppermann, C. (1976) Production of temperature signals in the peripherally denervated spinal cord of the dog. *Experientia (Basel)*, 32: 484–485.

Jessen, C., Simon, E. and Kullmann, R. (1968) Interaction of spinal and hypothalamic thermodetectors in body temperature regulation of the conscious dog. *Experientia (Basel)*, 24: 694–695.

Keil, R., Gerstberger, R. and Simon, E. (1994) Hypothalamic thermal stimulation modulates vasopressin release in hyperosmotically stimulated rabbits. *Am. J. Physiol.*, 267: R1089–R1097.

Kelso, S.R. and Boulant, J.A. (1982) Effect of synaptic blockade on thermosensitive neurons in hypothalamic tissue slices. *Am. J. Physiol.*, 243: R480–R490.

Kiyohara, T., Hirata, M., Hori, T. and Akaike, N. (1990) Hypothalamic warm-sensitive neurons possess a tetrodotoxin-sensitive sodium channel with a high Q_{10}. *Neurosci. Res.*, 8: 48–53.

Kleinebeckel, D. and Klussmann, F.W. (1990) Shivering. In: E. Schönbaum and P. Lomax (Eds.), *Thermoregulation: Physiology and Biochemistry*, Pergamon, Oxford, pp. 235–253.

Klussmann, F.W. (1964) The influence of temperature on the activity of spinal α- and γ-motoneurons. *Experientia (Basel)*, 20: 450.

Klussmann, F.W. and Pierau, F.-K. (1972) Extrahypothalamic deep body thermosensitivity. In: J. Bligh and R.E. Moore (Eds.), *Essays on Temperature Regulation*, North-Holland, Amsterdam, pp. 87–104.

Kobayashi, S. and Takahashi, T. (1993) Whole-cell properties of temperature-sensitive neurons in rat hypothalamic slices. *Proc. R. Soc. Lond. B*, 251: 89–94.

Kosaka, M., Simon, E. and Thauer, R. (1967) Shivering in intact and spinal rabbits during spinal cord cooling. *Experientia (Basel)*, 23: 385–387.

Kosaka, M., Simon, E., Thauer, R. and Walther, O.-E. (1969a) Effect of thermal stimulation of spinal cord on respiratory and cortical activity. *Am. J. Physiol.*, 217: 858–864.

Kosaka, M., Simon, E., Walther, O.-E. and Thauer, R. (1969b) Response of respiration to selective heating of the spinal cord below partial transection. *Experientia (Basel)*, 25: 36–37.

Lin, M.T. (1984) Hypothalamic mechanisms of thermoregulation in the rat: neurochemical aspects. In: J.R.S. Hales (Ed.), *Thermal Physiology*, Raven Press, New York, pp. 113–118.

Lin, M.T. and Simon, E. (1982) Properties of high Q_{10} units in the conscious duck's hypothalamus responsive to changes of core temperature. *J. Physiol. (Lond.)*, 322: 127–137.

Lin, M.T., Yin, T.H. and Chai, C.Y. (1972) Effects of heating and cooling of spinal cord on CV and respiratory responses and food and water intake. *Am. J. Physiol.*, 223: 626–631.

Murakami, N. (1973) Effects of iontophoretic application of 5-hydroxytryptamine, noradrenaline and acetylcholine upon hypothalamic temperature-sensitive neurons. *Jpn. J. Physiol.*, 23: 435–446.

Myers, R.D. (1975) An integrative model of monoamine and ionic mechanisms in the hypothalamic control of body temperature. In: P. Lomax, E. Schönbaum and J. Jacob (Eds.), *Temperature Regulation and Drug Action*, Karger, Basel, pp. 32–42.

Myers, R.D. and Lee, T.F. (1989) Neurochemical aspects of thermoregulation. In: L.C.H. Wang (Ed.), *Advances in Comparative and Environmental Physiology*, Springer, Berlin, pp. 161–203.

Myers, R.D. and Yaksh, T.L. (1969) Control of body temperature in the unanaesthetized monkey by cholinergic and aminergic systems in the hypothalamus. *J. Physiol. (Lond.)*, 202: 483–500.

Nakashima, T., Pierau, F.-K., Simon, E. and Hori, T. (1987) Comparison between hypothalamic thermoresponsive neurons from duck and rat slices. *Pflüg. Arch.*, 409: 236–243.

Nakayama, T., Eisenman, J.S. and Hardy, J.D. (1961) Single unit activity of anterior hypothalamus during local heating. *Science*, 134: 560–561.

Necker, R. (1975) Temperature-sensitive ascending neurons in the spinal cord of pigeons. *Pflüg. Arch.*, 353: 275–286.

Pehl, U. and Schmid, H.A. (1997) Electrophysiological responses of neurons in the rat spinal cord to nitric oxide. *Neuroscience*, 77: 563–573.

Pehl, U., Schmid, H.A. and Simon, E. (1994a) Local temperature sensitivity of spinal cord neurons recorded *in vitro*. In: K. Pleschka and R. Gerstberger (Eds.), *Integrative and Cellular Aspects of Autonomic Functions: Temperature and Osmoregulation*, John Libbey Eurotext, Paris, pp. 77–85.

Pehl, U., Schmid, H.A. and Simon, E. (1994b) Lamina-specific effects of nitric oxide on temperature sensitive neurons in rat spinal cord slices. In: E. Zeisberger, E. Schönbaum and P. Lomax (Eds.), *Thermal Balance in Health and Disease, Advances in Pharmacological Sciences*, Birkhäuser, Basel, pp. 45–51.

Pehl, U., Schmid, H.A. and Simon, E. (1997) Temperature sensitivity of neurones in slices of the rat spinal cord. *J. Physiol. (Lond.)*, 498: 483–495.

Perl, E.R. (1990) Central projections of thermoreceptors. In: J. Bligh and K. Voigt (Eds.), *Thermoreception and Temperature Regulation*, Springer, Berlin, pp. 89–106.

Pierau, F.-K., Klee, M.R. and Klussmann, F.W. (1969) Effects of local hypo- and hyperthermia on mammalian motoneurones. *Fed. Proc.*, 28: 1006–1010.

Pierau, F.-K., Klee, M.R. and Klussmann, F.W. (1976) Effect of temperature on postsynaptic potentials of cat spinal motoneurons. *Brain Res.*, 114: 21–34.

Pierau, F.-K., Torrey, P. and Carpenter, D.O. (1974) Mammalian cold receptor afferents: role of an electrogenic pump in sensory transduction. *Brain Res.*, 73: 156–160.

Pierau, F.-K., Torrey, P. and Carpenter, D.O. (1975) Effect of ouabain and potassium-free solution on mammalian thermosensitive afferents *in vitro*. *Pflüg. Arch.*, 359: 349–356.

Pierau, F.-K., Wurster, R.D., Neya, T., Yamasato, T. and Ulrich, J. (1980) Generation and processing of peripheral temperature signals in mammals. *Int. J. Biometeorol.*, 24: 243–252.

Pierau, F.-K., Schenda, J., Konrad, M. and Sann, H. (1994) Possible implications of the plasticity of temperature-sensitive neurons in the hypothalamus. In: E. Zeisberger, E. Schönbaum and P. Lomax (Eds.), *Thermal Balance in Health and Disease, Advances in Pharmacological Sciences*, Birkhäuser, Basel, pp. 31–36.

Puschmann, S. and Jessen, C. (1978) Anterior and posterior hypothalamus: effects of independent temperature displacements on heat production in conscious goats. *Pflüg. Arch.*, 373: 59–68.

Rautenberg, W. (1969) Die Bedeutung der zentralnervösen Thermosensitivität für die Temperaturregulation der Taube. *Z. vergl. Physiol.*, 62: 235–266.

Satinoff, E. (1978) Neural organization and evolution of thermal regulation in mammals. *Science*, 201: 16–22.

Sato, H. and Simon, E. (1988) Thermal characterization and transmitter analysis of single units in the preoptic and anterior hypothalamus of conscious ducks. *Pflüg. Arch.*, 411: 34–41.

Schmid, H.A. and Pierau, F.-K. (1993) Temperature sensitivity of neurons in slices of the rat PO/AH hypothalamic area: effect of calcium. *Am. J. Physiol.*, 264: R440–R448.

Schmid, H.A., Jansky, L. and Pierau, F.-K. (1993) Temperature sensitivity of neurons in slices of the rat PO/AH area: effect of bombesin and substance P. *Am. J. Physiol.*, 264: R449–R455.

Schmid, H.A., Pehl, U. and Simon, E. (1994) Temperature sensitivity of rat spinal cord neurons recorded *in vitro*. In:

A.S. Milton (Ed.), *Temperature Regulation, Advances in Pharmacological Sciences*, Birkhäuser, Basel, pp. 109–114.

Schmidt, I. (1978) Behavioral and autonomic thermoregulation in heat stressed pigeons modified by central thermal stimulation. *J. Comp. Physiol.*, 127: 75–87.

Scott, I.M. and Boulant, J.A. (1984) Dopamine effects on thermosensitive neurons in hypothalamic tissue slices. *Brain Res.*, 306: 157–163.

Simon, E. (1972) Temperature signals from skin and spinal cord converging on spinothalamic neurons. *Pflüg. Arch.*, 337: 323–332.

Simon, E. (1974) Temperature regulation: the spinal cord as a site of extrahypothalamic thermoregulatory functions. *Rev. Physiol. Biochem. Pharmacol.*, 71: 1–76.

Simon, E. (1981) Effects of CNS temperature on generation and transmission of temperature signals in homeotherms. A common concept for mammalian and avian thermoregulation. *Pflüg. Arch.*, 392: 79–88.

Simon, E. and Iriki, M. (1970) Ascending neurons of the spinal cord activated by cold. *Experientia (Basel)*, 26: 620–621.

Simon, E. and Iriki, M. (1971a) Ascending neurons highly sensitive to variations of spinal cord temperature. *J. Physiol. (Paris)*, 63: 415–417.

Simon, E. and Iriki, M. (1971b) Sensory transmission of spinal heat and cold sensitivity in ascending spinal neurons. *Pflüg. Arch.*, 328: 103–120.

Simon, E. and Nolte, P. (1990) Temperature dependence of thermal and nonthermal regulation: hypothalamic thermo- and osmoregulation in the duck. In: J. Bligh and K. Voigt (Eds.), *Thermoreception and Temperature Regulation*, Springer, Berlin, pp. 191–199.

Simon, E., Rautenberg, W., Thauer, R. and Iriki, M. (1963) Auslösung thermoregulatorischer Reaktionen durch lokale Kühlung im Vertebralkanal. *Naturwissenschaften*, 50: 337.

Simon, E., Rautenberg, W. and Jessen, C. (1965) Initiation of shivering in unanesthetized dogs by local cooling within the vertebral canal. *Experientia (Basel)*, 21: 476–477.

Simon, E., Hammel, H.T. and Oksche, A. (1977) Thermosensitivity of single units in the hypothalamus of the conscious Pekin duck. *J. Neurobiol.*, 8: 523–535.

Simon, E., Pierau, F.-K. and Taylor, D.C.M. (1986) Central and peripheral thermal control of effectors in homeothermic temperature regulation. *Physiol. Rev.*, 66: 235–300.

Simon-Oppermann, C., Simon, E., Jessen, C. and Hammel, H.T. (1978) Hypothalamic thermosensitivity in conscious Pekin ducks. *Am. J. Physiol.*, 235: R130–R140.

Vieth, E. (1989) Fitting piecewise linear regression functions to biological responses. *J. Appl. Physiol.*, 67: 390–396.

Walther, O.-E., Simon, E. and Jessen, C. (1971) Thermoregulatory adjustments of skin blood flow in chronically spinalized dogs. *Pflüg. Arch.*, 322: 323–335.

Watanabe, T., Morimoto, A. and Murakami, N. (1986) Effect of amine on temperature-responsive neuron in slice preparation of rat brain stem. *Am. J. Physiol.*, 250: R553–R559.

Wünnenberg, W. and Brück, K. (1968a) Single unit activity evoked by thermal stimulation of the cervical spinal cord in the guinea pig. *Nature*, 218: 1268–1269.

Wünnenberg, W. and Brück, K. (1968b) Zur Funktionsweise thermorezeptiver Strukturen im Cervicalmark des Meerschweinchens. *Pflüg. Arch.*, 299: 1–10.

Wünnenberg, W. and Brück, K. (1970) Studies on the ascending pathways from the thermosensitive region of the spinal cord. *Pflüg. Arch.*, 321: 233–241.

Wünnenberg, W. and Hardy, J.D. (1972) Response of single units of the posterior hypothalamus to thermal stimulation. *J. Appl. Physiol.*, 33: 547–552.

H.S. Sharma and J. Westman (Eds.)
Progress in Brain Research, Vol 115
© 1998 Elsevier Science BV. All rights reserved.

CHAPTER 4

Neuronal networks controlling thermoregulatory effectors

Kazuyuki Kanosue*, Takayoshi Hosono, Yi-Hong Zhang and Xiao-Ming Chen

Department of Physiology, School of Allied Health Sciences, Osaka University Faculty of Medicine, Yamadaoka 1-7, Suita, Osaka 565, Japan

Introduction

The body temperature of a homeothermic animal is regulated by multiple behavioral and autonomic effector responses, and the thermoreceptors responsible for these responses are distributed throughout the body. They are present not only in the skin and the hypothalamus, but also in other brain areas and deep in the body core (Simon et al., 1986). Although we know that this multiple-input/output system is controlled mainly by the nervous system, we still do not know much about the 'neuronal networks' for thermoregulation. That is, we know little about what kinds of neurons are responsible for each response, what areas in the brain these neurons are in, and where these neurons project. Why?

From the 1930s to the early 1960s, neurophysiologists concentrated on localizing the 'thermoregulatory center' by stimulating and ablating portions of the brain. These studies revealed the importance of the hypothalamus, especially its rostral part (Magoun et al., 1938; Clark et al., 1939). Some neural networks were also elucidated, although only roughly (Hemingway, 1963).

After thermosensitive neurons were discovered in the hypothalamus (Nakayama et al., 1961), neurophysiologists directed their efforts to the analysis of thermosensitive neurons. This trend seems to have been based on the belief that thermosensitive neurons would be found only where local thermal stimulation produces thermoregulatory responses. That is, a belief that thermosensitivity is a distinctive characteristic of neurons playing a role in the control of thermoregulation. Actually, however, signals from thermosensitive neurons could be recorded anywhere in the brain, even in the cerebral cortex (Barker and Carpenter, 1970). So in spite of the great number of single-unit studies that were made in the 1960s and 1970s (Boulant, 1980; Nakayama, 1985), the neurons playing a role in thermoregulation could not be clearly identified. Neurophysiologists then shifted their efforts into two major directions: the analysis of thermal afferent pathways, and the analysis of slice preparations. The analysis of the afferent pathways was accelerated by the finding of the 'scrotal system' (Hellon and Misra, 1973a, 1973b; Hellon and Mitchell, 1975). Sites along the thermal afferent pathways — such as the spinal cord, thalamus, somatosensory cortex, and hypothalamus — seemed to contain many neurons responding to scrotal warming, but the response of thalamic and hypothalamic neurons was eventu-

*Corresponding author. Tel: +81 6 8792612; fax: +81 6 8792619; e-mail: kanosue@sahs.med.osaka-u.ac.jp

ally found to be merely an activity change associated with change in EEG activity (Kanosue et al., 1984, 1985). The recording of neuronal activity in slice preparations, on the other hand, opened the door to the analysis of membrane mechanisms of thermosensitivity (Hori et al., 1980; Keslo et al., 1982) (for details, see chapters 1 and 5). But the severed input and output connections of this preparation meant that it would contribute little to network analysis.

Although the analysis of the thermoregulatory neuronal network thus almost halted at the level it had reached by the early 1960s, the last few years have brought new approaches that have started to break this stagnation. This review summarizes present knowledge about neuronal networks controlling thermoregulation, mainly knowledge about the efferent pathways from the hypothalamus. Pharmacological aspects will not be treated here because many other chapters in this volume are devoted to that topic.

Afferent pathways

Poulos wrote in the early 1980s that 'The anatomical pathways involved in the transmission of skin temperature information to regions such as the hypothalamus must be more clearly defined. Once the pathways are defined, electrophysiological analysis of the thermally sensitive neurons involved should reveal the kind of cutaneous thermal information made available to thermoregulatory neurons' (Poulos, 1981). But because there has been so little progress in this field, we will mention only a few recent topics. For general information about thermal afferent pathways, see other reviews (Hellon, 1983; Simon et al., 1986).

The subcoeruleus area and the nucleus raphe magnus had been thought to be important sites for conveying thermal information from the skin (Brück and Hinckel, 1980; Hinckel and Schroder-Rosenstock, 1981). Their importance, however, was called into question when it was found that when neurons in these area respond to the skin thermal stimulation, the responses are accompanied by changes in EEG activity (Grahn and Heller, 1989; Grahn et al., 1989), as had been found for the responses of thalamic and hypothalamic neurons to scrotal warming. These areas seem to be responsible for the modulation rather than the generation of thermal afferent information (Sato, 1993). The thermal response of dorsal horn cells, both warm-responsive and cold-responsive cells, is suppressed by electrical stimulation of the nucleus raphe magnus (Fig. 1) or the subcoeruleus area. This indicates that the raphe-spinal and subcoelureo-spinal descending pathways modulate the spinal transmission of warm and cold signals from the skin.

Also interesting is the modulation of skin thermal signals by the sympathetic nerve (Davies, 1985). The first-order and second-order cold-responsive neurons in the trigeminal system are facilitated by cervical sympathetic electrical stimulation at low frequencies, and this facilitation is blocked by phentolamine and mimicked by phenylephrine. There may thus be a direct α-receptor-mediated excitation of cold-receptive primary afferent fibers by the sympathetic system. The discoverer of this phenomenon speculated that the chill sensation felt in the early stages of fever is brought about by the sympathetic excitation of cold receptors.

Heat loss

Vasomotion

The preoptic area is widely known to be a thermosensitive site eliciting skin vasodilation when it is heated (Ishikawa et al., 1984). In rats this response is known to be elicited mainly by the activation of warm-sensitive neurons, since glutamate injection there produces vasodilation and procaine injection produce vasoconstriction (Zhang et al., 1995). Efferent pathways from the preoptic area descend through the medial forebrain bundle (Kanosue et al., 1994a). It seems that, for vasomotor control, in the lateral hypothalamus there is no synaptic connection at the level of the ventromedial hypothalamus (Shang et

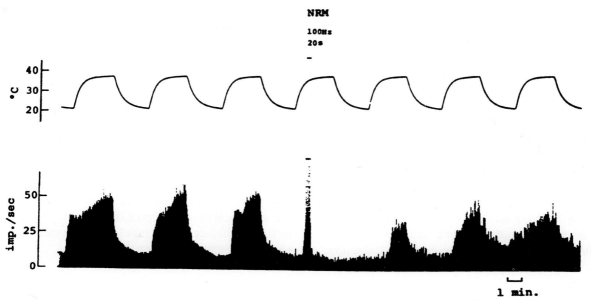

Fig. 1. The effect of electrical stimulation in the nucleus raphe magnus (NRM) on the temperature response of a warm-responsive dorsal horn cells evoked by repeating of warming and cooling of the scrotal skin. Upper trace is scrotal skin temperature and the lower trace is mean firing rate. Increase in firing rate during stimulation is artifact [from Sato et al. (1993), reprinted with kind permission of Elsevier Science Ltd, Kidlington, UK].

al., 1996). Two regions in the midbrain seem to participate in vasomotor control (Yamada et al., 1996). One extends from the most caudal edge of the lateral hypothalamus to the reticular formation ventrolateral to the periaqueductal grey: chemical stimulation of this region produces skin vasodilation and a knife cut there suppresses the skin vasodilation elicited by preoptic warming. The other region is the ventral tegmental area: stimulation there causes vasoconstriction of skin dilated by preoptic warming. The former region contains neurons excited by preoptic warming, and the latter region contains neurons inhibited by preoptic warming. The preoptic warm-sensitive neurons thus probably send excitatory signals to midbrain vasodilative neurons and inhibitory signals to midbrain vasoconstrictive neurons. It is not known yet where these vasodilative and vasoconstrictive neurons project.

The rostral ventrolateral medulla of a cat contains neurons projecting to the spinal cord, and presumably sending signals to the sympathetic preganglionic neurons, that are activated by body cooling (McAllen and Dampney, 1989). The activity of these premotor neurons, clustered around the ventromedial border of the subretrofacial nucleus (MacAllen and May, 1994), is suppressed by warming the preoptic area.

Direct recording of sympathetic nerve activities in man has revealed that skin sympathetic nerves contain vasoconstrictor and sudomotor fibers, and that cutaneous sympathetic nerve activity is not correlated with changes in blood pressure (Wallin, 1988). Skin vasoconstriction accompanying bursts of impulses has provided evidence of vasoconstrictor nerves, and the activity of such nerves increases in cold environments (Bini et al., 1980a,b; Okamoto et al., 1994). The activity (timing and strength of individual vasoconstrictor bursts) in a vasoconstrictor nerve innervating one skin area (such as a hand) is closely correlated with that recorded simultaneously in one innervating another skin area (such as a foot) (Bini et al., 1980a,b), suggesting that vasoconstrictor nerves are markedly influenced by a common signal. Vasodilation could be a result of this vaso-constrictive sympathetic tone being released, but active skin vasodilation is known to occur in man: skin blood flow increases transiently at high ambient temperatures, and this increase is eliminated by nerve blockade (Sugenoya et al., 1995). This vasodilation, however, is synchronized with sweat expulsion, and sympathetic bursts followed by a vasodilator response but not by sweat expulsion have not been observed. The active vasodilation is therefore probably elicited by sudomotor nerves. A vasodilator polypeptide such as VIP, which is released as a co-transmitter substance by the activation of sympathetic sudomotor nerve, might play an important role in this vasodilation.

Sweating

A naked skin well-supplied with sweat glands gives human beings an unusually high capacity to tolerate heat. And because the animals commonly used for physiological experiments (rats, cats, dogs, etc.) have fur on their body surface and do not sweat, most of our knowledge about the central nervous control of sweating has been obtained by examining patients with brain lesions (Appenzeller, 1990).

Signals from the rostral hypothalamus evidently descend through the zona incerta and prerubral field, and then through the dorsolateral part of the midbrain and pontine tegmentum (Carmel, 1968). At the level of the lower pons and the medulla oblongata, they seem to descend along the spinothalamic tract to reach the intermediolateral cell column in the spinal cord (Saito and Kogure, 1986). Some of the fibers in this descending pathway cross the midline but most do not (List and Peet, 1939). And although there must be several synapses between the hypothalamus and the sympathetic preganglionic neurons of the spinal cord, nothing is known about them. Fibers in this pathway from the hypothalamus facilitate sweating, but a pathway from the cerebral cortex contains inhibitory fibers. These inhibitory fibers cross at the level of the lower medulla, and uni-

lateral lesions in the cortex thus produce continuous hyperhidrosis on the contralateral side (Saito and Kogure, 1986).

Bursts of activity in the human cutaneous sympathetic nerve occur 2.4–3.0 s before sweat expulsion not only during thermal sweating but also during sweating in response to arousal stimuli (Sugenoya et al., 1990). The amplitude of this sudomotor activity is linearly related to the extent of the corresponding sweat expulsion, and the close correlation between sudomotor bursts recorded simultaneously from different nerves (the posterior cutaneous antebrachial nerve and the superficial radial nerve) (Bini et al., 1980a,b) indicates that common supraspinal signals influence sweat glands all over the body.

Salivary secretion and grooming

Rats in a hot environment increase their evaporative heat loss by spreading saliva on their fur (grooming) (Hainsworth and Stricker, 1970). Large amount of saliva are secreted in response to heat (thermally induced salivary secretion) (Nakayama et al., 1986), and the only brain sites at which warming induces salivary secretion are in the preoptic area and the anterior hypothalamus (Kanosue et al., 1990). Evaporative heat loss in a hot environment is suppressed by lesioning the lateral hypothalamus, so efferent signals from the preoptic area seem to descend through the medial forebrain bundle (Hainsworth and Stricker, 1970). The submaxillary and sublingual glands are important for thermally induced salivary secretion. Although they are innervated by both sympathetic and parasympathetic fibers, the parasympathetic fibers are the ones more important for thermoregulation (Hainsworth and Stricker, 1970). The preganglionic parasympathetic fibers (secretory fibers) innervating these glands are classified into two types — fibers activated by taste stimuli and fibers activated by noxious stimuli to the oral region — and thermally induced salivary secretion is elicited by activation of both types (Kanosue et al., 1986). The neural pathways between the hypothalamus and the medullary salivary neurons (preganglionic neurons) have not yet been identified.

Evaporative heat loss should be most effective when grooming behavior is coordinated with salivary secretion. Interestingly, however, the brain sites at which local warming elicits these responses are not the same. Grooming is induced by warming the posterior hypothalamus. Warming the preoptic area, which elicits salivary secretion, instead elicits another thermoregulatory behavior — body extension (Roberts and Mooney, 1974; Tanaka et al., 1986). Records of saliva secreted by freely moving rats in hot environments revealed that the threshold core temperatures for grooming and for thermally induced salivary secretion are very close to each other (Fig. 2), but there was no correlation between the incidence of the grooming and the rate of salivary flow (Yanase et al., 1991). This suggests that there is no coordination of the neural controls over grooming and salivary flow.

Heat production

Shivering

The preoptic area is of unquestionable importance in the control of shivering, which is elicited when this area is cooled and which is suppressed when this area is warmed. The efferent signals mediating these responses descend in the medial forebrain bundle (Kanosue et al., 1994b), and a recent study has indicated that most of them originate in warm-sensitive neurons (Fig. 3) (Zhang et al., 1995).

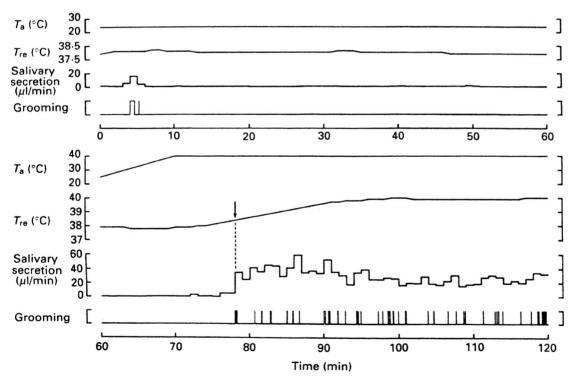

Fig. 2. Changes in rectal temperature (T_{re}), salivary secretion, and grooming behavior of an unrestrained rat when ambient temperature (T_a) was changed from 24 to 40°C. Note that salivary secretion and grooming started at very close to threshold T_{re} [from Yanase et al. (1991), reprinted with kind permission of Cambridge University Press, UK].

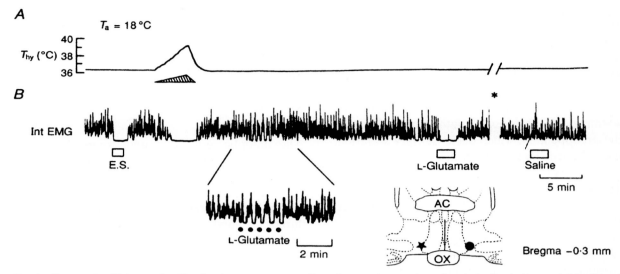

Fig. 3. Changes in thigh muscle shivering in response to unilateral preoptic warming, electrical stimulation, and injection of L-glutamate or control saline. Suppression of shivering by glutamate as well as warming indicates that preoptic warm-sensitive neurons mainly work for control shivering. (A) Local hypothalamic temperature (T_{hy}) record. The hatched bar roughly indicates the change in radio-frequency warming current. (B) Integrated EMG (Int EMG) of the thigh muscle. The filled circles under the time-expanded record mark injections of 0.2 μl of 0.2 mM glutamate. Open bars indicate electrical stimulation (E.S., 0.4 mA, 200 μs, 20 Hz), L-glutamate and control saline injection. The inset shows the location of electrode-thermocouple tip (●) and the tip of the injection cannula (★) [from Zhang et al. (1995), reprinted with kind permission of Cambridge University Press, UK].

The posterior hypothalamus has long been considered to be important for the control of shivering, and detailed stimulation and ablation studies have indicated that the dorsomedial region of the posterior hypothalamus is especially important (Stuart et al., 1961, 1962). The results of these earlier studies, largely done using cats, have also been confirmed by studies using rats (Halvorson and Thornhill, 1993). But because posterior hypothalamic lesions and electrical stimulations influence not only cell bodies but also passing fibers, it is not clear whether their effects are on neurons there that participate in the control of shivering or simply on fibers originating in other brain regions. The 'heat loss center' in the preoptic and anterior hypothalamus has been thought to suppress shivering by inhibiting the 'heat production center' in the posterior hypothalamus (Benzinger et al., 1961), but this has not been tested experimentally.

By the early 1960s a 'shivering pathway' had been inferred, mainly from the result of the stimulation and ablation studies (Hemingway, 1963). This pathway leaves the posterior hypothalamus and runs caudally through the midbrain area dorsolateral to the red nucleus. In the pons and medulla oblongata the pathway comes close to the ventrolateral surface and then to the lateral columns of the spinal cord.

Hori's group recorded the activity of electrophysiologically identified rubrospinal and reticulospinal neurons and tested the responses of these neurons to local and remote temperature changes (Fig. 4) (Asami et al., 1988a,b). In response to both local cooling and cooling of the preoptic area and skin, the proportion of the reticulospinal neurons increasing their activity was larger than that of the rubrospinal neurons. The reticulospinal neurons are in the reticular formation dorsolateral to the red nucleus, where applications of glutamate facilitated cold-induced shivering and applications of procaine suppressed it.

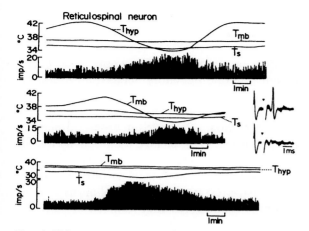

Fig. 4. Firing rate responses of a midbrain reticulospinal neuron to changes in local midbrain (T_{mb}), hypothalamic (T_{hyp}), and skin temperatures (T_s). Inset shows the antidromic responses to the stimulation of reticulospinal tract in the spinal cord with constant latency and their cancellation by spontaneous action potential [from Asami et al. (1988a), reprinted with kind permission of Elsevier Science, Inc., New York, USA].

These findings are strong evidence that reticulospinal neurons send efferent signals that control shivering, but whether the reticulospinal neurons receive synaptic input directly from the preoptic area or from the posterior hypothalamus is still an open question.

Nonshivering thermogenesis (NST)

The importance of the ventromedial hypothalamus in the control of NST has been well established (Thornhill and Halvorson, 1990; Perkins et al., 1994; Woods and Stock, 1994), and cooling of the preoptic area is also known to evoke increases in the temperature of brown adipose tissue (BAT) (Banet et al., 1978; Imai-Matsumura et al., 1984). We do not yet know, however, whether the signals driving this increase are due to the stimulation of cold-sensitive neurons or, like the signals driving shivering in response to preoptic cooling, to the inhibition of warm-sensitive neu-

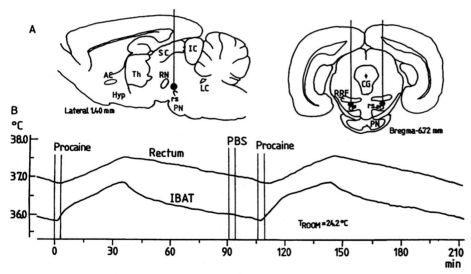

Fig. 5. Rise in rectal (Rectum) and interscapular brown adipose tissue (IBAT) temperature after bilateral procaine microinjection (10%, 1.0 μl/site) into upper-pontine reticular formation, indicating the existence of inhibitory system of nonshivering thermogenesis. (A) Procaine injection sites in the parasaggital (left) and coronal (right) sections of the rat brain. T_{ROOM}, room temperature. AC, anterior commissure; CG, central grey; Hyp, hypothalamus; IC, inferior colliculus; LC, locus coeruleus; PN, pontine nucleus; RN, red nucleus; RRF, retrorubral field; rs, rubrospinal tract; SC, superior colliculus; Th, thalamus. (B) PBS is control injection of phosphate buffer saline (1.0 μl/site) (Shibata et al., 1996).

rons. Nor do we know whether signals from the preoptic area are relayed in the ventromedial hypothalamus or descend directly to the lower brain structures.

Other hypothalamic nuclei such as the paraventricular nucleus and posterior hypothalamus seem to participate in the control of BAT thermogenesis, since electrical or chemical stimulation of these nuclei increases BAT thermogenesis (Freeman and Wellman, 1987; Holt et al., 1987; Amir, 1990a,b). And destruction or local anesthesia of the anterior or posterior hypothalamus facilitates BAT thermogenesis, suggesting that tonic signals from these areas inhibit BAT thermogenesis (Imai-Matsumura and Nakayama, 1987; Corbett et al., 1988; Woods and Stock, 1994).

The existence of a midbrain structure tonically inhibiting BAT thermogenesis has been indicated by the finding that BAT and rectal temperatures increase after a prepontine knife cut but not after a post-mammillary cut (Shibata et al., 1987). This structure has recently been localized to a lower midbrain region including the retrotubral field, pedunculopontine tegmental nucleus, and rubrospinal tract (Shibata et al., 1996). Procaine injected into these locations evokes a sudden increase in BAT thermogenesis (Fig. 5).

Although we know that BAT is innervated by sympathetic nerves, we know almost nothing about the relation between BAT thermogenesis and neural structures below the midbrain. Just as the neuroanatomy of the vasomotor system could be more easily analyzed after the premotor neurons of that system were identified, so would the analysis of the neuroanatomy of the system controlling BAT thermogenesis be facilitated by the identification of the neurons sending axons to the intermediolateral cell column in the spinal cord.

Behavioral regulation

Animals with preoptic and anterior hypothalamic lesions thermoregulate behaviorally as well as control animals do, even though they show severe deficits in autonomic regulation (Carlisle, 1969;

Satinoff and Rutstein, 1970). This does not, however, mean that the preoptic area does not participate in the control of behavioral regulation. Warming or cooling of the preoptic area elicits operant thermoregulatory behavior (Satinoff, 1964; Carlisle, 1966), indicating that this area works at least as a thermosensitive site for behavioral regulation. Preoptic neurons, especially thermosensitive ones, change their activity during thermoregulatory operant behavior (Hori et al., 1987). This change in activity is observed when rats are bar-pressing to obtain cool air in a warm environment and when they obtain cool air. The amount of the change was greater at higher rectal temperature. Destruction of the lateral hypothalamus impairs operant behavioral regulation (Satinoff and Shan, 1971) but also impairs other behaviors such as feeding, drinking, and shock avoidance. The deficits in behavioral thermoregulation might thus result from the destruction of a structure for motivation in general. It was noted above that warming of the posterior hypothalamus can elicit grooming in rats. But since thermal stimulation of the posterior hypothalamus also modulates operant thermoregulatory behavior (Refinetti and Carlisle, 1986), this region might not be related specifically to grooming.

The only part of the neocortex or limbic system that has been systematically investigated with regard to behavioral thermoregulation is the sulcal prefrontal cortex in the rat. Functional decortication accompanied by cortical spreading depression (CSD) has been found to inhibit cooling behavior and stimulate heating behavior (Shibata et al., 1983a,b), indicating that the frontal cortex normally produces signals driving behavior that lowers body temperature. In these experiments, one side of the preoptic and anterior hypothalamus (POAH) had been destroyed. Since the effect of CSD was observed only when CSD entered the frontal cortex contralateral to the lesioned POAH, the frontal cortex seems to participate in the behavioral thermoregulation through its connection with the ipsilateral POAH. Indeed, POAH warm-sensitive neurons were inhibited and cold-sensitive neurons were facilitated by the ipsilateral frontal CSD (Hori et al., 1984).

Laterality and independence

Recent investigations of the sharing of the control of three autonomic responses — shivering, vasomotion, and salivary secretion — between the right and left sides of the rat's brain have revealed that warming one side of the preoptic area changes shivering and vasomotor activity on both sides of the body (Kanosue et al., 1991). After unilateral transection of the hypothalamus just caudal to the anterior hypothalamus, unilateral preoptic warming of the intact side suppressed cold-induced shivering equally on both sides of the body but warming of the transected side had no effect on shivering (Fig. 6) (Kanosue et al., 1994b). It thus seems that no information for the control of shivering is exchanged between the left and right sides of the preoptic area and that efferent signals from the preoptic area cross the midline somewhere below the hypothalamus to equally innervate both sides of the body. The

vasodilation stimulated by unilateral preoptic warming of not only intact but also transected side, in contrast, was evident on both sides of the body — although the threshold stimulus temperature at which vasodilation was elicited was lower for the vasodilation on the intact side (Fig. 7) (Kanosue et al., 1994a). Information controlling thermoregulatory vasomotion is evidently exchanged between the left and right sides of the preoptic area, and efferent signals innervate skin blood vessels on both sides of the body, but the innervation is stronger for the ipsilateral side. Finally, unilateral stimulation of the preoptic area was found to stimulate the flow of saliva only from glands on the ipsilateral side (Fig. 8) (Kanosue et al., 1990), so signals for the control of salivary secretion are evidently not exchanged between the left and right sides of the preoptic area.

The fact that connections between the left and right sides of the preoptic area work for the control of thermoregulatory vasomotion but not

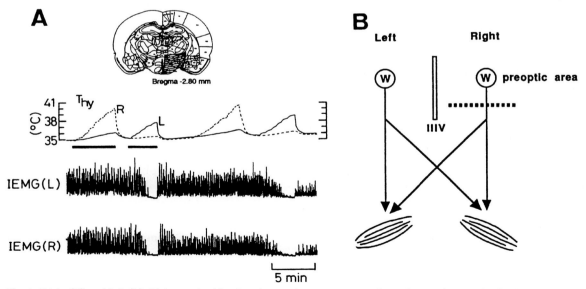

Fig. 6. Right (R) and left (L) thigh muscle shivering changes in response to unilateral preoptic warming in the rat with unilateral transection separating the preoptic area from the rest of the hypothalamus. (A) Solid and broken lines indicate left and right hypothalamic temperatures (T_{hy}). IEMG: integrated electromyogram. Inset: extent of microknife cut (hatching) [from Kanosue et al. (1994b), reprinted with kind permission of The American Physiological Society, Bethesda, MD, USA]. (B) Scheme showing the innervation of skeletal muscles by both sides of the preoptic area and the location of the transection (thick broken line).

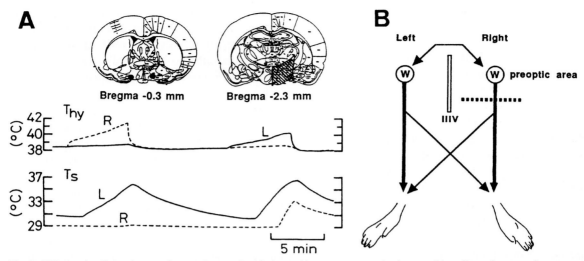

Fig. 7. Effects of unilateral preoptic warming on the hindpaw skin temperatures in the rat with unilateral transection separating the preoptic area from the rest of the hypothalamus. (A) T_{hy}: local hypothalamic temperature. T_s: paw skin temperature. Solid and broken lines indicate temperatures on the left (L) and right (R) sides. Inset: location of thermode tips (dots) and extent of microknife cut (hatched areas) [from Kanosue et al. (1994a), reprinted with kind permission of The American Physiological Society, Bethesda, MD, USA]. (B) Scheme illustrating the innervation of hindpaw skin blood vessels by both sides of the prepotic area and the location of the transection (thick broken line).

for the control of shivering indicates that the preoptic neurons sending efferent signals for these autonomic activities are different and function independently even though they are close to or even intermingled with each other. Likewise, even though salivation and vasodilation both increase

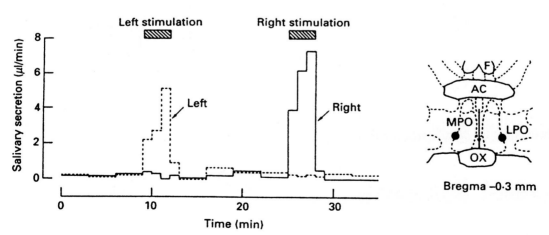

Fig. 8. Effects of unilateral electrical stimulation (0.3 mA, 1 ms, 20 Hz) of the preoptic area on secretion from the right and left submandibular and/or sublingual salivary glands. The sketch on the right shows where the tip of the electrodes were located. AC, anterior commissure; F, fornix; LPO, lateral preoptic area; MPO, medial preoptic area; OX, optic chiasma [from Kanosue et al. (1990), reprinted with kind permission of Cambridge University Press, UK].

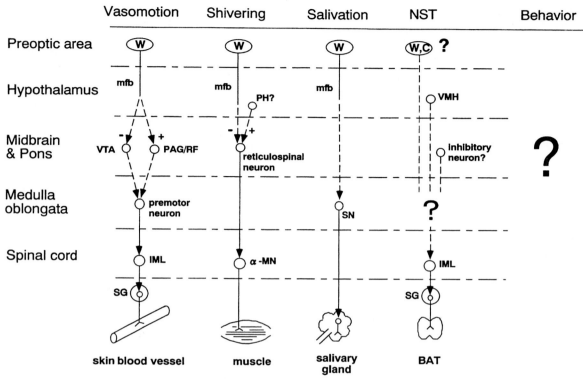

Fig. 9. Scheme illustrating efferent pathways from the preoptic area to each thermoregulatory effector. Continuous and broken lines indicate identified and unidentified connections, respectively. Neuronal network for behavioral thermoregulation is totally unknown. W, warm-sensitive neuron. C, cold-sensitive neuron. +, facilitaion. −, inhibition. IML, intermediolateral cell column; mfb, medial forebrain bundle; MN, motoneuron; PAG/RF, periaqueductal grey and reticular formation; PH, posterior hypothalamus; SG, sympathetic ganglion; SN, salivary nucleus; VMH, ventromedial hypothalamus; VTA, ventral tegmental area.

heat loss, preoptic neurons sending efferent signals for these activities are also different and function independently of each other. Furthermore, as noted above, preoptic neurons for salivary secretion send efferent signals independently of the posterior hypothalamic neurons for the control of grooming. All these data suggest that although different effector responses are functionally coordinated for thermoregulation, the preoptic area is merely an assembly of neuronal groups sending efferent signals to each effector and that these neuronal groups work without connections with each other or with the posterior hypothalamus (Roberts and Mooney, 1974; Satinoff, 1978; Yanase et al., 1991). This hypothesis should be extended to the control of other ther-

moregulatory effectors and also to other hypothalamic nuclei.

In summary, although some neurons in the thermoregulatory network have been identified, such as vasomotor neurons in the medula oblongata and reticulospinal neurons in the shivering pathway, our knowledge about thermoregulatory network is still fragmentary (Fig. 9). Pathways from the preoptic area to each effector must be traced, and the neurons along these pathways must be identified.

References

Amir, S. (1990a) Activation of brown adipose tissue thermogenesis by chemical stimulation of the posterior hypothalamus. *Brain Res.*, 534: 303–308.

Amir, S. (1990b) Stimulation of the paraventricular nucleus with glutamate activates interscapular brown adipose tissue thermogenesis in rats. *Brain Res.*, 508: 152–155.

Appenzeller, O. (1990) *The Autonomic Nervous System*, Elsevier, Amsterdam, pp. 117–140.

Asami, A., Asami, T., Hori, T., Kiyohara, T. and Nakashima, T. (1988a) Thermally-induced activities of the mesencephalic reticulospinal and rubrospinal neurons in the rat. *Brain Res. Bull.*, 20: 387–398.

Asami, T., Hori, T., Kiyohara, T. and Nakashima, T. (1988b) Convergence of thermal signals on the reticulospinal neurons in the midbrain, pons and medulla oblongata. *Brain Res. Bull.*, 20: 581–596.

Banet, M., Hensel, H. and Liebermann, H. (1978) The central control of shivering and non-shivering thermogenesis in the rat. *J. Physiol.*, 283: 569–584.

Barker, J.L. and Carpenter, D.O. (1970) Thermosensitivity of neurons in the sensorimotor cortex of the cat. *Science*, 169: 597–598.

Benzinger, T.H., Pratt, A.W. and Kitzinger, C. (1961) The thermostatic control of human metabolic heat production. *Proc. Natl. Acad. Sci. USA*, 47: 730–739.

Bini, G., Hagbarth, K., Hynninen, P. and Wallin, B. (1980a) Regional similarities and differences in thermoregulatory vaso- and sudomotor tone. *J. Physiol.*, 306: 553–565.

Bini, G., Hagbarth, K.-E., Nynninen, P. and Wallin, B.G. (1980b) Thermoregulatory and rhythm-genetating mechanisms governing the sudomotor and vasoconstrictor outflow in human cutaneous nerves. *J. Physiol.*, 306: 537–552.

Boulant, J.A. (1980) Hypothalamic control of thermoregulation. Neurophysiological basis. In: P.J. Morgane and J. Panksepp (Eds.), *Handbook of the Hypothalamus*, Vol. 3, Part A, Dekker, New York, pp. 1–82.

Bruck, K. and Hinckel, P. (1980) Thermoregulatory noradrenergic and serotonergic pathways to hypothalamic neurons. *J. Physiol.*, 304: 193–202.

Carlisle, H.Å. (1966) Behavioral significance of hypothalamic temperature-sensitive cells. *Nature*, 209: 1324–1325.

Carlisle, H. (1969) The effects of preoptic and anterior hypothalamic lesions on behavioral thermoregulation in the cold. *J. Comp. Physiol. Psychol.*, 69: 391–402.

Carmel, P. (1968) Sympathetic deficits following thalamotomy. *Arch. Neurol.*, 18: 378–387.

Clark, G., Magoun, H.W. and Ranson, S.W. (1939) Hypothalamic regulation of body temperature. *J. Neurophysiol.*, 2: 61–80.

Corbett, S.W., Kaufman, L.N. and Keesey, R.E. (1988) Thermogenesis after lateral hypothalamic lesion: contribution of brown adipose tissue. *Am. J. Physiol.*, 255: E708–E715.

Davies, S.N. (1985) Sympathetic modulation of cold-receptive neurones in the trigeminal system of the rat. *J. Physiol.*, 366: 315–329.

Freeman, P.H. and Wellman, P.J. (1987) Brown adipose tissue thermogenesis induced by low level electrical stimulation of hypothalamus in rats. *Brain Res. Bull.*, 18: 7–11.

Grahn, D.A. and Heller, H.C. (1989) Activity of most rostral ventromedial medulla neurons reflect EEG/EMG pattern changes. *Am. J. Physiol.*, 257: R1496–R1505.

Grahn, D.A., Radeke, C.M. and Heller, H.C. (1989) Arousal state vs. temperature effects on neuronal activity in subcoeruleus area. *Am. J. Physiol.*, 256: R840–R849.

Hainsworth, F.R. and Stricker, E.M. (1970) Salivary cooling by rats in the heat. In: J.D. Hardy, A.P. Gagge and J.A.J. Stolwijk (Eds.), *Physiological and Behavioural Temperature Regulation*, Thomas, Springfield, IL, pp. 611–626.

Halvorson, I. and Thornhill, J. (1993) Posterior hypothalamic stimulation of anesthetized normothermic and hypothermic rats evokes shivering thermogenesis. *Brain Res.*, 610(2): 208–215.

Hellon, R. and Misra, N. (1973a) Neurones in the dorsal horn of the rat responding to scrotal skin temperature changes. *J. Physiol.*, 232: 375–388.

Hellon, R. and Misra, N. (1973b) Neurones in the ventrobasal complex of the rat thalamus responding to scrotal skin temperature changes. *J. Physiol.*, 232: 389–399.

Hellon, R. and Mitchell, D. (1975) Convergence in a thermal afferent pathway in the rat. *J. Physiol.*, 248: 359–376.

Hellon, R. (1983) Central projections and processing of skin-temperature signals. *J. Therm. Biol.*, 8: 7–8.

Hemingway, A. (1963) Shivering. *Physiol. Rev.*, 43: 397–422.

Hinckel, P. and Schroder-Rosenstock, K. (1981) Responses of pontine units to skin-temperature changes in the guinea-pig. *J. Physiol.*, 314: 189–194.

Holt, S.J., Wheal, H.V. and York, D.A. (1987) Hypothalamic control of brown adipose tissue in Zucker lean and obese rats. Effects of electrical stimulation of the ventromedial nucleus and other hypothalamaic centres. *Brain Res.*, 405: 227–233.

Hori, T., Nakashima, T., Hori, N. and Kiyohara, T. (1980) Thermosensitive neurons in hypothalamic tissue slices *in vitro*. *Brain Res.*, 186: 203–207.

Hori, T., Shibata, M., Kiyohara, T. and Nakashima, T. (1984) Prefrontal cortical influences on behavioral thermoregulation and thermosensitive neurons. *J. Therm. Biol.*, 9: 27–31.

Hori, T., Kiyohara, T., Oomura, Y., Nishino, H., Aou, S. and Fujita, I. (1987) Activity of thermosensitive neurons of monkey preopic hypothalamus during thermoregulatory operant behavior. *Brain Res. Bull.*, 18: 649–655.

Imai-Matsumura, K., Matsumura, K. and Nakayama, T. (1984) Involvement of ventromedial hypothalamus in brown adipose tissue thermogenesis induced by preoptic cooling in rats. *Jpn. J. Physiol.*, 34: 939–943.

Imai-Matsumura, K. and Nakayama, T. (1987) The central efferent mechanism of brown adipose tissue thermogenesis induced by preoptic cooling. *Can. J. Physiol. Pharmacol.*, 65: 1299–1303.

Ishikawa, Y., Nakayama, T., Kanosue, K. and Matsumura, K. (1984) Activation of central warm-sensitive neurons and the tail vasomotor response in rats during brain and scrotal thermal stimulation. *Pflüg. Arch.*, 400: 222–227.

Kanosue, K., Nakayama, T., Ishikawa, Y. and Hosono, T. (1984) Threshold temperatures of diencephalic neurons responding to scrotal warming. *Pflüg. Arch.*, 400: 418–423.

Kanosue, K., Nakayama, T., Ishikawa, Y., Hosono, T., Kaminaga, T. and Shosaku, A. (1985) Responses of thalamic and hypothalamic neurons to scrotal warming in rats: Nonspecific responses? *Brain Res.*, 328: 207–213.

Kanosue, K., Matsuo, R., Tanaka, H. and Nakayama, T. (1986) Effect of body temperature on salivary reflexes in rats. *J. Auton. Nerv. Syst.*, 16: 233–237.

Kanosue, K., Nakayama, T., Tanaka, H., Yanase, M. and Yasuda, H. (1990) Modes of action of local hypothalamic and skin thermal stimulations on salivary secretion in rats. *J. Physiol.*, 424: 459–471.

Kanosue, K., Niwa, K., Andrew, P.D., Yasuda, H., Yanase, M., Tanaka, H. and Matsumura, K. (1991) Lateral distribution of hypothalamic signals controlling thermoregulatory vasomotor activity and shivering in rats. *Am. J. Physiol.*, 260: R485–R493.

Kanosue, K., Hosono, T. and Yanase-Fujiwara, M. (1994a) Hypothalamic network for thermoregulatory vasomotor activity. *Am. J. Physiol.*, 267: R283–R388.

Kanosue, K., Zhang, Y.-H., Yanase-Fujiwara, M. and Hosono, T. (1994b) Hypothalamic network for thermoregulatory shivering. *Am. J. Physiol.*, 267: R275–R282.

Keslo, S.R., Perlmutter, M.N. and Boulant, J.A. (1982) Thermosensitive single-unit activity of *in vitro* hypothalamic slices. *Am. J. Physiol.*, 242: R77–R84.

List, C. and Peet, M. (1939) Sweat secretion in man. *Arch. Neurol. Psychiatry*, 42: 1098–1127.

MacAllen, R. and May, C. (1994) Effects of preoptic warming on subretrofacial and cutaneous vasoconstrictor nerurons in anaesthetized cats. *J. Physiol.*, 481: 719–730.

Magoun, H.W., Harrison, F., Brobeck, J.R. and Ranson, S.W. (1938) Activation of heat loss mechanisms by local heating of the brain. *J. Neurophysiol.*, 1: 101–104.

McAllen, R. and Dampney, R. (1989) The selectivity of descending vasomotor control by subretrofacial neurons. *Prog. Brain Res.*, 81: 233–242.

Nakayama, T., Eisenman, J.S. and Hardy, J.D. (1961) Single unit activity of anterior hypothalamus during local heating. *Science*, 134: 560–561.

Nakayama, T. (1985) Thermosensitive neurons in the brain. *Jpn. J. Physiol.*, 35: 375–389.

Nakayama, T., Kanosue, K., Tanaka, H. and Kaminaga, T. (1986) Thermally induced salivary secretion in anesthetized rats. *Pflug. Arch.*, 406: 351–355.

Okamoto, T., Iwase, S., Sugenoya, J., Mano, T., Sugiyama, Y. and Yamamoto, K. (1994) Different thermal dependency of cutaneous sympathetic outflow to glabrous and hairy skin in humans. *Eur. J. Appl. Physiol.*, 68: 460–464.

Perkins, M.N., Rothwell, N.J., Stock, M.J. and Stone, T.W. (1994) Biphasic brown fat temperature responses to hypothalamic stimulation in rats. *Am. J. Physiol.*, 266: R328–R337.

Poulos, D. (1981) Central processing of cutaneous temperature information. *Fed. Proc.*, 40: 2825–2829.

Refinetti, R. and Carlisle, H. (1986) Effects of anterior and posterior hypothalamic temperature changes on thermoregulation in the rat. *Physiol. Behav.*, 36: 1099–1103.

Roberts, W.W. and Mooney, R.D. (1974) Brain areas controlling thermoregulatory grooming, prone extension, locomotion, and tail vasodilation in rats. *J. Comp. Physiol. Psychol.*, 86: 470–480.

Saito, H. and Kogure, K. (1986) Sudomotor deficits in unilateral brain stem lesions: studies on central sympathetic pathways. *J. Auton. Nerv. Syst.*, 23: 303–312 (Abstract in English).

Satinoff, E. (1964) Behavioral thermoregulation in response to local cooling of the rat brain. *Am. J. Physiol.*, 206: 1389–1394.

Satinoff, E. and Rutstein, J. (1970) Behavioral thermoregulation in rats with anterior hypothalamic lesions. *J. Comp. Physiol. Psychol.*, 71: 77–82.

Satinoff, E. and Shan, S. (1971) Loss of behavioral thermoregulation after lateral hypothalamic lesions in rats. *J. Comp. Physiol. Psychol.*, 77: 302–312.

Satinoff, E. (1978) Neural organization and evolution of thermal regulation in mammals. *Science*, 201: 16–22.

Sato, H. (1993) Raphe-spinal and subcoeruleo-spinal modulation of temperature signal transmission in rats. *J. Therm. Biol.*, 18: 211–221.

Shibata, M., Benzi, R.H., Seydoux, J. and Girardier, L. (1987) Hyperthermia induced by pre-pontine knifecut: evidence for a tonic inhibition of non-shivering thermogenesis in anaesthetized rat. *Brain Res.*, 436: 273–282.

Shibata, M., Hori, T., Kiyohara, T. and Nakashima, T. (1983a) Facilitation of thermoregulatory heating behavior by single cortical spreading depression in the rat. *Physiol. Behav.*, 31: 651–656.

Shibata, M., Hori, T., Kiyohara, T., Nakashima, T. and Osaka, T. (1983b) Impairment of thermoregulatory cooling behavior by single cortical spreading depression in the rat. *Physiol. Behav.*, 30: 599–605.

Shibata, M., Iriki, M., Arita, J., Kiyohara, T., Nakashima, T., Miyata, S. and Matsukawa, T. (1996) Procaine microinjection into the lower midbrain increases brown fat and body temperatures in anaesthetized rats. *Brain Res.*, in press.

Simon, E., Pierau, F.-K. and Taylor, D.C.M. (1986) Central and peripheral thermal control of effectors in homeothermic temperature regulation. *Physiol. Rev.*, 66: 235–300.

Stuart, D.G., Kawamura, Y. and Hemingway, A. (1961) Activation and suppression of shivering during septal and hypothalamic stimulation. *Exp. Neurol.*, 4: 485–506.

Stuart, D.G., Kawamura, Y., Hemingway, A. and Price, W.M. (1962) Effects of septal and hypothalamic lesions on shivering. *Exp. Neurol.*, 5: 335–347.

Sugenoya, J., Iwase, S., Mano, T. and Ogawa, T. (1990) Identification of sudomotor activity in cutaneous sympathetic nerves using sweat expulsion as the effector response. *Eur. J. Appl. Physiol.*, 61: 302–308.

Sugenoya, J., Ogawa, T., Jmai, K., Ohnishi, N. and Natsume, K. (1995) Cutaneous vasodilatation responses synchronize with sweat expulsions. *Eur. J. Appl. Physiol.*, 71: 33–40.

Tanaka, H., Kanosue, K., Nakayama, T. and Shen, Z.-W. (1986) Grooming, body extension, and vasomotor responses induced by hypothalamic warming at different ambient temperatures in rats. *Physiol. Behav.*, 38: 145–151.

Thornhill, J. and Halvorson, I. (1990) Brown adipose tissue thermogenetic responses of rats induced by central stimula-tion: effect of age and cold acclimation. *J. Physiol.*, 426: 317–333.

Wallin, B. (1988) Peripheral sympathetic neural activity in conscious humans. *Annu. Rev. Physiol.*, 50: 565–576.

Woods, A. and Stock, M. (1994) Biphasic brown fat temperature responses to hypothalamic stimulation in rats. *Am. J. Physiol.*, 266: R328–R337.

Yanase, M., Kanosue, K., Yasuda, H. and Tanaka, H. (1991) Salivary secretion and grooming behaviour during heat exposure in freely moving rats. *J. Physiol.*, 432: 585–592.

Zhang, Y.-H., Yanase-Fujiwara, M., Hosono, T. and Kanosue, K. (1995) Warm and cold signals from the preoptic area: which contribute more to the control of shivering in rats. *J. Physiol.*, 485: 195–202.

Zhang, Y.-H., Yamada, K., Hosono, T., Chen, X.-M., Shiosaka, S. and Kanosue, K. (1996) Efferent neuronal organization of thermoregulatory vasomotor control. *Ann. New York Acad. Sci.*, in press.

H.S. Sharma and J. Westman (Eds.)
Progress in Brain Research, Vol 115

CHAPTER 5

Plasticity of hypothalamic temperature-sensitive neurons

Friedrich-Karl Pierau*, Holger Sann, Krassimira S. Yakimova and Peter Haug

Max-Planck-Institute for Physiological and Clinical Research, William G. Kerckhoff-Institute, Parkstrasse 1, D-61231 Bad Nauheim, Germany

Introduction

Homeothermic animals maintain constant body temperatures between 36°C and 42°C in spite of substantial changes of environmental temperatures and extreme variability of endogenous heat production. Different parts of the central nervous system appear to be involved in the control of heat production and heat dissipation but the hypothalamus which is the integrative brain structure for most regulatory functions of the body seems to play the key role in converting multiple temperature signals into appropriate multiple effector responses (Simon, 1974; Satinoff, 1978). Within the hypothalamus, rostral areas appear to be particularly involved in the control of body temperature. Artificial modulation of the local temperature by implanted thermodes induces thermoregulatory responses only in the preoptic area and the anterior hypothalamus (PO/AH) but not in the posterior hypothalamus (Jessen, 1976; Puschmann and Jessen, 1978). Similarly, injection of various endogenous substances including endogenous pyrogens only change body temperature when applied into the rostral hypothalamus (Myers et al., 1974; Satinoff, 1979). Although recent conceptual models of temperature regulation assume a multiple thermostat system in which the controller function is achieved by integrating neuronal circuits in thermoresponsive and thermoreactive CNS areas within and outside the PO/AH, it is agreed that these compartments are hierarchically organized and that the PO/AH neurons play a prominent role (Boulant, 1980; Simon et al., 1986; Hori, 1991).

Interestingly, neuronal models of the central temperature controller were developed before neurophysiological investigations of hypothalamic neurons had been started (Hammel, 1965). In fact, the existence of three sets of neurons: warm-sensitive, cold-sensitive and temperature-insensitive neurons, which were later characterized in electrophysiological experiments by the slopes of their responses to local temperature changes, was already hypothesized at that time. The latter ones were, at least partially, regarded as reference neurons providing the reference temperature for the central controller, which is activated by deviations of the controlled variable from the reference temperature (Hardy, 1972). Since body temperature may change under various physiological and pathophysiological circumstances not connected to thermal challenge, e.g.

---

*Corresponding author. Tel: +49 6032 705251; fax: +49 6032 705211; email: fpierau@kerckhoff.mpg.de

circadian changes, hibernation, fever, the reference temperature or 'set point' is not a fixed value but is adjustable. Alterations of the set temperature have also been observed under thermal load (Hammel, 1968), and this alteration was associated with modulation of the temperature sensitivity of 'integrative' temperature sensitive neurons by signals from temperature sensors from the skin and the body core (Boulant and Bignall, 1973; Boulant and Hardy, 1974). Thus, variable properties of the set point and consequently of the neurons responsible for the generation of the reference signal are the inbuilt elements of plasticity in these neuronal models. In alternative models in which the load error which activates the controller is generated by comparing the feedback signals of two different sets of sensors, plasticity of the control system is provided by a variable gain or temperature sensitivity of hypothalamic neurons (Mitchell et al., 1970). Finally, in models in which the central controller is not activated by a load error but by a negative feedback signal generated by an odd number of negative input/output relations of multiple closed loop systems (steady state concept of thermoregulation, Werner, 1980), plasticity of the controller characteristics during fever or circadian fluctuations are supposed to result from changes of the gain and/or threshold of central neurons.

Electrophysiological investigations of hypothalamic neurons confirmed the existence of three populations of neurons in respect to their sensitivity to temperature changes (Boulant, 1980; Boulant and Dean, 1986). Numerous *in vivo* and *in vitro* experiments have revealed that approximately 40% of the PO/AH neurons are warm-sensitive, around 5% are cold-sensitive and the remaining are temperature-insensitive. However, to achieve discrimination with regard to neuronal temperature sensitivity certain conventions had to be introduced. Since most of the investigated neurons demonstrated a small increase of spontaneous activity with warming it was necessary to agree on a certain border line between warm-sensitive and temperature-insensitive neurons which was a temperature coefficient (TC = imp/s/°C)

of 0.6 or 0.8. Similarly, small increases in neuronal activity due to cooling posed the same problem and a TC of -0.6 was agreed upon to define a cold-sensitive neuron. Although there are some functional reasons for this classification (Boulant, 1996) it is unquestionably a convention and not accepted by all investigators (Glotzbach and Heller, 1984). The introduction of subpopulations particularly for temperature-insensitive neurons (Boulant, 1996; Griffin et al., 1996) made it even more obvious that the current definition is nothing more than a frame and is artificial as such frameworks usually are. Nevertheless, using this classification it was possible to compare investigations of different laboratories resulting in some insight to the function of the neuronal network possibly responsible for the control of body temperature.

Variability of temperature sensitivity of PO/AH neurons was to be expected from the many observations showing that these neurons also respond to stimuli relevant for non-thermal regulatory systems which are controlled as well in the hypothalamus, i.e. changes of osmotic pressure (Nakashima et al., 1985) glucose concentration (Silva and Boulant, 1986) or reproductive hormones, such as testosterone and estradiol (Silva and Boulant, 1984). However, these interactions were only tested with regard to tonic neuronal activity and possible changes in the degree of neuronal temperature sensitivity caused by the different types of non-thermal stimuli were not considered. At this time it was already known from investigations of Cabanac et al. (1968), Wit and Wang (1968) and Eisenman (1969) that the temperature sensitivity of PO/AH neurons may change after i.r. application of pyrogens. In their *in situ* preparation pyrogens reduced the slope of the temperature response of warm-sensitive neurons, whereas the TC of cold-sensitive and temperature-insensitive neurons was little or not affected. Although the introduction of brain slices (Hori et al., 1980a; Kelso and Boulant, 1982) permitted a better control of thermal and non-thermal parameters in comprehensive studies of neuronal temperature sensitivity, little attention has been paid to the variability of temperature sensitivity at the cellular level which certainly would contribute to the plasticity of the temperature controller.

Effects of pyrogens on thermosensitivity

It is generally agreed that during fever the body temperature is still regulated although at a higher level, implying that hypothalamic neurons are a major target for pyrogens. Microinjections of bacterial pyrogens into the PO/AH, indeed, induce characteristic fever reactions which are maximal and of short latency (Cooper et al., 1967; Rosendorff and Mooney, 1971). Electrophysiological studies of PO/AH neurons in intact animals demonstrated highly consistent changes of tonic activity of temperature-sensitive neurons after systemic or local application of bacterial or leucocyte pyrogens: more than 90% of the warm-sensitive neurons were inhibited whereas more than 90% of the cold-sensitive neurons were activated (Cabanac et al., 1968; Wit and Wang, 1968; Eisenman, 1969; Belyavskii and Abramova, 1975; Schoener and Wang, 1975). This action was specific for thermally-sensitive neurons since temperature-insensitive neurons, with a few exceptions, were not affected. The type of alterations of tonic activity observed in these investigations is in agreement with the concept that a reduced firing rate of warm-sensitive PO/AH neurons results in a decreased drive for heat loss effectors, while an increased activity of cold-sensitive neurons presumably increases the drive for heat production. In addition, in a number of neurons the decrease in firing rate was accompanied by a decrease in thermosensitivity (Eisenman, 1982), whereas the thermosensitivity of cold-sensitive neurons appeared not to be changed by pyrogens.

More recent investigations in hypothalamic slice preparations from guinea-pigs and rats confirmed that most of the temperature-insensitive neurons are insensitive to endogenous peptides. However, the effects on spontaneous activity of warm-sensitive neurons were not uniform in the slice preparations. Although in the majority of warm-sensitive neurons the firing rate decreased, increased

spontaneous activity was also observed, but possible changes of the temperature sensitivity were not investigated (Boulant and Scott, 1983; Ono et al., 1987). We have also observed variable effects of a bacterial pyrogen on the spontaneous activity of warm-sensitive neurons. In studies in which the experimental set-up permitted precise control of temperature changes in a sinusoidal fashion the tonic activity was only reduced in 10 of 25 warm-sensitive neurons, while the firing rate was not affected in 10 others (Fig. 1A) and even increased in the remaining five (Haug et al., unpublished data). In contrast, the TC of most warm-sensitive neurons was significantly reduced (20 out of 25) (Fig. 1A, Fig. 2). This effect on temperature sensitivity was independent of the change of spontaneous activity and could happen in neurons in which the tonic activity was increased. It usually outlasted the endotoxin perfusion by more than 30 min and resulted in a transformation of half of the warm-sensitive neurons into temperature-insensitive ones (Fig. 2). Temperature-insensitive neurons were only little affected by the pyrogen (Fig. 1B); tonic activity was only a little decreased in five out of 18 neurons and the TC was significantly reduced in only three neurons (Fig. 2).

Taken together, the data from intact animals and slice preparations clearly demonstrate the plasticity of warm-sensitive neurons under the influence of pyrogens. This could be interpreted as an indication for a change of the gain of the neuronal controller. How this is realized within the neuronal network is unknown. The transformation of warm-sensitive neurons into temperature-insensitive neurons reduces the number of the former and, consequently the transmission of warm-sensitive signals to the controller would be decreased and this might either change the threshold or the gain of the controller.

Effects of PGE$_2$

Although intrahypothalamic application of pyrogens induces a fever reaction and changes both the tonic activity and the temperature sensitivity of warm- and cold-sensitive hypothalamic neu-

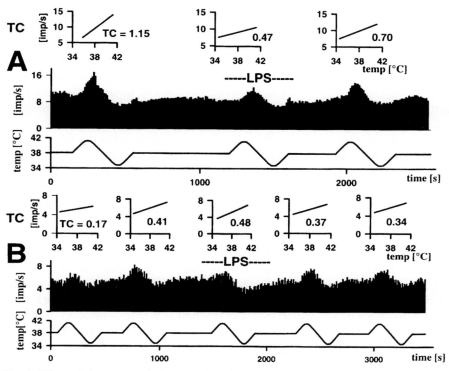

Fig. 1. Effect of the pyrogen LPS on tonic activity and temperature responses of a PO/AH warm-sensitive neuron (A) and a temperature-insensitive neuron (B) *in vitro*. The protocols show impulse activity (averaged over 10 s) and periodical changes of the slice temperature. Insets indicate the TC during the appropriate period of temperature change. LPS has only little effect on tonic activity of both types of neurons and on the TC of the temperature-insensitive neurons but distinctly decreases the TC of warm-sensitive neurons.

rons, the fever reaction is normally blood borne and the chain of events includes the activation of endogenous pyrogens such as leukotrienes and cytokines from macrophages and monocytes which in turn stimulate the production of prostaglandins via activation of arachidonic acid. Prostaglandins and in particular prostaglandin E_2 (PGE_2) are supposed to cross the blood–brain barrier and react with hypothalamic neurons. Indeed, application of PGE_2 into the PO/AH region induces a fever reaction very similar to the febrile response induced by exogenous pyrogens, suggesting a direct action of PGE_2 on hypothalamic neurons (Milton and Wendlandt, 1970; Feldberg and Saxena, 1971; Stitt, 1973). However, the changes of tonic activity of hypothalamic neurons after PGE_2

administration were quite variable in experiments carried out *in vivo* and *in vitro*. In most studies excitation of warm-sensitive PO/AH neurons was the predominant effect of PGE_2 (Boulant and Scott, 1986; Watanabe et al., 1987; Morimoto et al., 1988; Matsuda et al., 1992), but prevailing inhibition was also observed by a number of authors (Eisenman, 1969, 1982; Schoener and Wang, 1976; Gordon and Heath, 1980) in the preoptic area and in the ventromedial hypothalamus (Morimoto et al., 1988) and the organum vasculosum laminae terminalis (OVLT) (Matsuda et al., 1992). The latter observations were regarded as evidence for the assumption that these areas were more appropriate for the induction of fever, since PGE production might be induced by pyrogens in

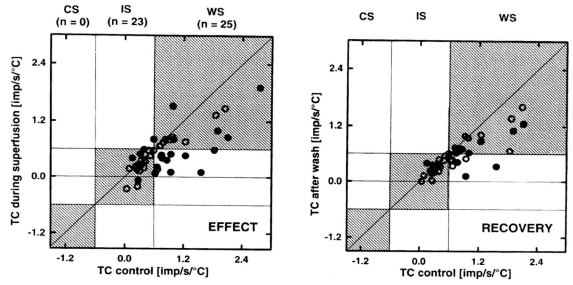

Fig. 2. Changes of the TC of individual neurons during superfusion of LPS (EFFECT) and after washing (about 20 min) (RECOVERY). The TC values of the single neurons during drug application or after the washing phase are plotted against their TC values during the control period. The distance of a circle from the line of identity indicates the degree of change. Circles in non-hatched areas represent neurons in which the TC changes were large enough to transform these neurons into another category (i.e. from warm-sensitive to temperature-insensitive, or vice versa). Filled circles represent significant changes; open circles = not significant. LPS decreases the TC of almost all warm-sensitive neurons while it has little or no affect on most of the temperature-insensitive neurons. CS = cold-sensitive; IS = temperature-insensitive; WS = warm-sensitive. LPS-concentration = 100 μg/ml.

brain areas in which the blood–brain barrier is permeable due to the fenestrated capillary endothelium.

Reevaluation of the PGE_2 effect on neurons of rat brain slices of anterior and posterior hypothalamic areas in close vicinity to the 3rd ventricle (nucl. periventricularis versus nucl. arcuatus) in our own studies confirmed the variability of the changes in tonic activity of neurons of both hypothalamic areas. The average frequency of all investigated warm-sensitive neurons was significantly decreased in both areas, while the average frequency of temperature-insensitive neurons was not changed (Fig. 3). This supports the interpretation of a special action of PGE_2 on the hypothalamic network rather than on single neurons. In contrast to the unambiguous decreasing effect of the bacterial pyrogen LPS on the TC of warm-sensitive neurons, PGE_2 increased as well as de-

creased individual TCs (Fig. 4). But again, evaluation of the averaged TC revealed a decrease of temperature sensitivity of the whole cell population. This might indicate that plasticity is not restricted to individual neurons but applies to the neuronal network and might change the gain of the controller. This reaction appears to be specific for warm-sensitive neurons since the average TC of temperature-insensitive neurons was not changed.

Effects of hyperthermic and hypothermic endogenous substances

GABA

A number of endogenous substances which reside in the hypothalamus have been shown to affect body temperature when exogenously applied ei-

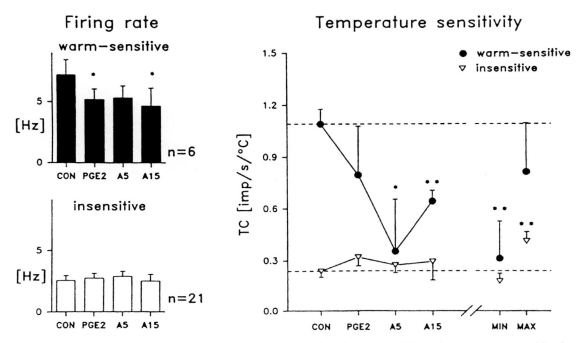

Fig. 3. Effect of PGE$_2$ on firing rate and temperature sensitivity of warm-sensitive and temperature-insensitive hypothalamic neurons *in vitro*. Only average firing rates and TC of warm-sensitive neurons are reduced; main effects occur during the first phase of washing, indicating a delayed action of PGE$_2$. CON = control; PGE2 = during superfusion of PGE$_2$; A5 = 5 min after superfusion; A15 = 15 min after superfusion; MIN, MAX = minimum or maximum TC calculated during the appropriate periods; Means ± S.E.M. Significant differences compared with control values: **$P < 0.01$; ***$P < 0.005$ [from Kulchitsky et al. (1994), reprinted with kind permission of John Libbey Eurotext, Paris, France].

ther into the preoptic area or systemically. One of the most interesting substances in this respect is GABA (Bligh, 1981) which has been demonstrated in relatively high concentrations in various hypothalamic nuclei, particularly in the PO/AH (Ottersen and Storm-Mathisen, 1984). GABA appears to be mainly associated with intrinsic hypothalamic neurons, thus, conforming to the hypothesis that GABA-ergic neurons form local neuronal networks modulating afferent temperature signals within the hypothalamus (Blatteis, 1981).

Administration of GABA or GABA agonists either centrally (intracerebroventricular, intrahypothalamic) or systemically (intraperitoneal, intravenous) usually induces hypothermia, whereas GABA antagonists produce hyperthermia. However, intensity, duration and direction of the ther-

moregulatory changes depend on the route and dose of application, animal species, ambient temperature and general conditions. More conclusive results were obtained from recent experiments in unanesthetized and unrestrained rats in which the hypothalamic actions of GABA agonists and GABA antagonists were systematically studied (Clark and Lipton, 1985; Serrano et al., 1985; Minano et al., 1989; Yakimova and Ovtcharov, 1989). The effect of GABA on temperature regulation appears to be mainly due to an activation of GABA$_B$-receptors, since the GABA-induced hypothermia could not be blocked by the GABA$_A$ antagonist bicuculline (Serrano et al., 1985). On the other hand, intraperitoneal as well as intraventricular application of the specific GABA$_B$ agonist baclofen does induce hypothermia in mice (Jackson and Nutt, 1991). According to our con-

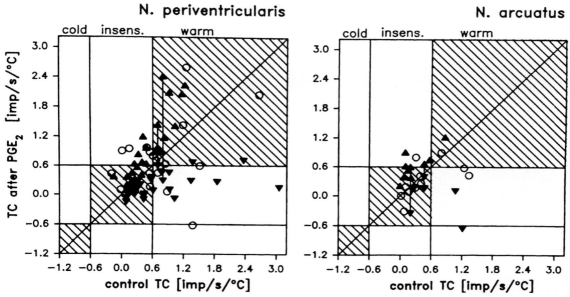

Fig. 4. PGE$_2$ effect on the TC of individual neurons of the anterior (Nucl. periventricularis) and the posterior hypothalamus (Nucl. arcuatus). The TC of individual neurons during the most pronounced PGE$_2$-induced change are plotted against their TC values during the control period. The distance from the line of identity indicates the degree of change. Triangles in non-hatched areas represent neurons in which the TC changes were large enough to transform these neurons into another category. Note the small number of warm-sensitive neurons in the posterior hypothalamus. Triangles represent significant changes ($P < 0.05$); open circles = not significant. Neurons showing both an increase and decrease of TC are connected with vertical lines. Cold = cold-sensitive; insens. = temperature-insensitive; warm = warm-sensitive [from Kulchitsky et al. (1994), reprinted with kind permission of John Libbey Eurotext, Paris, France].

cept that plasticity of thermal properties of hypothalamic neurons plays an important role in the adjustment of body temperature to different conditions, we anticipated that activation of GABA$_A$ and GABA$_B$ receptors would have different effects on PO/AH neurons and that this would become manifest particularly by an action on the temperature sensitivity.

Experiments in rat brain slices produced the expected different effects of substances binding specifically to GABA$_A$- or GABA$_B$-receptors of hypothalamic neurons. The GABA$_A$ agonist muscimol decreased the firing rate of warm-sensitive as well as temperature-insensitive neurons while the GABA$_A$ antagonist bicuculline had the opposite effect; the temperature sensitivity was not significantly changed in either population of neurons. The GABA$_B$ agonist baclofen also dose-dependently reduced the spontaneous activity of

warm-sensitive and temperature-insensitive PO/AH neurons (Fig. 5), but the GABA$_B$ antagonist phaclofen did not significantly change tonic activity (Fig. 6). In contrast to GABA$_A$ substances, however, baclofen specifically increased the TC of warm-sensitive PO/AH neurons. This effect was particularly impressive in experiments in which the neurons still responded to temperature changes, even when tonic activity had been completely abolished by baclofen (Fig. 5). The increase in temperature sensitivity by baclofen is particularly noteworthy for three reasons: (1) the increase of the TC is opposite in direction to the change of the tonic activity; (2) the effect on temperature sensitivity is specific for warm-sensitive neurons; (3) the effect is receptor specific, since the GABA$_B$ antagonist phaclofen completely prevented the baclofen-induced increase of the TC. Phaclofen itself decreased the TC of

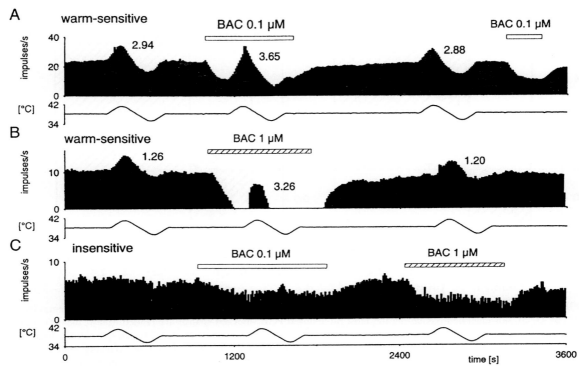

Fig. 5. Effect of the GABA$_B$ agonist baclofen (BAC) on two warm-sensitive (A, B) and one temperature-insensitive (C) PO/AH neuron. The protocols show impulse activity (averages of 10 s) and periodical changes of the slice temperature. Numbers in the protocol indicate the TC during the appropriate period of temperature change. Note: baclofen increases the temperature sensitivity of the warm-sensitive neuron demonstrated in B despite complete inhibition of tonic activity.

warm-sensitive neurons indicating that even in the slice preparation GABA is constantly released. Consequently, the temperature sensitivity of warm-senstivite PO/AH neurons might be continuously modulated by GABA under physiological conditions. An effect of phaclofen was not observed in temperature-insensitive neurons.

Effects of opioids

Opioids can have strong effects on body temperature, and the receptor specificity of their action became evident when experimental procedures were used in which the effects of anesthesia and stress on body temperature were avoided (Spencer et al., 1988; Handler et al., 1992). Intraventricular injection of different opioid agonists in unrestrained and unanesthetized rats revealed that μ-selective agonists induce hyperthermia while

κ-selective agonists induce hypothermia; each effect was prevented by pretreatment with the appropriate receptor-selective antagonists. Although the possible role of endogenous opioid peptides in thermoregulation is not clear, a modulatory effect on the transmission of thermal signals has been proposed (Stewart and Eikelboom, 1979; Clark, 1981). We have used different receptor-specific opioid agonists and antagonists to test the hypothesis that they might be specifically involved in the modulation of the hypothalamic controller of temperature regulation, taking the temperature sensitivity of PO/AH neurons and its plasticity, respectively, as an indicator.

Perfusion of hypothalamic slices with receptor-specific opioid agonists and antagonists revealed a new facet of the specific action of endogenous substances on the temperature sensitivity of PO/AH neurons. While the μ-opioid agonist

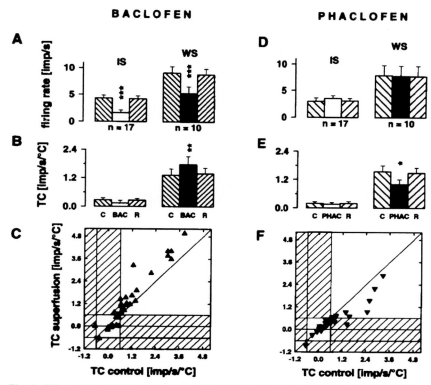

Fig. 6. Effect of the GABA$_B$ agonist baclofen and the GABA$_B$ antagonist phaclofen on firing rate (A; D), average TC (B; E) and individual TCs (C; F) of warm-sensitive (WS) and temperature-insensitive (IS) PO/AH neurons. Baclofen decreases tonic activity in both types of neurons but specifically increases the TC in warm-sensitive neurons. Phaclofen does not change tonic activity but specifically decreases the TC of warm-sensitive neurons. In C and F, the TC of individual neurons during superfusion of baclofen (C) and phaclofen (F) are plotted as a function of the TC during the control period. The distance from the line of identity indicates the degree of change. Triangles in hatched areas represent neurons in which the TC changes were large enough to transform these neurons into another category. C = control period, BAC or PHAC = test period, R = recovery period; Mean ± S.E.M. Significant differences to control values: $^*P < 0.05$; $^{**}P < 0.01$; $^{***}P < 0.005$ (from Pierau et al., 1997).

PL017 reduced tonic activity in most PO/AH neurons, regardless of whether they were temperature-sensitive or not, its effect on temperature sensitivity was rather distinct. At low concentrations between 0.5 and 10 nM, the temperature sensitivity was significantly decreased in warm-sensitive neurons only. At higher concentrations the TC of both populations of PO/AH neurons was decreased. Both actions were prevented by pre- and co-perfusion with the μ-opioid antagonist CTOP, but the antagonist did not affect tonic activity or temperature sensitivity by itself.

Similarly distinctive effects were observed after application of the κ-receptor agonist dynorphine

A_{1-17}. Only 54% of the PO/AH neurons were sensitive to dynorphine and, while the tonic activity of the majority of these neurons was increased at low concentrations (0.5 nM), it was predominantly decreased at higher doses in all types of neurons. In contrast, the effect of dynorphine A_{1-17} on temperature sensitivity was restricted to warm-sensitive neurons — and in this sense specific — but was different at low and high concentrations. A significant TC increase was observed after 0.5 nM, the TC did not significantly change after 5 and 10 nM, and a distinct decrease of temperature sensitivity was produced by 100 nM dynorphine A_{1-17} (Fig. 7). It is noteworthy, that

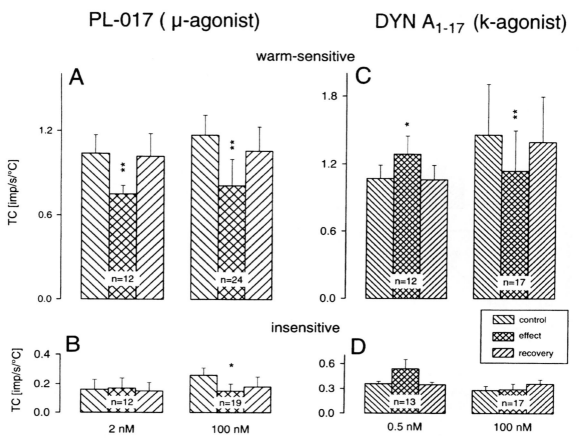

PL-017 (μ-agonist)

DYN A$_{1-17}$ (k-agonist)

Fig. 7. Differential effect of low and high concentrations of the μ-agonist (PL-017) and the κ-agonist (DYN A$_{1-17}$), respectively, on the temperature sensitivity of warm-sensitive and temperature-insensitive PO/AH neurons. The TC of warm-sensitive neurons is decreased by 2 nM and 100 nM concentrations of PL-017 (A), while the TC of temperature-insensitive neurons is only decreased at 100 nM (B). DYN A$_{1-17}$ increases the TC of warm-sensitive neurons at 0.5 nM but decreases it at 100 nM (C). The TC of temperature-insensitive neurons is only affected at the low concentration but not changed by the high concentration of DYN A$_{1-17}$ (D) [from Yakimova et al. (1996), reprinted with kind permission of Cambridge University Press, UK].

the κ-receptor antagonist nor-BNI only prevented the increase of the TC induced by 0.5 nM dynorphine A$_{1-17}$ but did not prevent the effect of higher agonist concentrations on temperature sensitivity or the effect on tonic activity in all concentrations.

It appears that the opioid effects on temperature regulation are only unambiguous at low concentrations and it is this range in which the μ-agonist as well as the κ-agonist specifically decrease or increase, respectively, the TC of warm-sensitive neurons and in which the receptor-

specific antagonists prevents this action. Thus, the specific concentration-dependent action of opioids on the temperature sensitivity of warm-sensitive neurons is a further indication that the plasticity of these neurons might be important for the control of body temperature and that the adjustment of the TC is very susceptible and might be modulated by small amounts of endogenous opioids according to the requirements of temperature regulation. The presented data would suggest that the hyperthermic effect of morphine is due to an activation of μ-receptors, which may decrease the gain or threshold of the temperature controller. Yet, opioids and pyrogens induce similar changes in body temperature but appear to do so by different cellular mechanisms, since antipyretics do not effect opioid-induced hyperthermia nor does naloxone prevent pyrogen-induced fever (Clark, 1981).

Effects of bombesin, substance P and thyrotropin releasing hormone

In general, endogenous substances which, upon intrahypothalamic or systemic application, change body temperature can be assumed to contribute to the adjustment or modulation of the temperature sensitivity of hypothalamic neurons involved

in temperature regulation. One of the substances which is of particular interest is bombesin, for which it has been demonstrated that the highest concentrations and the highest receptor densities within the CNS occur in the anterior hypothalamus. Central application of bombesin causes changes of body temperature, the direction of which depends on the environmental temperature; it was, therefore, assumed that bombesin makes the animals poikilothermic (Brown et al., 1977a; Nemeroff et al., 1979; Tache et al., 1980). However, careful studies in rabbits, in which the internal temperature was changed under constant ambient temperature conditions, revealed a decrease in the threshold temperature for the induction of cold defence and a reduced gain of the

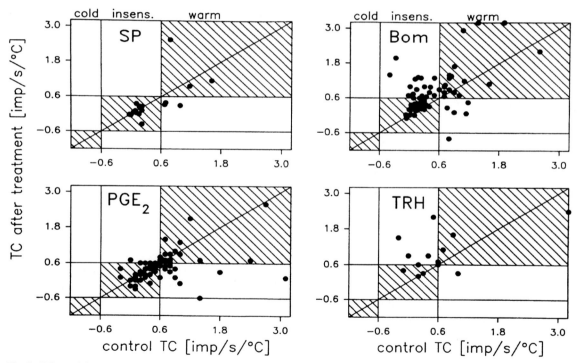

Fig. 8. Effect of SP, Bom, PGE$_2$ and TRH on the TC of individual PO/AH neurons. The TC during drug application is plotted as a function of the TC during the control period. The distance of a circle from the line of identity indicates the degree of change. Circles in non-hatched areas represent neurons in which the TC changes were large enough to transform these neurons into another category. SP and PGE$_2$ affect the TC of warm-sensitive neurons, while it is not affected in most of the temperature-insensitive neurons. Bom and TRH affect the TC of both neuronal populations. Transformation of temperature-insensitive neurons results in a recruitment of warm-sensitive neurons, while a decrease of warm-sensitive neurons results from a transformation into temperature-insensitive ones [from Pierau et al. (1994), reprinted with kind permission of Birkhäuser Verlag, Basel, Switzerland].

effector mechanisms (Jansky et al., 1987) indicating a specific action of the substance on the neuronal control of body temperature.

Another possible modulator which is present in high concentrations in the hypothalamus is substance P (SP) and participation of SP-containing central neurons in thermoregulation has been suggested (Szolcsányi, 1983; Hori et al., 1988a). Injection of SP into the hypothalamus, however, has little or no effect on body temperature (Bissette et al., 1976; Brown et al., 1977b). One would assume, therefore, that both substances have different actions on hypothalamic neurons, the prediction being that only bombesin specifically affects temperature sensitivity. Noteworthy, both peptides had similar effects on hypothalamic neurons when perfused to rat brain slices, in that they increased spontaneous activity of the majority of warm-sensitive and of two-thirds and one-half of temperature-insensitive neurons, respectively (Schmid et al., 1993). In the case of SP the number of sensitive neurons was higher than in similar experiments *in situ* (Shibata et al., 1988). It should also be noted that microiontophoretic application of bombesin to PO/AH neurons *in situ* inhibited the spontaneous activity of all neurons but an effect of the applied current cannot be excluded in these experiments (Hori et al., 1986). With respect to temperature sensitivity, however, both peptides induced different changes. Substance P, as a rule, decreased the TC of warm-sensitive neurons but did not affect the TC of temperature-insensitive neurons. In contrast, bombesin increased the TC in about half of the warm-sensitive neurons but decreased it in the other half (Fig. 8); thus, the average TC was not changed by bombesin. Instead, bombesin increased the TC of most of the temperature-insensitive neurons. The degree of the TC-increase was large enough to convert about half of the investigated neurons into warm-sensitive ones. Thus, the mechanism by which the hypothermic substance bombesin is affecting the central controller seems to be different from those responsible for the effects of all substances discussed previously in this paper and appears to consist in the recruitment of warm-sensitive neurons.

Although not immediately apparent, modulation of the TC also appears to account for the effect of thyrotropin releasing hormone (TRH) on body temperature. The TC was increased in some of the warm-sensitive neurons similarly as observed after bombesin while it was decreased in others. However, the TC of most of the temperature-insensitive neurons, was increased by TRH resulting in a recruitment of warm-sensitive neurons also similar to the effect observed after bombesin. At first glance, the direction of these TC changes is surprising, since TRH induces, in most animals, a hyperthermia upon injection into the hypothalamus, i.e. it changes body temperature in a direction opposite to that induced by bombesin. However, in the rat the TRH-induced hyperthermia is very short-lasting (5 min) and is followed by a long-lasting decrease in body temperature (Lin et al., 1980; Hori et al., 1988b). It was suggested that the increase of the TC in temperature-insensitive neurons corresponds to the hypothermic phase observed *in vivo*, since the TC changes became distinct not earlier than 10 min after the start of TRH superfusion in the slice preparation (Pierau et al., 1994). The recruitment of warm-sensitive neurons by bombesin and TRH suggests that the plasticity of the neuronal circuitry responsible for temperature regulation is accomplished by different mechanisms through which different mediators modulate body temperature.

In summary, a number of endogenous and exogenous substances which change body temperature have common effects on the temperature sensitivity of PO/AH neurons which can be categorized as two basically different mechanisms. One is related specifically to warm-sensitive neurons in that hypothermic substances induce an increase and hyperthermic substances a decrease of the TC of which the latter effect would imply a functional decrease of the number of warm-sensitive neurons and a recruitment of cold-sensitive ones. The other mechanism concerns temperature-insensitive neurons. Sufficient changes of their TC can result in a recruitment of temperature-sensitive neurons. So far, experimental evidence for such a mechanism exists only for hypothermic agents; in this case the number of warm-sensitive neurons is increased by the recruitment.

Effects of Ca^{2+}-concentration

Several *in vivo* studies suggest that changes of extracellular ionic concentrations (Nielsen, 1974) may affect temperature regulation. Changes of the ionic composition in the hypothalamus have been observed after central or peripheral temperature challenges or after intrahypothalamic injections of endogenous transmitter substances or pyrogens (Myers et al., 1976). At this time it had

been suggested that these different manipulations affect body temperature by an imbalance of extracellular ionic equilibrium which, in turn, results in the change of the set-point of the temperature controller. Indeed, changes of spontaneous activity of cerebral neurons *in vitro* after modulation of Ca^{2+}- and/or Mg^{2+}-concentrations were observed in various brain areas, e.g. in the guinea-pig cortex (Richards and Sercombe, 1970) and in hypothalamic slices (Pittmann et al., 1981). More recent experiments on hypothalamic slices demonstrated that not only spontaneous activity but also the temperature sensitivity of hypothalamic neurons could be changed by modulation of

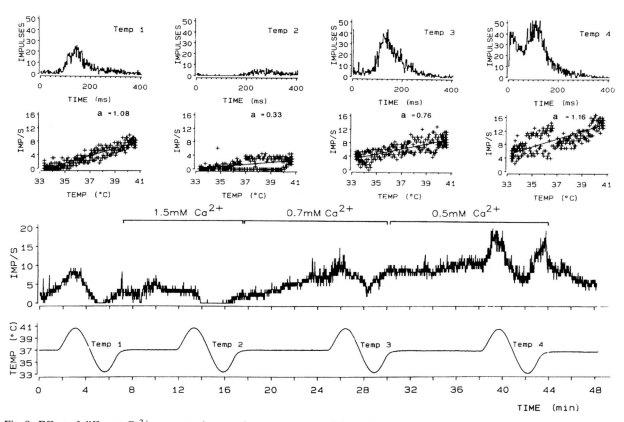

Fig. 9. Effect of different Ca^{2+}-concentrations on the spontaneous activity and temperature response of a warm-sensitive PO/AH neuron. The protocols show impulse activity (average of 10 s) and periodical changes of the slice temperature. The interval histograms and the frequency temperature relationships comprise the time periods of the four temperature cycles. The TC is indicated by the slope of the linear regression line (a) [from Schmid et al. (1993), reprinted with kind permission of The American Physiological Society, Bethesda, MD, USA].

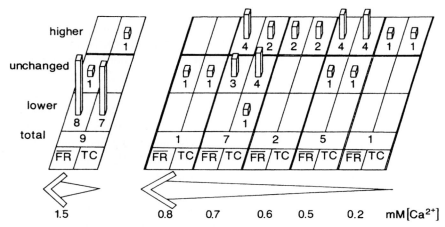

Fig. 10. Effect of different Ca^{2+}-concentrations on the average firing rate (FR) and TC of PO/AH neurons. Numbers represent neurons in the appropriate bars or total number of neurons. The CA^{2+}-concentration in the normal perfusion solution was 0.9 mM. An increase of the Ca^{2+}-concentration to 1.5 mM decreased the FR of eight and the TC of seven neurons; both parameters were increased at lower Ca^{2+}-concentrations [from Schmid et al. (1993), reprinted with kind permission of The American Physiological Society, Bethesda, MD, USA].

the extracellular Ca^{2+}-concentration (Schmid and Pierau, 1993). With Ca^{2+}-concentrations higher than 0.9 mM the TC of warm-sensitive as well as of temperature-insensitive neurons was usually decreased. Conversely, lowering the Ca^{2+}-concentration in the perfusate increased the temperature sensitivity of both cell populations resulting in part in a conversion of temperature-insensitive into warm-sensitive ones and, consequently, to a recruitment of warm-sensitive neurons (Figs. 9 and 10). These results should attract our attention to the possibility that changes of the extracellular ionic conditions can modulate body temperature by the plasticity of the central neuronal controller. The concentration of free Ca^{2+} varies between 0.75 and 1.5 mM in different brain areas (Heinemann et al., 1977; Nicholson et al., 1977) but sufficiently large changes may occur under physiological (Nicholson et al., 1977) or pathophysiological conditions (Heinemann et al., 1977). Mechanical stimulation of the cat's paw, for instance, decreases extracellular Ca^{2+}-concentration in the cortex from 1.3 to 0.7 mM. Similar effects on temperature sensitivity might occur from alterations of extracellular osmolality, since

a number of temperature-sensitive neurons also react to osmolality changes (Hori et al., 1989).

The fact that the temperature sensitivity of hypothalamic neurons depends on the local Ca^{2+}-concentration has also to be considered in investigations in which the synaptic activity is blocked by low Ca^{2+}- and high Mg^{2+}-concentrations (Kuno and Takahashi, 1986) to determine whether neuronal temperature sensitivity is inherent or depends on synaptic input (Hori et al., 1980b; Kelso and Boulant, 1982). In addition, the classification of neurons based on their temperature sensitivity might differ between various laboratories, since Ca^{2+}-concentrations between 0.9 and 2.4 mM were reported to be used in 'normal' CSF for perfusion of brain slices (Schmid and Pierau, 1993). The authors propose an optimal extracellular Ca^{2+}-concentration of 0.75 mM for the hypothalamic slice preparation, since complete inhibition of spontaneous activity was observed in many neurons after an elevation of extracellular Ca^{2+}-concentration to 1.26 mM.

Effects of local temperature changes

Changes of the milieu interieur result not only

from alterations of the extracellular ionic composition or osmolality but also from changes of the local hypothalamic temperature. Brain temperature in general and hypothalamic temperature in particular follow body temperature which may change under conditions of thermal load, stress, fever, and due to diurnal fluctuations (Hayward and Baker, 1968; Baker, 1972). However, considerable gradients of local brain temperature have been measured (Hayward, 1967), and temperature fluctuations might be attenuated in the beginning of heat and cold exposure (Kundt et al., 1957). In animals which possess a carotid rete, such as ruminants, dogs or cats, deviations of hypothalamic and body temperature occur under external or internal heat or cold stress (Finch and Robertshaw, 1979; Baker, 1982; Jessen et al., 1994). Consequently, the local temperature of the hypothalamic neuronal controller may change considerably and, consequently, the temperature sensitivity of neurons participating in the control circuit might change as it has been demonstrated for different variations of the milieu interieur.

In experiments in which rat brain slices were equilibrated at 36, 38 or 39°C for 10 min before neuronal temperature sensitivity was tested, the TC was stable at all temperatures in one-third of the investigated warm-sensitive neurons and in one-half of the temperature-insensitive neurons (Fig. 11) (Pierau et al., 1994). However, in most of the warm-sensitive neurons the TC was decreased at the lower equilibration temperature of 36°C, leading to a decrease in the number of warm-sensitive neurons (Fig. 12). The changes in temperature sensitivity were not so uniform after equilibration to 39°C, although in the majority of warm-sensitive neurons the TC was also decreased. The resulting conversion of some warm-sensitive neurons into temperature-insensitive neurons, however, was compensated by the transformation of a similar number of temperature-insensitive neurons into warm-sensitive ones (Fig. 12).

Although the results of these experiments should not be over-interpreted, since the equilibration time was only short, they indicate that the neuronal control of body temperature may vary

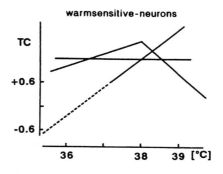

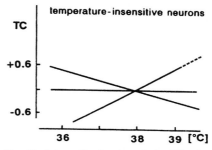

Fig. 11. Schematic drawing of the TC of warm-sensitive and temperature-insensitive PO/AH neurons at three different local temperatures. While the TCs of about one-third of the warm-sensitive neurons were stable they increased with increasing temperatures in most of the others; some neurons showed the highest TC at 38°C (upper diagram). Among the temperature-insensitive neurons about half of the neurons demonstrated identical TCs at the different temperatures; in most of the remaining neurons the TCs were increased but a few decreased with increasing temperatures (lower diagram). Broken lines indicate that some of the neurons were transformed into temperature-insensitive or warm-sensitive neurons, respectively.

under the influence of local temperature changes, again demonstrating the plasticity of the control system. Current investigations with temperature equilibrium times up to 20 min confirm this hypothesis (Haug, unpublished data).

Effects of acclimatisation

Acclimatisation to different ambient temperatures is characterized by a more efficient reaction of effector mechanisms and is assumed to involve changes of the central controller of temperature regulation (Bligh, 1973; Hensel, 1981). An involvement of thermoregulatory networks in the lower brain stem in thermal adaptation was suggested by Brück and Zeisberger (1978) and Brück and Hinckel (1982). Electrophysiological experiments revealed that the response of neurons of the midbrain raphe nuclei of rats to peripheral temperature stimulation was increased after cold adaptation in rats (Werner et al., 1981). In guinea-pigs, tonic activity of neurons in the nucleus raphe magnus and in the subcoeruleus region appeared to be changed after cold and warm adaptation (Hinckel and Schröder-Rosenstock, 1982; Hinckel and Perschel, 1987). In our own studies two different approaches were used to assess possible changes of the temperature sensitivity of hypothalamic neurons with the implication that the plasticity of the neuronal controller is part of adaptative processes (Konrad et al., 1993; Pierau et al., 1993).

The first approach was to compare the distribution of the two neuronal populations in rats adapted for 3–5 weeks to an ambient temperature of 5°C or 30°C, respectively, with the distribution of temperature-sensitive and tempera-ture-insensitive neurons of control rats. The most obvious result was that the relative number of warm-sensitive neurons was considerably changed in acclimated animals. While in control rats approximately 40% of the neurons were warm-sensitive this population was increased to 52% in cold-adapted rats but decreased to 29% in warm adapted rats (Fig. 13). The TC distribution of the warm-sensitive neurons was similar in control and cold adapted rats but high temperature coefficients were absent in warm adapted rats. Another clear difference was that about 20% of the warm-sensitive neurons in cold adapted rats had a TC in the range of 0.6–0.8 imp/s/°C while less than 8% of this neuronal population in warm adapted animals possessed a TC in this low range. Interpretation of these results can be only hypothetical. The larger number of warm-sensitive neurons in cold adapted rats could reflect the necessity to overcome the effect of increased heat insulation of the body shell by improving the drive for the different heat loss mechanisms in case of increased metabolic activity. Vice versa, a reduction of the drive for heat loss mechanisms might be necessary to conserve heat in warm

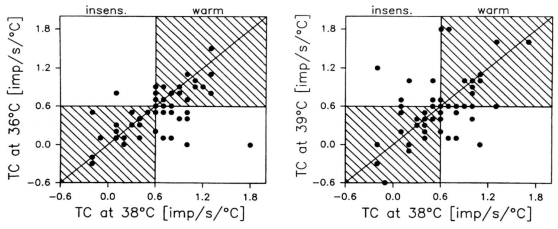

Fig. 12. Effect of different constant temperatures (short term adaptation) on individual TCs of PO/AH neurons. The TC at 36°C (left-hand diagram) and 39°C (right-hand diagram) is plotted as a function of the TC at 38°C. The distance of a circle from the line of identity indicates the degree of change. Circles in non-hatched areas represent neurons in which the TC changes were large enough to transform these neurons into another category [from Pierau et al. (1994), reprinted with kind permission of Birkhäuser Verlag, Basel, Switzerland].

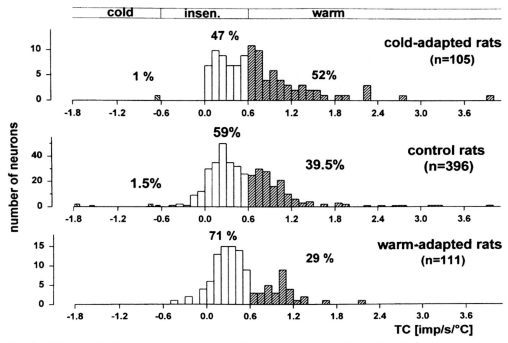

Fig. 13. Different distribution of temperature-sensitive and temperature-insensitive PO/AH neurons *in vitro* from rats adapted to 5°C (cold-adapted), 22°C (control), 30°C (warm-adapted) ambient temperature. Cold = cold-sensitive neurons; insen. = temperature-insensitive neurons; warm = warm-sensitive neurons. Relative numbers indicate percentage of the corresponding neuronal population.

adapted animals during exposure to cold environmental temperatures, e.g. during the night.

The second route of investigation was to explore the possibility of different reactions of hypothalamic neurons of acclimatized animals to endogenous mediators which are known to change the temperature sensitivity of PO/AH neurons. One of the most effective substances in this regard was bombesin, which predominantly increased the TC of temperature-insensitive neurons resulting in a recruitment of warm-sensitive neurons. An increase of the TC of temperature-insensitive neurons and their conversion into warm-sensitive ones was also the main effect of bombesin in rats adapted to warm or cold ambient temperatures. However, the relative number of recruited warm-sensitive neurons differed in the three neuronal populations, being lower in cold adapted and higher in warm adapted animals compared to the control group (Fig. 14). If mediators such as bombesin play a role in adaptation to acute regulatory demands or participate in the adjustment of physiological alterations of body temperature, e.g. in the course of circadian temperature deviations, a lower availability of recruited warm-sensitive neurons in cold adapted and a higher one in warm adapted animals could counteract the relative increase or decrease of warm-sensitive neurons in the different populations. This would, indeed, guarantee a very high degree of plasticity of the neuronal controller for body temperature and, consequently, improve stability of the regulated parameter.

Conclusion

This report summarizes the results of investigations which — proceeding from a few early hints

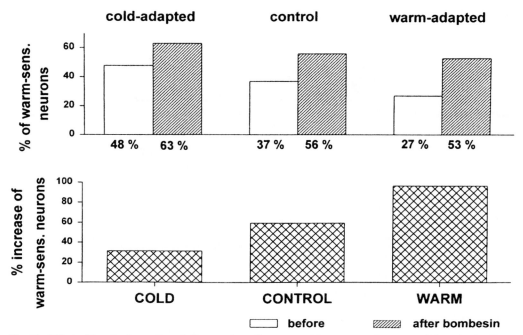

Fig. 14. Effect of bombesin on the relative number of warm-sensitive neurons (upper part) from brain slices of rats adapted to 5°C (cold-adapted), 22°C (control) and 30°C (warm-adapted) ambient temperature. The relative increase of warm-sensitive PO/AH neurons by bombesin was lower in cold-adapted and higher in warm-adapted rats compared to the control (lower part).

observed *in vivo* — have systematically assessed the plasticity of temperature coefficients of hypothalamic neurons as a new approach to the still enigmatic mechanisms, by which specific thermosensory signals and changes in thermoregulatory setpoint are somehow derived from a seemingly ubiquitous neuronal thermosensitivity. Using *in vitro* hypothalamic slice preparations from rats, the established convention to characterize temperature-sensitive and temperature-insensitive neurons was observed; however, the conversion of sensitive to insensitive neurons, and vice versa, was given particular attention. In the assessment of experimentally-induced changes of neuronal temperature coefficients, emphasis was put on the actions of those changes in the local environment of the slice preparation for which it is known that they may affect thermoregulation of the intact animal in a consistent fashion. In this way, pyrogens, GABA, neuropeptides, opioids and the corresponding pharmacological antagonists, were studied as well as changes of thermal and ionic parameters. Taken together, the results of these *in vitro* investigations have revealed reasonably consistent and thus encouraging relationships of the changes in temperature coefficients in general, and in the proportions of thermosensitive and -insensitive neurons in particular, to the changes in thermoregulatory control observed in intact animals under the influence of analogous procedures *in vivo*.

Acknowledgments

The authors wish to thank Professor E. Simon for discussing the manuscript. We are also grateful to N. Boll, V. Körber and K. Guckelsberger for technical assistance.

References

Baker, M.A. (1972) Influence of the carotid rete on brain temperature in cats exposed to hot environments. *J. Physiol.*, 220: 711–728.

Baker, M.A. (1982) Brain cooling in endotherms in heat and exercise. *Annu. Rev. Physiol.*, 44: 85–96.

Belyavskii, E.M. and Abramova, E.L. (1975) Effects of leucocyte pyrogen on thermosensitive neurons in the anterior hypothalamus. *Bull. Eksp. Biol. Med.*, 80: 17–20.

Bissette, G., Nemeroff, C.B., Loosen, P.T., Prange, A.J. Jr. and Lipton, M.A. (1976) Hypothermia and intolerance to cold induced by intracisternal administration of the hypothalamic peptide neurotensin. *Nature*, 262: 607–609.

Blatteis, C.M. (1981) Hypothalamic substances in the control of body temperature: general characteristics. *Fed. Proc.*, 40: 2735–2740.

Bligh, J. (1973) *Temperature Regulation in Mammals and other Vertebrates*, North-Holland, Amsterdam.

Bligh, J. (1981) Aminoacids as central synaptic transmitters or modulators in mammalian thermoregulation. *Fed. Proc.*, 40: 2746–2749.

Boulant, J.A. (1980) Hypothalamic control of thermoregulation. Neurophysiological basis. In: P.J. Morgane and J. Panksepp (Eds.), *Handbook of the Hypothalamus*, Vol. 3, Part A, Dekker, New York, pp. 1–82.

Boulant, J.A. (1996) Hypothalmic neurons regulating body temperature. In: M.J. Fregly and C.M. Blatteis (Eds.), *Handbook of Physiology, Environmental Physiology*, Oxford University Press, New York, Vol. 1, pp. 105–126.

Boulant, J.A. and Bignall, K.E. (1973) Hypothalamic neuronal responses to peripheral and deep-body temperatures. *Am. J. Physiol.*, 225: 1371–1374.

Boulant, J.A. and Hardy, J.D. (1974) The effect of spinal and skin temperatures on the firing rate and thermosensitivity of preoptic neurones. *J. Physiol. Lond.*, 240: 639–660.

Boulant, J.A. and Scott, I.M. (1983) Effect of leukocytic pyrogen on hypothalamic neurons in tissue slices. In: P. Lomax and E. Schönbaum (Eds.), *Environment, Drugs and Thermoregulation*, Karger, Basel, pp. 125–127.

Boulant, J.A. and Dean, J.B. (1986) Temperature receptors in the central nervous system. *Annu. Rev. Physiol.*, 48: 639–654.

Boulant, J.A. and Scott, I.M. (1986) Comparison of Prostaglandin E_2 and leukocytic pyrogen on hypothalamic neurons in tissue slices. In: K.E. Cooper, J. Lomax, E. Schönbaum and W.L. Veale (Eds.), *Homeostasis and Thermal Stress*, Karger, Basel, pp. 78–80.

Brown, M., Rivier, J. and Vale, W. (1977a) Bombesin: potent effects on thermoregulation in the rat. *Science*, 196: 998–1000.

Brown, M.R., Rivier, J. and Vale, W.W. (1977b) Bombesin affects the central nervous system to produce hyperglycemia in rats. *Life Sci.*, 21: 1729–1734.

Brück, K. and Zeisberger, E. (1978) Significance and possible central mechanisms of thermoregulatory threshold deviations in thermal adaptation. In: L.C.H. Wang and J.W. Hudson (Eds.), *Strategies in Cold: Natural Torpidity and Thermogenesis*, Academic Press, London, pp. 655–694.

Brück, K. and Hinckel, P. (1982) Thermoafferent systems and their adaptive modifications. *Pharmacol. Ther.*, 17: 357–381.

Cabanac, M., Stolwijk, J.A.J. and Hardy, J.D. (1968) Effect of temperature and pyrogens on single unit activity in the rabbit's brain stem. *J. Appl. Physiol.*, 24: 645–652.

Clark, W.G. (1981) Effects of opioid peptides on thermoregulation. *Fed. Proc.*, 40: 2754–2759.

Clark, W.G. and Lipton, J.M. (1985) Changes in body temperature after administration of amino acids, peptides, dopamine, neuroleptics and related agents. II. *Neurosci. Biobehav. Rev.*, 9: 299–371.

Cooper, K.E., Cranston, W.I. and Honour, J.A. (1967) Observations on the site and mode of action of pyrogens in the rabbit brain. *J. Physiol.*, 191: 325–338.

Eisenman, J.S. (1969) Pyrogen-induced changes in the thermosensitivity of septal and preoptic neurons. *Am. J. Physiol.*, 216: 330–334.

Eisenman, J.S. (1982) Electrophysiology of the hypothalamus: Thermoregulation and fever. In: A.S. Milton (Ed.), *Pyretics and Antipyretics*, Springer, Berlin, pp. 187–217.

Feldberg, W. and Saxena, P.N. (1971) Further studies on prostaglandin E_1 fever in cats. *J. Physiol.*, 219: 739–745.

Finch, V.A. and Robertshaw, D. (1979) Effect of dehydration on thermoregulation in eland and hartebeest. *Am. J. Physiol.*, 23: R192–R196.

Glotzbach, S.F. and Heller, C. (1984) Changes in the thermal characteristics of hypothalamic neurons during sleep and wakefulness. *Brain Res.*, 309: 17–26.

Gordon, C.J. and Heath, J.E. (1980) Effects of prostaglandin E_2 on the activity of thermosensitive and insensitive single units in the preoptic/anterior hypothalamus of unanesthetized rabbits. *Brain Res.*, 183: 113–121.

Griffin, J.D., Kaple, M.L., Chow, A.R. and Boulant, J.A. (1996) Cellular mechanisms for neuronal thermosensitivity in the rat hypothalamus. *J. Physiol.*, in press.

Hammel, H.T. (1965) Neurones and temperature regulation. In: W.S. Yamamoto and J.R. Brobeck (Eds.), *Physiological Controls and Regulations*, Saunders, Philadelphia, pp. 71–79.

Hammel, H.T. (1968) Regulation of internal body temperature. *Annu. Rev. Physiol.*, 30: 641–710.

Handler, C.M., Geller, E.B. and Adler, M.W (1992) Effect of μ-, κ- and δ-selective opioid agonists on thermoregulation in the rat. *Pharmacol. Biochem. Behav.*, 43: 1209–1216.

Hardy, J.D. (1972) Peripheral inputs to the central regulator of body temperature. In: S. Itoh, K. Ogata and H. Yoshimura (Eds.), *Advances in Climatic Physiology*, Igaku Shoin, Tokyo, pp. 3–21.

Hayward, J.N. (1967) Cerebral cooling during increased cerebral blood flow in the monkey. *Proc. Soc. Exp. Biol. Med.*, 124: 555–557.

Hayward, J.N. and Baker, M.A. (1968) The role of the cerebral arterial blood in the regulation of brain temperature in the monkey. *Am. J. Physiol.*, 515(2).

Heinemann, U., Lux, H.D. and Gutnick, M.J. (1977) Extracellular free calcium and potassium during paroxysmal activity in cerebral cortex of the cat. *Exp. Brain Res.*, 27: 237–243.

Hensel, H. (1981) *Thermoreception and Temperature Regulation*, Academic Press, London, pp. 219–234.

Hinckel, P. and Schröder-Rosenstock, K. (1982) Central thermal adaptation of lower brain stem units in the guinea-pig. *Pflüg. Arch.*, 395: 344–346.

Hinckel, P. and Perschel, W.T. (1987) Influence of cold and warm acclimation on neuronal responses in the lower brain stem. *Can. J. Physiol. Pharmacol.*, 65: 1281–1289.

Hori, T. (1991) An update on thermosensitive neurons in the brain: from cellular biology to thermal and non-thermal homeostatic functions. *Jpn. J. Physiol.*, 41: 1–22.

Hori, T., Nakashima, T., Hori, N. and Kiyohara, T. (1980a) Thermo-sensitive neurons in hypothalamic tissue slices *in vitro*. *Brain Res.*, 186: 203–207.

Hori, T., Nakashima, T., Kiyohara, T. and Hori, N. (1980b) Effect of calcium removal on thermosensitivity of preoptic neurons in hypothalamic slices. *Neurosci. Lett.*, 31: 171–175.

Hori, T., Yamasaki, M., Kiyohara, T. and Shibata, M. (1986) Responses of preoptic thermosensitive neurons to poikilothermia-inducing peptides — bombesin and neurotensin. *Pflüg. Arch.*, 407: 558–560.

Hori, T., Shibata, M., Kiyohara, T., Nakashima, T. and Asami, A. (1988a) Responses of anterior hypothalamic-preoptic thermosensitive neurons to locally applied capsaicin. *Neuropharmacology*, 27: 135–142.

Hori, T., Yamasaki, M., Asami, T., Koga, H. and Kiyohara, T. (1988b) Responses of anterior hypothalamic-preoptic thermosensitive neurons to thyrotropin releasing hormone and cyclo (his-pro). *Neuropharmacology*, 27: 895–901.

Hori, T., Kiyohara, T. and Nakashima, T. (1989) Thermosensitive neurons in the brain — the role in homeostatic functions. In: J.B. Mercer (Ed.), *Thermal Physiology*, Elsevier, Amsterdam, pp. 3–12.

Jackson, H.C. and Nutt, D.J. (1991) Inhibition of backlofen-induced hypothermia in mice by the novel $GABA_B$ antagonist CGP 35348. *Neuropharmacology*, 30: 535–538.

Jansky, L., Riedel, W., Simon, E., Simon-Oppermann, C. and Vybiral, S. (1987) Effect of bombesin on thermoregulation of the rabbit. *Pflüg. Arch.*, 409: 318–322.

Jessen, C. (1976) Two-dimensional determination of thermosensitive sites within the goat's hypothalamus. *J. Appl. Physiol.*, 40: 514–520.

Jessen, C., Laburn, H.P., Knight, M.H., Kuhnen, G., Goelst, K. and Mitchell, D. (1994) Blood and brain temperatures of free-ranging black wildebeest in their natural environment. *Am. J. Physiol.*, 267: R1528–R1536.

Kelso, S.R. and Boulant, J.A. (1982) Effect of synaptic blockade on thermosensitive neurons in hypothalamic tissue slices. *Am. J. Physiol.*, 243: R480–R490.

Konrad, M., Pierau, Fr.-K. and Sann, H. (1993) Adaptive changes of hypothalamic neurons in rat brain slices after cold and warm adaptation. *Pflüg. Arch. Suppl.*, 422: R58.

Kulchitsky, V., Sann, H. and Pierau, F.K. (1994) Effects of prostaglandin E_2 on the thermosensitivity of anterior and posterior hypothalamic neurones *in vitro*. In: K. Pleschka and R. Gerstberger (Eds.), *Integrative and cellular aspects of autonomic functions: temperature and osmoregulation*. John Libbey Eurotext, Paris 1994, pp. 37–46.

Kundt, H.W., Brück, K. and Hensel, H. (1957) Hypothalamustemperatur und Hautdurchblutung der nichtnarkotisierten Katze. *Pflüg. Arch. ges. Physiol.*, 264: 97–106.

Kuno, M. and Takahashi, T. (1986) Effects of calcium and magnesium on transmitter release at synapses of rat spinal motoneurones *in vitro*. *J. Physiol. Lond.*, 376: 543–553.

Lin, M.T., Chandra, A., Chern, Y.F. and Tsay, B.L. (1980) Effects of thyrotropin-releasing hormone (TRH) on thermoregulation in the rat. *Experientia*, 36: 1077–1078.

Matsuda, T., Hori, T. and Nakashima, T. (1992) Thermal and PGE_2 sensitivity of the organum vasculosum lamina terminalis region and preoptic area in rat brain slices. *J. Physiol.*, 454: 197–212.

Milton, A.S. and Wendlandt, S. (1970) A possible role for prostaglandin E_1 as a modulator for temperature regulation in the central nervous system of the cat. *J. Physiol.*, 207: 76–77P.

Minano, F.J., Serrano, J.S., Sancibrian, M. and Myers, R.D. (1989) Effects of central administration of GABA on thermoregulation. In: P. Lomax and E. Schönbaum (Eds.), *Thermoregulation: Research and Clinical Applications*, Karger, Basel, pp. 184–186.

Mitchell, D., Snellen, J.W. and Atkins, A.R. (1970) Thermoregulation during fever: change of set-point or change of gain. *Pflüg. Arch.*, 321: 293–302.

Morimoto, A., Murakami, N. and Watanabe, T. (1988) Effect of prostaglandin E_2 on thermoresponsive neurones in the preoptic and ventromedial hypothalamic regions of rats. *J. Physiol.*, 405: 713–725.

Myers, R.D., Rudy, T.A. and Yaksh, T.L. (1974) Fever produced by endotoxin injected into the hypothalamus of the monkey and its antagonism by salicylate. *J. Physiol.*, 243: 167–193.

Myers, R.D., Simpson, C.W., Higgins, D., Nattermann, R.A., Rice, J.C., Redgrave, P. and Metcalf, G. (1976) Hypothalamic Na and Ca ions and temperature set-point: new mechanisms of action of a central or peripheral thermal challenge and intrahypothalamic 5-NT, NE, PGE1 and pyrogen. *Brain Res. Bull.*, 1: 301–327.

Nakashima, T., Hori, T., Kiyohara, T. and Shibata, M. (1985) Osmosensitivity of preoptic thermosensitive neurons in hypothalamic slices *in vitro*. *Pflüg. Arch.*, 405: 112–117.

Nemeroff, C.B., Osbahr III, A.J., Manberg, P.J., Ervin, G.N. and Prange, A.J. Jr. (1979) Alterations in nociception and body temperature after intracisternal administration of neurotensin, β-endorphin, other endogenous peptides, and morphine. *Proc. Natl. Acad. Sci. USA,* 76: 5368–5371.

Nicholson, C., ten Bruggencate, G., Steinberg, R. and Stöckle, H. (1977) Calcium modulation in brain extracellular microenvironment demonstrated with ion-sensitive micropipette. *Proc. Natl. Acad. Sci. USA,* 74: 1287–1290.

Nielsen, B. (1974) Actions of intravenous Ca^{2+} and Na^+ on body temperature in rabbits. *Acta Physiol. Scand.,* 90: 445–450.

Ono, T., Morimoto, A., Watanabe, T. and Murakami, N. (1987) Effects of endogenous pyrogen and prostaglandin E_2 on hypothalamic neurons in guinea pig brain slices. *J. Appl. Physiol.,* 63: 175–180.

Ottersen, O.P. and Storm-Mathisen, J. (1984) Neurons containing or accumulating transmitter amino acids. In: A. Björklund, T. Hökfelt and M.J. Kuhar (Eds.), *Handbook of Chemical Neuroanatomy, Classical Transmitters and Transmitter Receptors in the CNS,* Part II, Elsevier, Amsterdam, pp. 141–246.

Pierau, Fr.-K., Schenda, J., Tzschentke, B., Konrad, M. and Sann, H. (1993) Adaptive changes of hypothalamic thermosensitive neurons after exposure to cold environmental temperature. In: C. Carey, G.L. Florant, B.A. Wunder and B. Horwitz (Eds.), *Life in the Cold, Ecological, Physiological and Molecular Mechanisms,* Westview Press, Boulder, pp. 323–329.

Pierau, Fr.-K., Schenda, J., Konrad, M. and Sann, H. (1994) Possible implications of the plasticity of temperature-sensitive neurons in the hypothalamus. In: E. Zeisberger, E. Schönbaum and P. Lomax (Eds.), *Thermal Balances in Health and Disease, Advances in Pharmacological Sciences,* Birkhäuser, Basel, pp. 31–36.

Pierau, Fr.-K., Yakimova, K.S., Sann, H. and Schmid, H.A. (1997) Specific action of $GABA_B$ ligands on the temperature sensitivity of hypothalamic neurons. *Ann. NY Acad. Sci.,* 813: 146–155.

Pittmann, Q.J., Hatton, J.D. and Bloom, F.E. (1981) Spontaneous activity in perfused hypothalamic slices: dependence on calcium content of the perfusate. *Exp. Brain Res.,* 42: 49–52.

Puschmann, S. and Jessen, C. (1978) Anterior and posterior hypothalamus: effects of independent temperature displacements on heat production in conscious goats. *Pflüg. Arch.,* 373: 59–68.

Richards, C.D. and Sercombe, R. (1970) Calcium, magnesium and the electrical activity of guinea-pig olfactory cortex *in vitro. J. Physiol. Lond.,* 211: 571–584.

Rosendorff, C. and Mooney, J.J. (1971) Central nervous system sites of action of a purified leucocyte pyrogen. *Am. J. Physiol.,* 220: 597–603.

Satinoff, E. (1978) Neural organization and evolution of thermal regulation in mammals. *Science,* 201: 16–22.

Satinoff, E. (1979) Drugs and thermoregulatory behavior. In: P. Lomax and E. Schönbaum (Eds.), *Body Temperature: Regulation, Drug Effects and Therapeutic Implications,* Dekker, New York, pp. 151–181.

Serrano, J.S., Minano, F.J., Sancibrian, M. and Duran, J.A. (1985) Involvement of bicuculline-insensitive receptors in the hypothermic effect of GABA and its agonists. *Gen. Pharmacol.,* 16: 505–508.

Schmid, H.A. and Pierau, Fr.-K. (1993) Temperature sensitivity of neurons in slices of the rat PO/AH hypothalamic area: effect of calcium. *Am. J. Physiol.,* 264: R440–R448.

Schmid, H.A., Jansky, L. and Pierau, Fr.-K. (1993) Temperature sensitivity of neurons in slices of the rat PO/AH area: effect of bombesin and substance P. *Am. J. Physiol.,* 264: R449–R455.

Schoener, E.P. and Wang, S.C. (1975) Leucocytic pyrogen and sodium acetylsalicylate on hypothalamic neurons in the cat. *Am. J. Physiol.,* 229: 185–190.

Schoener, E.P. and Wang, S.C. (1976) Effects of locally administered prostaglandin E_1 on anterior hypothalamic neurons. *Brain Res.,* 117: 157–162.

Shibata, M., Hori, T., Kiyohara, T., Nakashima, T. and Asami, T. (1988) Responses of anterior hypothalamic-preoptic thermosensitive neurons to substance P and capsaicin. *Neuropharmacology,* 27: 143–148.

Silva, N.L. and Boulant, J.A. (1984) Effects of osmotic pressure, glucose, and temperature on neurons in preoptic tissue slices. *Am. J. Physiol.,* 247: R335–R345.

Silva, N.L. and Boulant, J.A. (1986) Effects of testosterone, estradiol, and temperature on neurons in preoptic tissue slices. *Am. J. Physiol.,* 250: R625–R632.

Simon, E. (1974) Temperature regulation: the spinal cord as a site of extrahypothalamic thermoregulatory functions. *Rev. Physiol. Biochem. Pharmacol.,* 71: 1–16.

Simon, E., Pierau, F.K. and Taylor, D.C.M. (1986) Central and peripheral thermal control of effectors in homeothermic temperature regulation. *Physiol. Rev.,* 66: 253–300.

Spencer, R.L., Hruby, V.J. and Burks, T.F. (1988) Body temperature response profiles for selective Mu, Delta and Kappa opioid agonists in restrained and unrestrained rats. *J. Pharmacol. Exp. Ther.,* 246: 92–101.

Stewart, J. and Eikelboom, R. (1979) Stress masks the hypothermic effect of naloxone in rats. *Life Sci.,* 25: 1165–1171.

Stitt, J.T. (1973) Prostaglandin E_1 fever induced in rabbits. *J. Physiol.,* 232: 163–179.

Szolcsányi, J. (1983) Disturbances of thermoregulation induced by capsaicin. *J. Therm. Biol.,* 8: 207–212.

Tache, Y., Pittman, Q. and Brown, M. (1980) Bombesin-induced poikilothermy in rats. *Brain Res.,* 188: 525–530.

Watanabe, T., Morimoto, A. and Murakami, N. (1987) Effect of PGE$_2$ on preoptic and anterior hypothalamic neurones using brain slice preparation. *J. Appl. Physiol.*, 63: 918–922.

Werner, J. (1980) The concept of regulation for human body temperature. *J. Therm. Biol.*, 5: 75–82.

Werner, J., Schingnitz, G. and Hensel, H. (1981) Influence of cold adaptation on the activity of thermoresponsive neurons in thalamus and midbrain of the rat. *Pflüg. Arch.*, 391: 327–330.

Wit, A. and Wang, S.C. (1968) Temperature-sensitive neurons in preoptic anterior hypothalamic region: Actions of pyrogen and acetylsalicylate. *Am. J. Physiol.*, 215: 1160–1169.

Yakimova, K. and Ovtcharov, R. (1989) Central temperature effects of the transmitter amino acids. *Acta Physiol. Pharmacol. Bulg.*, 15: 50–54.

Yakimova, K., Sann, H., Schmid, H.A. and Pierau, F-K. (1996) Effects of GABA agonists and antagonists on temperature-sensitive neurones in the rat hypothalamus. *J. Physiol.*, 494.1: 217–230.

Yakimova, K.S., Pierau, Fr.-K. and Sann, H. (1997) Effects of opioids on thermosensitivity of rat hypothalamic neurons. *Ann. NY Acad. Sci.*, 813: 156–165.

SECTION II

Pharmacological aspects

H.S. Sharma and J. Westman (Eds.)
Progress in Brain Research, Vol 115
© 1998 Elsevier Science BV. All rights reserved.

CHAPTER 6

Role of nitric oxide in temperature regulation

Herbert A. Schmid*, Walter Riedel and Eckhart Simon

Max-Planck-Institute for Physiological and Clinical Research, William G. Kerckhoff-Institute, Parkstrasse 1, D-61231 Bad Nauheim, Germany

Introduction

Soon after the anion nitrate had been shown to be a physiological metabolite in mammals (Green et al., 1981a,b), it was observed that fever in humans or application of the exogenous pyrogen lipopolysaccharide (LPS) to rats greatly stimulated urinary nitrate excretion (Wagner et al., 1983) and that macrophages were the site of LPS-induced nitrate synthesis (Stuehr and Marletta, 1985). After the identity of the endothelium-derived relaxing factor (Furchgott and Zawadzki, 1980) as nitric oxide (NO) (Ignarro et al., 1987; Palmer et al., 1987) and its synthesis in endothelial cells (Palmer et al., 1988) had been discovered, it was shown for macrophages that these cells also generated nitrogen oxides from L-arginine and that the radical NO was, indeed, formed as the presumably relevant intermediate (Marletta et al., 1988; Stuehr et al., 1989). It is now established that NO is synthesized peripherally and by nervous elements from L-arginine as the natural precursor. Nitric oxide synthase (NOS) are either constitutive (cNOS), which is Ca^{2+}/calmodulin dependent, or inducible (iNOS), which is Ca^{2+}/calmodulin independent. NOS isoforms require FAD, FMN, heme and tetrahydrobiopterin as cofactors and display NADPH-di-

aphorase activity (Nathan, 1992; Griffith and Stuehr, 1995). NO exerts most of its physiological actions by activating a soluble guanylate cyclase as the second messenger, but direct interactions of NO with enzymes and superoxide anions are also considered (Nathan, 1992; Mayer et al., 1993).

In the central nervous system (CNS) the function of NO first identified was that of an intercellular messenger involved in the regulation of cGMP levels in response to stimulation of especially the N-methyl-D-aspartate (NMDA) subtype of glutamate receptors (Garthwaite et al., 1988). NO is assumed to be synthesized in the brain on demand and to leave a neuron or its terminals by diffusion and, therefore, its messenger function must be regulated differently from those of classical transmitters/modulators stored in presynaptic vesicles (Zhang and Synder, 1995). As a further consequence, the range of action of NO as a diffusible messenger considerably exceeds the dimensions of a synapse or even of a single neuron (Garthwaite and Boulton, 1995). Staining of the NOS by means of immunocytochemistry or by histochemical detection of its NADPH-diaphorase activity (Dawson et al., 1991; Hope et al., 1991) have revealed the widespread presence of 'nitroxidergic' (or 'nitrergic') neurons in the CNS, as well as in the periphery. Although some reservation was recently expressed that neuronal NADPH-diaphorase might not only represent NOS (Brüning et al., 1994; Traub et al., 1994), a very high degree of colocalization of the NOS and

---

*Corresponding author. E-mail: hschmid@kerckhoff.mpg.de

NADPH-diaphorase reactions was reported for the hypothalamus (Jurzak et al., 1994) and autonomic and enteric neurons (Rand and Li, 1995a).

Assessment of messenger functions of NO in temperature regulation

The putative role of NO in temperature regulation has only recently attracted interest. In the periphery, the ubiquity of NO generating cells, like the vascular endothelium and the phagocytic elements of the reticulo-endothelial system cells, almost necessarily implies that the widespread actions of NO somehow interfere with thermoregulatory activities. In the CNS, the presence of nitroxidergic neurons in hypothalamic nuclei and circumventricular organs associated with salt and fluid balance (Arévalo et al., 1992; Pow, 1992; Vincent and Kimura, 1992; Jurzak et al., 1994) and gonadotropin regulation (Bhat et al., 1995) does not exclude that such neurons are also incorporated into the structurally less well defined hypothalamic thermoregulatory control system. In the short-term control activities of physiological temperature regulation, changes in activity of the cNOS may be most relevant. In the longer lasting pathophysiological process of fever and associated humoral and cellular defence activities, the additional involvement of iNOS induced by LPS or by cytokines with a delay in the order of hours has to be considered. However, recent evidence suggests that some degree of activity of iNOS may exist in apparently normal conditions, including the possibility of pre-existing cryptic stimulation by subliminal degrees of cytokine activation (Nathan and Xie, 1994).

For the experimental evaluation of NO effects of thermoregulatory relevance, a variety of pharmacological NO-donors, in addition to the physiological precursor L-arginine, and several pharmacological analogs inhibiting NOS are available. The role of NO as a peripheral or central messenger in the control of single thermoregulatory effectors as well as in the coordination of the multiple, metabolic, vasomotor, sudomotor, and respiratory response components of thermoregulation are being analyzed in this way. Endogenous NO formation in defined conditions of thermoregulatory control may be evaluated by determining the generation of nitrite and nitrate anions as indicators for NO in biological fluids (Stuehr et al., 1989). Methods to measure NO quantitatively were recently reviewed (Archer, 1993).

NO as a peripheral messenger in temperature regulation

Since NO is a vasodilator, systemic application of NO-donors cause decreases in mean arterial blood pressure (MAP) and reflex-mediated increases in heart rate (HR), while NOS-inhibitors cause opposite responses. For these reasons, it is difficult to judge the thermoregulatory specificity of accompanying changes in skin blood flow. In a first systematic study (Gerstberger et al., 1994) on chronically instrumented, conscious rabbits, MAP, HR and rectal temperature (T_{rec}) were recorded, and oxygen consumption ($\dot{V}_{O_2}$), respiratory frequency (RF), respiratory evaporative water loss (REWL) and ear skin temperature (T_{ear}) were monitored (Fig. 1). These parameters served as indicators for metabolic heat production, evaporative heat loss and blood flow to the skin. Most measurements were carried out at ambient thermoneutrality (24°C), but in exploratory studies ambient temperature was elevated to 31.5°C to impose a peripheral heat load, or lowered to 5°C to impose a peripheral cold load. At thermoneutrality, i.v. infusion over 15 min of 3–15 μg/kg/min of the NO-donors SNAP (S-nitroso-N-acetyl-penicillamine) or SIN-1 (3-morpholino-sydnonimine-hydrochloride) induced the expected hypotensive and tachycardic circulatory effects which reflected general vasodilatation and, therefore, precluded a safe conclusion on the thermoregulatory origin of the simultaneously observed rise in T_{ear}. Significant increases of RF and REWL at an unchanged oxygen consumption, however, seemed to represent true heat loss

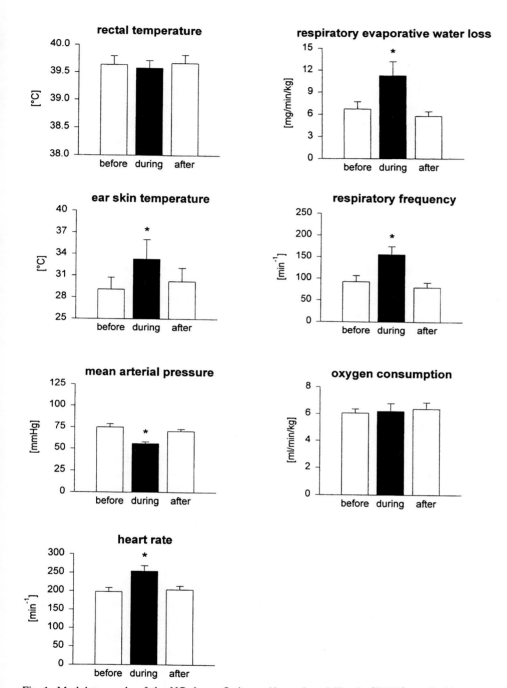

Fig. 1. Modulatory role of the NO-donor *S*-nitroso-*N*-acetyl-penicillamin (SNAP), applied intravenously at a concentration of 15 μg/min/kg for 20 min to conscious rabbits exposed to 24°C environmental temperature. Shown are the peak effects with the S.E.M. of the respective responses of six animals significant changes vs. the control (modified according to Gerstberger et al., 1994).

responses. Partially opposite effects were induced by bolus injections of 10 mg/kg of the NOS-inhibitor L-NAME (N^G-nitro-L-arginine-methylester) which increased MAP and decreased HR and significantly reduced RF and REWL, while T_{ear} remained unchanged. At warm ambient conditions L-NAME caused a more pronounced reduction of evaporative heat loss and a significant decrease in T_{ear}, both indicating a stimulation of heat conserving mechanisms by NOS-inhibition. However, at thermoneutrality oxygen consumption decreased rather than rose, as one would have expected for a coordinated cold defence response. Further, at cold ambient conditions, in which an elevated oxygen consumption indicated enhanced metabolic heat production, oxygen consumption was also clearly depressed by L-NAME. Taken together this first analysis of a potential thermoregulatory relevance of peripheral NO-generating systems provided some evidence for a supportive role of NO in the stimulation of heat loss responses but no corresponding inhibitory action on metabolic heat production.

A specific role of peripherally acting NO in the control of thermogenic mechanisms is also denied by studies on the sympathetic control of heat generation in the brown adipose tissue (BAT) which is a specific thermoregulatory effector of metabolic cold defence responsible for the non-shivering thermogenesis (NST). In anesthetized rats, intraperitoneal injections of the NOS-inhibitor L-NAME reduced the activity in sympathetic branches innervating the BAT and decreased its oxygen consumption (De Luca et al., 1995). These reactions were opposite to those to be expected, if NO acted as a peripheral mediator which not only enhanced heat loss but also suppressed metabolic heat production in a coordinated fashion. Instead, NO seems to exert a thermogenic action in the BAT. In line with this conclusion seems to be the notion 'that NO may be a signalling molecule for an enhanced NST in cold acclimation' (Kuroshima, 1995).

Less clear were the results of a recent study on rabbits in which SNP (sodium nitroprusside) was i.v. applied as a NO-donor and its actions were compared with those of arginine vasopressin in normothermia and fever (Gagalo et al., 1995). In normothermic animals continuously infused SNP induced a distinct hypothermia which was associated, contrary to the well established vasodilatory effect of SNP, with a decrease in T_{ear}. Since the applied SNP dose was strongly hypotensive, the reduction in ear skin blood flow indicated by the course of T_{ear} may have been secondary to the general hemodynamic effect of the NO-donor.

Nerves whose transmitter is neither noradrenaline nor acetylcholine (NANC) form an important component of the autonomic innervation of smooth muscle in the gut and circulation. In line with the impression of a supportive role of peripheral NO in the activation of heat loss are recent studies on vascular areas of known thermoregulatory significance as heat dissipating areas in which vasodilatation is at least in part accomplished by activation of NANC autonomic efferents in addition to the decrease in adrenergic vasoconstrictor tone; this applies to ear skin of rabbits (Gregor et al., 1976). In a study on conscious rabbits, which had been chronically instrumented to measure arterial pressure and heart rate, to monitor ear blood flow velocity by Doppler ultrasound, and to apply drugs topically via the lingual artery, large increases in ear blood flow velocity were induced by whole body heating (Taylor and Bishop, 1993). Intraarterial application of the NOS-inhibitor L-NNA (N^ω-nitro-L-arginine) virtually abolished heat-induced vasodilatation with a slow onset and a persistence for more than 30 min. An effect secondary to the general circulatory effect of the NOS-inhibitor could be excluded. Infusion of the natural NO-donor L-arginine restored the dilator response. Acetylcholine did not seem to be involved as a transmitter. In a further study an unimpaired local formation of NO, most likely in the endothelium, was shown to be a necessary prerequisite for heat-induced vasodilatation in the rabbit ear skin, but the involvement of an additional, unidentified transmitter, different from NO, had to be postulated (Farrell and Bishop, 1995).

In the canine nasal mucosa, thermoregulatory control of blood flow is predominant, and vasodilatation as a heat loss response involves reduction of vasoconstrictor tone, as well as NANC vasodilatation (Sugahara and Pleschka, 1992). In an in vitro study on tissue specimens from the canine nasal mucosa kept in Krebs solution, the transmitter involved in NANC blood vessel relaxation was analyzed (Watanabe et al., 1995). After pharmacological blockade of cholinergic and adrenergic transmission and partial contraction induced by ergotamine, the vessels reacted to transmural electrical stimulation with a relaxation. Adding the NOS-inhibitor L-NNA to the bath fluid abolished blood vessel relaxation in response to electrostimulation and thereby suggested that NO was the transmitter for NANC vasodilatation in this vascular region.

While the reported results provide evidence for the involvement of NO in the local control of blood flow in heat dissipating tissue surfaces, the specificity of NO as a transmitter of NANC vasodilatation during thermoregulatory responses remains to be established. In particular, the results cannot be generalized, since in a study on humans, heat-induced NANC vasodilatation in the forearm was not suppressed by intraarterial infusion of the NOS-inhibitor L-NMMA (N^{G}-monomethyl-L-arginine) at a dose which abolished vasodilatation induced by intraarterial infusion of acetylcholine (Dietz et al., 1994).

NO as a central messenger in temperature regulation

Injections into the lateral cerebral ventricles, into the 3rd ventricle or directly into the hypothalamic neural tissue are established techniques to evaluate the thermoregulatory specificity of central nervous messengers. In the case of NO, studies are emerging which suggest a central thermolytic function with coordinated, stimulatory effects on heat dissipating mechanisms and inhibitory effects on heat generating mechanisms.

In a study on rats, either recovering from hypothermia of about 25°C or being overheated in a hot environment of 37°C, the influence of i.c.v. injections of the NO-donor N-(ethoxycarbonyl)-3-(4-morpholinyl)-sydnonimine and of the NOS-inhibitor L-NA (N-nitro-L-arginine) on the course of the core temperature were followed up (Gourine, 1994). The NO-donor significantly delayed the recovery from hypothermia, suggesting an inhibition of heat conserving and generating mechanisms, while recovery in animals treated with the NOS-inhibitor of rats did not differ from that of untreated rats. During heat exposure, the hyperthermic rise of core temperature was enhanced by i.c.v. application of the NOS-inhibitor, suggesting the suppression of a NO-dependent activation of heat dissipating mechanisms, while the course of core temperature in animals treated with the NO-donor did not differ from that of untreated rats.

A preliminary study on chronically instrumented, conscious rabbits, although carried out on only three animals, was most informative, because all relevant thermoregulatory effectors (T_{rec}, T_{ear}, V_{O_2}, RF, REWL), MAP and HR were simultaneously monitored in a thermoneutral environment to assess the thermoregulatory specificity of the central NO action (Helmqvist et al., unpublished data). Infusion of the NO-donor SIN-1 into the 3rd cerebral ventricle for 20 min at a dose of 2 μg/min/kg and at a rate of 2 μl/min elicited a coordinated heat loss response with a fall in T_{rec}, a rise in T_{ear}, and parallel increases in RF and REWL (Fig. 2). The general circulatory effect of the centrally applied NO-donor consisted in a rise in MAP and a decrease in HR, i.e. reactions opposite to those induced by peripherally acting NO, and, thus, indicated that the cutaneous vasodilatory response to centrally acting NO, as indicated by the rise in T_{ear}, was a specific thermoregulatory reaction, rather than secondary to the general hemodynamic effect.

Support for the hypothesis that NO acts centrally as a specific thermolytic messenger in hypothalamic control of body temperature is especially provided by studies on rats in which sympathetic control and thermogenesis in the BAT were analyzed (De Luca et al., 1995; Monda et al., 1995a). Unlike its action in the periphery, the NOS-inhibitor L-NAME, when applied i.c.v., enhanced sympathetic activity in branches innervating the BAT and significantly increased oxygen consumption, i.e. blockade of hypothalamic NO

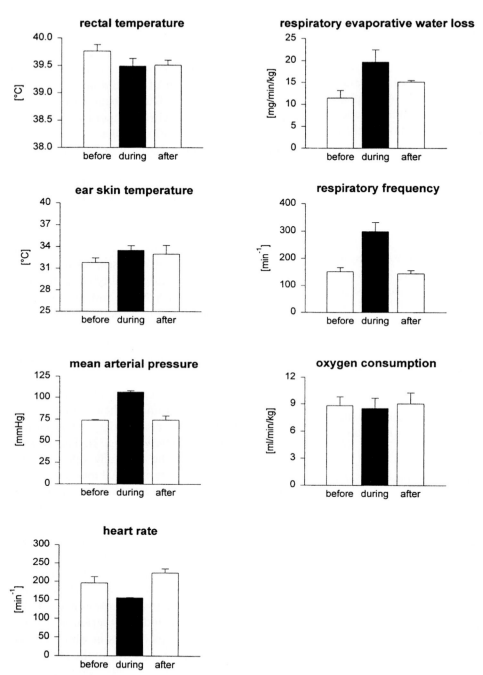

Fig. 2. Modulatory role of the NO-donor SIN-1 applied into the 3rd cerebral ventricle for 20 min at a dose of 2 μg/min/kg and at a rate of 2 μl/min to conscious rabbits exposed to 24°C environmental temperature. Shown are the peak effects with the S.E.M. of the respective responses of three animals (from pilot experiments of Eriksson et al., 1997).

formation removed a messenger suppressing metabolic heat production. In line with this observation, both the acute hyperthermic effect induced by lateral hypothalamic lesioning and the associated increase in activity of sympathetic innervation of the BAT, were attenuated or abolished, when L-arginine and SNP were i.c.v. injected as NO-donors (Monda et al., 1995a).

Role of NO in fever

Fever is the normal reaction of homeothermic animals to the intrusion of a multitude of agents which are recognized as alien by elements of the RES. As a model compound in experimental fever, LPS, after entering the extracellular space, activates a multitude of reticulo-endothelial system responses. It rapidly activates in mobile or sessile macrophages the membrane-bound respiratory burst (NADPH) oxidase, which causes, within minutes, the release of free oxygen radicals (Badwey and Karnovsky, 1980; Rossi, 1986; Segal, 1989; Thelen et al., 1993). A similar fast response of the reticulo-endothelial system to LPS is the release of cytokines, of which tumor necrosis factor α (TNFα), interleukin-1 (IL-1), interleukin-6 (IL-6), and interferon γ (IFNγ) have been considered as the putative endogenous mediators of fever (Dinarello et al., 1986; Blatteis, 1990; Kluger, 1991). Binding of LPS to the endothelium stimulates arachidonic acid metabolism with the synthesis of vasodilatory acting prostaglandin E_2 (PGE$_2$) and prostacyclin as the primary eicosanoids formed (Renzi and Flynn, 1992). Traditionally, PGE$_2$ is believed to act centrally as the obligatory mediator of fever (Dinarello et al., 1988; Coceani, 1991; Rothwell, 1992).

That NO might play a role in fever is an intriguing assumption. The presence of nitroxidergic neurons and nerve fibres in circumventricular organs, where a blood–brain barrier is missing, suggests the possibility that exogenous pyrogens, cytokines and prostaglandins may interact with nitroxidergic neurons, especially in the organum vasculosum laminae terminalis (OVLT) as the most important blood-to-brain interface in the generation of fever (Blatteis, 1992). In addition, enhanced NO synthesis following the induction of iNOS, especially by the endogenous pyrogens, the cytokines IL-1, TNFα and IFNγ may be important for host-defence activities (Nathan, 1992). The contribution of NO in the fever pathway is, however, complicated, as NO mutually interacts with, and inactivates, superoxide anions (McCall et al., 1989). On the other hand, NO produced by cNOS has been shown by Salvemini et al. (1994) to stimulate directly PGE$_2$ synthesis via constitutive cyclooxygenase (COX-1), while iNOS augments PGE$_2$ production via activation of inducible cyclooxygenase (COX-2). Oxygen radicals, particularly superoxide anions, have been determined by Feng et al. (1995) to be potent inducers of COX-2. Thus, NO acts, on the one hand, as a stimulator of PGE$_2$ synthesis and, as a free radical scavenger, inhibits PGE$_2$ synthesis on the other. In other words, fever depends both on the activity of the respiratory burst (NADPH) oxidase and on the time course of NO production, complicating thereby the evaluation of its specific contribution (Nathan, 1992; Rand and Li, 1995b).

It is, therefore, not surprising that reports on effects of NO on prostaglandin-induced hyperthermia or febrile reactions show a great variability. In urethane-anesthetized rats, the temperature rise in the BAT as an indicator for NST and the hyperthermic reaction following i.c.v. injection of PGE$_2$, the presumed central mediator of fever, were attenuated by co-injection of the NOS-inhibitor L-NMMA, suggesting an enhancing role of NO on PGE-induced heat generation (Amir et al., 1991). Conversely, also in urethane-anesthetized rats, prostaglandin E_1 (PGE$_1$) applied i.c.v. induced a hyperthermic response, a rise in BAT temperature and enhanced activity in sympathetic filaments innervating BAT, but all these responses were reduced when L-arginine was co-injected with PGE$_1$ (Monda et al., 1995b). The proper interpretation of these seemingly divergent results is, however, only possible in connection with details of the actual activity of NOS

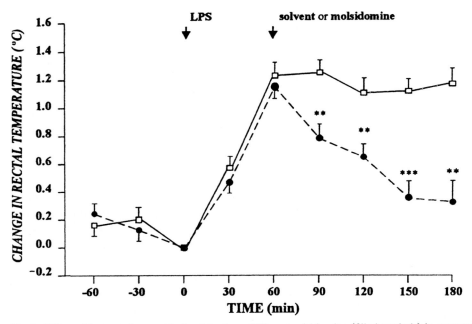

Fig. 3. Effect of intracerebroventricular injection of 75 μg molsidomine (filled symbols) in comparison to controls (open symbols) on febrile response induced by intravenous injection of 0.5 μg/kg *S. typhosa* lipopolysaccharide (LPS) in rabbits. **, *** ($P < 0.01$, $P < 0.001$) denotes significant differences from control (from Gourine, 1995, reprinted with kind permission of Elsevier Science Inc., New York, USA).

and the knowledge of possible side effects of the pharmacological tools by which it is manipulated.

More conclusive results suggesting an endogenous antipyretic role for NO were provided by Gourine (1995). Intravenous (i.v.) application of the NO-donor molsidomine 60 min after LPS-induced fever in rabbits caused an immediate fall of core temperature, which was, as to be expected, mainly elicited by peripheral vasodilatation. Interestingly, the i.c.v. application of molsidomine 60 min after i.v. injection of LPS (Fig. 3) was immediately followed by cutaneous vasodilatation associated with a fall of core temperature. This finding suggests that within the first hours following LPS NO is not produced, apparently by inhibition of cNOS as shown by MacNaul and Hutchinson (1993). On the other hand, if iNOS is activated, as known to occur in pyrogenic tolerance, then i.c.v. application of L-NNA, an inhibitor of NOS, augments fever (Gourine, 1995).

These findings provide evidence that NO acts centrally as an antipyretic.

Similar conclusions on an antipyretic role of NO in fever can be drawn from experiments in rabbits where the time course of NO production following i.v. injection of LPS and IL-1β was evaluated by measuring plasma nitrate levels, and the level of oxygen radical formation by estimating malondialdehyde (MDA) as the peroxidative reaction product of lipids with oxygen radicals (Das and Engelman, 1990), together with PGE$_2$ and prostaglandin F$_{2\alpha}$ (PGF$_{2\alpha}$), and TNFα. As shown in Fig. 4, LPS caused a fever associated with an increase of MDA, a rise of TNFα, and a fall of plasma nitrate, which confirms that cNOS is acutely inhibited by LPS. Plasma PGF$_{2\alpha}$ and PGE$_2$ levels increased about fourfold. Compared with the LPS effects on core temperature, MDA, PGF$_{2\alpha}$, PGE$_2$ and nitrate, no statistically significant difference was found when IL-1β was

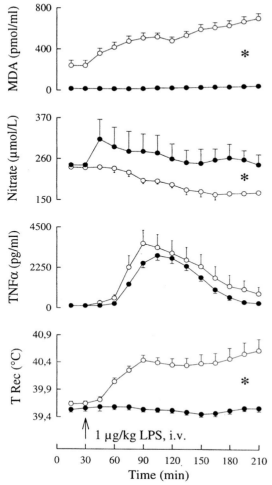

Fig. 4. Abolition of fever induced by i.v. lipopolysaccharide (LPS) injection (1 μg/kg) in rabbits treated with a continuous i.v. infusion of 5 mg/kg/h methylene blue starting 30–45 min prior to LPS injection (closed symbols) in comparison to controls receiving only LPS (open symbols): time courses of core temperatures (T_{Rec}), plasma TNFα, nitrate and malondialdehyde (MDA). Values are means ± S.E. (n = 10); significant differences in the time courses between control and treated animals (modified from Weihrauch and Riedel, 1997, reprinted with kind permission of the New York Academy of Science, USA).

administered, except that no detectable increase of TNFα occurred within 3 h (Weihrauch and Riedel, 1997).

Pretreatment of the rabbits with methylene blue

totally prevented LPS or IL-1β fever without altering TNFα and PGE_2 secretion (Fig. 4). Methylene blue, which has been shown to prevent superoxide anion generation (Keaney et al., 1994), lowered MDA levels and LPS and IL-1β caused a rise of nitrate under these experimental conditions. It seems, therefore, that the combination of increased free oxygen radical formation and a reduced synthesis of NO following exposure of the reticulo-endothelial system to LPS and IL-1β is associated with fever. Elevated plasma levels of PGE_2 and $PGF_{2\alpha}$ of normal and methylene blue-treated rabbits indicate that LPS and IL-1β stimulate the synthesis of these cyclooxygenase products independently from the development of fever, and, secondly, that methylene blue exerts its antipyretic action not by inhibition of cyclooxygenase activity as shown for aspirin (Milton, 1982). Even more interesting is the finding that an elevation of NO, as indicated by rising nitrate levels, was associated with the abolition of prostaglandin pyrogenicity. The same assumption can be made for the effects of a second dose of LPS in pyrogenic tolerant rabbits. At elevated PGE_2 levels, antipyresis with cutaneous vasodilatation and panting, starts only when plasma nitrate levels rise (Weihrauch and Riedel, 1997). Taking all these data, then one could conclude that PGE_2 and NO interact with each other in stimulating or inhibiting, at the central level, the action of the final, still unknown endogenous pyrogenic mechanism.

It is conceivable that the reported plasma levels of prostaglandins also mirror, in a way, the time course of PG synthesis at the central level, as can be deduced from similar PGE values obtained from third ventricle of rabbits (Philipp-Dormston and Siegert, 1974; Bernheim et al., 1980) following LPS. This allows the conclusion that in the experiments of Gourine (1995) the i.c.v. released NO did not alter cyclooxygenase activity but interacted rather with PGE_2 in altering its pyrogenicity, corroborating the results of Monda et al. (1995b).

NO has been implicated as a principal mediator of catecholamine-resistant vasodilation in septic shock. Among the cytokines, only TNFα has been found to be positively correlated with plasma nitrite/nitrate levels, conforming to its known effect on inducing iNOS (Barthlen et al., 1994). These authors also found a significant negative correlation of body temperature with plasma nitrate in 84 patients, that is, the patients with the highest fever apparently exhibited a reduced capability of NO synthesis. This observation corresponds to the inverse relationship between body temperature and plasma nitrate observed during LPS fever and would be in line with an antipyretic action of NO. Whether this correlation reflects a cause-and-effect relationship due to a peripheral or central action of NO has to be further elucidated.

Neurobiological aspects of NO as a putative central messenger in thermoregulation

In temperature regulation, the preoptic and anterior hypothalamus (PO/AH) represent the highest level of integration in the control of mechanisms by which heat is dissipated or conserved, or extra heat is generated, with the aim to maintain a constant deep body temperature. In addition, hypothalamic as well as spinal structures contribute importantly as thermosensors to mammalian and avian temperature regulation (Simon et al., 1986). The thermoregulatory functions of the hypothalamus cannot be associated with particular hypothalamic nuclei, but rather seem to be accomplished by neuronal networks that have remained ill-defined despite numerous efforts to attribute certain functions to particular types of hypothalamic neurons (Boulant, 1996; Simon et al., 1997, this volume). Further, no transmitter/receptor systems are known for which thermoregulatory specificity could be claimed. In this respect the thermoregulatory system differs fundamentally from phylogenetically older, hypothalamic control systems in which defined functions can be attributed to particular nuclei and circumventricular structures which are, moreover, identifiable by demonstrating the presence of neuropeptides and of peptide receptors, respec-

tively, with well-established specific regulatory functions. Examples for the involvement of nitroxidergic neurons in structurally well-defined hypothalamic control systems are salt and fluid balance (Arévalo et al., 1992; Pow, 1992; Vincent and Kimura, 1992; Jurzak et al., 1994) and gonadotropin regulation (Bhat et al., 1995). The information about the distribution of nitroxidergic neurons obtained in these studies cannot be directly related to the hypothalamic thermoregulatory control system as a more or less diffuse neuronal network. However, they also do not exclude the relevance of nitroxidergic neurons in temperature regulation, at least, with respect to the multiple interactions known to exist between thermoregulation and body fluid control (Mack and Nadel, 1996).

Effects of systemic NO-donors on central thermosensitive neurons

With respect to NO acting from the systemic circulation, evidence for a modulatory action on central nervous thermosensitivity has remained indirect, so far. When recording single unit activity in the PO/AH region of rats, Koga et al. (1987) found that i.v. infusion of 1–5 μg SNP activated 53% of the warm-sensitive neurons and inhibited 46% of the cold-sensitive units; however, these neuronal responses were apparently caused by the SNP-induced decrease in blood pressure (5–30 mmHg), because the same effects could be observed when similar degrees of arterial hypotension were induced by withdrawing 0.5–3 ml of blood. Although this result does not assign peripheral NO a specific role as a modulator of thermosensitivity, it suggests a particular mode by which application of NO-donors might indirectly affect temperature regulation, besides their well described peripheral vasodilatory effect (Ignarro et al., 1987; Gerstberger et al., 1994; Gagalo et al., 1995). In line with this assumption, Koga et al. (1987) deduced from their observation that arterial hypotension might favor a hypothermic response, e.g. by inhibiting shivering (Ishii and Ishii, 1960; Brendel, 1962; Hori et al.,

1987). On the other hand, a biochemical study using cGMP immunohistochemistry suggested that peripheral application of SNP might also affect certain neurons by direct NO actions, because perfusion of SNP (30–40 ml/min, 10 μmol for 15 min) caused an increase in cGMP levels in regions located outside the blood–brain barrier (Berkelmans et al., 1989).

Histological demonstration of NOS in the spinal cord and PO / AH

According to histological studies, neuronal somata containing NOS seem to be scarce in the PO/AH itself, but NADPH-diaphorase positive neurons scattered along the wall of the third ventricle and NOS containing fibers can readily be observed throughout this region (Vincent and Kimura, 1992; Schmid et al., unpublished data). Within the spinal cord, as a second central nervous region of thermoregulatory relevance, large amounts of NOS containing cell bodies and nerve terminals have been reported in laminae I + II and X of the dorsal horn using NOS-immunohistochemistry (Dun et al., 1992; Valtschanoff et al., 1992b; Wu et al., 1994; Bernardi et al., 1995) and NADPH-diaphorase techniques (Anderson, 1992; Valtschanoff et al., 1992a; Simon et al., 1997, this volume). Another region with strong NADPH-diaphorase staining is the intermediolateral cell column (IML) at the thoracal level of the rat spinal cord, where preganglionic sympathetic neurons are primarily located (Valtschanoff et al., 1992a). The specificity of the NADPH-diaphorase technique to label NO synthesizing neurons was demonstrated by Wu et al. (1994) and Anderson (1992), showing that immunoreactive NOS, NADPH diaphorase and neuronal NOS messenger RNA (using in situ hybridization) were colocalized in rat spinal cord neurons. Neurons which respond to NO are presumably not identical with the neurons which contain NOS, but should be located in close proximity, as suggested by the short half-life of NO ($\approx$ 5 s) in oxygen containing solutions (Garthwaite and Boulton, 1995). The exclusive occurrence of NOS containing and NO

responsive neurons must be concluded from biochemical experiments which showed that the formation of NO from L-arginine requires Ca^{2+}, due to the known Ca^{2+} (Garthwaite, 1991) and calmodulin dependence (Bredt and Snyder, 1990) of neuronal NOS. Because the half-maximal stimulation of NOS is achieved at about 160 nM Ca^{2+} and the soluble guanylate cyclase, as the prime target for NO, is half-maximally inhibited by 120 nM Ca^{2+}, it has been regarded unlikely that the same cells which produce NO should also respond to it with an elevation of cGMP (Knowles et al., 1989; Vincent and Hope, 1992; Schmidt et al., 1993; Garthwaite and Boulton, 1995).

Electrophysiological studies on the effect of NO on neurons in the spinal cord and PO / AH

According to classical concepts of thermoregulation (Hammel, 1968; Bligh, 1972; Simon, 1974) the activation or inhibition of heat loss and heat gain mechanisms, which ultimately result in a change in body temperature, are caused by the stimulation or inhibition of thermosensitive elements, located in thermophysiologically relevant regions of the CNS. Thus, a specific involvement of NO in thermoregulation might be derived from investigating direct effects of NO on the activity and temperature sensitivity of neurons located in the PO/AH and/or the spinal cord, because for these two CNS regions the thermophysiological relevance has been clearly demonstrated in vivo (Hammel, 1968; Simon, 1974; Boulant and Dean, 1986; Simon et al., 1986). Due to the fact that specific criteria are still missing to classify PO/AH neurons and spinal cord neurons as being specifically involved in temperature regulation (Simon et al., 1997, this volume) and in view of recent evidence showing that the temperature sensitivity of neurons is not an unchangeable property, but one that can be induced or diminished by neurotransmitters (Yakimova et al., 1996), neuropeptides (Schmid et al., 1993), prostaglandins (Kulchitsky et al., 1994), or by changing the extracellular calcium concentration (Schmid and

Pierau, 1993), the effect of NO on temperature sensitive as well as temperature insensitive neurons has to be taken into consideration when determining a possible specific involvement of NO in temperature regulation at the cellular level.

A detailed investigation of the NO effects on thermosensitive neurons in vitro has so far only been carried out in the spinal cord by recording extracellularly from neurons in a slice preparation (Pehl et al., 1994a; Schmid et al., 1994). In these studies, no correlation could be found between the thermosensitivity of spontaneously active spinal cord neurons and their reactivity to NO (Table 1). As summarized in Table 1, superfusion with SNP excited the majority (96%; $n = 72$) of SNP-responsive neurons in lamina X (i.e. the area around the central canal), but inhibitions prevailed (67%; $n = 88$) among the SNP-responsive neurons of laminae I + II (i.e. the superficial dorsal horn, an area where peripheral thermoreceptors terminate). The inhibitory as well as the excitatory effect of SNP could be mimicked by other NO-donors (SIN-1 and SNAP), both effects were dose-dependent, with a threshold concentration of 10^{-6} M SNP and could be mimicked by application of 8Br-cGMP, the membrane permeable analog of cGMP which has been identified as the second messenger for NO in many neuronal and non-neuronal systems (Schmidt et al., 1993; Lipton et al., 1994; Garthwaite and Boulton, 1995). The NO induced excitations as well as the

inhibitions persisted in an extracellular recording solution containing 0.3 mM Ca^{2+} and 9.0 mM Mg^{2+}, known to block synaptic transmission. These experiments exclude the possibility that either of the two responses is due to an effect on inhibitory interneurons and furthermore suggest that the NO-mediated changes in firing rate (FR) are caused by a direct action on the responsive neurons rather than a modulatory effect of NO on synaptic transmission (Pehl and Schmid, 1997). Even under our in vitro slice conditions, endogenous NOS produced sufficient amounts of NO to cause a reduction of the spontaneous activity of those neurons which could be inhibited by SNP, because application of the NOS inhibitor L-NMMA was able to increase the activity of these cells and this effect could be reversed by L-arginine, the natural substrate of the NOS. Furthermore, it could be demonstrated that the temperature coefficient (TC) of those spinal cord neurons which were inhibited by SNP or L-arginine decreased (Fig. 5), while the TC of those neurons which were excited by SNP increased (Fig. 6). Again, this effect was equally observed on temperature sensitive as well as on insensitive neurons (Schmid and Pehl, 1996). The effect of the NO-donor or the NOS blocker on the TC of neurons could result in a loss of thermosensitivity of formerly warm sensitive neurons (in case of an inhibitory effect on the FR) or it could convert formerly temperature insensitive neurons into

TABLE 1

Response of neurons to SNP

	Response to SNP									Total
	Warm sensitive			Cold sensitive			Temperature sensitive			
	Excited	Inhibited	No	Excited	Inhibited	No	Excited	Inhibited	No	
Laminae I + II	24	31	16	1		1	4	28	8	113
Lamina X	56	2	2	1	1	1	12		1	76
PO/AH		7						10		17

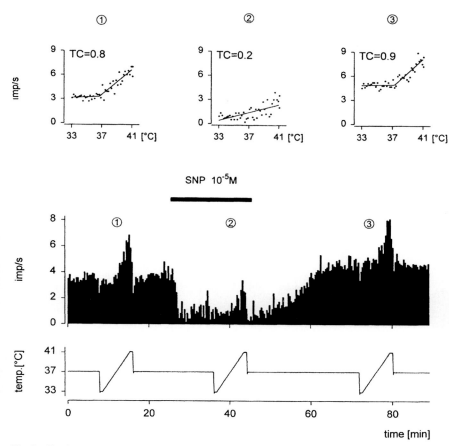

Fig. 5. Continuous rate meter recording of a spontaneously active neuron from lamina II of a rat spinal cord slice. Superfusion with SNP (10^{-5} M) results in a reversible inhibition of the activity. Determination of the temperature coefficient (TC) before (1), during (2) and after (3) superfusion with SNP shows that this warm-sensitive neuron reversibly lost its temperature sensitivity during superfusion with the NO-donor.

warm-sensitive ones (in case of an excitatory effect on the FR), thus confirming the statement (Schmid et al., 1993) that the temperature sensitivity of neurons is not an immutable property of neurons, but can be induced or converted by factors in the extracellular environment.

With regard to the effects of NO on PO/AH neurons, only two preliminary investigations have been conducted so far (Gourine et al., 1995; Schmid, unpublished data). In the study of Gourine et al. (1995), i.c.v. application of the NO-donors molsidomine and isosorbiddinitrat

(ISDN) and the NOS blocker L-NMMA caused excitatory and inhibitory effects on PO/AH neurons with the same frequency, although the small number of neurons studied (2–5 neurons in each category) may still preclude a predominant effect of NO on a certain group of neurons, of which the temperature sensitivity was not determined in this study. Two neurons which were inhibited by the NO-donor were excited by subsequent application of interleukin 1β (IL-1β) and one neuron which was excited by NO could be inhibited by IL-1β. The authors conclude that this antagonis-

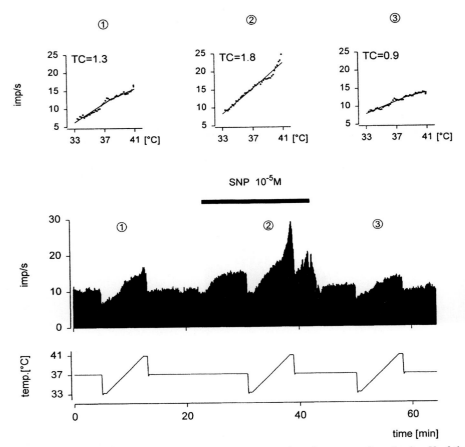

Fig. 6. Continuous rate meter recording of a spontaneously active neuron from lamina X of the rat spinal cord. Superfusion with SNP (10^{-5} M) results in a reversible excitation of the activity. Determination of the temperature coefficient (TC) before (1), during (2) and after (3) superfusion with SNP shows that this warm-sensitive neuron strongly increased its temperature sensitivity during superfusion with the NO-donor.

tic effect of NO and IL-1β might represent the cellular basis for the antipyretic effect of NO on endotoxin-induced fever (Gourine et al., 1995).

In a preliminary study on PO/AH slices (Schmid, unpublished data) 17 out of 17 PO/AH neurons recorded under identical conditions as described before for spinal cord slices (Pehl et al., 1994a; Schmid et al., 1994) were reversibly inhibited by superfusion with SNP (10^{-5}–10^{-4} M). Application of SNP (10^{-4} M; 3 ml; 2 min) reduced the spontaneous activity for 6–25 min by $73 \pm 2\%$ ($n = 12$) compared to the respective baseline, eight neurons ceased firing completely

for 5–18 min. Seven neurons were warm-sensitive and 10 were temperature insensitive according to their TC > or < 0.6 imp/s/°C (Table 1). The inhibitory effects of SNP (Fig. 7) could be mimicked by superfusion with another NO-donor (SIN-1, 10^{-4} M) on a neuron which was inhibited previously by SNP and by application of the membrane permeable 8Br-cGMP in both neurons tested. In contrast, SNP had no effect on the activity of neurons ($n = 5$) in the area of the nucleus of the vertical limb of the diagonal band of Broca (Paxinos and Watson, 1986), located 100–500 μm rostrally to the PO/AH, thus underlining the specificity of the observed effect of SNP on PO/AH neurons.

In summary, the available electrophysiological data on slices suggest an exclusively (in case of the PO/AH) or predominantly (in case of the laminae I + II of the spinal cord) inhibitory effect of NO on spontaneously active neurons in both regions of the CNS that are relevant in temperature regulation, without showing a correlation with the thermosensitivity of the investigated neurons. While these two regions belong to

an afferent, sensory pathway in thermoregulation, many neurons in lamina X of the lumbar spinal cord are known to belong to the central autonomic nucleus (Hancock and Peveto, 1979; Strack et al., 1988) and might thus serve efferent sympathetic functions, where NO has been shown to play a major role in ongoing electrical activity (Hakim et al., 1995). Assuming a similar function for neurons in the intermediolateral nucleus (IML) and in the central autonomic nucleus, the primarily excitatory effect of NO on neurons in

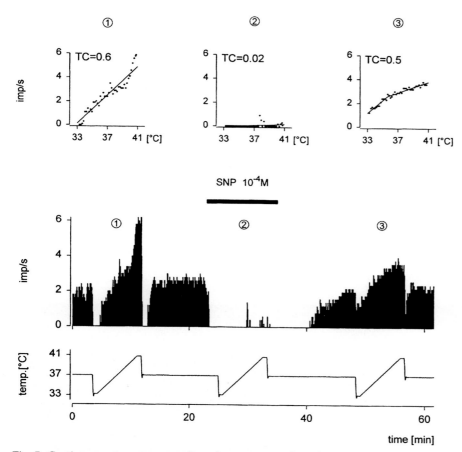

Fig. 7. Continuous rate meter recording of a spontaneously active neuron from the PO/AH. Superfusion with SNP (10^{-4} M) results in a reversible inhibition of the activity. Determination of the temperature coefficient (TC) before (1), during (2) and after (3) superfusion with SNP shows that this warm-sensitive neuron reversibly lost its temperature sensitivity during superfusion with the NO-donor.

lamina X is in line with a predominantly excitatory effect of intrathecally applied NO on IML neurons as observed by Hakim et al. (1995) monitoring renal sympathetic nerve activity. Thus in terms of thermoregulatory function, the release of NO in the spinal cord should facilitate sympathetic effector mechanisms, while it should exert primarily inhibitory effects on thermosensory afferent signals.

NO-dependent rise in cGMP concentration in the PO / AH and spinal cord

As already mentioned, many of the NO-mediated effects are due to the activation of the guanylate cyclase resulting in an elevated level of cGMP in the responsive cells (Schmidt et al., 1993; Garthwaite and Boulton, 1995). Using an antibody which had been designed to directly stain cGMP (De Vente et al., 1987, 1989; De Vente and Steinbusch, 1992), we could show that the level of cGMP strongly increased in discrete areas in 500-μm thick slices of the spinal cord and in the PO/AH after incubation with an NO-donor. Fig. 8 shows a representative section of the lumbar region of the rat spinal cord, which had been incubated in vitro for 10 min in 10^{-4} M SNP

under otherwise identical conditions as described for slices used for electrophysiological recordings from spinal cord neurons in vitro (Pehl et al., 1994b; Schmid and Pehl, 1996). Fig. 9 shows a representative section of the PO/AH at the level of the anterior commissure taken from a 500-μm thick slice of the rat hypothalamus after incubating the slice in SNAP (10^{-4} M). Qualitatively similar results could be obtained when incubating the slices in SNP or SIN-1 for the same time and at equimolar doses, although the intensity of the staining was consistently lower with SIN-1 compared with the other two NO-donors. Taking the results of the electrophysiological and immunocytochemical experiments together, these data suggest that the excitatory as well as the inhibitory effect of NO observed in the spinal cord and the inhibitory effect of NO observed in the PO/AH may be mediated by a NO dependent rise in cGMP.

Apart from the physiological implications, a more general conclusion from these data is that a biochemically detected rise in intracellular cGMP does not allow any predictions as to whether a neurotransmitter or neuromodulator like NO which stimulates guanylate cyclase has an excitatory or inhibitory effect on the FR of neurons in different regions of the spinal cord.

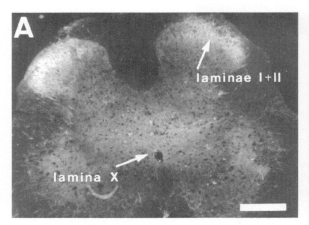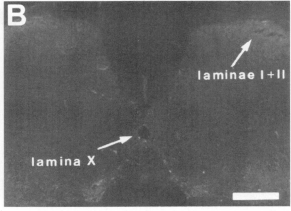

Fig. 8. Immunohistochemical demonstration of cGMP in a section of the lumbar rat spinal cord. (A) After incubation of the spinal cord slice for 10 min in SNP (10^{-4} M). (B) Control section without SNP. Bar = 200 μm.

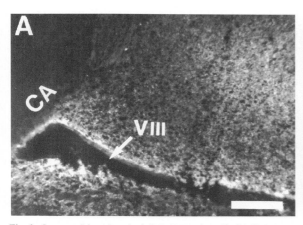 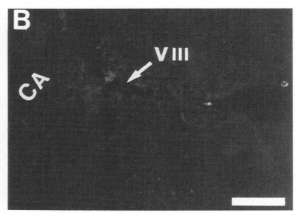

Fig. 9. Immunohistochemical demonstration of cGMP in a section of the PO/AH at the level of the anterior commissure (CA). (A) After incubation of the PO/AH slice for 10 min in SNAP (10^{-4} M). (B) Control section without SNAP. VIII marks the 3rd ventricle. Bar = 200 μm.

Possible transduction mechanisms of NO

Only relatively few studies have characterized direct effects of NO on the electrical activity of neurons with a similar approach to that which we have used in our investigations on slices from the spinal cord and from the PO/AH. In these studies, which had not been conducted to clarify possible thermoregulatory functions of NO, purely or predominantly excitatory effects of NO-donors or the natural substrate for NOS, L-arginine, were described for neurons of the rat dorsal motor nucleus of the vagus (Travagli and Gillis, 1994) and for neurons of the nucleus tractus solitarius (Tagawa et al., 1994; Ma et al., 1995). Purely inhibitory effects of NO-donors were described in spontaneously active subfornical organ neurons (Schmid et al., 1995), and similarly, NOS-inhibitors increased the spontaneous activity in neurons of the carotid body (Prabhakar et al., 1993).

Numerous studies have characterized the effect of NO on synaptic transmission (Williams et al., 1993; Lin and Bennett, 1994; Zhuo et al., 1994; Garthwaite and Boulton, 1995; Sandor et al., 1995). Notably in phenomena such as long-term potentiation (LTP) or long-term depression (LTD), NO is thought to play a major role as a retrograde messenger from the postsynaptic neuron to the presynaptic terminal. A large body of electrophysiological evidence on slices (mainly from the hippocampus) exists showing that LTP could not be produced in the presence of NOS-inhibitors and this effect could be reversed by L-arginine. (Böhme et al., 1991; Haley et al., 1992; Schuman, 1995). Furthermore, LTP could not be evoked if the NO-scavenger hemoglobin was present in the extracellular medium of hippocampal slices or if NOS blockers were applied directly into the postsynaptic neurons (Schuman and Madison, 1991; O'Dell et al., 1991). A physiologically relevant involvement of NO in LTP has recently been questioned by the group of Bliss et al. (Bliss and Collingridge, 1993; Williams et al., 1993) by showing that NO-dependent LTP can only be evoked in slices from young animals and when the experiments were performed at room temperature; at higher, more physiological temperatures (29°C) the LTP was independent from NO. In slices from the cerebellum, NO has been shown to reduce excitatory synaptic potentials (EPSPs), an effect which may underlie phenomena like LTD (Crepel and Jaillard, 1990; Daniel et al., 1993).

In the retinal system, NO has been shown to

activate a cGMP-gated unspecific cation channel (Ahmad et al., 1994), which is similar to the well characterized cGMP-gated channel in retinal rod outer segments (Fesenko et al., 1985) and olfactory receptor cilia (Nakamura and Gold, 1987). Apart from a direct action of NO mediated through cGMP-gated channels, the NO/cGMP pathway has been shown to modulate other ionic conductances, possibly by phosphorylation or dephosphorylation of ion channels. In different neuronal tissues, cGMP dependent increases (Chen and Schofield, 1995) and decreases (Khurana and Bennett, 1993) of Ca^{2+} currents have been reported, as well as an activation (Robertson et al., 1993) and inhibition of Ca^{2+}-dependent K^+-currents (Cetiner and Bennett, 1993; Fagni et al., 1995).

Despite those cGMP mediated effects, recent studies suggest that NO can also exert direct effects on ion channels without requiring the involvement of cGMP. A recent single channel recording study on salamander olfactory neurons provided evidence that NO, in one of its redox states, can directly activate cyclic nucleotide gated channels in inside-out-patches (Broillet and Firestein, 1996). Activation of these channels in the intact cell would lead to an influx of Na^+ and Ca^{2+} ions which might ultimately result in membrane depolarization. In the study of Fagni et al. (1995) NO has been shown to cause a direct inhibitory effect on the NMDA receptor, probably by interacting with divalent cations in the channel pore and thus causing an inhibition of excitatory synaptic transmission.

In summary, these electrophysiological studies provide evidence that NO can exert both excitatory and inhibitory effects on neuronal activity as well as on synaptic transmission, mainly by cGMP-dependent but also by cGMP-independent mechanisms in different regions of the CNS. The diversity of NO evoked neuronal responses precludes a generalization of the NO action in the CNS and suggests different transduction mechanisms for the observed effects. Although extracel-

lular recordings, as conducted in the PO/AH and in the spinal cord, can never provide direct information about the cellular mechanisms by which NO could alter the firing rate of neurons, our data suggest that NO exerts a primarily inhibitory action on thermosensitive- as well as thermoinsensitive-neurons, located in thermoregulatory relevant areas of the CNS, via a cGMP-mediated action.

Concluding remarks

As an ubiquitous systemic mediator, NO has been shown to facilitate thermolytic mechanisms, mainly due to its circulatory action. At the current and probably still early state of knowledge, it does not seem to affect the multitude of thermoregulatory effectors in a manner coordinated sufficiently to attribute a specific messenger function in the control of body temperature. On the other hand, a consistent inverse relationship seems to exist between body temperature and systemic NO action in fever. At the central level, in vivo experiments have suggested a more coordinated function for NO as a thermolytic mediator in thermoregulation and fever. Generally, the distribution of NO producing and NO responsive neurons in central nervous regions of thermoregulatory relevance, like the PO/AH and the spinal cord, suggests the involvement of NO in temperature signal transmission. However, the observed inhibitory effect of NO on the majority of neurons in the PO/AH and spinal laminae I + II is presently at variance with the prevailing thermolytic effects of central NO observed in the in vivo experiments, if one follows the assumption that activity changes of thermosensitive neurons consequently mean equidirectional changes in thermosensory input. Due to the fact that NO generating and NO responsive neurons are present almost ubiquitously in the CNS, more detailed investigations with a higher spatial resolution than i.c.v. applications are needed (e.g. microapplication of NO-donors or NOS-inhibitors directly into the PO/AH or the spinal cord, or measuring NO production in these areas) in order to attribute site-specific functions to central neurons susceptible to NO.

Addendum

Since the submission of this review early in 1996, the assessment of effects of NO-donors or of inhibitors of NO-synthase applied via different routes on thermoregulatory activities and on fever have considerably proceeded. These most recent studies have, so far, added to the impression that the role of NO, especially as a centrally acting mediator in temperature regulation, lacks general consistency. However, from a summary of the available data, as it is listed in Table 2, the impression may be gained that the site-specificity of NO actions as well as species differences may account for part of the observed diversity. For instance, the comparison of observations suggesting that NO actions at a receptive brain site, the OVLT, were hyperthermic or hyperpyretic (Lin and Lin, 1996), whereas its actions following applications into the 3rd cerebral ventricle, i.e. close to thermointegrative structures, rather were hypothermic and antipyretic (Eriksson et al., 1997; Gourine, 1995), suggests the working hypothesis that receptive and integrative functions may be oppositely influenced by NO. A hyperthermic NO action at thermoreceptive sites would be in line with the electrophysiological data according to which neurons in the superficial dorsal horn, where spinal warm signals are assumed to originate (Table 1), as well as neurons in the POAH region, where hypothalamic warm signals are generated (Schmid, unpublished), were predominantly inhibited by NO. Accordingly, the new data seem to endorse those concluding remarks which expect the elucidation of the site-specificity of NO actions in the thermoregulatory system from studies aiming at a higher degree of spatial resolution of local NO effects within the brain.

TABLE 2

Sites of application of NO-donors or of inhibitors of NOS in different species, where they affected body temperature or single thermoregulatory effectors in ways indicating either a hypothermic or a hyperthermic NO action

Animal species	Site of application	Mode of NO-action	References
A: effects on normal temperature regulation			
Rat	POAH	(−)	Amir et al., 1991
Rat	i.p.	hyper	De Luca et al., 1995
Rat	i.c.v.	hypo	De Luca et al., 1995
Rat	i.v.	hyper	Scammell et al., 1996
Rabbit	i.v.	hypo	Farrell and Bishop, 1995
Rabbit	OVLT	hyper	Lin and Lin, 1996
Rabbit	i.v.	hypo	Mathai et al., 1997
Rabbit	i.c.v.	hypo	Eriksson et al., 1997
Horse	i.v.	hypo	Mills et al., 1997
B: effects on fever (induced by LPS, IL-1 or PGE)			
Rat	POAH	hyper	Amir et al., 1991
Rat	i.p.	hyper	Reimers et al., 1994
Rat	i.c.v.	hypo	Monda et al., 1995b
Rat	i.v.	hyper	Scammell et al., 1996
Rabbit	i.c.v.	(−)	Kapas et al., 1994
Rabbit	i.v.	hypo	Gagalo et al., 1995
Rabbit	i.c.v.	hypo	Gourine, 1995
Rabbit	OVLT	hyper	Lin and Lin, 1996
Cat	i.v./i.c.v.	(−)	Redford et al., 1995

Explanations: hypo: presumed hypothermic, thermolytic, antipyretic action; hyper: presumed hyperthermic, thermogenic, pyretic action; (−): no effect. Sites of application: i.v. intravenous, i.p. intraperitoneal, i.c.v. intracerebroventricular (3rd or lateral ventricle), OVLT organum vasculosum laminae terminalis, POAH preoptic and anterior hypothalamic region. Pyrogenic agents: LPS lipopolysaccharide, IL-1 interleukin 1, PGE prostaglandin E.

Acknowledgments

The authors thank Dr J. De Vente for the cGMP antibody used in this study. The research of E. Simon and H.A. Schmid was supported by DFG grants (Si 230/8-1 and 2).

References

Ahmad, I., Leinders-Zufall, T., Kocsis, J.D., Shepherd, G.M., Zufall, F. and Barnstable, C.J. (1994) Retinal ganglion cells express a cGMP-gated cation conductance activable by nitric oxide donors. *Neuron*, 12: 155–165.

Amir, S., De Blasio, E. and English, A.M. (1991) N^G-Monomethyl-L-arginine co-injection attenuates the thermogenic and hyperthermic effects of E_2 prostaglandin microinjections into the anterior hypothalamic preoptic area in rats. *Brain Res.*, 556: 157–160.

Anderson, C.R. (1992) NADPH diaphorase-positive neurons in the rat spinal cord include a subpopulation of autonomic preganglionic neurons. *Neurosci. Lett.*, 139: 280–284.

Archer, S. (1993) Measurement of nitric oxide in biological models. *FASEB J.*, 7: 349–360.

Arévalo, R., Sanchez, F., Alonso, J.R., Carretero, J., Vásquez, R. and Aijón, J. (1992) NADPH-diaphorase activity in the hypothalamic magnocellular neurosecretory nuclei. *Brain Res. Bull.*, 28: 599–603.

Badwey, J.A. and Karnovsky, M.L. (1980) Active oxygen species and the functions of phagocytic leukocytes. *Annu. Rev. Biochem.*, 49: 695–726.

Barthlen, W., Stadler, J., Lehn, N.L., Miethke, T., Bartels, H. and Siewert, J.R. (1994) Serum levels of end products of nitric oxide synthesis correlate positively with tumor necrosis factor α and negatively with body temperature in patients with postoperative abdominal sepsis. *Shock*, 2: 398–401.

Bernardi, P.S., Valtschanoff, J.G., Weinberg, R.J., Schmidt, H.H.H.W. and Rustioni, A. (1995) Synaptic-interactions between primary afferent terminals and gaba and nitric oxide-synthesizing neurons in superficial laminae of the rat spinal-cord. *J. Neurosci.*, 15: 1363–1371.

Bernheim, H.A., Gilbert, T.M. and Stitt, J.T. (1980) Prostaglandin E levels in third ventricular cerebrospinal fluid of rabbits during fever and changes in body temperature. *J. Physiol. (Lond.)*, 301: 69–78.

Berkelmans, H.S., Schipper, J., Hudson, L., Steinbusch, H.W.M. and De Vente, J. (1989) cGMP immunocytochemistry in aorta, kidney, retina and brain tissues of the rat after perfusion with nitroprusside. *Histochemistry*, 93: 143–148.

Bhat, G.K., Mahesh, V.B., Lamar, C.A., Ping, L., Aguan, K. and Brann, D.W. (1995) Histochemical localization of nitric-oxide neurons in the hypothalamus — association with gonadotropin releasing hormone neurons and colocalization with N-methyl-D-aspartate receptors. *Neuroendocrinology*, 62: 187–197.

Blatteis, C.M. (1990) Cytokines as endogenous pyrogens. In: A. Nowotny, J.J. Spitzer and E.J. Ziegler (Eds.), *Cellular and Molecular Aspects of Endotoxin Reactions*, Excerpta Medica, Amsterdam, pp. 447–454.

Blatteis, C.M. (1992) Role of the OVLT in the febrile response to circulating pyrogens. In: A. Ermisch, R. Landgraf and H.J. Rühle (Eds.), *Circumventricular Organs and Brain Fluid Environment. Progress in Brain Research*, Vol. 91, Elsevier, Amsterdam, pp. 409–412.

Bligh, J. (1972) Neuronal models of mammalian temperature regulation. In: J. Bligh and R. Moore (Eds.), *Essays on Temperature Regulation*, North-Holland, Amsterdam, pp. 105–120.

Bliss, T.V.P. and Collingridge, G.L. (1993) A synaptic model of memory: long-term potentiation in the hippocampus. *Nature*, 361: 31–39.

Böhme, G.A., Bon, C., Stutzmann, J.-M., Doble, A. and Blanchard, J.-C. (1991) Possible involvement of nitric oxide in long-term potentiation. *Eur. J. Pharmacol.*, 199: 379–381.

Boulant, J.A. (1996) Hypothalamic neurons regulating body temperature. In: M.J. Fregly and C.M. Blatteis (Eds.), *Handbook of Physiology, Section 4, Environmental Physiology*, Oxford University Press, Oxford, pp. 105–126.

Boulant, J.A. and Dean, J.B. (1986) Temperature receptors in the central nervous system. *Annu. Rev. Physiol.*, 48: 639–654.

Bredt, D.S. and Snyder, S.H. (1990). Isolation of nitric oxide synthetase, a calmodulin requiring enzyme. *Proc. Natl. Acad. Sci. USA*, 87: 682–685.

Brendel, W. (1962) Die Bedeutung der Hirntemperatur für die Kältegegenregulation: II. Der Einfluss der Hirntemperatur auf den respiratorischen Stoffwechsel des Hundes unter Kältebelastung. *Pflüg. Arch.*, 270: 628–647.

Broillet, M.-C. and Firestein, S. (1996) Direct activation of the olfactory cyclic nucleotide-gated channel through modification of sulfhydryl groups by NO compounds. *Neuron*, 16: 377–385.

Brüning, G., Funk, U. and Mayer, B. (1994) Immunocytochemical localization of nitric oxide synthase in the brain of the chicken. *NeuroReport*, 5: 2425–2428.

Cetiner, M. and Bennett, M.R. (1993) Nitric oxide modulation of calcium-activated potassium channels in postganglionic neurones of avian cultured ciliary ganglia. *Br. J. Pharmacol.*, 110: 995–1002.

Chen, C. and Schofield, G.G. (1995) Nitric oxide donors enhanced Ca^{2+} currents and blocked noradrenaline-induced Ca^{2+} current inhibition in rat sympathetic neurons. *J. Physiol. (Lond.)*, 482: 521–531.

Coceani, F. (1991) Prostaglandins and fever. Facts and controversies. In: P. Mackowiak (Ed.), *Fever: Basic Mechanisms and Management*, Raven Press, New York, pp. 59–70.

Crepel, F. and Jaillard, D. (1990) Protein kinases, nitric oxide and long-term depression of synapses in the cerebellum. *NeuroReport*, 1: 133–136.

Daniel, H., Hemart, N., Jaillard, D. and Crepel, F. (1993) Long-term depression requires nitric oxide and guanosine 3′-5′ cyclic monophosphate production in rat cerebellar Purkinje cells. *Eur. J. Neurosci.*, 5: 1079–1082.

Das, D.K. and Engelman, R.M. (1990) Mechanism of free radical generation during reperfusion of ischemic myocardium. In: D.K. Das and W.B. Essman (Eds.), *Oxygen Radicals: Systemic Events and Disease Processes*, Karger, Basel, pp. 97–128.

Dawson, T.M., Bredt, D.S., Fotuhi, M., Hwang, P.M. and Snyder, S.H. (1991) Nitric oxide synthase and neuronal NADPH diaphorase are identical in brain and peripheral tissues. *Proc. Natl. Acad. Sci. USA,* 88: 7797–7801.

De Luca, B., Monda, M. and Sullo, A. (1995) Changes in eating behavior and thermogenic activity following inhibition of nitric oxide formation. *Am. J. Physiol.,* 268: R1533–R1538.

De Vente, J. and Steinbusch, H.W. (1992) On the stimulation of soluble and particulate guanylate cyclase in the rat brain and the involvement of nitric oxide as studied by cGMP immunocytochemistry. *Acta Histochim.,* 92: 13–38.

De Vente, J., Steinbusch, H.W. and Schipper, J. (1987) A new approach to immunocytochemistry of 3′,5′-cyclic guanosine monophosphate: preparation, specificity, and initial application of a new antiserum against formaldehyde-fixed 3′,5′-cyclic guanosine monophosphate. *Neuroscience,* 22: 361–373.

De Vente, J., Schipper, J. and Steinbusch, H.W. (1989) Formaldehyde fixation of cGMP in distinct cellular pools and their recognition by different cGMP-antisera. An immunocytochemical study into the problem of serum specificity. *Histochemistry,* 91: 401–412.

Dietz, N.M., Rivera, J.M., Warner, D.O. and Joyner, M.J. (1994) Is nitric oxide involved in cutaneous vasodilatation during body heating in humans? *J. Appl. Physiol.,* 76: 2047–2053.

Dinarello, C.A., Cannon, J.G., Wolff, S.M., Bernheim, H.A., Beutler, B., Cerami, A., Figari, I.S., Palladino, M.A. and O'Connor, J.V. (1986) Tumor necrosis factor (Cachectin) is an endogenous pyrogen and induces production of interleukin 1. *J. Exp. Med.,* 163: 1433–1450.

Dinarello, C.S, Cannon, J.G. and Wolff, S.M. (1988) New concepts on the pathogenesis of fever. *Rev. Infect. Dis.,* 10: 168–189.

Dun, N.J., Dun, S.L., Förstermann, U. and Tseng, L.F. (1992) Nitric oxide synthase immunoreactivity in rat spinal cord. *Neurosci. Lett.,* 147: 217–220.

Eriksson, S., Hjelmqvist, H., Keil., R. and Gerstberger, R. (1997) Central application of a nitric oxide donor activates heat defense in rabbits. *Brain Res.* (in press).

Fagni, L., Olivier, M., Lafon-Cazal, M. and Bockaert, J. (1995) Involvement of divalent ions in the nitric oxide-induced blockade of *N*-methyl-D-aspartate receptors in cerebellar granule cells. *Mol. Pharmacol.,* 47: 1239–1247.

Farrell, D.M. and Bishop, V.S. (1995) Permissive role for nitric oxide in active thermoregulatory vasodilatation in rabbit ear. *Am. J. Physiol.,* 269: H1613–H1618.

Feng, L., Xia, Y., Garcia, G.E., Hwang, D. and Wilson, C.B. (1995) Involvement of reactive oxygen intermediates in cyclooxygenase-2 expression induced by interleukin-1, tumor necrosis factor-α, and lipopolysaccharide. *J. Clin. Invest.,* 95: 1669–1675.

Fesenko, E.E., Kolesnikov, S.S. and Lyubarsky, A.L. (1985) Direct action of cGMP on the conductance of retinal rod plasma membrane. *Biochim. Biophys. Acta,* 856: 661–671.

Furchgott, R.F. and Zawadzki, J.V. (1980) The obligatory role of endothelial cells in the relaxation of arterial smooth muscle by acetylcholine. *Nature,* 228: 373–376.

Gagalo, I.T., Hac, E.E., Matuszek, M.T., Rekowski, P., Kupryszewski, G. and Korolkiewicz, K.Z. (1995) Thermoregulatory activity of sodium nitroprusside and arginine vasopressin. *Gen. Pharmacol.,* 26: 393–397.

Garthwaite, J. (1991) Glutamate, nitric oxide and cell-cell signalling in the nervous system. *Trends Neurosci.,* 14: 60–67.

Garthwaite, J. and Boulton, C.L. (1995) Nitric oxide signalling in the central nervous system. *Annu. Rev. Physiol.,* 57: 683–706.

Garthwaite, J., Charles, S.L. and Chess-Williams, R. (1988) Endothelium-derived relaxing factor release on activation of NMDA receptors suggests role as intercellular messenger in the brain. *Nature,* 336: 385–388.

Gerstberger, R., Hjelmqvist, H. and Keil, R. (1994) Nitric oxide modulates thermoregulatory effector mechanisms in the conscious rabbit. In: E. Zeisberger, E. Schönbaum and P. Lomax (Eds.), *Thermal Balance in Health and Disease: Advances in Pharmacological Sciences*, Birkhäuser, Basel, pp. 485–490.

Gourine, A.V. (1994) Does central nitric oxide play a role in thermoregulation? In: E. Zeisberger, E. Schönbaum and P. Lomax (Eds.), *Thermal Balance in Health and Disease: Advances in Pharmacological Sciences*, Birkhäuser, Basel, pp. 491–495.

Gourine, A.V. (1995) Pharmacological evidence that nitric oxide can act as an endogenous antipyretic factor in endotoxin-induced fever in rabbits. *Gen. Pharmacol.,* 26: 835–841.

Gourine, A.V., Kulchitsky, V.A. and Gourine, V.N. (1995) Nitric oxide affects the activity of neurones in the preoptic/anterior hypothalamus of anaesthetized rats: interaction with the effects of centrally administered interleukin-1. *J. Physiol. (Lond.)* 483, 72P (Abstract).

Green, L.C., Ruiz de Luzuriaga, K., Wagner, D.A., Rand, W., Istfan, N., Young, V.R. and Tannenbaum, S.R. (1981a) Nitrate biosynthesis in man. *Proc. Natl. Acad. Sci. USA,* 78: 7764–7768.

Green, L.C., Tannenbaum, S.R. and Goldman, P. (1981b) Nitrate synthesis in the germfree and conventional rat. *Science,* 212: 56–58.

Gregor, M., Jänig, W. and Riedel, W. (1976) Response pattern of cutaneous postganglionic neurones to the hindlimb on spinal cord heating and cooling in the cat. *Pflüg. Arch.,* 363: 135–140.

Griffith, O.W. and Stuehr, D.J. (1995) Nitric oxide synthases: properties and catalytic mechanism. *Annu. Rev. Physiol.*, 57: 707–736.

Hakim, M.A., Hirooka, Y., Coleman, M.J., Bennett, M.R. and Dampney, R.A.L. (1995) Evidence for a critical role of nitric-oxide in the tonic excitation of rabbit renal sympathetic preganglionic neurons. *J. Physiol. (Lond.)*, 482: 401–407.

Haley, J.E., Wilcox, G.L. and Chapman, P.F. (1992) The role of nitric oxide in hippocampal long-term potentiation. *Neuron*, 8: 211–216.

Hammel, H.T. (1968) Regulation of internal body temperature. *Annu. Rev. Physiol.*, 30: 641–710.

Hancock, M.B. and Peveto, C.A. (1979) A preganglionic autonomic nucleus in the dorsal gray comissure of the lumbar spinal cord of the rat. *J. Comp. Neurol.*, 183: 65–72.

Hope, G.T., Michael, G.J., Knigge, K.M. and Vincent, S.R. (1991) Neuronal NADPH diaphorase is a nitric oxide synthase. *Proc. Natl. Acad. Sci. USA*, 88: 2811–2814.

Hori, T., Kiyohara, T., Nakashima, T., Shibata, M. and Koga, H. (1987) Multimodal responses of preoptic and anterior hypothalamic neurons to thermal and nonthermal homeostatic parameters. *Can. J. Physiol. Pharmacol.*, 65: 1290–1298.

Ignarro, L.J., Buga, G.M., Wood, K.S., Byrns, R.E. and Chaudhuri, G. (1987) Endothelium-derived relaxing factor produced and released from artery and vein is nitric oxide. *Proc. Natl. Acad. Sci. USA*, 84: 9265–9269.

Ishii, K. and Ishii, K. (1960) Relation of blood pressure to shivering. *Tohoku J. Exp. Med.*, 72: 237–242.

Jurzak, M., Schmid, H.A. and Gerstberger, R. (1994) NADPH-diaphorase staining and NO-synthase immunoreactivity in circumventricular organs of the rat brain. In: K. Pleschka and R. Gerstberger (Eds.), *Integrative and Cellular Aspects of Autonomic Functions: Temperature and Osmoregulation*, John Libbey Eurotext, Paris, pp. 451–459.

Kapas, L., Shibata, M., Kimura, M. and Krueger, J.M. (1994) Inhibition of nitric oxide synthesis suppresses sleep in rabbits. *Am. J. Physiol.* 266: R151–R157.

Keaney, J.F., Puyana, J.C., Francis, S., Loscalzo, J.F., Stamler, J.S. and Loscalzo, J. (1994) Methylene blue reverses endotoxin-induced hypotension. *Circ. Res.*, 74: 1121–1125.

Khurana, G. and Bennett, M.R. (1993) Nitric oxide and arachidonic acid modulation of calcium currents in postganglionic neurones of avian cultured ciliary ganglia. *Br. J. Pharmacol.*, 109: 480–485.

Kluger, M.J. (1991) Fever: Role of pyrogens and cryogens. *Physiol. Rev.*, 71: 93–127.

Knowles, R.G., Palacios, M., Palmer, R.M.J. and Moncada, S. (1989) Formation of nitric oxide from L-arginine in the central nervous system: A transduction mechanism for stimulation of the soluble guanylate cyclase. *Proc. Natl. Acad. Sci. USA*, 86: 5159–5162.

Koga, H., Hori, T., Inoue, T., Kiyohara, T. and Nakashima, T.

(1987) Convergence of hepatoportal osmotic and cardiovascular signals on preoptic thermosensitive neurons. *Brain Res. Bull.*, 19: 109–113.

Kulchitsky, V., Sann, H. and Pierau, F.K. (1994) Effects of prostaglandin E2 on the thermosensitivity of anterior and posterior hypothalamic neurones in vitro. In: K. Pleschka and R. Gerstberger (Eds.), *Integrative Aspects of Autonomic Functions: Temperature and Osmoregulation*, John Libbey Eurotext, Paris, pp. 37–46.

Kuroshima, A. (1995) Regulation of thermoregulatory thermogenesis. *Hokkaido J. Med. Sci.*, 70: 1–8.

Lin, Y.-Q. and Bennett, M.R. (1994) Nitric oxide modulation of quantal secretion in chick ciliary ganglia. *J. Physiol. (Lond.)*, 481: 385–394.

Lin, J.H. and Lin M.T (1996) Nitric oxide synthase-cyclooxygenase pathways in organum vasculosum laminae terminalis: possible role in pyrogenic fever in rabbits. *British J. Pharmacol.* 118: 179–185.

Lipton, S.A., Singel, D.J. and Stamler, J.S. (1994) Nitric oxide in the central nervous system. *Prog. Brain Res.*, 103: 359–364.

Ma, S.X., Abboud, F.M. and Felder, R.B. (1995) Effects of L-arginine-derived nitric oxide synthesis on neuronal activity in nucleus tractus solitarius. *Am. J. Physiol.*, 37: R487–R491.

Mack, G.W. and Nadel, E.R. (1996) Body fluid balance during heat stress in humans. In: M.L. Fregly and C.M. Blatteis (Eds.), *Handbook of Physiology, Section 4, Environmental Physiology*, Oxford University Press, Oxford, pp. 187–214.

MacNaul, K.L. and Hutchinson, N.I. (1993) Differential expression of iNOS and cNOS mRNA in human vascular smooth muscle cells and endothelial cells under normal and inflammatory conditions. *Biochem. Biophys. Res. Commun.*, 196: 1330–1334.

Marletta, M.A., Yoon, P.S., Iyengar, R., Leaf, C.D. and Wishnok, J.S. (1988) Macrophage oxidation of L-arginine to nitrite and nitrate: nitric oxide is an intermediate. *Biochemistry*, 27: 8706–8711.

Mathai, M.L., Hjelmqvist, H., Keil, R. and Gerstberger, R. (1997) Nitric oxide increases cutaneous and respiratory heat dissipation in conscious rabbits. *Am. J. Physiol.* 272: R1691–R1697.

Mayer, B., Brunner, F. and Schmidt, K. (1993) Inhibition of nitric oxide synthesis by methylene blue. *Biochem. Pharmacol.*, 45: 367–374.

McCall, T.B., Boughton-Smith, N., Palmer, R.M.J., Whittle, B.J.R. and Moncada, S. (1989) Synthesis of nitric oxide from L-arginine by neutrophils. *Biochem. J.*, 261: 293–296.

Mills, P.C., Marlin, D.J., Scott, C.M. and Smith, N.C. (1997) Nitric oxide and thermoregulation during exercise in the horse. *J. Appl. Physiol.* 82: 1035–1039.

Milton, A.S. (1982) Prostaglandins in fever and the mode of action of antipyretic drugs. In: A.S. Milton (Ed.), *Pyretics and Antipyretics*, Springer, Berlin, pp. 257–303.

Monda, M., Amaro, S., Sullo, A. and De Luca, B. (1995a) Nitric oxide reduces the thermogenic changes induced by lateral hypothalamic lesions. *J. Physiol. (Paris)*, 88: 347–352.

Monda, M., Amaro, S., Sullo, A. and De Luca, B. (1995b) Nitric oxide reduces body temperature and sympathetic input to brown adipose tissue during PGE_1 hyperthermia. *Brain Res. Bull.*, 38: 489–493.

Nakamura, T. and Gold, G.H. (1987) A cyclic nucleotide-gated conductance in olfactory receptor cilia. *Nature*, 325: 442–444.

Nathan, C. (1992) Nitric oxide as a secretory product of mammalian cells. *FASEB J.*, 6: 3051–3064.

Nathan, C. and Xie, Q.-W. (1994) Regulation of biosynthesis of nitric oxide. *J. Biol. Chem.*, 269: 13725–13728.

O'Dell, T.J., Hawkins, R.D., Kandel, E. and Arancio, O. (1991). Tests for the roles of two diffusible substances in long-term potentiation: evidence for nitric oxide as a possible early retrograde messenger. *Proc. Natl. Acad. Sci. USA*, 88: 11285–11289.

Palmer, R.M.J., Ferrige, A.G. and Moncada, S. (1987) Nitric oxide release accounts for the biological activity of endothelium-derived relaxing factor. *Nature*, 327: 524–526.

Palmer, R.M.J., Ashton, D.S. and Moncada, S. (1988) Vascular endothelial cells synthesize nitric oxide from L-arginine. *Nature*, 333: 664–666.

Paxinos, G. and Watson, C. (1986) *The Rat Brain in Stereotaxic Coordinates*, Academic Press, Sydney.

Pehl, U. and Schmid, H.A. (1997) Electrophysiological responses of neurons in the rat spinal cord to nitric oxide. *Neuroscience*, 77: 563–573.

Pehl, U., Schmid, H.A. and Simon, E. (1994a) Lamina-specific effects of nitric oxide on temperature-sensitive neurons in rat spinal cord slices. In: E. Zeisberger, E. Schönbaum and P. Lomax (Eds.), *Thermal Balance in Health and Disease*, Birkhäuser, Basel, pp. 45–52.

Pehl, U., Schmid, H.A. and Simon, E. (1994b) Local temperature sensitivity of spinal cord neurons recorded in vitro. In: K. Pleschka and R. Gerstberger (Eds.), *Integrative and Cellular Aspects of Autonomic Functions: Temperature and Osmoregulation,* John Libbey Eurotext, Paris, pp. 77–86.

Philipp-Dormston, W.K. and Siegert, R. (1974) Prostaglandins of the E and F series in rabbit cerebrospinal fluid during fever induced by newcastle disease virus, E. coli-endotoxin, or endogenous pyrogen. *Med. Microbiol. Immunol.*, 59: 279–284.

Pow, D.A. (1992) NADPH-diaphorase (nitric oxide synthase) staining in the rat supraoptic nucleus is activity-dependent; possible functional implications. *J. Neuroendocrinol.*, 4: 377–380.

Prabhakar, N.R., Kumar, G.K., Chang, C.H., Agani, F.H. and Haxhiu, M.A. (1993) Nitric oxide in the sensory function of the carotid body. *Brain Res.*, 625: 16–22.

Rand, M.J. and Li, C.G. (1995a) Nitric oxide in the autonomic and enteric nervous systems. In: S.R. Vincent (Ed.), *Neuroscience Perspectives: Nitric Oxide in the Nervous System*, Academic Press, London, pp. 227–279.

Rand, M.J. and Li, C.G. (1995b) Nitric oxide as a neurotransmitter in peripheral nerves: Nature of transmitter and mechanisms of transmission. *Annu. Rev. Physiol.*, 57: 659–682.

Redford, J., Bishai, I. and Coceani, F. (1995) Pyrogen-prostaglandin coupling in the pathogenesis of fever—evidence against a role for nitric-oxide. *Can. J. Physiol. Pharmacol.*, 73: 1466–1474.

Reimers, J.I., Bierre, U., Mandrup-Poulsen, T. and Nerup, J. (1994) Interleukin 1β induces diabetes and fever in normal rats by nitric oxide via induction of different nitric oxide syntheses. *Cytokine* 6: 512–520.

Renzi, P.M. and Flynn, J.T. (1992) Endotoxin enhances arachidonic acid metabolism by cultured rabbit microvascular endothelial cells. *Am. J. Physiol.*, 263: H1213–H1221.

Robertson, B.E., Schubert, R., Hescheler, J. and Nelson, M.T. (1993) cGMP-dependent protein kinase activates Ca-activated K channels in cerebral artery smooth muscle cells. *Am. J. Physiol.*, 265: C299–C303.

Rossi, F. (1986) The O_2-forming NADPH oxidase of the phagocytes: nature, mechanisms of activation and function. *Biochim. Biophys. Acta*, 853: 65–89.

Rothwell, N.J. (1992) Eicosanoids, thermogenesis and thermoregulation. *Prostaglandins Leukotrienes Essent. Fatty Acids*, 46: 1–7.

Salvemini, D., Seibert, K., Masferrer, J.L., Misko, T.P., Currie, M.G. and Needelman, P. (1994) Endogenous nitric oxide enhances prostaglandin production in a model of renal inflammation. *J. Clin. Invest.*, 93: 1940–1947.

Sandor, N.T., Brassai, A., Puskas, A. and Lendvai, B. (1995) Role of nitric-oxide in modulating neurotransmitter release from rat striatum. *Brain Res. Bull.*, 36: 483–486.

Scammell, T.E., Elmquist, J.K. and Saper, C.B. (1996) Inhibition of nitric oxide synthase produces hypothermia and depresses lipopolysaccharide fever. *Am. J. Physiol.*, 271: R333–R338.

Schmid, H.A. and Pierau, F.-K. (1993) Temperature sensitivity of neurons in slices of the rat PO/AH hypothalamic area: effect of calcium. *Am. J. Physiol.*, 264: R440–R448.

Schmid, H.A. and Pehl, U. (1996) Regional specific effects of nitric oxide donors and cGMP on the electrical activity of neurons in the rat spinal cord. *J. Chem. Neuroanat.*, 10: 197–201.

Schmid, H.A., Jansky, L. and Pierau, F.-K. (1993) Temperature sensitivity of neurons in slices of the rat PO/AH area: effect of bombesin and substance P. *Am. J. Physiol.*, 264: R449–R455.

Schmid, H.A., Pehl, U. and Simon, E. (1994) Temperature sensitivity of rat spinal cord neurons recorded in vitro. In: A.S. Milton (Ed.), *Temperature Regulation*, Birkhäuser, Basel, pp. 109–115.

Schmid, H.A., Schäfer, F. and Simon, E. (1995) Opposite effects of angiotensin II and nitric oxide on neurons in the duck subfornical organ. *Neurosci. Lett.*, 187: 149–152.

Schmidt, H.H.H.W., Lohmann, S.M. and Walter, U. (1993) The nitric oxide and cGMP signal transduction system: regulation and mechanism of action. *Biochim. Biophys. Acta*, 1178: 153–175.

Schuman, E.M. (1995) Nitric oxide signalling, long-term potentiation and long-term depression. In: S.R. Vincent, (Ed.), *Nitric Oxide in the Central Nervous System*, Academic Press, London, pp. 125–150.

Schuman, E.M. and Madison, D.V. (1991) A requirement for the intercellular messenger nitric oxide in long-term potentiation. *Science*, 254: 1503–1506.

Segal, A.W. (1989) The electron transport chain of the microbicidal oxidase of phagocytic cells and its involvement in the molecular pathology of chronic granulomatous disease. *J. Clin. Invest.*, 83: 1785–1793.

Sehic, E., Gerstberger, R. and Blatteis, C.M. (1997) The effect of intravenous lipopolysaccharide on NADPH-diaphorase staining (= nitric oxide synthase activity) in the *Organum Vasculosum Laminae Terminalis* of guinea pigs. *Ann. N.Y. Acad. Sci.*, 813: 383–391.

Simon, E. (1974) Temperature regulation: The spinal cord as a site of extrahypothalamic thermoregulatory functions. *Rev. Physiol. Biochem. Pharmacol.*, 71: 1–76.

Simon, E., Pierau, F.-K. and Taylor, D.C.M. (1986) Central and peripheral thermal control of effectors in homeothermic temperature regulation. *Physiol. Rev.*, 66: 235–300.

Simon, E., Schmid, H.A. and Pehl, U. (1997) Spinal neuronal thermosensitivity in vivo and in vitro in relation to hypothalamic neuronal thermosensitivity. In: H.S. Sharma and J. Westman (Eds.), *Brain Functions in Hot Environment: Basic and Clinical Perspectives*, Elsevier, Amsterdam, this volume.

Strack, A.M., Sawyer, W.B., Marubio, L.M. and Loewy, A.D. (1988) Spinal origin of sympathetic preganglionic neurons in the rat. *Brain Res.*, 455: 187–191.

Stuehr, D.J. and Marletta, M.A. (1985) Mammalian nitrate biosynthesis: mouse macrophages produced nitrite and nitrate in response to *Escherichia coli* lipopolysaccharide. *Proc. Natl. Acad. Sci. USA*, 82: 7738–7742.

Stuehr, D.J., Gross, S.S., Sakuma, I., Levi, R. and Nathan, C.F. (1989) Activated murine macrophages secrete a metabolite of arginine with the bioactivity of endothelium-derived relaxing factor and the chemical reactivity of nitric oxide. *J. Exp. Med.*, 169: 1011–1020.

Sugahara, M. and Pleschka, K. (1992) Nutrient and shunt flow responses to vidian nerve stimulation in nasal and facial tissues of the dog. *Eur. Arch. Otolaryngol.*, 249: 79–84.

Tagawa, T., Imaizumi, T., Harada, S., Endo, T., Shiramoto, M., Hirooka, Y. and Takeshita, A. (1994) Nitric-oxide influences neuronal-activity in the nucleus-tractus-solitarius of rat brain-stem slices. *Circ. Res.*, 75: 70–76.

Taylor, W.F. and Bishop, V.S. (1993) A role for nitric oxide in active thermoregulatory vasodilatation. *Am. J. Physiol.*, 264: H1355–H1359.

Thelen, M., Dewald, B. and Baggiolini, M. (1993) Neutrophil signal transduction and activation of the respiratory burst. *Physiol. Rev.*, 73: 797–821.

Traub, R.J., Solodkin, A., Meller, S.T. and Gebhart, G.F. (1994) Spinal cord NADPH-diaphorase histochemical staining but not nitric oxide synthase immunoreactivity increases following carrageenan-produced hindpaw inflammation in the rat. *Brain Res.*, 668: 204–210.

Travagli, R.A. and Gillis, R.A. (1994) Nitric oxide-mediated excitatory effect on neurons of dorsal motor nucleus of vagus. *Am. J. Physiol.*, 266: G154–G160.

Valtschanoff, J.G., Weinberg, R.J. and Rustioni, A. (1992a) NADPH diaphorase in the spinal cord of rats. *J. Comp. Neurol.*, 321: 209–222.

Valtschanoff, J.G., Weinberg, R.J., Rustioni, A. and Schmidt, H.H.H.W. (1992b) Nitric oxide synthase and GABA colocalize in lamina II of rat spinal cord. *Neurosci. Lett.*, 148: 6–10.

Vincent, S.R. and Hope, B.T. (1992) Neurons that say NO. *Trends. Neurol. Sci.*, 15: 108–113.

Vincent, S.R. and Kimura, H. (1992) Histochemical mapping of nitric oxide synthase in the rat brain. *Neuroscience*, 46: 755–784.

Wagner, D.A., Young, V.B. and Tannenbaum, S.R. (1983) Mammalian nitrate biosynthesis: incorporation of 15NH3 into nitrate is enhanced by endotoxin treatment. *Proc. Natl. Acad. Sci. USA*, 80: 4518–4521.

Watanabe, H., Tsuru, H., Kawamoto, H., Yajin, K., Sasa, M. and Harada, Y. (1995) Nitroxidergic vasodilator nerve in the canine nasal mucosa. *Life Sci.*, 57: 109–112.

Weihrauch, D. and Riedel, W. (1997) Nitric oxide (NO) and oxygen radicals, but not prostaglandins, modulate fever. *Ann. New York Acad. Sci.*, 813: 373–382.

Williams, J.H., Li, Y.G., Nayak, A., Errington, M.L., Murphy, K.P.S.J. and Bliss, T.V.P. (1993) The suppression of long-term potentiation in rat hippocampus by inhibitors of nitric-oxide synthase is temperature and age-dependent. *Neuron*, 11: 877–884.

Wu, W., Liuzzi, F.J., Schinco, F.P., Depto, A.S., Li, Y., Mong, J.A., Dawson, T.M. and Snyder, S.H. (1994) Neuronal nitric-oxide synthase is induced in spinal neurons by traumatic injury. *Neuroscience*, 61: 719–726.

Yakimova, K., Sann, H., Schmid, H.A. and Pierau, F.-K. (1996) Effects of GABA agonists and antagonists on temperature sensitive neurones in the rat hypothalamus. *J. Physiol. (Lond.)*, 494.1: 217–230.

Zhang, J. and Synder, S.H. (1995) Nitric oxide in the central nervous system. *Annu. Rev. Pharmacol. Toxicol.*, 35: 213–233.

Zhuo, M., Kandel, E.R. and Hawkins, R.D. (1994) Nitric oxide and cGMP can produce either synaptic depression or potentiation depending on the frequency of presynaptic stimulation in the hippocampus. *NeuroReport*, 5: 1033–1036.

H.S. Sharma and J. Westman (Eds.)
Progress in Brain Research, Vol 115

CHAPTER 7

Pathophysiology of opioids in hyperthermic states

Andrej A. Romanovsky[1,*] and Clark M. Blatteis[2]

[1]*Thermoregulation Laboratory, Legacy Research, Legacy Holladay Park Medical Center, Portland, OR 97208-3950, USA*
[2]*Department of Physiology and Biophysics, University of Tennessee, Memphis, TN 38163, USA*

Introduction

Among the disorders characterized by a body temperature (T_b) rise, fever and heat stroke are, without doubt, the most important from the clinical point of view. Occurring as a sign of systemic inflammation (typically infection), fever is perhaps the most ancient and widely known hallmark of disease. For much of history, the word 'fever' has been used almost synonymously with disease itself as various epidemics have ravaged the civilizations of East and West alike (Atkins and Bodel, 1972). Heat stroke, although much less common, also has played a noticeable and sad role in human history. This role can be illustrated by numerous examples: from the failure of a Roman military expedition to North Africa due to an outbreak of heat stroke in 24 BC to recent reports of athletes, miners, urban dwellers, and soldiers all suffering a significant morbidity during periods of heat stress (for review, see Shibolet et al., 1976; Delaney and Goldfrank, 1990). A frightening number of deaths caused by heat stroke is associated with Makkah Hajj, the annual 7-day pilgrimage to Mecca, where some 2 million people are squeezed into a small area at an ambient temperature (T_a) usually between 35°C and 50°C (Hales, 1983). In 1959 and 1960, heat stroke caused 800 deaths among pilgrims (Eichler et al., 1969). In 1982, more than a thousand pilgrims were successfully treated for heat stroke, but several hundred others died before they could reach special heat illness treatment centers organized by the Saudi Arabian government (Al-Marzoogi et al., 1983). Although the incidence of heat disorders during Makkah Hajj is rather extreme, heat-related illness remains a significant cause of mortality in many countries. During hot summers in the United States, an average of 820 deaths are caused by heat injury, with at least 10 times more due to cardiovascular problems exacerbated by heat stress (Anderson et al., 1983).

Despite the apparent clinical significance of the hyperthermic disorders, the arsenal of therapeutic measures used in both heat stroke and fever to control the patient's T_b is usually limited to physical cooling and/or administration of 'traditional' antipyretics [viz, inhibitors of prostaglandin (PG) synthesis]. It is no surprise, therefore, that, over the last few decades, many pharmacological substances that had traditionally been used in non-thermoregulatory disorders, have been intensively screened for their potential therapeutic effects in fever and heat stroke. Among those substances are opiates, drugs known to man for a long time

---
*Corresponding author. Tel: +1 503 4132086; fax: +1 503 4134942; e-mail: aromanov@lhs.org

due to their analgesic, euphoric, antidiarrheal, cough-suppressing, and addictive effects (Brownstein, 1993; Foley, 1993). Without doubt, some other effects of opiates [e.g. cardiovascular (Holaday, 1983)] have also been known to the user and abuser of these substances for several centuries. Yet other of their effects have been discovered only recently. Among them are findings suggesting that opioids may be involved in the mechanisms of both fever (Blatteis et al., 1991; Milton et al., 1994; Romanovsky et al., 1994) and heat stroke (Appenzeller et al., 1986; Panjwani et al., 1991; Romanovsky and Blatteis, 1996). Elucidating the role of endogenous opioid agonists in hyperthermic disorders is the purpose of the present paper.

Opioids: a brief overview

Opioid ligands and receptors

There are three separate families of natural (endogenous) peptides that can be characterized as opioid receptor ligands: enkephalins, endorphins, and dynorphins (for detailed characteristics, see Pleuvry, 1991). They are derived from three different prohormones, i.e. proenkephalin, pro-opiomelanocortin, and prodynorphin, which are coded by three separate genes (Fig. 1). In a single species, the three families of opioids differ in their distribution, receptor selectivity, and biological roles (Khachaturian et al., 1985; Pleuvry, 1991); yet their selectivity is relative, distribution is partly overlapping, and roles are somewhat interchangeable. *In vivo*, multiple opioid ligands act in the organism upon multiple opioid receptor types. The first classification of the latter included three types, μ, κ, and σ, which were defined based on the activity of three exogenous ligands (morphine, ketocyclazocine, and N-allylnormetazocine, respectively) in the spinal dog (Martin et al., 1976). Since this original classification, there have been several attempts to introduce additional receptor types and subtypes such as μ_1, μ_2, δ_1, δ_2, κ_1, κ_2, κ_3, and ϵ (for reviews, see Pleuvry, 1991; Foley, 1993; Pasternak, 1993). Yet, only

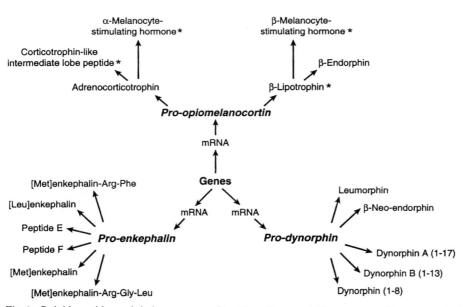

Fig. 1. Opioid peptides and their precursors. Peptides with no opioid receptor activity are marked with an asterisk [from Pleuvry et al. (1991), reprinted with kind permission of BMJ Publishing Group, London, UK].

three classes of receptors (μ, δ, and κ) have endured and are firmly established now; by the same token, both μ- and κ-sites have been confirmed to be pharmacologically heterogeneous (Pleuvry, 1991). As for the rest of the proposed types (including one of the originally proposed — σ), the data on either their existence or specificity (or both) are controversial. Noteworthily, interconversions between μ and δ receptors have been demonstrated (Bowen et al., 1981); the idea of a complex allosteric receptor has been proposed (Barnard and Demoliou-Mason, 1983); and the notion has been advanced that both μ and δ receptors exist in two forms, i.e. separate and complexed together (Heyman et al., 1989; Rothman et al., 1990). To make the picture more complete, we should add that most of the endogenous opioid agonists can bind to several receptor types, and that most of the antagonists available today are also only relatively selective. Finally, it should be noted that, in the central nervous system, enkephalins and endorphins are found often to coexist with 'classical' neurotransmitters such as noradrenaline and serotonin (Cooper et al., 1986). Although the full significance of such coexistence awaits elucidation, the co-transmitters are thought to modulate both the release and action of opioid peptides, and vice versa.

Opioids in temperature regulation: pharmacological analysis

Taking into consideration the above characteristics of opioid receptors and their ligands, it is not surprising that the biological effects of exogenously administered opioids depend on a large number of factors. In the case of thermoregulatory effects, these factors include, but are not limited to, the route of administration and dose of the drug, species used, age, circadian rhythm, degree of stress (restraint), and ambient temperature (for review, see Clark, 1979; Adler et al., 1988). The development of tolerance, which is characteristic of many opioid substances, also influences the thermoregulatory effect of a drug (Ary and Lomax, 1979; Adler et al., 1988). The

complexity of the opioidergic system, variability of biological effects of opioid agonists and antagonists, and limitations of the available pharmacological tools (most of the opioid substances that have been used possess relatively low selectivity) have made the pharmacological analysis of the thermoregulatory effects of opioids an extremely difficult task. Not surprisingly, therefore, pharmacological studies often do not result in a definitive answer. A recent example is given by Mayfield and D'Alecy (1992, 1994), who have demonstrated that naloxone, a nonselective opioid antagonist, blocked the hypoxic conditioning-induced decrease in T_b. The authors attempted to delineate the potential contributions of major opioid receptor types to this response by using selective μ, δ, and κ antagonists, none of which appeared to be effective. The authors hypothesized that, in some cases, more than one of the opioid receptor types have to be blocked in order to affect an opioid-mediated T_b response (Mayfield and D'Alecy, 1994). Nevertheless, certain results have been achieved in pharmacological studies. Importantly, a consensus has been reached in regard to the rat — the most widely used laboratory species. Although with some reservations (Spencer et al., 1990), it is generally agreed that, in the rat, central μ receptors are likely to be involved in responses that result in heat gain, peripheral κ receptors mediate heat-loss responses, and that activation of δ sites probably has no direct thermoregulatory consequence (Adler et al., 1988).

Pathophysiological approach

Whereas pharmacological studies concentrate on the further search for thermally active opioid substances and characterization of the particular type of opioid receptor involved in a given thermoregulatory response, the emphasis of this review will be on physiological or — more precisely — pathophysiological studies. The latter seek to answer three major questions.

1. Is any particular thermoregulatory response opioid-mediated (regardless of which opioid receptor subtype is involved)?

2. What specific mechanisms of this response involve participation of endogenous opioid peptides (are these mechanisms located within or outside the central nervous system? Is this effect due to a direct or indirect action of opioids on T_b regulation, etc.)?

3. Could the observed experimental phenomenon have a potential for clinical application?

Below, we will try to answer some of these questions in respect to potential roles of endogenous opioids in fever and heat stroke. The two central subjects of our discussion will be the phenomenon of naloxone-induced antipyresis (Blatteis et al., 1991; Milton et al., 1994; Romanovsky et al., 1994) and the complex thermoregulatory effect of naltrexone in an experimentally-induced heat disorder (Romanovsky and Blatteis, 1996).

Fever

Are opioids involved?

In addition to the well-known pyrogenic mediators, cytokines and PGs of the E-series, several neuropeptides have been recently proposed to participate in the genesis of fever. The list of new candidates includes somatostatin (Lin et al., 1989), substance P (Blatteis et al., 1994), cholecystokinin (Szelényi et al., 1994), and opioid peptides — the subject of the present paper. The possible involvement of opioids (particularly, μ-receptor agonists such as β-endorphin and met-enkephalin) in fever production has been suggested by several reports. Thus, elevations of plasma, cerebrospinal fluid, and hypothalamic levels of β-endorphin have been found during bacteremia and in both lipopolysaccharide (LPS)- and endogenous pyrogen-induced fevers (Carr et al., 1982; Murphy et al., 1983; Leshin and Malven, 1984; Knigge et al., 1994). One of the primary endogenous pyrogens, interleukin (IL)-1, has been shown to induce β-endorphin secretion by pituitary cells (Fagarasan et al., 1990) and to modulate opioid receptor

binding in the brain (Ahmed et al., 1988; Wiederman, 1989). Another pyrogenic cytokine, interferon (IFN)-α, both binds to opioid receptors in the brain and possesses opioid-like activity (Blalock and Smith, 1981; Menzies et al., 1992). Naloxone, a wide spectrum opioid receptor antagonist with strong anti-μ activity, prevents the effects of the pyrogenic cytokines IL-6 (Xin and Blatteis, 1992) and IFN-α (Nakashima et al., 1987, 1988; Hori et al., 1991) on the activity of hypothalamic thermosensitive neurons in slice preparations. Importantly, autoradiographic studies involving highly selective opioid ligands have shown that the density of μ receptors is especially high in the preoptic/anterior hypothalamus (Desjardins et al., 1990), the key brain structure in T_b regulation. Furthermore, both peripheral and central injections of β-endorphin and the prototypic μ-receptor agonist morphine cause fever-like (i.e. ascribed to an increase in the thermoregulatory balance point) hyperthermia, whereas opioid antagonists, particularly naloxone and naltrexone, block this hyperthermia and produce hypothermia by themselves when injected either centrally or peripherally (Ary and Lomax, 1979; Clark, 1979; Yehuda and Kastin, 1980; Kandasamy and Williams, 1983a, 1983c; Adler et al., 1988). Opioids are also thought to participate in the mechanisms of stress hyperthermia, which is similar to fever in respect to both the thermoregulatory changes and mediators apparently involved (cytokines, PGs); naloxone and naltrexone substantially attenuate this response (Blasig et al., 1978; Pae et al., 1985).

Despite these lines of evidence, several attempts to block fever by administration of naloxone in cats (Clark and Harris, 1978), rabbits (Kandasamy and Williams, 1983a; Hellon et al., 1985; Davidson et al., 1987; Kapás and Krueger, 1993), and guinea pigs (Kandasamy and Williams, 1983c) were unsuccessful. Naloxone-induced antipyresis was, however, observed in several other studies: in humans (Norman et al., 1986), rats (Zawada et al., 1992), and rabbits (Milton et al., 1994). In addition, naltrexone has also been reported to attenuate INF-α-induced fever in rats

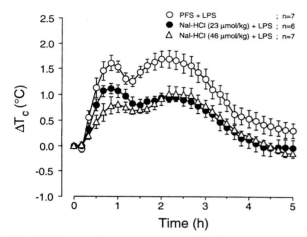

Fig. 2. Changes in colonic temperature (ΔT_c) induced by subcutaneous injection of naloxone-hydrochloride (Nal-HCl; doses indicated) or pyrogen-free saline (PFS) just before intravenous injection of *S. enteritidis* lipopolysaccharide (LPS; 2 μg/kg) at time *0* to conscious, lightly restrained guinea pigs. The data are presented as mean ± standard error; *n*, number of experiments [modified from Romanovsky et al. (1994), reprinted with kind permission of The American Physiological Society, Bethesda, MD, USA].

(Nakashima et al., 1992), and another opioid antagonist, β-chlornaltrexamine, to block the T_b response to LPS in mice (Kozak et al., 1995). In our experiments, naloxone reproducibly blocked febrile responses of guinea pigs to intravenous LPS (Fig. 2; see also Ahokas et al., 1985; Blatteis et al., 1991; Romanovsky et al., 1994), IL-6, INF-α, and tumor necrosis factor (TNF)-α (Blatteis et al., 1991). It is tempting to conclude, therefore, that endogenous opioids, perhaps β-endorphin, do participate in fever production. The recent results of Xin et al. (1996) strongly support this conclusion.

Naloxone antipyresis: a central or a peripheral effect?

In order to examine the role of opioids in the genesis of fever, we made an attempt to clarify the mechanisms of the antipyretic action of naloxone (Blatteis and Romanovsky, 1994; Romanovsky et al., 1994). Since the commonly used preparation of naloxone (naloxone hydrochloride) readily crosses the blood–brain barrier, it was first necessary to differentiate whether the attenuation of LPS fever by the subcutaneous injection of this antagonist is due to its peripheral or central action. To address this issue, we conducted a study using two quaternary ammonium derivatives of naloxone, naloxone methiodide and naloxone methobromide (Romanovsky et al., 1994).

Quaternary opioid antagonists do not cross the blood–brain barrier and, when administered peripherally, are presumed to exert their actions at peripheral sites only (Panerai et al., 1983; Valentino et al., 1983; Katovich et al., 1986; Milne et al., 1990; De Simoni et al., 1993). Their receptor binding and antagonistic properties are 10–100 times lower than those of their relatively nonpolar tertiary counterparts (Valentino et al., 1983), but when administered at relatively high doses in vivo, under circumstances providing access to either their central targets (peripheral administration in spinalized animals, central administration in intact animals) or their peripheral targets (peripheral administration), their biological effects are similar to those of their parent tertiary compounds (Panerai et al., 1983; Milne et al., 1990).

In our study (Romanovsky et al., 1994), we compared the thermal response of unanesthetized guinea pigs to subcutaneous naloxone hydrochloride (has both peripheral and central actions), intracerebroventricular naloxone hydrochloride (has a central action only), and subcutaneous naloxone methiodide and naloxone methobromide (have peripheral actions only). It appeared that the quaternary salts of naloxone, injected subcutaneously, attenuated both the first and second phases of the characteristically biphasic LPS-induced fever, similarly to their parent compound. We concluded, therefore, that naloxone affected both phases of fever by acting on peripheral rather than central receptors. In the same study (Romanovsky et al., 1994), we further supported this conclusion by finding that no attenuation of the febrile response occurred when naloxone hydrochloride (two different doses, 0.25 and 1.25 μmol) was injected intracerebroventricularly. The inability of naloxone to prevent or attenuate fever when administered into one of the brain ventricles (either before or after administration of a pyrogen) was also reported previously in crude leukocytic pyrogen-induced fever in cats (Clark and Harris, 1978) and rabbits (Davidson et al., 1987), IFN-α-induced fever in rats (Zawada et al., 1992), and LPS-fever and PGE_2-hyperthermia in rabbits (Kandasamy and Williams, 1983a). Yet even the dose of 100 μg (equal to approximately 0.25 μmol, i.e. the lowest dose used in our experiments) of naloxone hydrochloride administered intracerebroventricularly has been shown to effectively antagonize the T_b rise produced by a centrally delivered opiate agonist in guinea pigs (Kandasamy and Williams, 1983b). Therefore, the failure of the intracerebroventricular naloxone to induce antipyresis is unlikely to be due to species differences, insufficient dose, or inadequate time of administration in relation to LPS.

A priori, the peripherally mediated attenuation of LPS fever by naloxone may be attributed to its action(s) on one or several of the following peripheral stages in fever genesis: (1) synthesis and release of endogenous pyrogens; (2) activation of thermoregulatory effectors; and/or (3) translation of the pyrogenic signal from the periphery to the brain.

What stage of fever production is affected by naloxone?

A literature analysis leads us to the conclusion that the mechanism of the antipyretic effect of naloxone is unlikely to involve the blockade of the production of endogenous pyrogens. Although μ-opioid agonists can influence the synthesis and/or release of various cytokines (Yang and Li, 1989; Carr, 1991), and although some processes leading to cytokine release are naloxone-sensitive [e.g. systemic IL-6 induction by central IL-1 (De Simoni et al., 1993)], subcutaneous naloxone does not block the acute phase proteinemic response to intravenous LPS (as determined by elevations in plasma copper and N-acetyl-neuraminic acid levels), implying that endogenous pyrogen production is not impeded by

naloxone (Ahokas et al., 1985). Furthermore, naloxone still exerted an obvious antipyretic effect when fever was induced by cytokines (IFN-α, TNF-α, and IL-6) instead of exogenous pyrogens, thus bypassing the stage of endogenous pyrogen production (Blatteis et al., 1991). The inability of naloxone to affect the production or release of IL-1 has also been demonstrated by direct measurements (Yang and Li, 1989).

The next logical question to ask would be: Does naloxone attenuate fever through its direct action upon thermoregulatory effectors? The answer to this question is not a simple one. When administered peripherally at high doses, most pyrogens (including LPS) induce a biphasic fever (for review, see Kluger, 1991) with the two phases differing from each other in their biochemical mediation, thermoregulatory mechanisms, and perhaps even biological significance (Vybíral et al., 1987; Romanovsky and Blatteis, 1995; Romanovsky et al., 1996a). Although naloxone attenuated the two phases of LPS fever to a comparable extent (Fig. 2; also see Blatteis et al., 1991; Romanovsky et al., 1994), the mechanisms of the two phenomena are apparently different. The dose-dependent attenuation by naloxone of the first (early) phase of LPS fever is likely to reflect a thermolytic rather than a truly antipyretic action of the drug. Indeed, this effect is very similar (in both its magnitude and duration) to the hypothermia induced by naloxone in afebrile animals (Fig. 3). Moreover, both the hypothermic response to naloxone under the afebrile conditions and the attenuation of the first febrile phase by the drug were associated with ear skin vasodilation (Blatteis and Romanovsky, 1994; Romanovsky et al., 1994). Since various vascular beds contain opiate receptors (Altura et al., 1980), and since morphine has been shown to possess naloxone-sensitive vasoconstrictor action *in vitro* (El-Sharkawy et al., 1991), it is likely that the thermolytic action of peripheral naloxone is, at least partly, due to a decrease in cutaneous vasomotor tone, although potential alterations in heat production could not be excluded a priori.

In contrast to the attenuation of the first phase, the naloxone-induced decrease in T_b during the

---

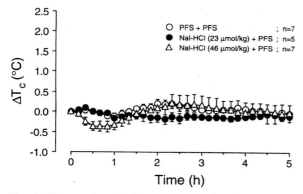

Fig. 3. Changes in colonic temperature (ΔT_c) induced by subcutaneous injection of naloxone-hydrochloride (Nal-HCl; doses indicated) or pyrogen-free saline (PFS) just before intravenous injection of PFS at time *0* to conscious, lightly restrained guinea pigs. The data are presented as mean ± standard error; *n*, number of experiments [modified from Romanovsky et al. (1994), reprinted with kind permission of The American Physiological Society, Bethesda, MD, USA].

second febrile phase is probably separate from the thermolytic action. Indeed, it would seem unlikely that a relatively short-lasting (1 h) and mild (0.5°C) thermolytic effect of naloxone under the afebrile conditions (Fig. 3) could have ac-

counted for a substantial (1°C), 5-h-long attenuation of the second phase (Fig. 2). In a separate study (Romanovsky and Blatteis, 1995), we demonstrated that a prolonged attenuation of the second febrile phase is not a direct consequence of the preceding attenuation of the first phase. To do this, we mimicked the thermolytic action of naloxone by applying intraperitoneal cooling throughout the first phase of LPS fever in guinea pigs and determined the effect of such a procedure on the second phase. Although the intraperitoneal cooling was sufficient to completely block the first febrile T_b rise, it did not result in any attenuation of the second phase (Fig. 4). We suggest, therefore, that in contrast to the attenuation by naloxone of the first febrile phase, the attenuation of the second phase of fever is not due to a direct, thermolytic action of the drug on thermoregulatory effectors. This perhaps represents a truly antipyretic effect. Surprisingly, as the results with quaternary naloxone derivatives have shown, this antipyretic effect is due to an action of naloxone on some targets that are not separated from the blood by the blood–brain barrier. What sites could these be?

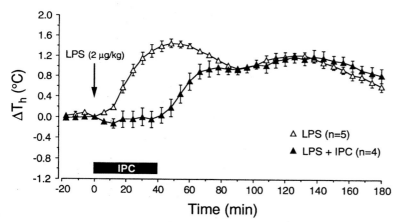

Fig. 4. Changes in hypothalamic temperature (ΔT_h) caused by intraperitoneal cooling (IPC) applied to conscious, lightly restrained guinea pigs during the first phase (0–40 min after pyrogen administration) of a biphasic fever. The fever was induced by intravenous *S. enteritidis* lipopolysaccharide (LPS; dose indicated). IPC was performed by perfusing water at a constant rate of heat withdrawal (11.6 ± 1.2 mW/g) through an implanted silicone thermode. The data are presented as mean ± standard error; *n*, number of experiments [modified from Romanovsky and Blatteis (1995), reprinted with kind permission of The American Physiological Society, Bethesda, MD, USA].

Opioids interfere with the pyrogenic signal transduction from the periphery to the brain

Since the antipyretic effect of naloxone is mediated through its action outside the blood–brain barrier and involves neither the blockade of the production of endogenous pyrogens nor the direct alteration of thermoregulatory effectors, we propose that naloxone initiates antipyresis at a peripheral site (or at a central site lacking the blood–brain barrier). The involvement of peripheral opiates in centrally-mediated responses has been documented; e.g. both opioid agonists and antagonists modulate luteinizing hormone secretion in the hypophysis by acting outside the blood–brain barrier (Forman et al., 1983; Panerai et al., 1983). As for the antipyretic action of naloxone, it is not yet clear exactly where opiates interfere with the peripherally initiated and centrally mediated process of fever. It is difficult to find the answer to this question, because we do not yet know how the pyrogenic signal per se crosses the blood–brain barrier.

The currently prevalent concept is the one originally proposed by Blatteis et al. (1983) and further developed by Stitt (1985), Blatteis et al. (1987a,b), Shibata and Blatteis (1991), Hunter et al. (1994), and others (for review, see Blatteis, 1992; Moltz, 1993; Blatteis and Sehic, 1997a,b). According to this concept, the pyrogenic signal reaches the brain through one of the circumventricular organs, which lack a blood–brain barrier, specifically, the *organum vasculosum laminae terminalis* (OVLT). The exact scenario of this process is not clear and it is not known what substance or cascade of substances (an exogenous pyrogen → pyrogenic cytokines → PGs of the E-series) plays the key role in it. If cytokines enter the perivascular spaces of the OVLT and find their target cells within these spaces, opioids could potentially interfere with this process. Indeed, circumventricular structures, including the OVLT, have been shown to contain opioid receptors (Young et al., 1980; Moskowitz and Goodman, 1984; Mansour et al., 1987). Moreover, pyro-genic cytokines have been shown to influence the specific binding of opioid agonists in the central nervous system (Ahmed et al., 1988; Wiederman, 1989). Furthermore, the action of opioid agonists on neurons located in and/or around the OVLT has been shown to result in some physiological effects such as polydipsia (Hattori et al., 1991). This is in addition to a body of other circumstantial evidence supporting the hypothesis that β-endorphin (and possibly enkephalins) may gain access to autonomic centers in the brain via circumventricular sites (Holaday et al., 1978; Faden and Holaday, 1980; Holaday, 1983).

Another, currently emerging, concept of the pathogenesis of fever postulates that the pyrogenic signal reaches the brain through the vagus nerve. This concept is based on the fact that electrical activity of the rat vagus is increased following hepatoportal injection of IL-1β (Niijima, 1992), whereas desensitization of the abdominal afferents with capsaicin in the rat (Székely et al., 1995) as well as subdiaphragmatic vagotomy in the rat (Watkins et al., 1995a,b; Romanovsky et al., 1997a,b) and guinea pig (Sehic and Blatteis, 1996) all result in attenuation of the thermal response to a peripherally administered pyrogen. A single injection of a pyrogen causes not only changes in T_b, but also alterations in nociception, motor activity, and other autonomic and behavioral functions, thus forming the dose-dependent and time-specific pattern — sickness syndrome (Romanovsky et al., 1996a). Vagotomy appears to block not only the febrile response to a pyrogen, but also several other symptoms of the sickness syndrome such as depression of social investigation (Bluthé et al., 1994) and hyperalgesia (Watkins et al., 1994). Moreover, the LPS-induced expression of IL-1β mRNA in the brain of vagotomized mice (Layé et al., 1995) and the rise in PGE_2 concentration in the brain of vagotomized guinea pigs (Sehic and Blatteis, 1996) were also attenuated. It could be concluded, therefore, that abdominal vagal afferents are likely to constitute a pathway to the central nervous system for pyrogenic signals originating in the periphery. If this is the case, endogenous opioid agonists can interfere with this pathway.

Indeed, Young et al. (1980) have demonstrated that the vagus nerve contains opiate receptors that are transported along axons from cell bodies in the nodose ganglia in both centripetal and centrifugal directions. Peripherally administered alkaloid opiates and perhaps endogenous μ-opioid opioids induce several effects (bradycardia, hypotension) that are mediated through brainstem actions, but can be blocked by vagotomy (Wei et al., 1980; Holaday, 1983).

Several other hypotheses on how information about systemic inflammation reaches the brain have been recently proposed (for review, see Watkins et al., 1995b). Which one is the most productive? The answer to this question will probably determine the most successful line of further investigations of the role of opioids in fever genesis.

Opioids and fever: additional interactions

The fact that naloxone attenuates fever through a peripheral rather than a central action does not, however, exclude the potential existence of another opioid-mediated mechanism of fever production located within the brain. Indeed, naloxone has been reported to prevent the effects of IFN-α (reviewed by Hori et al., 1991) and IL-6 (Xin and Blatteis, 1992) on the activities of thermosensitive neurons in slice preparations of the rat and guinea pig preoptic area, a hypothalamic structure with a very high density of μ receptors (Desjardins et al., 1990). However, any results obtained in vitro should be interpreted with caution from the point of view of their *in vivo* implications. Thus, *in vivo*, intracerebroventricular naloxone does not alter the hyperthermic response to intracerebroventricular IFN-α (Zawada et al., 1992), despite the *in vitro* effects already mentioned. Moreover, subcutaneous naloxone attenuates fever induced by both intravenous (Blatteis et al., 1991) and intracerebroventricular (Zawada et al., 1992) IFN-α and the changes in sleep evoked by intracerebroventricular administration of the same cytokine (Birmanns et al., 1990).

Finally, opioids may be involved in fever not only by directly interfering with the 'major pyrogenic cascade' (an exogenous pyrogen $\rightarrow$ pyrogenic cytokines $\rightarrow$ PGE), but also by affecting the synthesis, release, transport, degradation, and/or action of other substances — various modulators of the febrile response. As an example, opioids have been shown to inhibit the release of norepinephrine from noradrenergic nerve endings (Kohno et al., 1983), whereas hypothalamic norepinephrine has been implicated as both a febrigenic (Cox and Lee, 1982) and an antipyretic (Shido et al., 1993) mediator. Due to their complexity, however, such interactions are difficult to study, and their biological significance remains speculative.

Heat stroke

Are opioids involved?

Although the number of studies assessing the role of opioids in heat stroke is small, the data reported suggest that these substances may participate in the mechanisms of heat-induced disorders. Thus, naloxone has been reported to substantially increase the survival time in rats exposed to heat (Panjwani et al., 1991) and to prevent hyperthermia-induced convulsions in rat pups (Puig et al., 1986). In our recent study (Romanovsky and Blatteis, 1996), we induced heat stroke in guinea pigs by applying intensive and prolonged intraperitoneal heating through a preimplanted thermode; naltrexone completely eliminated the mortality in this model of heat stroke. A fourfold increase in the plasma level of β-endorphin/β-lipotropin has been recorded in Mecca pilgrims with heat stroke (Appenzeller et al., 1986).

Although the protective effect of naloxone and naltrexone in animal models of heat stroke is obvious, it is not clear whether this effect is due to a thermoregulatory or a cardiovascular action. Besides directly affecting T_b regulation (vide supra) and participating in the mechanisms of heat adaptation (Holaday et al., 1978; Thornhill et al., 1980), opioids have also been proposed to play a role in the pathogenesis of shock (for a review, see Holaday, 1983). Opioid agonists, even in small doses, induce hypotension (Holaday, 1983). Opioid antagonists, e.g. naltrexone and naloxone, lessen the severity of shock of various etiologies, including endotoxin shock (Faden and Holaday, 1980; Wright and Weller, 1980). As demonstrated by Faden and Holaday (1979, 1980) and Faden et al. (1980) in animal models of

endotoxemic, hemorrhagic, and so-called spinal shock, naloxone not only prolongs survival, but also attenuates hypotension in all these models.

In our previous study in guinea pigs (Romanovsky and Blatteis, 1994), intensive and prolonged intraperitoneal heating caused a pathologic sequela characterized by high mortality (heat stroke). This heat disorder was accompanied by two 'paradoxical' thermoregulatory phenomena (Fig. 5). First, although ear skin vasodilation read-

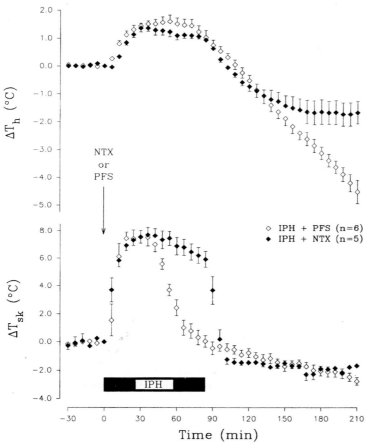

Fig. 5. Effects of the subcutaneous injection of naltrexone (NTX; 50 μmol/kg) or pyrogen-free saline (PFS) on thermoregulatory signs of heat stroke induced by intraperitoneal heating (IPH) in conscious, lightly restrained guinea pigs. IPH was performed by perfusing water (45°C, 50 ml/min, 80 min) through an implanted silicone thermode; IPH was started immediately after the injection. ΔT_h, changes in hypothalamic temperature; ΔT_{sk}, changes in ear skin temperature. The data are presented as mean $\pm$ standard error; n, number of experiments. Note that NTX prevented the development of the hyperthermia-induced vasoconstriction and attenuated the hyperthermia-induced hypothermia [modified from Romanovsky and Blatteis (1996) Heat Stroke: Opioid-Mediated Mechanisms. *J. Appl. Physiol.*, 81(6): 2565–2570].

ily occurred at the onset of the hyperthermia, it later changed to vasoconstriction, despite the continuing intraperitoneal heating and a high T_b; we termed this phenomenon 'hyperthermia-induced vasoconstriction.' Second, when intraperitoneal heating was stopped, the initial hyperthermia was followed by not just a return of T_b to its pre-heating level, but by its fall to below this level; we termed this phenomenon 'hyperthermia-induced hypothermia.' Since opioids can potentially participate in the mechanisms of heat stroke by acting upon both the thermoregulatory and cardiovascular systems, we investigated the effect of naloxone on the two complex phenomena described above.

Hyperthermia-induced vasoconstriction

During heat exposure, water-consuming heat-defense responses (in guinea pigs, polypnea) and thermoregulatory redistribution of blood toward the skin eventually lead to dehydration and/or hypovolemia; both have been shown to increase the threshold T_b for cutaneous vasodilation (Nadel et al., 1980; Proppe, 1990). This results in the development of skin vasoconstriction at high T_bs that, under usual conditions (euhydration and normovolemia), are associated with skin vasodilation. Indeed, skin vasoconstriction has been mentioned as a potential response to an excessive heat load in humans; if this happens, it could be attributed to decreased blood volume and central venous pressure (Khogali, 1987). In addition, the hyperthermia-induced vasoconstriction may be related to the selective loss of splanchnic vasculature constrictive ability. Splanchnic vasoconstriction constitutes an adaptive response to hyperthermia and readily occurs in hyperthermic subjects, thus allowing a larger portion of the cardiac output to be directed to the skin (for review, see Johnson and Proppe, 1996). In severe hyperthermia, however, the splanchnic vasculature becomes unresponsive to constrictor stimuli, presumably due to the release of nitric oxide into the splanchnic circulation (Hall et al., 1994). This lessens the proportion of the cardiac output available to the skin and precipitates skin vasoconstriction. The idea that circulatory collapse in heat stroke is triggered by splanchnic vasodilation was first proposed by Kielblock et al. (1982) and further developed by Kregel et al. (1988), Hall et al. (1994), and others.

We have demonstrated that the hyperthermia-induced vasoconstriction is opioid-dependent because naltrexone prevented its occurrence (Fig. 5; see also Romanovsky and Blatteis, 1996). Although the specific action of endogenous opioid agonists in the mechanism of the hyperthermia-induced vasoconstriction remains to be elucidated, the participation of opioids in this phenomenon is in general agreement with the literature. Thus, opioid peptides are released into the blood in response to various stressors, including heat; exogenous opioid agonists, even in small doses, induce hypotension; and opioid antagonists block hemodynamic alterations in various models of shock (for review, see Holaday, 1983). We also can conclude that, at least in some cases, opioids can influence thermoregulatory responses to heat through their cardiovascular actions or, more specifically, by preventing the recruitment of one of the effector mechanisms (skin vasoconstriction) in heat defense.

Hyperthermia-induced hypothermia

Among the symptoms that have traditionally been used to define heat stroke is high ($> 40.6°C$) T_b. This criterion should not, however, be considered obligatory because many patients with severe exertional heat stroke have a lower T_b, presumably due to the progression of time from the actual heat overload (Delaney and Goldfrank, 1990). In fact, if the heat exposure is followed by an exposure to a near-thermoneutral environment, hypothermia rather than hyperthermia is likely to occur. In our experiments (Romanovsky and Blatteis, 1994, 1996), the hyperthermia induced by intraperitoneal heating in guinea pigs was succeeded not by just a return of T_b to its pre-heating level, but by marked hypothermia. This phenomenon (hyperthermia-induced hypothermia) has been demonstrated in various experimental models and in different animal species. Thus, whole body heat exposure in guinea pigs (Adolph, 1947), rats (Lord et al., 1984), mice (Wright, 1976; Wilkinson et al., 1988) and cats (Adolph, 1947), as well as intraperitoneal heating in rats (Shido et al., 1991), all result in a T_b fall occurring after the heating is stopped. Moreover, the longer and more intensive the initial heat exposure was, the deeper and longer was the consequent hypothermia (Wilkinson et al., 1988; Romanovsky and Blatteis, 1994).

A priori, the thermoregulatory mechanisms of the hyperthermia-induced hypothermia could involve: (1) inhibition of metabolism; (2) excessive heat loss (e.g. generalized peripheral vasodilation); (3) regulation of T_b at a new, decreased level (parallel shifts of thermoeffector thresholds to a lower T_b); (4) a substantially decreased precision of T_b regulation (development of the wide dead-band, poikilothermic type of control) when T_a is below thermoneutrality; or (5) partial contributions of several of the mechanisms listed above. It has been demonstrated that hyperthermia-induced hypothermia occurs at low, but not high, T_as (Wilkinson et al., 1988). It has also been shown that this phenomenon is associated with the widening of the interthreshold zone (poikilothermia), probably as a result of a decrease of the threshold T_b for cold thermogenesis (unpublished observations; see also Romanovsky and Blatteis, 1994). We speculate, therefore, that this metabolic inhibition and the consequent widening of the interthreshold zone constitute the major autonomic mechanisms of hyperthermia-induced hypothermia. It is worth noting that these are exactly the same mechanisms that have been recently found to underlie the hypothermia of endotoxin shock (Romanovsky et al., 1996b). Perhaps, the hyperthermia-induced hypothermia is also relative to hypothermic/hypometabolic responses to a wide range of insults, including trauma, hypoxia, exposure to different toxicants, etc. (for review, see Gordon, 1996). The phenomena of hyperthermia-induced hypothermia and LPS-induced hypothermia (endotoxin shock) are both opioid-dependent, because naltrexone significantly attenuated the former (Fig. 5; also see Romanovsky and Blatteis, 1996) whereas naloxone blocked the latter (Wright and Weller, 1980). If our concept of the thermoregulatory mechanisms of these phenomena is correct, this would imply that endogenous opioids mediate the proposed metabolic inhibition. Existing literature supports this hypothesis. Indeed, opioids are known to inhibit metabolism and cause hypothermia at T_as below thermoneutral (Lin and Su, 1979; Egawa et al., 1993).

Conclusions

Opioids in hyperthermic states: multiple actions on multiple targets

It is generally appreciated that interactions between the opioidergic system and thermoregulation are complex, and that a thermoregulatory effect of a particular opioid substance often depends on a large number of factors, including the route of administration and dose of the drug, the degree of stress, the ambient temperature, etc. (for review, see Ary and Lomax, 1979; Clark, 1979; Adler et al., 1988). One of the reasons for such variability is that any particular opioid agonist or antagonist can act simultaneously on multiple, mutually independent targets, and that the resultant effect on T_b represents the sum of these actions. Although the discussed effects of naloxone on fever and of naltrexone on heat stroke demonstrate this statement, we reviewed only some, selected mechanisms from the wide spectrum of opioid-dependent responses that can contribute to T_b regulation.

Opioids: pathophysiological rather than physiological regulators

When evaluating thermoregulatory effects of exogenous opioid antagonists, one finds that these drugs do not significantly influence T_b under normal conditions (Fig. 3). It can be concluded, therefore, that endogenous opioids are unlikely to contribute noticeably to 'normal' thermoregulation (Clark, 1979). In contrast to the minimal effects of opioid antagonists on T_b under physiological conditions, these drugs markedly affect the pathophysiological thermoregulatory responses, as we illustrated in the present paper for the cases of fever and heat stroke (Figs. 2 and 5). Interestingly, the role of endogenous opioids in normal cardiovascular homeostasis is also questionable, whereas the involvement of these substances in pathophysiological cardiovascular responses is widely recognized (Holaday, 1983; Sirén and Feuerstein, 1992). In this regard, there is little doubt that the analgesic effects of opioids are of much greater importance in pathological rather than physiological situations.

Opioids in thermoregulatory disorders: potential clinical significance

The apparent involvement of opioids in pathological rather than physiological responses contributes to the keen interest of physicians in opiate antagonists, particularly naloxone (Chamberlain and Klein, 1994). Potent therapeutic effects of this drug, including a drastic reduction in mortality, have been observed in several experimental models of hyperthermic disorders (Puig et al., 1986; Panjwani et al., 1991; Romanovsky and Blatteis, 1996). This would suggest that naloxone and perhaps some other opioid antagonists may find new clinical applications in patients with hyperthermic disorders.

References

Adler, M.W., Geller, E.B., Rosow, C.E. and Cochin, J. (1988) The opioid system and temperature regulation. *Annu. Rev. Pharmacol. Toxicol.*, 28: 429–449.

Adolph, E.F. (1947) Tolerance of heat and dehydration in several species of mammals. *Am. J. Physiol.*, 151: 564–575.

Ahmed, M.S., Llanos-Q, J., Dinarello, C.A. and Blatteis, C.M. (1988) Interleukin 1 reduces opioid binding in guinea pig brain. *Peptides*, 6: 1149–1154.

Ahokas, R.A., Seydoux, J., Llanos-Q, J., Mashburn Jr., T.A. and Blatteis, C.M. (1985) Hypothalamic opioids and the acute-phase glycoprotein response in guinea pigs. *Brain Res. Bull.*, 15: 603–608.

Al-Marzoogi, A., Khogali, M. and El-Ergesus, A. (1983) Organizational set up: detection, screening, treatment and follow-up to heat disorders. In: M. Khogali and J.R.S. Hales (Eds.), *Heat Stroke and Temperature Regulation*, Academic Press, Sydney, pp. 31–39.

Altura, B.M., Altura, B.T., Carella, A., Turlapaty, P.D.M.D. and Weinberg, J. (1980) Vascular smooth muscle and general anesthetics. *Fed. Proc.*, 39: 1584–1591.

Anderson, R.J., Reed, G. and Knockhel, J. (1983) Heatstroke. *Adv. Intern. Med.*, 28: 115–140.

Appenzeller, O., Khogali, M., Carr, D.B., Gumaa, K., Mustafa, M.K.Y., Jamjoom, A. and Skipper, B. (1986) Makkah Hajj: heat stroke and endocrine responses. *Ann. Sport Med.*, 3: 30–32.

Ary, M. and Lomax, P. (1979) Influence of narcotic agents on temperature regulation. In: H.H. Loh and D.H. Ross (Eds.), *Neurochemical Mechanisms of Opiates and Endorphins* (Adv. Biochem. Psychopharmacol., Vol. 20), Raven Press, New York, pp. 429–451.

Atkins, E. and Bodel, E. (1972) Fever. *New Engl. J. Med.*, 286: 27–34.

Barnard, E.A. and Demoliou-Mason, C. (1983) Molecular properties of opioid receptors. *Br. Med. Bull.*, 39: 37–45.

Birmanns, B., Saphier, D. and Abramsky, O. (1990) α-Interferon modifies cortical EEG activity: dose-dependence and antagonism by naloxone. *J. Neurol. Sci.*, 100: 22–26.

Blalock, J.E. and Smith, E.M. (1981) Human leukocyte interferon (HuINF-α): potent endorphin-like opioid activity. *Biochem. Biophys. Res. Commun.*, 101: 472–478.

Blasig, J., Hollt, V., Bauerle, U. and Herz, A. (1978) Involvement of endorphins in emotional hyperthermia of rats. *Life Sci.*, 23: 2525–2531.

Blatteis, C.M. (1992) Role of the OVLT in the febrile response to circulating pyrogens. *Prog. Brain Res.*, 91: 409–412.

Blatteis, C.M. and Romanovsky, A.A. (1994) Endogenous opioids and fever. In: E. Zeisberger, E. Shönbaum and P. Lomax (Eds.), *Thermal Balance in Health and Disease: Recent Basic Research and Clinical Progress*, Birkhäuser, Basel, pp. 435–441.

Blatteis, C.M. and Sehic, E. (1997a) Fever: how may circulating pyrogens signal the brain? *News Physiol. Sci.*, 12: 1–9.

Blatteis, C.M. and Sehic, E. (1997b) Prostaglandin E2: a putative fever mediator. In: P.A. Mackowiak (Ed.), *Fever: Basic Mechanisms and Management*, Lippincott-Raven, Philadelphia, 2nd edn., pp. 117–145.

Blatteis, C.M., Bealer, S.L., Hunter, W.S., Llanos-Q, J., Ahokas, R.A. and Mashburn, Jr., T.A. (1983) Suppression of fever after lesions of the anteroventral third ventricle in guinea pigs. *Brain Res. Bull.*, 11: 519–526.

Blatteis, C.M., Hales, J.R.S., McKinley, M.J. and Fawcett, A.A. (1987a) Role of the anteroventral third ventricle region in fever in sheep. *Can. J. Physiol. Pharmacol.*, 65: 1255–1260.

Blatteis, C.M., Hunter, W.S., Wright, J.M., Ahokas, R.A., Llanos-Q., J. and Mashburn, Jr., T.A. (1987b) Thermoregulatory responses of guinea pigs with anteroventral third ventricle lesions in guinea pigs. *Can. J. Physiol. Pharmacol.*, 65: 1261–1266.

Blatteis, C.M., Xin, L. and Quan, N. (1991) Neuromodulation of fever: apparent involvement of opioids. *Brain Res. Bull.*, 26: 219–223.

Blatteis, C.M., Xin, L. and Quan, N. (1994) Neuromodulation of fever: a possible role for substance P. *Ann. New York Acad. Sci.*, 741: 162–173.

Bluthé, R.-M., Walter, V., Parnet, P., Layé, S., Lestage, J., Verrier, D., Poole, S., Stenning, B.E., Kelley, K.W. and Dantzer, R. (1994) Lipopolysaccharide induces sickness behavior in rats by a vagal mediated mechanism. *C. R. Acad. Sci. Paris, Sciences de la vie*, 317: 499–503.

Bowen, W.D., Gentleman, S., Herkenham, M. and Pert, C.B. (1981) Interconverting μ and δ forms of the opiate receptor in rat striatal patches. *Proc. Natl. Acad. Sci. USA*, 78: 4818–4822.

Brownstein, M.J. (1993) A brief history of opiates, opioid peptides, and opioid receptors. *Proc. Natl. Acad. Sci. USA*, 90: 5391–5393.

Carr, D.B., Bergland, R., Hamilton, A., Blume, H., Kasting, N., Arnold, M., Martin, J.B. and Rosenblatt, M. (1982) Endotoxin-stimulated opioid secretion: two secretory pools and feedback control *in vivo*. *Science*, 217: 845–848.

Carr, D.J.J. (1991) The role of endogenous opioids and their receptors in the immune system. *Proc. Soc. Exp. Biol. Med.*, 198: 710–720.

Chamberlain, J.M. and Klein, B.L. (1994) A comprehensive review of naloxone for the emergency physician. *Am. J. Emerg. Med.*, 12: 650–660.

Clark, W.G. (1979) Influence of opioids on central thermoregulatory mechanisms. *Pharmacol. Biochem. Behav.*, 10: 609–613.

Clark, W.G. and Harris, N.F. (1978) Naloxone does not antagonize leukocytic pyrogen. *Eur. J. Pharmacol.*, 49: 301–304.

Cooper, J.R., Bloom, F.E. and Roth, R.H. (1986) Neuroactive peptides. In: *The Biochemical Basis of Neuropharmacology*, 5th edn., Oxford University Press, Oxford, pp. 352–387.

Cox, B. and Lee, T.F. (1982) Role of central neurotransmitters in fever. In: A.S. Milton (Ed.), Pyretics and Antipyretics, Springer, Berlin, pp. 125–150.

Davidson, J., Milton, A.S. and Rotondo, D. (1987) A study of the involvement of opioid receptor sub-types in normal thermoregulation and during fever in the rabbit. *Br. J. Pharmacol.*, 91: 494P.

Delaney, K.A. and Goldfrank, L.R. (1990) The metabolic aspects of hyperthermia. In: R.D. Cohen, B. Lewis, K.G.M.M. Alberti and A.M. Denman (Eds.), *The Metabolic and Molecular Basis of Disease*, Vol. 2, Baillière Tindall, London, pp. 381–402.

De Simoni, M.G., De Luigi, A., Gemma, L., Sironi, M., Manfridi, A. and Ghezzi, P. (1993) Modulation of systemic interleukin-6 induction by central interleukin-1. *Am. J. Physiol.*, 265: R739–R742.

Desjardins, G.C., Brawer, J.R. and Beaudet, A. (1990) Distribution of μ, δ, and κ opioid receptors in the hypothalamus of the rat. *Brain Res.*, 536: 114–123.

Egawa, M., Yoshimatsu, H. and Bray, G.A. (1993) Effect of β-endorphin on sympathetic nerve activity to interscapular brown adipose tissue. *Am. J. Physiol.*, 264: R109–R115.

Eichler, A.C., McFee, A.S. and Root, H.D. (1969) Heatstroke. *Am. J. Surg.*, 118: 855–861.

El-Sharkawy, T.Y., Al-Shireida, M.F. and Pilcher, C.W.T. (1991) Vascular effects of some opioid receptor agonists. *Can. J. Physiol. Pharmacol.*, 69: 846–851.

Faden, A. and Holaday, J.W. (1979) Opiate antagonists: a role in the treatment of hypovolemic shock: stereospecificity of physiologic and pharmacologic effects in the rat. *Science*, 205: 317–318.

Faden, A. and Holaday, J.W. (1980) Naloxone treatment of endotoxin shock: stereospecificity of physiologic and pharmacologic effects in the rat. *J. Pharmacol. Exp. Ther.*, 212: 441–447.

Faden, A., Jacobs, T.P. and Holaday, J.W. (1980) Endorphin-parasympathetic interactions in spinal shock. *J. Auton. Nerv. Syst.*, 2: 295–304.

Fagarasan, M.O., Aiello, F., Muegge, K., Durum, S. and Axelrod, J. (1990) Interleukin 1 induces β-endorphin secretion via Fos and Jun in AtT-20 pituitary cells. *Proc. Natl. Acad. Sci. USA*, 87: 7871–7874.

Foley, K.M. (1993) Opioids. *Neurol. Clin.*, 11: 503–522.

Forman, L.J., Sonntag, W.E. and Meites, J. (1983) Elevation of plasma LH in response to systemic injection of β-endorphin antiserum in adult male rats. *Proc. Soc. Exp. Biol. Med.*, 173: 14–16.

Gordon, C.J. (1996) Homeothermy: does it impede the response to cellular injury? *J. Therm. Biol.*, 21: 29–36.

Hall, D.M., Buettner, G.R., Matthes, R.D. and Gisolfi, C.V. (1994) Hyperthermia stimulates nitric oxide formation: electron paramagnetic resonance detection of ·NO-heme in blood. *J. Appl. Physiol.*, 77: 548–553.

Hales, J.R.S. (1983) Preface. In: M. Khogali and J.R.S. Hales (Eds.), *Heat Stroke and Temperature Regulation*, Academic Press, Sydney, pp. xi–xii.

Hattori, Y., Katafuchi, T. and Koizumi, K. (1991) Characterization of opioid-sensitive neurons in the anteroventral third ventricle region of polydipsic inbred mice *in vivo*. *Brain Res.*, 538: 283–288.

Hellon, R.F., Townsend, Y. and Cranston, W.I. (1985) Naloxone does not influence a pyrogen fever in rabbits. *Pflüg. Arch.*, 404: 290–291.

Heyman, J.S., Jiang, Q., Rothman, R.B., Mosberg, H.I. and Porreca, F. (1989) Modulation of μ mediated antinociception by δ agonists: characterization with antagonists. *Eur. J. Pharmacol.*, 169: 43–52.

Holaday, J.W. (1983) Cardiovascular effects of endogenous opiate systems. *Annu. Rev. Pharmacol. Toxicol.*, 23: 541–594.

Holaday, J.W., Wei, E., Loh, H.H. and Li, C.H. (1978) Endorphins may function in heat adaptation. *Proc. Natl. Acad. Sci. USA*, 75: 2923–2927.

Hori, T., Nakashima, T., Take, S., Kaizuka, Y., Mori, T. and Katafuchi, T. (1991) Immune cytokines and regulation of body temperature, food intake and cellular immunity. *Brain Res. Bull.*, 27: 309–313.

Hunter, W.S., Sehic, E. and Blatteis, C.M. (1994) Fever and the *Organum vasculosum laminae terminalis*: another look. In: A.S. Milton (Ed.), *Temperature Regulation: Recent Physiological and Pharmacological Advances*, Birkhäuser, Basel, pp. 75–79.

Johnson, J. and Proppe, D.W. (1996) Cardiovascular adjustments to heat stress. In: M.J. Fregly and C.M. Blatteis (Eds.), *Handbook of Physiology. Environmental Physiology*, Section 4, Vol. I, Oxford University Press, New York, pp. 215–243.

Kandasamy, S.B. and Williams, B.A. (1983a) Central effects of some peptide and non-peptide opioids and naloxone on thermoregulation in the rabbit. In: P. Lomax and E. Shönbaum (Eds.), *Environment, Drugs and Thermoregulation*, Karger, Basel, pp. 98–100.

Kandasamy, S.B. and Williams, B.A. (1983b) Hyperthermic effects of centrally injected (D-ala^2, N-Me-Phe^4, Met-(O)^5-ol)-enkephalin (FK 33-824) in rabbits and guinea pigs. *Neuropharmacology*, 22: 1177–1181.

Kandasamy, S.B. and Williams, B.A. (1983c) Hyperthermic responses to central injections of some peptide and non-peptide opioids in the guinea pig. *Neuropharmacology*, 22: 621–628.

Kapás, L. and Krueger, J.M. (1993) Effects of naloxone on pretreatment on interleukin 1-induced sleep and fever. *Sleep Res.*, 22: 435.

Katovich, M.J., Simpkins, J.W. and O'Mera, J. (1986) Effects of opioid antagonists and their quaternary analogs on temperature changes in morphine-dependent rats. *Life Sci.*, 39: 1845–1854.

Khachaturian, H., Lewis, M.E., Schafer, M.K.-H. and Watson, S.J. (1985) Anatomy of the CNS opioid systems. *Trends Neurosci.*, 8: 111–119.

Khogali, M. (1987) Heat stroke: an overview with particular reference to the Makkah pilgrimage. In: J.R.S. Hales and D.A.B. Richards (Eds.), *Heat Stress: Physical Exertion and Environment*, Excerpta Medica, Amsterdam, pp. 21–36.

Kielblock, A.J., Strydom, N.B., Burger, F.J., Pretorius, P.J. and Manjoo, M. (1982) Cardiovascular origins of heatstroke pathology: an anesthetized rat model. *Aviat. Space Environ. Med.*, 53: 171–178.

Kluger, M.J. (1991) Fever: role of pyrogens and cryogens. *Physiol. Rev.*, 71: 93–127.

Knigge, U., Kjaer, A., Jørgensen, A., Garbarg, M., Ross, C., Rouleau, A. and Warberg, J. (1994) Role of hypothalamic histaminergic neurons in mediation of ACTH and beta-endorphin responses to LPS endotoxin *in vivo*. *Neuroendocrinology*, 60: 243–251.

Kohno, Y., Tanaka, M., Haaki, Y. and Nagasaki, N. (1983) Differential modification by opioid agents in acutely enhanced noradrenaline release in discrete brain regions. *Eur. J. Pharmacol.*, 92: 265–268.

Kozak, W., Conn, C.A. and Kluger, M.J. (1995) Body temperature, motor activity, and feeding behavior of mice treated with β-chlornaltrexamine. *Physiol. Behav.*, 58: 353–362.

Kregel, K.C., Wall, P.T. and Gisolfi, C.V. (1988) Peripheral vascular responses to hyperthermia in the rat. *J. Appl. Physiol.*, 64: 2582–2588.

Layé, S., Bluthé, R.-M., Kent, S., Combe, C., Médina, C., Parnet, P., Kelley, K.W. and Dantzer, R. (1995) Subdiaphragmatic vagotomy blocks the induction of IL-1β mRNA in mice brain in response to peripheral LPS. *Am. J. Physiol.*, 268: R1327–R1331.

Leshin, L.S. and Malven, P.V. (1984) Bacteremia-induced changes in pituitary hormone release and effect of naloxone. *Am. J. Physiol.*, 247: E585–E591.

Lin, M.T. and Su, C.Y. (1979) Metabolic, respiratory, vasomotor and body temperature responses to β-endorphin and morphine in rabbits. *J. Physiol. (Lond.)*, 295: 179–189.

Lin, M.T., Uang, W.-N and Ho, L.-T. (1989) Hypothalamic somatostatin may mediate endotoxin-induced fever in the rat. *Arch. Pharmacol.*, 339: 608–612.

Lord, P.F., Kapp, D.S., Hayes, T. and Weshler, Z. (1984) Production of systemic hyperthermia in the rat. *Eur. J. Cancer Clin. Oncol.*, 20: 1079–1085.

Mansour, A., Khachaturian, H., Lewis, M.E., Akil, H. and Watson, S.J. (1987) Autoradiographic differentiation of mu, delta, and kappa opioid receptors in the rat forebrain and midbrain. *J. Neurosci.*, 7: 2445–2464.

Martin, W.R., Eades, C.G., Thomson, J.A., Huppler, R.E. and Gilbert, P.E. (1976) The effect of morphine and nalorphine-like drugs in the nondependent and morphine dependent chronic spinal dog. *J. Pharmacol. Exp. Ther.*, 197: 517–532.

Mayfield, K.P. and D'Alecy, L.G. (1992) Role of endogenous opioid receptors in the acute adaptation to hypoxia. *Brain Res.*, 582: 226–231.

Mayfield, K.P. and D'Alecy, L.G. (1994) *Delta*-1 opioid receptor dependence of acute hypoxic adaptation. *J. Pharmacol. Exp. Ther.*, 268: 74–77.

Menzies, R.A., Patel, R., Hall, N.R.S., O'Grady, M.P. and Rier, S.E. (1992) Human recombinant interferon alpha inhibits naloxone binding to rat brain membranes. *Life Sci.*, 50: 227–232.

Milne, R.J., Coddington, J.M. and Gambe, G.D. (1990) Quaternary naloxone blocks morphine analgesia in spinal but not intact rats. *Neurosci. Lett.*, 114: 259–264.

Milton, A.S., Eastmond, N.C. and Davidson, J. (1994) Peripheral administration of the opiate antagonist naloxone attenuates the febrile response to polyinosinic: polycytidilic acid. In: E. Zeisberger, E. Shönbaum and P. Lomax (Eds.),

Thermal Balance in Health and Disease: Recent Basic Research and Clinical Progress, Birkhäuser, Basel, pp. 427–432.

Moltz, H. (1993) Fever: causes and consequences. *Neurosci. Biobehav. Rev.*, 17: 237–267.

Moskowitz, A.S. and Goodman, R.R. (1984) Light microscopic autoradiographic localization of μ and δ opioid binding sites in the mouse central nervous system. *J. Neurosci.*, 4: 1331–1342.

Murphy, M.T., Koenig, J.I. and Lipton, J.M. (1983) Changes in central concentration of β-endorphin in fever. *Fed. Proc.*, 42: 464.

Nadel, E.R., Fortney, S.M. and Wenger, C.B. (1980) Effect of hydration state on circulatory and thermal regulations. *J. Appl. Physiol.*, 49: 715–721.

Nakashima, T., Hori, T., Kuriyama, K. and Kiyohara, T. (1987) Naloxone blocks the interferon-α induced changes in hypothalamic neuronal activity. *Neurosci. Lett.*, 82: 332–336.

Nakashima, T., Hori, T., Kuriyama, K. and Matsuda, T. (1988) Effects of interferon-α on the activity of preoptic thermosensitive neurons in tissue slices. *Brain Res.*, 454: 361–367.

Nakashima, T., Kiyohara, T. and Hori, T. (1992) Effect of naltrexone on interferon α fever. *Neurosci. Res.*, S17: 156.

Niijima, A. (1992) The afferent discharges from sensors for interleukin-1beta in hepatoportal system in the anesthetized rat. *J. Physiol. (Lond.)*, 446: 236P.

Norman, D.C., Lin, J.H., Morley, J.E. and Yoshikawa, T.T. (1986) Aging and fever: naloxone blocks the thermogenic effect of interleukin-1. *Clin. Res.*, 34: 87.

Pae, Y.S., Lai, H. and Horita, A. (1985) Hyperthermia in the rat from handling stress blocked by naltrexone injected into the preoptic-anterior hypothalamus. *Pharmacol. Biochem. Behav.*, 22: 337–339.

Panerai, A.E., Martini, A., Casanueva, F., Petraglia, F., Di Giulio, A.M. and Mantegazza, P. (1983) Opiates and their antagonists modulate luteinizing hormone acting outside the blood brain barrier. *Life Sci.*, 32: 1751–1756.

Panjwani, G.D., Mustafa, M.K., Muhailan, A., Aneja, I.S. and Owunwanne, A. (1991) Effect of hyperthermia on somatosensory evoked potentials in anaesthetized rat. *Electroencephalogr. Clin. Neurophysiol.*, 80: 384–391.

Pasternak, G.W. (1993) Progress in opioid pharmacology. In: C.R. Chapman and K.M. Foley (Eds.), *Advances in Pain Research and Therapy. Current and Emerging Issues in Cancer Pain: Research and Practice*, Raven Press, New York, pp. 113–127.

Pleuvry, B.J. (1991) Opioid receptors and their ligands: natural and unnatural. *Br. J. Anaesth.*, 66: 370–380.

Proppe, D.W. (1990) Effect of hyperosmolarity and diuretics on baboon limb vasodilation during heating. *Am. J. Physiol.*, 258: R309–R317.

Puig, M.M., Miralles, F. and Laorden, L. (1986) Naloxone prevents hyperthermia induced convulsions in immature rats. *Methods Find. Exp. Clin. Pharmacol.*, 8: 649–653.

Romanovsky, A.A. and Blatteis, C.M. (1994) Elevation of body temperature per se induces the late phase syndrome. In: A.S. Milton (Ed.), *Temperature Regulation: Recent Physiological and Pharmacological Advances*, Birkhäuser, Basel, pp. 41–46.

Romanovsky, A.A. and Blatteis, C.M. (1995) Biphasic fever: what triggers the second temperature rise? *Am. J. Physiol.*, 269: R280–R286.

Romanovsky, A.A. and Blatteis, C.M. (1996) Heat stroke: opioid-mediated mechanisms. *J. Appl. Physiol.*, 81: 2565–2570.

Romanovsky, A.A., Shido, O., Ungar, A.L. and Blatteis, C.M. (1994) Peripheral naloxone attenuates lipopolysaccharide fever in guinea pigs by an action outside the blood–brain barrier. *Am. J. Physiol.*, 266: R1824–R1831.

Romanovsky, A.A., Kulchitsky, V.A., Akulich, N.V., Koulchitsky, S.V., Simons, C.T., Sessler, D.I. and Gourine, V.N. (1996a) The first and second phases of biphasic fever: two sequential stages of the sickness syndrome? *Am. J. Physiol.*, 271: R244–R253..

Romanovsky, A.A., Shido, O., Sakurada, S., Sugimoto, N. and Nagasaka, T. (1996b) Endotoxin shock: thermoregulatory mechanisms. *Am. J. Physiol.*, 270: R693–R703.

Romanovsky, A.A., Kulchitsky, V.A., Simons, C.T., Sugimoto, N. and Székely, M. (1997a) Febrile responsiveness of vagotomized rats is suppressed even in the absence of malnutrition. *Am. J. Physiol.*, 273: R777–R783.

Romanovsky, A.A., Simons, C.T., Székely, M. and Kulchitsky, V.A. (1997b) The vagus nerve in the thermoregulatory response to systemic inflammation. *Am. J. Physiol.*, 273: R407–413.

Rothman, R.B., Lon, J.B., Bykov, V., Jacobson, A.C., Rice, K.C. and Holaday, J.W. (1990) Pretreatment of rats with the irreversible μ receptor antagonist β-FNA, fails to prevent naltrexone-induced upregulation of μ opioid receptors. *Neuropharmacology*, 29: 805–810.

Sehic, E. and Blatteis, C.M. (1996) Blockade of lipopolysaccharide-induced fever by subdiaphragmatic vagotomy in guinea pigs. *Brain Res.*, 726: 160–166.

Shibata, M. and Blatteis, C.M. (1991) Human recombinant tumor necrosis factor and interferon affect the activity of neurons in the *organum vasculosum laminae terminalis*. *Brain Res.*, 562: 323–326.

Shibolet, S., Lancaster, M.C. and Danon, Y. (1976) Heat stroke: a review. *Aviat. Space Environ. Med.*, 47: 280–301.

Shido, O., Yoneda, Y. and Nagasaka, T. (1991) Shifts in the hypothalamic temperature of rats acclimated to direct internal heat load with different schedules. *J. Therm. Biol.*, 16: 276–271.

Shido, O., Romanovsky, A.A., Ungar, A.L. and Blatteis, C.M. (1993) Role of intrapreoptic norepinephrine in endotoxin-induced fever in guinea pigs. *Am. J. Physiol.*, 265: R1369–R1375.

Sirén, A.-L. and Feuerstein, G. (1992) The opioid system in circulatory control. *News Physiol. Sci.*, 7: 26–30.

Spencer, R.L., Hruby, V.J. and Burks, T.F. (1990) Alteration of thermoregulatory set point with opioid agonists. *J. Pharmacol. Exp. Ther.*, 252: 696–704.

Stitt, J.T. (1985) Evidence for the involvement of the *organum vasculosum laminae terminalis* in the febrile response of rabbits and rats. *J. Physiol. (Lond.)*, 368: 501–511.

Székely, M., Balaskó, M. and Romanovsky, A.A. (1995) Capsaicin-sensitive neural afferents in fever pathogenesis. *Pflüg. Arch.*, 430 (suppl.): R61.

Szelényi, Z., Barthó, L., Székely, M. and Romanovsky, A.A. (1994) Cholecystkinin octapeptide (CCK-8) injected into a cerebral ventricle induces a fever-like thermoregulatory response mediated by type B CCK-receptors in the rat. *Brain Res.*, 638: 67–77.

Thornhill, J.A., Cooper, K.E. and Veale, W.L. (1980) Core temperature changes following administration of naloxone and naltrexone to rats exposed to hot and cold ambient temperatures. Evidence for the physiological role of endorphins in hot and cold acclimatization. *J. Pharm. Pharmacol.*, 32: 427–430.

Valentino, R.J., Katz, J.L., Medzihradsky, F. and Woods, J.H. (1983) Receptor binding, antagonist, and withdrawal precipitating properties of opiate antagonists. *Life Sci.*, 32: 2887–2896.

Vybíral, S., Székely, M., Janský, L. and Černý, L. (1987) Thermoregulation of the rabbit during the late phase of endotoxin fever. *Pflüg. Arch.*, 410: 220–222.

Watkins, L.R., Wiertlak, E.P., Goehler, L.E., Smith, K.P., Martin, D. and Maier, S.F. (1994) Characterization of cytokine-induced hyperalgesia. *Brain Res.*, 664: 15–26.

Watkins, L.R., Goehler, L.E., Relton, J.K., Tartaglia, N., Silbert, L., Martin, D. and Maier, S.F. (1995a) Blockade of interleukin-1 induced hyperthermia by subdiaphragmatic vagotomy: evidence for vagal mediation of immune-brain communication. *Neurosci. Lett.*, 183: 27–31.

Watkins, L.R., Maier, S.F. and Goehler, L.E. (1995b) Cytokine-to-brain communication: a review & analysis of alternative mechanisms. *Life Sci.*, 57: 1011–1026.

Wei, E.T., Lee, A. and Chang, J.K. (1980) Cardiovascular effects of peptides related to enkephalins and beta-casomorphin. *Life Sci.*, 26: 1517–1522.

Wiederman, C.J. (1989) Interleukin-1 interaction with neuroregulatory systems: selective enhancement by recombinant human and mouse interleukin-1 *in vitro* opioid receptor binding in rat brain. *J. Neurosci. Res.*, 22: 172–180.

Wilkinson, D.A., Burholt, D.R. and Srivastava, P.N. (1988) Hypothermia following whole-body heating of mice: effect of heating time and temperature. *Int. J. Hyperthermia*, 4: 171–182.

Wright, C.L. (1976) Critical thermal maximum in mice. *J. Appl. Physiol.*, 40: 683–687.

Wright, D.J.M. and Weller, M.P.I. (1980) Inhibition by naloxone of endotoxin-induced reactions in mice. *Br. J. Pharmacol.*, 70: 99.

Xin, L. and Blatteis, C.M. (1992) Hypothalamic neuronal responses to interleukin-6 in tissue slices: effects of indomethacin and naloxone. *Brain Res. Bull.*, 29: 27–35.

Xin, L., Geller, E.B. and Adler, M.W. (1996) Involvement of opioid and prostaglandin systems in interleukin-1 β-induced fever in rats. *FASEB J.*, 10: A120.

Yang, S.-X. and Li, X.I. (1989) Enhancement of interleukin-1 production in mouse peritoneal macrophages by methionine-enkephalin. *Acta Pharmacol. Sin.*, 10: 266–270.

Yehuda, S. and Kastin, A.J. (1980) Peptides and thermoregulation. *Neurosci. Biobehav. Rev.*, 4: 459–471.

Young, W.S., Wamsley, J.K., Zarbin, M.A. and Kuhar, M.J. (1980) Opiate receptors undergo axonal flow. *Science*, 210: 76–77.

Zawada, W.M., Clarke, J. and Ruwe, W.D. (1992) Systemic and central administration of naloxone (NLX): differential alteration of fevers induced by intracerebroventricular (ICV) endogenous pyrogens (EPs). *FASEB J.*, 6: A1199.

H.S. Sharma and J. Westman (Eds.)
Progress in Brain Research, Vol 115

CHAPTER 8

Prostaglandins and fever

A.S. Milton

Department of Pharmacology, University of Cambridge, Tennis Court Road, Cambridge, CB2 1QJ, UK

Introduction

Fever is a major manifestation of the acute phase of the immune response to infection caused by a variety of micro-organisms and viruses. The actions of exogenous pyrogens such as bacterial endotoxin (lipopolysaccharide) and muramyl dipeptide, and synthetic pyrogens such as the ribonucleotide polyinosinic:polycytidylic acid (Poly I:C) are thought to be mediated through a number of cytokines including interleukin 1, 6 and 8, and interferon γ which are released from cells of the reticuloendothelial system. These cytokines are thought to, in turn, activate the synthesis of prostaglandins, which may be regarded as the final common mediators.

That prostaglandins have a role in fever was first intimated by Milton and Wendlandt (1970) when they reported that prostaglandin E_1 when injected into the cerebral ventricles of the conscious cat produced a rise in deep body temperature. The rise in temperature was accompanied by shivering, piloerection, vasoconstriction and with the animals taking up a 'curled up' position. These effects produced by the injection of prostaglandin E_1 (PGE_1) were almost identical with those observed following the injection of bacterial pyrogen. The main differences being that the effect of the prostaglandin was short lasting and the response was monophasic whereas the effects of bacterial pyrogens were long lasting and biphasic. The most important observation made by Milton and Wendlandt on the effects of i.c.v. injection of

PGE_1 was that they were neither prevented nor abolished by the administration of the antipyretic, non-steroidal anti-inflammatory drug, paracetamol (4-acetamidophenol). This was in direct contrast to the effects of paracetamol on bacterial pyrogen fever (Milton and Wendlandt, 1968).

It was as a result of these observations that Milton and Wendlandt stated, 'it is possible to speculate that PGE_1 may be acting as a modulator in temperature regulation and that the action of antipyretics may be to interfere with the release of PGE_1'.

In 1971, Vane published a paper in which he showed that the synthesis of the prostaglandins could be inhibited by aspirin-like drugs. He proposed that all three actions of these drugs, namely, antipyretic, analgesic and anti-inflammatory were mediated by the inhibition of prostaglandin synthesis. The interference in release of PGE_1 as proposed by Milton and Wendlandt, could now be correctly explained as an inhibition of synthesis. The end result of course being the same, that PGE_1 was responsible for fever, and in its absence, produced by inhibition of synthesis, rather than inhibition of release, then fever could not occur.

Prostaglandins of the E series

In their first experiments, Milton and Wendlandt (1970) had injected PGE_1, as this was the only one available to them at that time; subsequently they administered PGE_2, and compared its effects with PGE_1 (Milton and Wendlandt, 1971). They were found to be approximately equipotent, with both producing a rise in body temperature which was unaffected by the antipyretic paracetamol. The threshold dose for PGE_1 was in the order of 10 ng (2.8×10^{-11} M) which made it the most potent substance then known to produce a rise in body temperature. The effects of PGE_1 were dose-dependent. In contrast PGA_1, $PGF_{1\alpha}$ and $PGF_{2\alpha}$ were without effect on body temperature at the same dose level. In 1971, Feldberg and Saxena located the site of action of PGE_1 to the pre optic area of the anterior hypothalamus (PO/AH).

In 1970, Milton and Wendlandt reported that a prostaglandin-like substance had been found in cat cerebral spinal fluid, and in 1973, Feldberg and Gupta obtained cerebrospinal fluid (csf) from the third ventricle of the conscious cat and assayed it for contractile activity using the rat fundus strip preparation. They found that in csf from afebrile animals, contractile activity was very low or absent, whereas during fever produced by injecting pyrogen directly into the third cerebral ventricle, the contractile activity of the csf was considerably greater. On administration of paracetamol which produced defervescence, the activity was again low. Feldberg et al. (1973) collected csf from the cisterna magna of the conscious cat and measured this for prostaglandin like activity. They found that the O-somatic antigen of *Shigella dysenteriae* produced a fever when given intravenously and at the same time increased the PG like activity in the csf. They also observed that the three different antipyretic actions, aspirin, paracetamol and indomethacin all abolished the fever and at the same time the PG like activity of the csf fell. Thin layer chromatography of the csf samples followed by bioassay and radio immunoassay indicated that the prostaglandin present in the csf was PGE_2.

Prostaglandins of the F series

In the experiments of Milton and Wendlandt (1971), the thermoregulatory activity of the F prostaglandins was very low compared with PGE_2. In 1976, Ewen et al. reinvestigated the ther-

moregulatory effects of $PGF_{2\alpha}$ and showed that its thermoregulatory activity was approximately 1/27 that of PGE_2. Milton et al. (1993a) measured simultaneously circulating blood levels of PGE_2 and $PGF_{2\alpha}$ during Poly I:C induced fever. They found that PGE_2 levels rose from about 45 ng/l to 250 ng/l, whereas $PGF_{2\alpha}$ levels increased from 850 ng/l to over 2.5 μg/l. At these levels $PGF_{2\alpha}$ could be contributing to the febrile response. Of particular interest was that, though the PGE_2 blood levels showed two peaks corresponding to the first and second peaks of the febrile response, the changes in $PGF_{2\alpha}$ were monophasic, reaching a maximum during the development of the second febrile peak. The nonsteroidal anti-inflammatory drug Ketoprofen, reduced the circulating levels of both PGE_2 and $PGF_{2\alpha}$ to undetectable levels.

Mode of action of prostaglandins

Prostaglandins increase body temperature by increasing heat production and decreasing heat loss. In their first experiments, Milton and Wendlandt (1971) report that when PGE_1 and PGE_2 are injected into the lateral ventricles of cats, the animals shiver (increased heat production), vasoconstrict, piloerect and curl up in a ball (decreased heat loss). They also showed that in the rabbit the ears became vasoconstricted thus reducing heat loss. The mechanisms were comprehensively investigated by Bligh and Milton (1973) when they infused PGE_1 into the lateral ventricles of Welsh mountain sheep maintained at different ambient temperatures. They measured deep body temperature, respiratory rate, ear skin temperature and shivering. The sheep was chosen as the experimental animal for this study because of its ability to maintain a constant deep body temperature when exposed to a wide range of ambient temperatures, varying from below freezing to well above its deep body temperature. It does this by regulating both heat gain and heat loss mechanisms. Bligh and Milton used three different ambient temperatures, namely 10, 18 and 45°C and the animals were shorn to circumvent the insulation provided by the wool. PGE_1 was infused at a rate of 2.5 μg/min. When the ambient temperature was cold (10°C), respiratory rate was low, minimizing heat loss, and the ear skin temperature was the same as the ambient temperature, indicating vasoconstriction. Occasional bursts of electrical activity recorded from a thigh muscle indicated sporadic shivering (heat production). These results showed that the sheep were maintaining deep body temperature by minimizing heat loss and occasionally increasing heat production. When the PGE_1 infusion was started there was no change in ear skin temperature, the respiratory rate dropped slightly and vigorous shivering was recorded. This resulted in an immediate rise in deep body temperature. The elevated temperature was maintained for as long as the infusion was continued. However, as soon as the infusion was stopped the animals began to pant, shivering stopped and the body began to lose heat until deep body temperature had returned to the pre-infusion level. In contrast when the animals were maintained at an ambient temperature of 45°C, that is above deep body temperature, the ear blood vessels were fully dilated, and vigorous panting was observed with no sign of shivering. The animals were, therefore, actively preventing deep body temperature from rising by evaporative heat loss. Under these conditions when the PGE_1 infusion was started the respiratory rate dropped dramatically; but there was no vasoconstriction and no shivering. Deep body temperature rose rapidly due to the inhibition of the evaporative heat loss produced by panting, and the animals being unable to lose heat in the presence of a high ambient temperature. Immediately the PGE_1 infusion was stopped, panting recommenced and rose well above the pre-infusion level. This elevated panting was maintained until the deep body temperature had returned to normal. When the sheep were maintained at 18°C, the ear skin temperature was between deep body temperature and air temperature, indicating controlled vasomotor tone. There was no shivering but an elevated respiratory rate. It should be noted that though

the animals were at 'room temperature', a temperature of 18°C is considerably greater than that normally experienced during a summer day in the mountains. The PGE_1 infusion produced a fall in respiratory rate, a decrease in ear skin temperature, indicating vasoconstriction and an occasional burst of shivering (heat production). When the infusion was stopped, shivering ceased, ear skin temperature rose (vasodilatation) and the respiratory rate rose (evaporative heat loss). The deep body temperature soon returned to normal. In a further series of experiments, Milton et al. (1981, 1983) showed that in the endotoxin resistant MFI mouse, injection of PGE_2 intracerebroventricularly produced a coordinated increase in oxygen consumption, vasoconstriction and a rise in deep body temperature.

Prostaglandins and the 'set point'

The experiments on the effects of PGE_1 and PGE_2 show quite clearly that prostaglandins raise body temperature by a coordinated increase in heat production and a decrease in heat loss. Body temperature rises until a new equilibrium has been reached. Similarly on removal of the prostaglandin, deep body temperature actively falls until the previous equilibrium is reached. Extrapolating this to fever and antipyresis, fever produced by an increase in prostaglandin production equates to the reaching of a new equilibrium and antipyresis, produced by drugs which inhibit the synthesis and hence availability of prostaglandins, is a return of the elevated febrile temperature to normal. There is no need to postulate that fever is an elevation of 'set point' or antipyresis a resetting of the 'set point' to normal. Indeed the idea of 'set point' is as unnecessary as postulating that there is a 'barostat' setting blood pressure, or 'glucostat' setting blood sugar levels. One should not forget Claude Bernard and the *milieu interior*.

Source of prostaglandins producing fever

There is no evidence that either bacterial endotoxin or interleukin-1 can cross the blood–brain barrier. It has been shown that radiolabelled lipopolysaccharide given peripherally is not detected in csf collected from the cisterna magna whilst being able to produce fever, indicating that the lipopolysaccharide does not cross the blood–brain barrier (Dascombe and Milton, 1979). Similarly, purified natural [^{125}I]IL-1 and recombinant [^{125}I]IL-1 have been administered peripherally and it has been demonstrated that no IL-1 enters the brain parenchyma (Dinarello et al., 1978; Blatteis et al., 1989). In addition no interleukin-1 can be detected in the csf of cats after the i.v. injection of endotoxin (Coceani et al., 1988). In their study the IL-1 content of csf was measured during both the rising phase of the endotoxin fever and at the peak of the febrile response. No IL-1 could be found in the csf at any time indicating that the increase in body temperature did not occur in response to centrally acting IL-1. However as was first reported by Feldberg et al. (1973), pyrogens increase the level of PGE_2 in the csf during pyrogen-induced fever.

Hashimoto et al. (1991) showed that circulating colloidal gold-labelled IL-1β did not cross the endothelium of brain blood vessels in rabbits whilst retaining its pyrogenic activity. The prostaglandins responsible for fever may, therefore, reach the PO/AH either by crossing the blood–brain barrier from the peripheral circulation, or by being synthesized within the CNS by the action of pyrogens triggering events outside the blood–brain barrier. A possible site for such an action of the pyrogens is the OVLT.

In 1988, Rotondo et al. showed that during fever produced by three different pyrogens, bacterial endotoxin, the pyrogenic interferon inducer polyinosinic:polycytidylic acid (PolyI:C) and interleukin-1, the circulating levels of PGE_2 in the blood mirrored the changes in body temperature. The non-steroidal drug ketoprofen when administered at the height of the fevers produced an immediate defervescence and a simultaneous decrease in plasma PGE_2 levels. When ketoprofen was administered before the pyrogens, there were no rises in body temperature nor increases in

circulating levels of PGE_2. When the experimental animals were subjected to an environmental temperature of 34°C, a hyperthermia was observed without any changes in the blood PGE_2 levels. The authors conclude that the increases in circulating PGE_2, following pyrogen administration are responsible for the febrile response.

In a recent publication, Abul et al. (1996) have shown that PGE_2 enters the brain following stimulation of the acute phase immune response by pyrogen. They showed that the levels of PGE_2 in samples of csf collected by push–pull perfusion of the third cerebral ventricle during the first peak of the febrile response to bacterial pyrogen increased almost eight times that from csf of control animals receiving saline. A similar increase was observed during a fever produced by Poly I:C.

In order to ascertain whether changes in the levels of PGE_2 in csf samples were associated with the entry of PGE_2 from the peripheral circulation, animals were administered [^{125}I]PGE_2 i.v. followed by sampling csf by push–pull perfusion and measuring the levels of radioactivity. Animals were given either LPS or Poly I:C and subsequently a bolus injection of [^{125}I]PGE_2 5 min before the peak increase in body temperature followed by sampling of csf during the peak changes in body temperature. Radioactivity measured from csf samples collected from saline-treated animals was indistinguishable from the background level. However, the radioactivity collected during the peak of the febrile response was considerably elevated. The authors conclude from their experiments that either PGE_2 enters the CNS only in the presence of immunomodulators activated outwith the CNS by pyrogens, or that the pyrogens directly facilitate the entry of PGE_2 into the CNS from the periphery. The authors are of the opinion that the second of these two alternatives is the most likely. The experiments by Davidson et al. (1991) that lipocortin is antipyretic would also support the view that peripherally derived prostaglandins are responsible for fever. Lipocortin, being a protein, is a large molecule and would not be expected to cross the blood–brain barrier, and therefore must be inhibiting prostaglandin synthesis peripherally not centrally.

Antipyresis

Non-steroidal anti-inflammatory antipyretic drugs

One of the most important observations made by Milton and Wendlandt (1968) was that whereas the fever produced by bacterial endotoxin was completely abolished or prevented by the non-steroidal antipyretic paracetamol (4-acetamidophenol), the fever produced by PGE_1 was unaffected. These results indicated that if prostaglandins were involved in fever, then antipyretic drugs must act between the action of the endotoxin and the action of the prostaglandins. At the time, how this could be achieved was not known. However, in 1971, Vane showed that aspirin-like drugs acted by inhibiting the enzyme system responsible for the synthesis of the prostaglandins. At that time, it was usually referred to as PG-synthetase, but is now known as cyclo-oxygenase which exits in at least two forms: COX-1 which is normally present in the various tissues, and an inducible form COX-2 (a discussion of these two enzymes is outside the scope of this chapter, but has been concisely reviewed by Vane (1994)). Suffice it to say that the synthesis of prostaglandins following activation of the system by pyrogens, both exogenous and endogenous, is completely inhibited by the non-steroidal anti-inflammatory antipyretic drugs. These drugs, when administered before the pyrogen completely inhibit any febrile response, whereas, when administered during the febrile response produce immediate defervescence. This inhibition of the fever occurs at all stages, both during the rising phase and at the first and second peaks. These observations indicate that prostaglandins are involved throughout all the phases of fever. At one time it had been suggested that the first phase was due to a prostaglandin whereas the second phase was due to some other agent, for example 5-hydroxytryptamine. The action of the antipyretics would

not support this view, unless one can believe that the COX inhibitors have two entirely different actions, both which are antipyretic. This is difficult to believe. What is more probable is that during the various phases of the febrile response the source of the prostaglandins changes, as perhaps different cells of the reticuloendothelial system are activated at different times. Another possibility is that if both PGE_2 and $PGF_{2\alpha}$ are involved, the proportion of each synthesized during the febrile response varies. One scenario is that PGE_2 is involved in the first phase and $PGF_{2\alpha}$ in the second. A third possibility is that the cytokines involved are different in the various phases, and this again could be linked to the cells involved. In addition different cytokines may be involved in activation of PGE_2 and $PGF_{2\alpha}$.

Steroidal anti-inflammatory drugs

The anti-inflammatory actions of the glucocorticoid steroids is generally accepted to be mediated by a phospholipase A_2 inhibitor known as lipocortin. Steroids are thought to stimulate messenger RNA to stimulate the production of lipocortin which is a protein and which in turn inhibits the cell membrane phospholipase A_2 (PLA_2). PLA_2 is responsible for the mobilization of arachidonic from membrane phospholipids. Arachidonic is the precursor of the eicosanoids including the prostaglandins. Inhibition of PLA_2 will therefore result in inhibition of prostaglandin synthesis, though at a stage earlier than the non-steroidal anti-inflammatories. Therefore, one would expect the glucocorticoids to be antipyretic though clinically they are not usually used for this purpose.

Abul et al. (1987) studied the antipyretic action of dexamethasone in great detail. Dexamethasone is a synthetic glucocorticoid with an anti-inflammatory potency some 25-fold greater than hydrocortisone. Abul et al. (1987) found that dexamethasone significantly reduced the febrile response to pyrogens, both exogenous and endogenous. However, the time course was of particular interest. A maximum effect was seen when the dexamethasone was administered 1 h before the pyrogen, with no effect when it was administered 6–72 h previously. When the pyrogen and steroid were administered together there was no inhibition of fever, and when given after the pyrogen a potentiation occurred. No explanation of this latter effect has yet been made. The dose response curve to dexamethasone showed that a maximum was seen with 3 mg/kg, with a lesser effect with 6 mg. In contrast to the aspirin like antipyretics which produce 100% inhibition of fever, with dexamethasone a maximum of 50% inhibition was seen.

Since lipocortin is though to be involved in the action of the steroids, Davidson et al. (1991) investigated the action of human recombinant

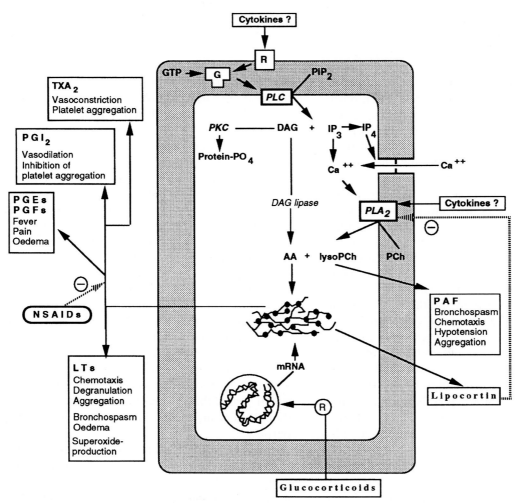

Fig. 1. Summary of the interrelationship between the cytokines, eicosanoids and antipyretic agents. NSAIDs, Non steroidal Anti-inflammatory Drugs; TXA$_2$, Thromboxane A$_2$; PGI$_2$, Prostacyclin; PGES, Prostaglandins of E series; PGFs, Prostaglandins of F series; LTs, Leukotrienes; PAF, Platelet Aggregating Factor; PLA$_2$, Phospholipase A$_2$; AA, Arachidonic Acid; R, Receptor; G, G-protein; PLC, Phospholipase C; IP3, Inositol triphosphate; IP4, Inositol 4 phosphate; PKC, Phosphokinase C; DAG, Diacyl glycerol; PCh, Phosphatidylcholine; GTP, Guanosine triphosphate [from Milton and Rotondo (1989), reprinted with kind permission of Karger AG, Basel, Switzerland].

lipocortin-1, and showed that it had antipyretic activity.

A summary of the interrelationship of the cytokines, prostaglandins and antipyretic agents is given in Fig. 1 (Milton and Rotondo, 1989).

Hypothalamic pituitary adrenal axis and prostaglandins

It is now generally accepted that fever is just one part of the response to infection and bacterial endotoxin, which *in toto* forms the acute phase of the immune response. This response involves the hypothalamus, pituitary and adrenal glands. Milton et al. (1992, 1993a,b,c) and Milton and Milton (1992) investigated the interrelationship between circulating prostaglandins, cortisol, ACTH and arginine vasopressin, and Davidson et al. (1992) reported on the effects of α-MSH on fever and circulating levels of PGE_2.

Milton et al. demonstrated the ability of pyrogens to activate the HPA axis as measured by increases in circulating immunoreactive cortisol at the same time as eliciting rises in body temperature and circulating prostaglandins. The activation of the HPA axis was shown to be CRF-41 dependent by the use of specific immunoneutralization. Using monoclonal anti-CRF-41 antibodies administered intravenously prior to administration of the pyrogen, poly I:C, the ir-cortisol response was abolished, suggesting a major role for CRF-41 in the HPA axis activation. AVP, another potent stimulus for ACTH *in vivo* which also has synergistic actions with CRF-41 in many stress responses (Gillies et al., 1982), does not appear to be a major component of the observed increases in circulating ir-cortisol. The AVP (V1) receptor antagonist, previously demonstrated to antagonize ACTH responses (Plotsky et al., 1985), had no effect on the poly I:C stimulated rises in circulating ir-cortisol. The observed increase in circulating ir-cortisol after poly I:C administration in animals pre-treated with the anti-inflammatory drug ketoprofen, which prevents the temperature rise plus the normally observed stimulation of both $irPGE_2$ and $irPGF_{2\alpha}$, suggests

that the stimulatory activity of poly I:C has a component independent of the elevated body temperature and prostaglandins. In conclusion therefore, poly I:C activates the HPA via a CRF-41 dependent and prostaglandin independent mechanism. Whether poly I:C activates the HPA directly or via a secondary mediator is unknown. Poly I:C itself activates cytokines and prostaglandins, two groups of compounds activated in immune challenge and by other pyrogens. The observations that poly I:C and the cytokines IL-1 and interferon (INF), known to be induced by poly I:C, fail to stimulate CRF-41 release from the rat hypothalamus *in vitro* (Milton et al., 1993d) suggests that the HPA axis activation by poly I:C may involve other mediators.

The cortisol and ACTH responses showed different time courses with cortisol levels raised after 90 min whilst ACTH was not raised. The elevation of ACTH after cortisol suggests that this may be a secondary activation of ACTH. The results suggest that rises in circulating ACTH levels during the febrile response to poly-I:C are not accompanied by rises in circulating CRF-41 and AVP levels and are independent of the changes in body temperature. The ACTH response occurs after the onset of temperature rises and between the two body temperature peaks.

It is suggested that peripheral AVP and CRF-41 have a modulatory role in the febrile response. The dose of Poly I:C used to induce fever was sub-maximal (Rotondo et al., 1987), to enable either inhibition or potentiation of the responses to be measured. The ability of peripheral immunoneutralization or CRF-41 receptor antagonism to attenuate the febrile response suggests that endogenous peripheral CRF-41 has a propyretic role in this system. Likewise peripheral AVP V1 receptor antagonism caused an attenuation of the febrile response suggesting that endogenous peripheral AVP has a pro-pyretic role in this system.

The results from this study show that antagonism of peripheral CRF-41 using either anti-CRF-41 antibodies or a CRF-41 receptor antagonist significantly reduced the Poly I:C-stimulated rises in circulating $irPGF_{2\alpha}$ and $irPGE_2$. The dose of CRF-41 antagonist used was similar to those reported to inhibit the cardiovascular but not the adrenocorticotrophin-inducing activities of CRF-41 (Fisher et al., 1991). Previous *in vitro* studies have shown that CRF-41 can stimulate release of PGE_2, but not PGD_2 or $PGF_{2\alpha}$, from the anterior pituitary gland (Vlaskovska et al., 1984). The observation that CRF-41 antagonism inhibits both the temperature and PG responses suggests that CRF-41 and PGs have roles in the febrile state. The marked reduction in the $PGF_{2\alpha}$ response by CRF-41 antagonism contrasts with a detectable, if reduced, febrile response suggesting that $PGF_{2\alpha}$ is not itself directly responsible for the fever. Previous studies have suggested that PGE_2 is the PG responsible for activation of the hypothalamic thermoregulatory centres (Milton and Wendlandt, 1971) and the results for CRF-41 receptor antagonism show a reduced but intact $irPGE_2$ response, in parallel with the effects on the febrile response. The time-course for the rises in core body temperature are paralleled by increases in circulating $irPGE_2$. However, the increases in $irPGF_{2\alpha}$ show a longer lag phase and reach a peak after the initial peaks in both core body temperature and $irPGE_2$. $PGF_{2\alpha}$ has been shown to have 1/27th of the potency of PGE_2 when tested for its ability to cause fevers (Milton and Wendlandt, 1971) and the role of $PGF_{2\alpha}$ in the febrile response to Poly I:C is unknown. The results for CRF-41 actions on PG production and release may provide an explanation of the mechanism underlying CRF-41 modulation of immune function (Jain et al., 1991).

The reduction in the febrile response to poly-I:C caused by administration of the AVP V1-antagonist was accompanied by an abolition of the circulating $irPGE_2$ response. The reduction in the $irPGF_{2\alpha}$ response to poly-I:C caused by administration of the V1-antagonist was less marked and only significant at the peak 2.5-h measurement. Poly-I:C induced temperature rises are PG dependent (Rotondo et al., 1987) and the observed antipyresis caused by the V1-antagonist may therefore be the result of inhibition of PGs. The specificity of the effects of the V1-antagonist on poly-I:C stimulated PGs, with effects on PGE_2 but not $PGF_{2\alpha}$, may provide an explanation for the partial inhibition of the febrile response. These differential effects of the AVP V1-antagonist on PGE_2 and $PGF_{2\alpha}$ responses may reflect different sites of PG production or an action of AVP which specifically modifies the PGE_2 response. Both PGE_2 and $PGF_{2\alpha}$ are pyrogenic when administered centrally (Milton and Wendlandt, 1971) and antipyretic drugs act by inhibition of arachidonic acid conversion to PGs (Vane, 1971). The results from this study suggest that the observed antipyresis with a V1-antagonist may be due to specific inhibition of PGE_2, which is the most potent fever-inducing prostaglandin (Milton and Wendlandt, 1971). The observation that the V1-antagonist pretreatment resulted in only a partially reduced febrile response to poly-I:C and a complete blockade of the observed PGE_2 response, suggests that another PG, possibly $PGF_{2\alpha}$, may be responsible for the observed rises in body temperature. Whilst the original studies by Milton and Wendlandt (1971) demonstrated that PGE_2 was the most potent prostaglandin with a potency 27 times that of $PGF_{2\alpha}$, the results from this study show poly-I:C stimulated levels of circulating $PGF_{2\alpha}$ are 10–15 times those of circulating PGE_2, suggesting that $PGF_{2\alpha}$ may be present at sufficient concentrations to elicit effects.

The suggestion that the pro-pyretic actions of AVP could be mediated via stimulatory actions on interferon production (Johnson et al., 1982; Johnson and Torres, 1985) are not incompatible with the results suggesting an involvement with PGE_2 since interferon fevers are PG dependent (Dinarello et al., 1984). This leads to the suggestion that poly-I:C induces an interferon, which in turn stimulates PGE_2, and that production of this interferon is modulated by peripheral AVP.

The significant reduction in the thermoregulatory index (TRI5) for the response to poly-I:C when animals were pre-treated with an AVP V1-antagonist was accompanied by a change in the

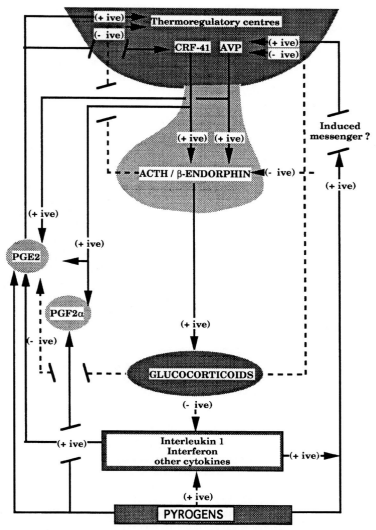

Fig. 2. Schematic diagram of the relationships between the hypothalamic pituitary axis, prostaglandins and fever. CRF-41, Corticotrophin Releasing Factor 41; ACTH, Adrenocorticotrophic Hormone; PGE_2, Prostaglandin E_2; $PGF_{2\alpha}$, Prostaglandin $F_{2\alpha}$; AVP, Arginine Vasopressin [from Milton (1994), reprinted with kind permission of Birkhäuser Verlag, Basel, Switzerland].

pattern of poly-I:C stimulated temperature rises. This change in the pattern of poly-I:C fever, from biphasic to monophasic, when the AVP V1-antagonist was administered peripherally, suggests either that AVP modulates the initial rises in body temperature or that the drop in body temperature could be due to stimulation of AVP,

which is producing a transient antipyretic effect. The previous observations of AVP induced antipyresis mediated via central AVP V1-receptors (Cooper et al., 1987) is consistent with the suggestion that the biphasic temperature change pattern could be due to transient AVP induced antipyresis.

A schematic diagram of the relationship between the HPA axis, prostaglandins and fever is given in Fig. 2 (Milton, 1994).

Acknowledgement

The author is in receipt of a Leverhulme Emeritus Fellowship.

References

Abul, H.T., Davidson, J., Milton, A.S. and Rotondo, D. (1987) Dexamethasone pre-treatment is antipyretic toward polyinosinic:polycytidylic acid, lipopolysaccharide and interleukin-1/endogenous pyrogen. *Naunyn-Schmiedberg's Arch. Pharmacol.*, 336: 332–341.

Abul, H.T., Davidson, J., Milton, A.S. and Rotondo, D. (1996) Prostaglandin E_2 enters the brain following stimulation of the acute phase immune response. In: C. Blatteis (Ed.), *Thermoregulation: Recent Progress and New Frontiers*, New York Academy of Science, New York.

Blatteis, C.M., Dinarello, C.A., Shibata, M., Lanos-Q, J.L., Quan, N. and Busija, D.W. (1989) Does circulating IL-1 enter the brain? In: J.B. Mercer (Ed.), *Thermal Physiology 1989*, Elsevier, Amsterdam, pp. 385–390.

Bligh, J. and Milton, A.S. (1973) The thermoregulatory effects of prostaglandin E_1 when infused into a lateral cerebral ventricle of the Welsh mountain sheep at different ambient temperatures. *J. Physiol. (Lond.)*, 229: 30–31P.

Coceani, F., Lees, J. and Dinarello, C.A. (1988) Occurrence of interleukin-1 in the cerebrospinal fluid of the conscious cat. *Brain Res.*, 446: 245.

Cooper, K.E., Naylor, A.M. and Veale, W.L. (1987) Evidence supporting a role for endogenous vasopressin in fever suppression in the rat. *J. Physiol. (Lond.)*, 387: 163–172.

Dascombe, M.J. and Milton, A.S. (1979) Study on the possible entry of bacterial endotoxin and prostaglandin E_2 into the central nervous system from the blood. *Br. J. Pharmacol.*, 66: 565–572.

Davidson, J., Flower, R.J., Milton, A.S., Peers, S. and Rotondo, D. (1991) Antipyretic actions of human recombinant lipocortin-1. *Br. J. Pharmacol.*, 102: 7–9.

Davidson, J., Milton, A.S. and Rotondo, D. (1992) α-Melanocyte-stimulating hormone suppresses fever and increases in plasma levels of prostaglandin E_2 in the rabbit. *J. Physiol. (Lond.)*, 451: 491–502.

Dinarello, C.A., Weiner, P. and Wolff, S.M. (1978) Radiolabelling and disposition in rabbits of purified human leucocytic pyrogen. *Clin. Res.*, 26: 522A.

Dinarello, C.A., Bernheim, H.A., Duff, G.W., Le, H.V., Nagabhushan, T.L., Hamilton, N.C. and Coceani, F. (1984) Mechanisms of fever induced by recombinant human interferon. *J. Clin. Invest.*, 74: 906–913.

Ewen, L., Milton, A.S. and Smith, S. (1976) Effects of prostaglandin $F_{2\alpha}$ and prostaglandin D_2 on the body temperature of conscious cats. *J. Physiol. (Lond.)*, 258: 121–122P.

Feldberg, W. and Gupta, K.P. (1973) Pyrogen fever and prostaglandin activity in cerebrospinal fluid. *J. Physiol. (Lond.)*, 228: 41–53.

Feldberg, W. and Saxena, P.N. (1971) Fever produced by prostaglandin E_1. *J. Physiol. (Lond.)*, 217: 547–556.

Feldberg, W., Gupta, K.P., Milton, A.S. and Wendlandt, S. (1973) Effect of pyrogen and antipyretics on prostaglandin activity in cisternal CSF of unanaesthetized cats. *J. Physiol. (Lond.)*, 234: 279–303.

Fisher, L., Rivier, C., Rivier, J. and Brown, M. (1991) Differential agonist activity of α-helical corticotropin releasing factor 9-41 in three bioassay systems. *Endocrinology*, 129: 1312–1316.

Gillies, G.E., Linton, E.A. and Lowry, P.J. (1982) Corticotropin releasing activity of the new CRF is potentiated several times by vasopressin. *Nature*, 299: 355–357.

Hashimoto, M., Ishikawa, Y.S., Yokota, S., Goto, F., Bando, T., Sakakibara, Y. and Iriki, M. (1991) Action site of circulating interleukin-1 on the rabbit brain. *Brain Res.*, 540: 217–223.

Jain, R., Zwicker, D., Hollander, C.S., Brand, H., Saperstein, A., Hutchinson, B., Brown, C. and Audhya, T. (1991) Corticotropin-releasing factor modulates the immune response to stress in the rat. *Endocrinology*, 128: 1329–1336.

Johnson, H.M. and Torres, B.A. (1985) Regulation of lymphokin production by arginine vasopressin and oxytocin: modulation of lymphocyte function by neurohypophyseal hormones. *J. Immunol.*, 135: 743s–745s.

Johnson, H.M., Farrar, W.L. and Torres, B.A. (1982) Vasopressin replacement of Interleukin-2 requirement in gamma interferon production: lymphokine activity of a neuroendocrine hormone. *J. Immunol.*, 129: 983–986.

Milton, A.S. and Milton, N.G.N. (1992) The modulatory role of peripheral corticotrophin-releasing factor (CRF) in the febrile response to polyinosinic:polycytidylic acid (poly-I:C). In: P. Lomax and E. Schönbaum (Eds.), *Thermoregulation: The Pathophysiological Basis of Clinical Disorders*, Karger, Basel, pp. 25–27.

Milton, A.S. and Wendlandt, S. (1968) The effect of 4-acetamidophenol in reducing fever produced by the intracerebral injection of 5-hydroxytryptamine and pyrogen in the conscious cat. *Br. J. Pharmacol.*, 34: 215–216P.

Milton, A.S. and Wendlandt, S. (1970) A possible role for prostaglandin E_1 as a modulator for temperature regulation in the central nervous system of the cat. *J. Physiol. (Lond.)*, 207: 76–77P.

Milton, A.S. and Wendlandt, S. (1971) Effects on body temperature of prostaglandins of the A, E and F series on injection into the third ventricle of unanaesthetized cats and rabbits. *J. Physiol. (Lond.)*, 218: 325–336.

Milton, A.S., Pertwee, R.G. and Todd, D.A. (1981) The effects of prostaglandin E_2 and pyrogen on thermoregulation in the MFI mouse. *J. Physiol. (Lond.)*, 322: 59P.

Milton, A.S., Pertwee, R.G. and Todd, D.A. (1983) Prostaglandin hyperthermia in mice: effects of ambient temperature. In: P. Lomax and E. Schönbaum (Eds.), *Environment, Drugs and Thermoregulation*, Karger, Basel, pp. 150–152.

Milton, I.H. and Rotondo, D. (1989) Cover Illustration. In: P. Lomax and E. Schönbaum (Eds.), *Thermoregulation: Research and Clinical Applications*, Karger, Basel.

Milton, N.G.N. (1994) Effect of peripheral corticotrophin-releasing factors on febrile responses. In: A.S. Milton (Ed.), *Temperature Regulation. Advances in Pharmacological Sciences*, Birkhäuser, Basel, pp. 1–10.

Milton, N.G.N., Hillhouse, E.W. and Milton, A.S. (1992) Activation of the hypothalamo-pituitary-adrenocortical axis in the conscious rabbit by the pyrogen polyinosinic:polycytidylic acid is dependent on corticotrophin releasing factor-41. *J. Endocrinol.*, 135: 69–75.

Milton, N.G.N., Hillhouse, E.W. and Milton, A.S. (1993a) Modulation of the prostaglandin response of conscious rabbits to the pyrogen polyinosinic: polycytidylic acid by corticotrophin-releasing factor-41. *J. Endocrinol.*, 138: 7–11.

Milton, N.G.N., Hillhouse, E.W. and Milton, A.S. (1993b) A possible role for endogenous peripheral corticotrophin-releasing factor-41 in the febrile response of conscious rabbits. *J. Physiol. (Lond.)*, 465: 415–425.

Milton, N.G.N., Hillhouse, E.W. and Milton, A.S. (1993c) Does endogenous peripheral arginine vasopressin have a role in the febrile response of conscious rabbits? *J. Physiol. (Lond.)*, 469: 525–534.

Milton, N.G.N., Self, C.H. and Hillhouse, E.W. (1993d) Effects of pyrogenic immunomodulators on the release of corticotrophin-releasing factor-41 and prostglandin E_2 from the intact rat hypothalamus *in vitro. Br. J. Pharmacol.*, 109: 88–93.

Plotsky, P.M., Bruhn, T.O. and Vale, W. (1985) Hypophysiotropic regulation of adrenocorticotropin secretion in response to insulin-induced hypoglycemia. *Endocrinology*, 117: 323–329.

Rotondo, D., Abul, H.T., Milton, A.S. and Davidson, J. (1987) The pyrogenic actions of the interferon-inducer polyinosinic: polycytidylic acid are antagonised by ketoprofen. *Eur. J. Pharmacol.*, 137: 257–260.

Rotondo, D., Abul, T., Milton, A.S. and Davidson, J. (1988) Pyrogenic immunomodulators increase the level of prostaglandin E_2 in the blood simultaneously with the onset of fever. *Eur. J. Pharmacol.*, 154: 145–152.

Vane, J.R. (1971) Inhibition of prostaglandin synthesis as a mechanism of action for aspirin-like drugs. *Nature New Biol.*, 23: 232–235.

Vane, J.R. (1994) Towards a better aspirin. *Nature*, 367: 215.

Vlaskovska, M.A., Hertting, G. and Knepel, W. (1984) Adrenocorticotropin and β-endorphin release from the rat adenohypophysis *in vitro*: inhibition by prostaglandin E_2 formed locally in response to vasopressin and corticotropin-releasing factor. *Endocrinology*, 115: 895–903.

H.S. Sharma and J. Westman (Eds.)
Progress in Brain Research, Vol 115
© 1998 Elsevier Science BV. All rights reserved.

CHAPTER 9

Brain eicosanoids and LPS fever: species and age differences

Vadim Fraifeld and Jacob Kaplanski*

Department of Clinical Pharmacology, Faculty of Health Sciences, Ben-Gurion University of the Negev, P.O.B. 653, Beer-Sheva 84105, Israel

Introduction

Fever is thought to be one of the important non-specific mechanisms of host defence against infections, being involved in so called 'acute phase response' (Kluger, 1986). The widely accepted paradigm of the concept of fever considers the critical role of prostaglandin E_2 (PGE_2), as a final central mediator of various pyrogens, in inducing a fever by resetting the hypothalamic thermoregulatory 'set point' to a new higher level. The possible involvement of several other eicosanoids (ESs) has been also suggested (for review, see Rothwell, 1992).

The role of brain ESs in the central mechanisms of fever gained support from three lines of observations: (1) a number of exogenously ESs, when administered i.c.v. or into certain brain regions, exert a considerable pyrogenic effect; (2) various systemically or intracerebrally administered pyrogens induce the increase in brain ES production; and (3) specific inhibitors of prostanoid synthesis are able to prevent or attenuate fever response to most pyrogens. However, regardless of numerous data accumulated in this area, the role of PGE_2, as well as ESs in general,

continues to be debatable (Coceani, 1991), up to the opinion that they are neither obligatory nor essential factors for the expression of pyrogen fever (Simpson et al., 1994).

The pyrogen applied traditionally in studies of fever is bacterial endotoxin (lipopolysaccharide, LPS), obtained from various pathogenic gram-negative bacteria. They express on their surface substrates (endotoxins) which are essential for bacterial growth and survival. Chemically, endotoxins are lipopolysaccharides composed of polysaccharide and lipid component, termed lipid A. The last one is responsible for the induction of endotoxin effects (for review, see Seydel et al., 1994). If released from the bacterial cell, endotoxins induce, in higher organisms, a variety of pathophysiological effects known as 'acute phase response', one of the most prominent manifestations of which are thermoregulatory alterations known as fever (Kluger, 1986). Being administered systemically or intracerebroventricularly (i.c.v.), LPS induces fever response in a variety of endothermic species (mice, rats, hamsters, guinea pigs, rabbits, cats, dogs, monkeys, chickens, pigeons) and induces also behavioral changes promoting an elevation in body temperature in ectotherms by preferring higher ambient temperature. The LPS exerts its pyrogenic features by inducing cascade of changes which effect on thermosensitive neurons in hypothalamic thermoregu-

_____

* Corresponding author.

latory center promoting them to a new level of functional activity (set point elevation).

It has been considered that the LPS can act directly on the thermoregulatory center in the hypothalamus or indirectly, by inducing the synthesis of endogenous pyrogens (cytokines), which also act on the hypothalamus to induce fever. Most of these cytokines stimulate the production of ESs in CNS, which (mainly prostaglandins of E series, and perhaps $PGF_{2\alpha}$) are considered to be responsible for thermoregulatory 'set point' elevation with subsequent manifestation of fever (for review, see Dinarello et al., 1988; Milton, 1989; Kluger, 1991; Rothwell, 1992, 1994; Saper and Breder, 1992).

Two aspects of the problem, i.e. species and age differences in the central mechanisms of fever, have received relatively less attention, although such information could be considerably valuable for understanding the role of brain ESs in pyrogenesis. Hence, it remains unclear if there are the common central mechanisms of fever across various species of endotherms, i.e. mammals and avians. In particular, little is known concerning the involvement of brain ESs in avian fever, as well as in pyrogen-induced thermoregulatory modifications in small mammals, which often develop hypothermia rather than hyperthermia in response to pyrogen. The impact of age on the relationship between pyrogen-induced synthesis of brain ESs and febrile response also has not yet been critically established, especially in developing and aged animals.

In the present study, the data obtained at our laboratory in the last few years on rodents, including rats of a wide age range, and birds will be presented. It should be emphasized that these investigations have been based on the common methodological approaches, that facilitate a comparison and interpretation of the results obtained on different strains and species. It seems that, at least in part, the existing controversies are related to certain difficulties in the interpretation of the data obtained on various species by using different methodologies. The pyrogenic effects of exogenous ESs will be mentioned briefly, focusing mainly on the effects of bacterial endotoxin on brain prostanoid production and body temperature in regard to (i) species, and (ii) age differences.

Pyrogenic effects of exogenous eicosanoids

The pyrogenic effects of exogenously administered ESs have been previously reviewed by Clark and Lipton (1985), Murphy and Pearce (1988), Coceani (1991) and Rothwell (1992). Here, the data obtained in various species and with various routes of administration are briefly summarized in Table 1.

As has been shown in numerous studies, the prostaglandins (PGs) of E series (both E_1 and E_2) are extremely potent hyperthermic agents, and their action has been observed across various mammalian species examined so far (rat, rabbit, cat, monkey, pig), as well as in birds (broilers).

$PGF_{2\alpha}$ appears to be almost equipotent with PGs of E series in developing fever. Moreover, it has been suggested that PGE_2 and $PGF_{2\alpha}$ may act via different mechanisms, since their maximal effects on fever and thermogenesis in rat are additive. Only $PGF_{2\alpha}$ but not PGE_2 appears to depend on CRF for its action (Rothwell, 1992; Coelho et al., 1995).

In regard to PGD_2, the data obtained so far are rather mixed: depending on the species studied, dose and route of administration, and, perhaps, arousal state, PGD_2 may exert mild or weak hyperthermic effects (Kantha et al., 1994), or even hypothermic (Ueno et al., 1982). Inhibition of the brain PGD_2 synthesis caused by inorganic selenium compounds (inhibitors of prostaglandin D synthase) was accompanied by a decrease in brain temperature during the nocturnal period (Takahata et al., 1993), when it increases generally, pointing at possible involvement of PGD_2 in thermoregulation.

Controversial results have also been reported for PGI_2. Ueno et al. (1982) failed to find any effect of intra-AH/POA PGI_2 administration on body temperature, while recently, it has been demonstrated that its stable analogue, iloprost,

TABLE 1

Effect of i.c.v. or intrahypothalamic (AH/POA, OVLT, PH) administration of exogenous eicosanoids on body temperature

Eicosanoids	Species	Effect	References
PGE_2	Rabbit	Hyperthermia	Lipton and Ticknor, 1979; Morimoto et al., 1990; Krueger et al., 1992; Watanabe et al., 1994
	Rat	Hyperthermia	Ueno et al., 1982; Amir et al., 1991; Morimoto et al., 1990, 1991
	Pig[a]	Hyperthermia	Parrott et al., 1995
	Broilers	Hyperthermia	Macari et al., 1993
PGE_1	Rabbit	Hyperthermia	Ruwe et al., 1988
	Rat	Hyperthermia	Stitt, 1991
	Monkey	Hyperthermia	Simpson et al., 1994
$PGF_{2\alpha}$	Rabbit	Hyperthermia	Watanabe et al., 1994
	Rat	Hyperthermia	Ueno et al., 1982
PGI_2	Rat	No effect	Splawinski et al., 1978; Ueno et al., 1982
	Rat[b]	Hyperthermia	Akarsu and Ayhan, 1993
PGD_2	Rabbit	Hyperthermia	Krueger et al., 1992
	Rat	Hyperthermia	Kantha et al., 1994
		Hypothermia	Ueno et al., 1982
	Cat	Hyperthermia	Ewen et al., 1976
	Monkey	Hyperthermia	Hayaishi, 1991
TXA_2	Rat	No effect	Splawinski et al., 1978
LTC_4, D_4, E_4	Rat	No effect	O'Rourke and Rudy, 1984; Kantha et al., 1994
LXA_4	Rat	No effect	Kantha et al., 1994
LXB_4	Rat	Hyperthermia	Kantha et al., 1994

AH/POA, preoptic area of anterior hypothalamus; OVLT, organum vasculosum laminae terminalis; PH, posterior hypothalamus.
[a] i.v. administration.
[b] Iloprost, a stable analogue of PGI_2.

can potentiate hyperthermic effects of PGE_2 (Akarsu and Ayhan, 1993).

Thromboxanes and leukotriens seem to be inactive in inducing fever (Splawinski et al., 1978; Hynes et al., 1991; Kantha et al., 1994). However, their indirect involvement cannot be excluded, in particular, via increasing the permeability of the blood–brain barrier for endogenous pyrogens.

Lipoxins may have a small hyperthermic effect, which has been found so far only for LXB_4 but not for LXA_4 (Kantha et al., 1994).

Hence, this set of data show that minute doses of certain ESs, examined so far, when administered near or intra putative site of thermoregulatory center, can exhibit thermoregulatory, predominantly, hyperthermic effects, and hence point at and support the idea of a possible implication of brain ESs, due to their thermoregulatory properties, in the central mechanisms of fever.

Effect of LPS on brain eicosanoid production and body temperature in endotherms

The studies conducted in the past (Feldberg and Gupta, 1973; Feldberg et al., 1973; Lipton and Ticknor, 1979; Bernheim et al., 1980; Coceani et al., 1983; and others) and also in recent years (Hynes et al., 1991; Coelho et al., 1995) on different laboratory mammals demonstrated that the concentration of certain ESs in CSF increased considerably in response to systemic or i.c.v. LPS administration. The effect was also observed on the hypothalamus, *in vivo* (Sirco et al., 1989) or ex vivo (Hadas et al., 1989; Kaplanski et al., 1989a,b, 1992, 1993, 1995, 1996a,b; Fraifeld and Kaplanski, 1993; Fraifeld et al., 1995b), and on ex vivo incubated frontal cortex (Weidenfeld et al., 1993). The elevation of PGs occurred in a dose-dependent manner and preceded the increase in body temperature. Noteworthy, LPS was found to cause an elevation of those ESs, which consistently exhibited a clear hyperthermic effect after their i.c.v. or intrahypothalamic administration, i.e. PGs of E series and $PGF_{2\alpha}$. Concerning the other ESs, our knowledge is still incomplete, and only sporadic data exist in literature. In particular, no detectable elevation of TXB_2 in CSF (Coceani et al., 1983), TXA_2 production by ex vivo incubated hypothalamus (Kaplanski et al., 1992), or leukotriens' concentration in CSF (Hynes et al., 1991) was observed in febrile animals.

The ability of different sites in CNS to produce ESs is now under intensive investigation. Cerebral endothelial cells (Wahl and Schilling, 1993; Spatz et al., 1994; De Vries et al., 1995) and glial cells (Murphy et al., 1988; Brenner et al., 1992; Nam et al., 1995) are considered to be the main sources of brain eicosanoids (for review, see Murphy and Pearce, 1988), although neurons in certain brain regions have also been shown to produce a considerable amount of eicosanoids. Recently, a distribution of inducible cyclooxygenase (COX 2) in

the neurons of the ovine (Breder et al., 1992) and rat brain (Breder et al., 1995) has been characterized in detail. The authors found that the brain regions involved in stress response (hippocampus, amigdala, hypothalamus, neocortex, but not cerebellum) contain the greatest amount of COX 2. Significantly, a considerable concentration of the PGE_2 binding sites in post-mortem human brain was found in the hypothalamus and limbic system, but no significant binding was observed in cerebellar nuclei and cortex (Watanabe et al., 1985). Somewhat consistent with these studies, are our data on ex vivo incubated brain slices from LPS-treated mice: a considerable elevation in PGE_2 production was observed in hypothalamus, hippocampus, frontal cortex but not significant in cerebellum (unpublished data). Furthermore, it should be noted that, in addition to involvement in mechanisms of pyrogenesis, ESs may also be involved in elaboration of autonomic, endocrine, and behavioral responses, which to a certain extent may be associated with a fever response. A number of brain regions can also be implicated in thermoregulatory responses and even take a function of thermoregulatory center, when the hypothalamus or its conductive pathways are destroyed. However, in the present study, we focused on the hypothalamus as the major CNS region involved in the control of thermal homeostasis (Rothwell, 1994).

In view of the continuing debates in regard to putative permeability of the blood–brain barrier for exo- (e.g. LPS) and endogenous pyrogens, it appears to be of principal importance that the hypothalamus per se is a site of cytokine generation (for review, see Spangelo and Gorospe, 1995): a considerable increase of pyrogenic cytokine (IL-1β or IL-6) production in response to systemic or *in vitro* LPS administration was noted in rabbits (Nakamori et al., 1994), guinea pigs (Roth et al., 1993), rats (Spangelo et al., 1990; Hillhouse and Mosley, 1993; Navarra et al., 1993), mice (Takao et al., 1993), and pigs (Molenaar et al., 1990).

To investigate the role of hypothalamic ESs in response to bacterial pyrogen, for several years we have applied a method of ex-vivo incubation of hypothalamus from LPS-treated animals. This method was described in detail elsewhere (Kaplanski et al., 1989a, 1992; Fraifeld et al., 1995a,b). Briefly, various doses of LPS from *Escherichia coli* Serotype 0127:B8 (Sigma, USA), dissolved in saline, were injected intraperitoneally (i.p.). Control animals were injected i.p. with pyrogen-free (0.1 ml in mice; 0.4–0.5 ml in rats and chickens). At different post-injection periods, animals were decapitated and their hypothalami were quickly excised. Each hypothalamus was incubated in a vial with Krebs–Henseleit buffer solution containing 0.2% glucose for 3 h at 37°C, 95% O_2 and 5% CO_2, and pH 7.35–7.40. The buffer samples were harvested to tubes containing 20 μg of indomethacin (Sigma, USA) in 100 μl of 2% $NaHCO_3$ solution to stop prostaglandin synthesis, centrifuged to eliminate any remaining tissue, and then stored at -20°C, until assayed. The content of ESs in samples was determined by radioimmunoassay, using specific antibodies (Bio-Makor, Rehovot, Israel).

Rodents

The studies on fever in small rodents conducted in the past have led to rather conflicting results, showing that mice and rats in contrast to larger animals usually do not become febrile in response to LPS, rather they tend to develop hypothermia (for review, see Kluger, 1991). The relationship between hypothalamic prostaglandins and body temperature in rodents, especially in mice, has not yet been carefully examined. Therefore, we compared the effects of LPS on body temperature and hypothalamic prostanoid (PGE_2 and 6-keto-$PGF_{1\alpha}$, stable metabolite of PGI_2, and PGD_2) production in mice (CD-1 or ICR) and rats (Sprague–Dawley or Wistar).

Basal level

The basal level of hypothalamic PGE_2 production in male young adult mice was significantly higher than that in male rats of the same age (Fig. 1), whereas no significant differences in hypothalamic prostanoid production between the

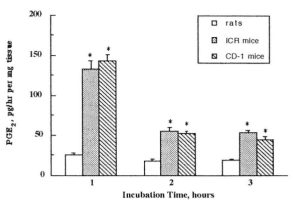

Fig. 1. Basal level of PGE_2 production by incubated hypothalamus of rodents. $^*P < 0.05$, mice vs. rats.

two strains of mice were observed at each period of incubation. Similar data were observed in regard to 6-keto-$PGF_{1\alpha}$ (data are not shown). Whereas average values of body (colonic) temperature in mice and rats measured before excising the hypothalami were at similar magnitude (within 37.0–37.4°C), the basal level of PGE_2 and 6-keto-$PGF_{1\alpha}$ in mouse hypothalamus was approximately threefold greater than in rats, apparently due to a higher metabolic level and, hence, a more rapid generation and turnover of arachidonic acid products. Another attractive possibility could suggest an existence of the relationship between thermogenesis and a constitutive production of thermoregulatory prostanoids, so that the maintenance of thermoregulatory 'set point' at normothermic level in smaller animals (e.g. mice) requires enhanced values of hypothalamic prostanoid production, as compared with larger animals (e.g. rats). Consistent with these considerations, are also the data of Romero et al. (1984) who have found that in cats and dogs, the concentrations of several prostanoids, including PGE_2 and PGI_2, were several-fold higher than in humans.

LPS-induced changes in hypothalamic prostanoid production and body temperature

Both in rats and mice, systemic injection of

LPS resulted in an elevation in hypothalamic prostanoid production and changes in T_b. However the order and magnitude of these alterations, the relationship between hypothalamic prostanoid production and T_b response, as well as between different prostanoids, were rather specific and differed in rats and mice. Moreover, the two murine lines also displayed different patterns of LPS-induced effects.

LPS-treated rats developed hyperthermia preceded with several hours of hypothermic phase (Fig. 2A). In contrast to rats, mice were unable to develop hyperthermia in response to LPS, and were actually hypothermic (Fig. 3A). A significant difference was also observed between ICR and CD-1 mice. As compared with ICR mice, CD-1 mice exhibited more pronounced hypothermia

that lasted for a longer time. As shown in Fig. 3A, T_b of LPS-treated ICR mice returned to the control level by 6 h post-injection, whereas T_b of the CD-1 mice remained hypothermic during almost the entire period measured.

An approximately twofold increase in hypothalamic prostanoid (PGE_2 and 6-keto-$PGF_{1\alpha}$) production was found in LPS-treated rats in both early (hypothermic) and late (hyperthermic) phases of febrile response (Fig. 2B,C). Relatively less elevation occurred in the production of PGD_2, which was observed only in the early phase of febrile response (Fig. 2D). Interestingly, a correlation between 6-keto-$PGF_{1\alpha}$ level and T_b was found within the first few hours post LPS administration ($R = 0.78$; $P < 0.05$), but not in the late phase, while for PGE_2 such a correlation ($R =$

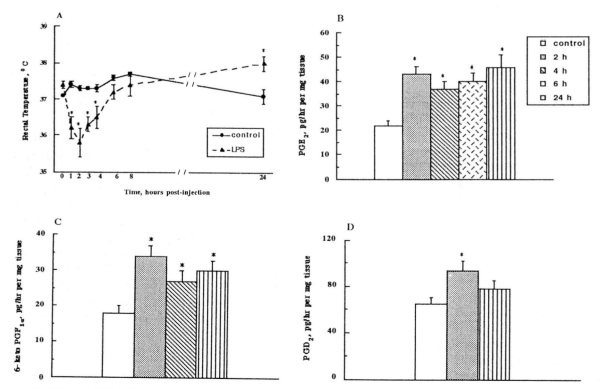

Fig. 2. Effect of LPS (100 μg per rat, i.p.) on body temperature (A) and hypothalamic prostanoid production (B–D) in rats. $^*P < 0.05$ vs. control.

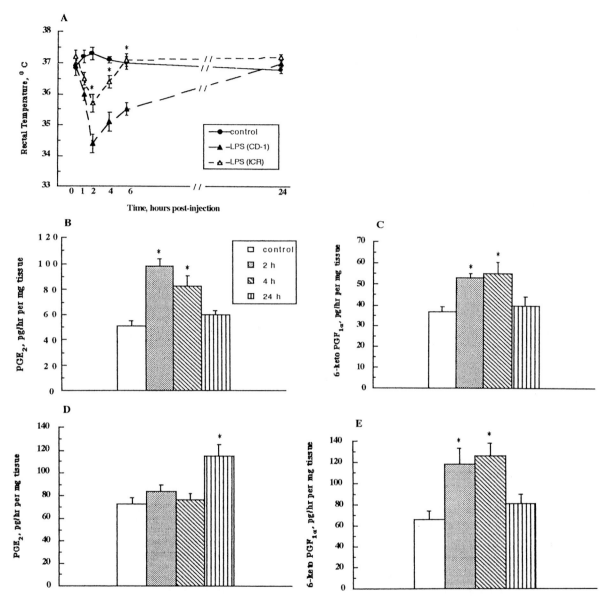

Fig. 3. Effect of LPS (25 μg per mouse, i.p.) on body temperature (A) and hypothalamic prostanoid production (B–E) in two strains of mouse: CD-1 (B–C) and ICR (D–E). *P < 0.05 vs. control (B–E) or ICR vs. CD-1 (A).

0.72; P < 0.05) was found only in hyperthermic phase. In mice, LPS also caused a considerable increase in hypothalamic prostanoid production, and this increase occurred in a time-dependent manner. The CD-1 mice responded by elevation

in PGE_2 and 6-keto-$PGF_{1\alpha}$ levels only at the early phase but not at the late one (Fig. 3B,C), while in ICR mice, the elevation in PGE_2 production occurred later, than in CD-1 mice, and was preceded by that of 6-keto-$PGF_{1\alpha}$ (Fig. 3D,E).

Thus, in mice, the relationship between LPS-induced hypothalamic prostanoid production and T_b response is dependent upon the mouse strain.

Taken together, the data obtained on rodents and other mammals investigated so far, indicate that changes in T_b induced by systemic administration of bacterial endotoxin are accompanied by significant, although species-specific activation of prostanoid synthesis in hypothalamus. It should also be taken into account that LPS-induced elevation in hypothalamic prostanoid production might be a secondary or resultant effect of pyrogen. To elucidate if these changes are significant for induction and development of fever response, our second step was to apply the inhibitors of eicosanoid synthesis.

Effects of inhibitors of eicosanoid synthesis

The antipyretic action of eicosanoid synthesis inhibitors is well-known and has been observed in a variety of endotherm species. As follows from our data, in rodents, the elevation in hypothalamic prostanoid production in response to LPS occurred also in the hypothermic phase of febrile response. Therefore, to complete the picture and examine the possible relationship between ESs and T_b, we focused on the effects of ES synthesis on short-term response to LPS.

The inhibitor of cyclooxygenase, indomethacin administered i.p. 2 h before LPS injection in a dose (5 mg/kg) that does not affect T_b of untreated rodents, efficaciously prevented the elevation in hypothalamic prostanoid production and the drop in T_b of the rats at each point measured in the hypothermic phase (Fig. 4A,B). In contrast, in mice, indomethacin even potentiated the hypothermic effect of LPS (Fig. 4C), regardless of the concomitant inhibition of PGE_2 production (Fig. 4D).

Dexamethasone (5 mg/kg i.p.) injected 48, 24, and 2 h before LPS administration prevented any LPS-associated changes in T_b and the activation of prostanoid production both in rats (Fig. 5A,B) and mice (Fig. 5C,D).

Indomethacin interferes with production of prostanoids, while dexamethasone, via inhibition of phospholipase A_2, inhibits generation of both prostanoids and leukotrienes (Weidenfeld et al., 1993). Besides, the anti-LPS action of glucocorticoids could be mediated by reducing the release of CRF and, as well, the synthesis of pyrogenic cytokines (Coelho et al., 1995). Hence, it seems likely that in rats, LPS-induced hypothermia can be mediated by prostanoids, while in mice, the prostanoids play a minor, if any, role and rather leukotrienes or some other factors involving steroid interference play a major role in this phenomenon.

LPS-induced changes in hypothalamic prostanoid production and body temperature in developing and aged rats

During early post-natal period, the thermoregulatory system of newborn endotherms undergoes considerable alterations. Newborn endotherms, in contrast to adult animals, are actually poikilothermic (Teisner and Haahr, 1974), and this provides a unique possibility to investigate the role of natural age-related poikilothermia in mammals on the effects of pyrogens. However, the mechanisms of fever response in developing animals remain largely unclear. Recently, we examined T_b and hypothalamic PGE_2 response to various doses of LPS in 3-, 6-, 14-, and 21-day-old Sprague–Dawley rat pups (Kaplanski et al., 1996b). It was found that in rat pups LPS stimulates hypothalamic PGE_2 production in a similar way to adult rats, while their T_b response was rather age-specific. Weaning rats (21 days old) responded to LPS by elevation in T_b, suckling 2-week-old rats were unable to evoke hyperthermia, and the youngest groups developed considerable hypothermia. It seems that peripheral rather than central thermoregulatory mechanisms are responsible for specificity of T_b response to LPS in developing animals. In particular, endotoxin caused an increase in VO_2 of newborn rabbits without elevation in the colonic temperature (Hull et al., 1993).

The ability to develop fever in response to pyrogenic stimuli is compromised by aging (Lipton and Ticknor, 1979; Norman et al., 1985; Ruwe

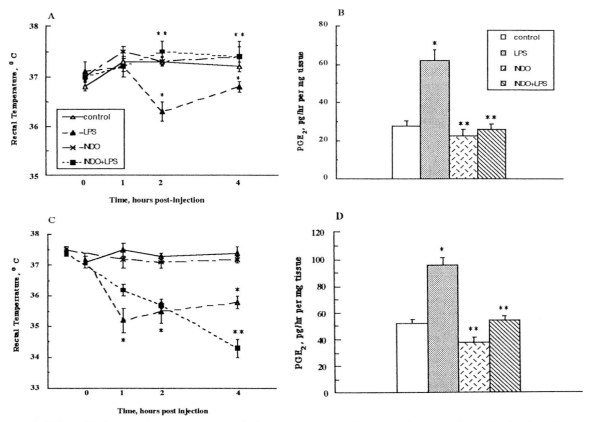

Fig. 4. Effect of indomethacin pretreatment on body temperature and hypothalamic prostanoid production in LPS-treated rats (A–B) and CD-1 mice (C–D). *$P < 0.05$ vs. control. **$P < 0.05$, INDO + LPS vs. LPS.

et al., 1988; Foster et al., 1992; Scarpace et al., 1992; Fraifeld and Kaplanski, 1993; Strijbos et al., 1993; Kaplanski et al., 1994; Fraifeld et al., 1995b). The importance of this observation follows from the idea which considers the beneficial role of fever in host defence against infections (Kluger, 1986). Hence, a reduced febrile response is considered to contribute, at least in part, to increased mortality and prolonged recovery from infections in the elderly (Norman et al., 1985).

The mechanisms of age-associated changes in febrile response remain largely unclear. The reduced ability of the hypothalamus to produce PGE_2 has been suggested as one of the possibilities (Grahn et al., 1987). The authors demonstrated decreased PGE_2 production by *in vitro*

LPS-stimulated homogenates of brain hemisphere from old rats as compared to young rats. Recently, we have shown that in aging, the reduced febrile response to *in vivo* LPS administration is not associated with an inability of the hypothalamus of old animals to produce PGE_2 (Kaplanski et al., 1994; Fraifeld et al., 1995b). The difference between our results and those reported by Grahn et al. (1987) could be accounted in part by methodological differences: hypothalamus vs. all brain tissue; *in vivo* vs. in vitro LPS-administration. Both at the peak of T_b response (Kaplanski et al., 1994) and at the initial phase of febrile response (Fraifeld et al., 1995b), which was found to be generally delayed in aged animals (Lipton and Ticknor, 1979; Ruwe et al., 1988; Foster et

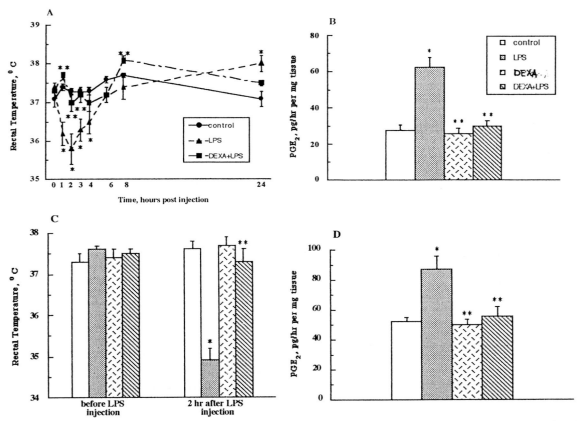

Fig. 5. Effect of dexamethasone pretreatment on body temperature and hypothalamic prostanoid production in LPS-treated rats (A–B) and CD-1 mice (C–D). $^*P < 0.05$ vs. control. $^{**}P < 0.05$, DEXA + LPS vs. LPS.

al., 1992; Scarpace et al., 1992; Strijbos et al., 1993), the hypothalamus of old Wistar rats produced as much PGE_2 as the young rats, and no age-dependent differences were observed in hypothalamic PGE_2 production either in LPS-treated, or in control rats. Regardless of the lack of age difference in hypothalamic PGE_2 production, the latent period of T_b elevation, in response to LPS, was shorter in young rats as compared to old ones. Moreover, when T_b started to increase in the younger group, old rats were actually hypothermic. The apparent discrepancy between unaltered hypothalamic PGE_2 production and delayed febrile response in old rats may be related to decreased sensitivity of thermosensi-

tive neurons to PGE_2, or/and to an inability of peripheral mechanisms to reach a new thermoregulatory level. This suggestion is supported by data from Ueno et al. (1985), who demonstrated a pronounced decrease of the synaptic membrane binding sites for PGE_2 in rat brain during maturation and aging, and by data of Lipton and Ticknor (1979) and Ruwe et al. (1988), who found a reduced febrile response in aged rabbits to i.c.v. PGE_2 (Lipton and Ticknor, 1979) or intrahypothalamic PGE_1 (Ruwe et al., 1988) administration. Another possibility may consider the role for endogenous lipocortin-1 (Strijbos et al., 1993) or for IL-8, which exerts pyrogenic features via PG-independent mechanisms

(Rothwell et al., 1990; Zampronio et al., 1994) and was found to be over-produced in response to LPS in male elderlies, as compared with the young population (Clark and Peterson, 1994).

Birds

Information on avian fever is limited. However, a number of data indicate the similarity of mechanisms of fever in birds and mammals, including the involvement of brain prostanoids: (i) as well as mammals, birds are able to evoke fever in response to living (D'Alecy and Kluger, 1975) or dead pathogenic bacteria (D'Alecy and Kluger, 1975; Jones et al., 1982), systemic (Artunkal et al., 1977a; Johnson et al., 1993a; Macari et al., 1993; Fraifeld et al., 1995a) or i.c.v. administration of LPS (Johnson et al., 1993b; Macari et al., 1993), i.c.v. injection of endogenous (IL-1) pyrogen (Macari et al., 1993); (ii) inhibitors of cyclooxygenase, sodium salicylate (D'Alecy and Kluger, 1975) or indomethacin (Johnson et al., 1993a; Macari et al., 1993), effectively attenuated a febrile response to pyrogens both in birds and mammals; (iii) small doses of PGE_1 administered i.v. (Artunkal et al., 1977a), PGE_2 injected i.c.v. (Macari et al., 1993), or PGs of E series injected into the hypothalamus (Artunkal et al., 1977b) caused a significant increase in body temperature both in birds and mammals.

Hence, these data fit at least two of the three requirements mentioned above for likely involvement of PGs in mechanisms of pyrogenesis. Furthermore, the question arises whether hypothalamic PGE_2 is also involved in central mechanisms of avian fever as it is in a variety of mammals. If so, in addition to the observations of hyperthermic effect of PGE_2 i.c.v. administration and the ability of cyclooxygenase inhibitors' pretreatment to block LPS fever, the increased hypothalamic PGE_2 production in response to LPS should also be found. However, in our recent study on male broilers (Fraifeld et al., 1995a), we failed to observe such an effect: hyperthermia following LPS i.p. administration was not accompanied by elevation in hypothalamic PGE_2 pro-duction, neither in early nor in later phases of the febrile response.

Hence, it seems likely that (i) prostanoids, other than PGE_2 may be involved in central mechanisms of avian fever, and (ii) hyperthermia induced by PGE_2 i.c.v. administration reflects its pharmacological rather than pathophysiological effects.

Summary

The results of the present study, summarized in Table 2, demonstrate that different species and strains of rodents (rats and mice) and birds (chickens) exhibit rather specific fever response. Systemic administration of LPS caused monophasic elevation in T_b of chickens, biphasic changes in T_b of rats (initial drop followed by an increase in T_b), whereas mice failed to develop hyperthermia and responded by a decreased T_b. The LPS-induced alterations in hypothalamic prostanoid synthesis were also rather species-specific and differ markedly even between the two strains of mice.

We failed to find a common direct correlation between LPS-induced changes in T_b and hypothalamic prostanoid production in rodents (rats and mice). This observation is supported by our recent study on age-related changes in fever response in rats, where we found that hypothalami of LPS-treated old and young adult rats produced similar amounts of PGE_2 and PGI_2, in spite of more pronounced and prolonged hypothermia, and a delayed elevation in T_b of old rats, as compared with young (Fraifeld et al., 1995b). Moreover, the hypothalamus of febrile chickens did not display any detectable activation of PGE_2 production, suggesting that PGE_2 is not a common central mediator of fever in homeotherms (Fraifeld et al., 1995a). Apparently, the actual body temperature not always reflects the functional state of central thermostat, and increased PGE_2 production in hypothalamus would not directly, at least in rodents, lead to body temperature elevation. Furthermore, peripheral effects, including PG-mediated ones, of pyrogens can interfere and even

TABLE 2

Summary of results: Effects of LPS on T_b and ex-vivo hypothalamic prostanoid production in rodents and chickens

Species	Effect on T_b	Effect on hypothalamic PGs
[a] Rats		
Newborn	Long-lasting hypothermia	Elevation in PGE_2 and 6-keto-$PGF_{1\alpha}$
Weaning	Long-lasting hyperthermia	Elevation in PGE_2 and 6-keto-$PGF_{1\alpha}$
Young adult	Initial short-lasting hypothermia followed by hyperthermia	Elevation in PGE_2 and 6-keto-$PGF_{1\alpha}$
Old	Prolonged hypothermia and delayed hyperthermia	No differences from young adults
CD-1 mice	Long-lasting hypothermia	Elevation in PGE_2 and 6-keto-$PGF_{1\alpha}$ only in the early (hypothermic) phase of fever response
[b] ICR mice	Short-lasting hypothermia	Elevation in PGE_2 only in the late phase preceded by elevation in 6-keto-$PGF_{1\alpha}$ in the early (hypothermic) phase
[c] Chickens	Long-lasting hyperthermia	No significant changes in PGE_2 production

[a] Indomethacin and dexamethasone prevent both hypo- and hyperthermia.
[b] Dexamethasone, but not indomethacin, prevents LPS-induced hypothermia. At subthermoneutral zone (22°C), mice failed to develop hyperthermia. However, at thermoneutral zone (30°C), mice did evoke hyperthermia few hours following LPS injection.
[c] Inhibitors of cyclooxygenase exert antipyretic effect (D'Alecy and Kluger, 1975; Macari et al., 1993).

overcome their centrally-mediated effects (Morimoto et al., 1991; Burysek et al., 1993). Previously, we have shown that no additional elevation in hypothalamic PGE_2 production occurs in response to doses of LPS over 10 μg in rats and 25 μg in mice, while the increased doses led to further changes in T_b response (Kaplanski et al., 1993). Morimoto et al. (1991) have considered that PGE_2 acts centrally to cause fever and peripherally to cause hypothermia, and, hence, these opposing actions, both being induced by LPS, may act together to determine the final thermoregulatory response. Other possibilities could be related to counterbalance of endogenous antipyretics (Kluger, 1991; Kozak et al., 1995), that may occur not only at the level of thermoregulatory center but also outside the CNS (Klir et al., 1995), and to the existence of PG-independent mechanisms of LPS fever. The latter have been shown for IL-8 (Rothwell et al., 1990; Zampronio et al., 1994) and MIP-1 (Davatelis et al., 1989; Minano et al., 1990; Hayashi et al., 1995; Lopez-Valpuesta and Myers, 1995), which are, apparently, mediated via CRF (Strijbos et al., 1992; Zampronio et al., 1994), and INF-α, mediated via the opioid receptor mechanisms (Hori et al., 1991, 1992). However, it has been shown recently that in different species the same pyrogenic cytokines (IL-8) may induced fever via different, PG-independent (in rats; Zampronio et al., 1994) or PG-dependent (in rabbits; Zampronio et al., 1995) mechanisms.

It should be noted that fever response is not always accompanied by an elevation in T_b. The final effect of pyrogens on body temperature depends upon the balance between heat production and heat loss, which in turn is highly dependent upon body size and ambient temperature, especially in small animals. Perhaps, the hypothermic response observed in our mice and rats at 22°C may be in part attributed to ambient temperature, which was below a thermoneutral zone. The reduced febrile response is considered, at least in part, to contribute to an increased mortality and prolonged recovery from infections (Kluger, 1986). From this point, it is difficult to suggest whether the hypothermia observed in our mice and rats could be of somewhat adaptive significance. It has been shown that at the ambient temperature of 30°C, Swiss Webster mice can respond to LPS by T_b elevation (Kozak et al., 1994). We have obtained a similar result on LPS-treated CD-1 mice kept at thermoneutral zone (unpublished data). Moreover, it has been reported that LPS-treated mice preferred a higher ambient temperature in a thermal gradient, suggesting the important role of behavioral activity in the development of fever in small rodents (Akins et al., 1991; Goujon et al., 1995). In view of the wide spectrum of ESs effects, it may be speculated that behavioral alterations could also be mediated by LPS-induced prostanoid production in CNS. However, the mechanisms of hypothermic response to bacterial endotoxin in small rodents remain largely unclear. Recently, Derijk et al. (1994) has demonstrated that not only increased heat loss but rather reduced thermogenesis may be responsible for hypothermia in rats after LPS administration. The involvement of antipyretic products released from macrophages has also been suggested (Derijk et al., 1994). The data concerning the role of prostaglandins are controversial (Derijk et al., 1994; Kozak et al., 1994; Kaplanski et al., 1995), being based mainly on indirect approaches, such as applying nonspecific inhibitors of prostanoid or eicosanoid synthesis. In the present study, we looked for the production of hypothalamic PGE_2 and 6-keto-$PGF_{1\alpha}$ in rodents at different times

after i.p. injection of LPS. We found that, in rats, LPS induced a considerable increase in hypothalamic PGE_2 production both in early (hypothermic) and late (hyperthermic) phases of fever response. In contrast, in ICR mice, the increase in PGE_2 production was observed only at 24 h, while in CD-1 mice during the first few hours post LPS injection, when the ICR mice were actually normothermic and CD-1 mice were hypothermic, respectively. We have obtained data pointing at the possible involvement of PGI_2 in the mechanisms of fever in rodents (Abramovich et al., 1995). In particular, a reciprocal relationship between PGE_2 and PGI_2 production was observed in the hypothalamus of LPS-treated ICR mice. In rats, the correlations between hypothalamic PGE_2 or PGI_2 production and T_b have been found to be dependent upon the phase of fever response. The thermoregulatory role of PGD_2 is still controversial (Table 1). However, in view of its probable hypothermic action, its elevation in rats during the early phase post LPS injection and, on the other hand, the preventive effect of indomethacin-pretreatment, may point at an involvement of PGD_2 in the development of LPS hypothermia in rats.

Thus, having been considered rather 'clear' in the past, the role of brain ESs in pyrogenesis, nowadays, appears to be more and more complicated. It seems that at least part of the controversies could be obviated by recognizing the two components of LPS fever: (a) the major, PG-dependent component, and (b) an additional, PG-independent component. A contribution of each of these two components may differ between various species determining species-dependent specificity of central mechanisms of fever. In addition, it appears that no single ES (e.g. PGE_2) is responsible for fever induction, but complicated interrelationships exist between different ESs, so that some may possess the role of major central mediators/inducers of fever (PGE_2, PGE_1, $PGF_{2\alpha}$), others might play a modulatory role (PGI_2, and probably PGD_2 and lipoxins), while thromboxanes and leukotrienes might possess indirect influence via their action on permeability of the blood–brain barrier for endogenous pyrogens. On the whole, the problem is far from being resolved, and a lot of questions have still to be answered.

References

Abramovich, L., Fraifeld, V. and Kaplanski, J. (1995) Elevation of prostacyclin synthesis precedes the increase in PGE_2 production in mouse hypothalamus during the febrile response. *Pflüg. Arch.*, 430, Suppl. R133, Abstr. 493.

Akarsu, E.S. and Ayhan, I.H. (1993) Iloprost, a stable analogue of PGI_2, potentiates the hyperthermic effect of PGE_2 in rats. *Pharmacol. Biochem. Behav.*, 46: 383–389.

Akins, C., Thiessen, D. and Cocke, R. (1991) Lipopolysaccharide increases ambient temperature preference in C57BL/6J adult mice. *Physiol. Behav.*, 50: 461–463.

Amir, S., de Blasio, E. and English, A.M. (1991) NG-monomethyl-L-arginine co-injection attenuates the thermogenic and hyperthermic effects of E_2 prostaglandin microinjection into the anterior hypothalamic preoptic area in rats. *Brain Res.*, 556: 157–160.

Artunkal, A.A., Marley, E. and Stephenson, J.D. (1977a) Some effects of intravenous prostaglandin E_1 and endotoxin in young chickens. *Br. J. Pharmacol.*, 61: 29–37.

Artunkal, A.A., Marley, E. and Stephenson, J.D. (1977b) Some effects of intravenous prostaglandin E_1 and E_2 and of endotoxin injected into the hypothalamus of young chicks: dissociation between endotoxin fever and the effects of prostaglandins. *Br. J. Pharmacol.*, 61: 39–46.

Bernheim, H.A., Gilbert, T.M., Stitt, J.T. (1980) Prostaglandin E levels in third ventricular cerebrospinal fluid of rabbits during fever and changes in body temperature. *J. Physiol.*, 301: 69–78.

Breder, C.D., Smith, W.L., Raz, A., Masferrer, J.L., Seibert, K., Needleman, P. and Saper, C.B. (1992) The distribution and characterization of cyclooxygenase-like immunoreactivity in the ovine brain. *J. Comp. Neurol.*, 322: 409–438.

Breder, C.D., Dewitt, D. and Kraig, R.P. (1995) Characterization of inducible cyclooxygenase in rat brain. *J. Comp. Neurol.*, 355: 296–315.

Brenner, T., Bohen, A., Shohami, E., Abramsky, O. and Weidenfeld, J. (1992) Glucocorticoid regulation of eicosanoid production by glial cells under basal and stimulated conditions. *J. Neuroimmunol.*, 40: 237–280.

Burysek, L., Tvrdik, P. and Houstek, J. (1993) Expression of interleukin-1α and interleukin-1 receptor type I genes in murine grown adipose tissue. *FEBS Lett.*, 334: 229–232.

Clark, W.G. and Lipton, J.M. (1985) Changes in body temperature after administration of acetylcholine, histamine, morphine, prostaglandins and related agents: II. *Neurosci. Biobehav. Rev.*, 9: 479–552.

Clark, J.A. and Peterson, T.C. (1994) Cytokine production and aging; overproduction of IL-8 in the elderly males in response to lipopolysaccharide. *Mech. Ageing Dev.*, 77: 127–139.

Coceani, F. (1991) Prostaglandins and fever: Facts and controversies. In: P. Mackowiak (Ed.), *Fever: Basic Mechanisms and Management*, Raven Press, New York, pp. 59–83.

Coceani, F., Bishai, I., Dinarello, C.A. and Fitzpatrick, F.A. (1983) Prostaglandin E_2 and thromboxane B_2 in cerebrospinal fluid of afebrile and febrile cat. *Am. J. Physiol.*, 244: R785–R793.

Coelho, M.M., Luheshi, G., Hopkins, S.J., Pela, I.R. and Rothwell, N.J. (1995) Multiple mechanisms mediate antipyretic action of glucocorticoids. *Am. J. Physiol.*, 269: R527–R535.

D'Alecy, L.G. and Kluger, M.J. (1975) Avian febrile response. *J. Physiol. (Lond.)*, 253: 223–232.

Davatelis, G., Wolpe, S.D., Sherry, B., Dayer, J.-M., Chicheportiche, R. and Cerami, A. (1989) Macrophage inflammatory protein-1: a prostaglandin-independent endogenous pyrogen. *Science*, 243: 1066–1068.

Derijk, R.H., van Kampen, M. and van Rooijen, N. (1994) Hypothermia to endotoxin involves reduced thermogenesis, macrophage-dependent mechanisms, and prostaglandins. *Am. J. Physiol.*, 266: R1–R8.

De Vries, H.E., Hoogendoorn, K.H., van Dijk, J., Zijlstra, F.J., van Dam, A.M., Breimer, D.D., van Berkel, T.J., de Boer, A.G. and Kuiper, J. (1995) Eicosanoid production by rat cerebral endothelial cells: stimulation by lipopolysaccharide, interleukin-1 and interleukin-6. *J. Neuroimmunol.*, 59: 1–8.

Dinarello, C.A., Cannon, J.G. and Wolf, S.M. (1988) New concepts of the pathogenesis of fever. *Rev. Infect. Dis.*, 10: 168–189.

Ewen, L., Milton, A.C. and Smith, S. (1976) Effects of prostaglandin $F_{2\alpha}$ and prostaglandin D_2 on the body temperature of conscious cats. *J. Physiol. (Lond.)*, 258: 121P–122P.

Feldberg, W. and Gupta, K.P. (1973) Pyrogen fever and prostaglandin-like activity in cerebrospinal fluid. *J. Physiol.*, 228: 41–53.

Feldberg, W., Gupta, K.P., Milton, A.S. and Wendlandt, S. (1973) Effect of pyrogen and antipyretics on prostaglandin activity in cisternal C.S.F. of unanesthetized cats. *J. Physiol.*, 234: 279–303.

Foster, K.D., Conn, C.A. and Kluger, M.J. (1992) Fever, tumor necrosis factor, and interleukin-6 in young, mature, and aged Fischer 344 rats. *Am. J. Physiol.*, 262: R211–R215.

Fraifeld, V. and Kaplanski, J. (1993) Fever and aging: putative role of hypothalamic prostaglandins and endogenous antipyretics. *Probl. Aging Longevity (Kiev)*, 3: 269–278.

Fraifeld, V., Blaicher-Kulick, R., Degen, A.A. and Kaplanski, J. (1995a) Is hypothalamic prostaglandin E_2 involved in avian fever? *Life Sci.*, 56: 1343–1346.

Fraifeld, V., Abramovich, L. and Kaplanski, J. (1995b) Delayed febrile response in old rats is not associated with an inability of hypothalamus to produce prostaglandin E_2. *Mech. Ageing Dev.*, 79: 137–140.

Goujon, E., Parnet, P., Aubert, A., Goodall, G. and Dantzer, R. (1995) Corticosterone regulates behavioral effects of lipopolysaccharide and interleukin-1β in mice. *Am. J. Physiol.*, 269: R154–R159.

Grahn, D., Norman, D.C. and Yoshikava, T.T. (1987) Fever and aging: central nervous system prostaglandin E_2 in response to endotoxin. *Exp. Gerontol.*, 22: 249–255.

Hadas, H., Sod-Moriah, U.A. and Kaplanski, J. (1989) The effect of lipopolysaccharide on fever and thermoregulation in rats. In: J.B. Mercer (Ed.), *Thermal Physiology*, Elsevier, Amsterdam, pp. 395–400.

Hayaishi, O. (1991) Molecular mechanisms of sleep-wake regulation: roles of prostaglandin D_2 and E_2. *FASEB J.*, 5: 2575–2581.

Hayashi, M., Luo, Y., Laning, J., Strieter, R.M. and Dorf, M.E. (1995) Production and function of monocyte chemoattractant protein-1 and other β-chemokines in murine glial cells. *J. Neuroimmunol.*, 60: 143–150.

Hillhouse, E.W. and Mosley, K. (1993) Peripheral endotoxin induces hypothalamic immunoreactive interleukin-1β in the rat. *Br. J. Pharmacol.*, 109: 289–290.

Hori, T., Nakashima, T., Take, S., Kaizuka, Y., Mori, T. and Katafuchi, T. (1991) Immune cytokines and regulation of body temperature, food intake and cellular immunity. *Brain Res. Bull.*, 27: 309–313.

Hori, T., Kiyohara, T., Nakashima, T., Mizuno, K., Muratani, H. and Katafuchi, T. (1992) Effects of temperature and neuroactive substances on hypothalamic neurons *in vitro*: possible implications for the induction of fever. *Physiol. Res.*, 41: 77–81.

Hull, D., McIntyre, J. and Vinter, J. (1993) Age-related changes in endotoxin sensitivity and the febrile response of newborn rabbits. *Biol. Neonate*, 63: 370–379.

Hynes, N., Bishai, I., Lees, J. and Coceani, F. (1991) Leukotrienes in brain: natural occurrence and induced changes. *Brain. Res.*, 553: 4–13.

Johnson, R.W., Curtis, S.E., Dantzer, R. and Kelley, K.W. (1993a) Central and peripheral prostaglandins are involved in sickness behavior in birds. *Physiol. Behav.*, 53: 127–131.

Johnson, R.W., Curtis, S.E., Dantzer, R., Bahr, J.M. and Kelley, K.W. (1993b) Sickness behavior in birds caused by peripheral or central injection of endotoxin. *Physiol. Behav.*, 53: 343–348.

Jones, C.A., Edens, F.W. and Denbow, D.M. (1982) Peripherally administered cations do not modify febrile responses induced in chickens by *Escherichia coli*. *Poult. Sci.*, 61: 1322–1328.

Kantha, S.S., Matsumura, H., Kubo, E., Kawase, K., Takahata, R., Serhan, C.N. and Hayaishi, O. (1994) Effects of prostaglandin D_2, lipoxins and leukotrienes on sleep and brain temperature of rats. *Prostaglandins Leukotrienes Essent. Fatty Acids*, 51: 87–93.

Kaplanski, J., Hadas, H. and Sod-Moriah, U. (1989a) Effect of indomethacin on hyperthermia induced by lipopolysaccharide or high ambient temperature in rats. In: E. Schonbaum and P. Lomax (Eds.), *Thermoregulation: Research and Clinical Applications*, Karger, Basel, pp. 176–178.

Kaplanski, J., Hadas, H. and Sod-Moriah, U. (1989b) Effect of dexamethasone on fever and thermoregulation in acutely heat-exposed rats. In: J.B. Mercer (Ed.), *Thermal Physiology*, Elsevier, Amsterdam, pp. 407–412.

Kaplanski, J., Hadas, H. and Sod-Moriah, U. (1992) Effects of various doses of indomethacin and dexamethasone on rectal temperature and hypothalamic prostanoids in febrile rats. In: E. Schonbaum and P. Lomax (Eds.), *Thermoregulation: The Pathophysiological Basis of Clinical Disorders*, Karger, Basel, pp. 33–36.

Kaplanski, J., Fraifeld, V. and Abramovich, L. (1993) The effect of LPS on hypothalamic prostaglandins and rectal temperature: species and gender differences. In: A.S. Milton (Ed.), *Thermal Physiology*, Aberdeen, p. 61.

Kaplanski, J., Fraifeld, V. and Abramovich, L. (1994) Effect of LPS on body temperature and hypothalamic PGE_2 production in young and old rats. *Can. J. Physiol. Pharmacol.*, 72 Suppl. 1: 283 (Abstr. P10.5.5).

Kaplanski, J., Abramovich, L. and Fraifeld, V. (1995) Effect of LPS and inhibitors of eicosanoid synthesis on short term fever response and production of hypothalamic PGE_2. In: E. Zeisberger, E. Schonbaum and P. Lomax (Eds.), *Thermal Balance in Health and Disease*, Birkhauser, Basel, pp. 379–383.

Kaplanski, J., Abramovich, L. and Fraifeld, V. (1996a) Effect of lipopolysaccharides on rectal temperature and hypothalamic prostanoids of rodents. In: *Rodents and Space*, Actes Editions, Rabat (in press).

Kaplanski, J., Rubin, M. and Fraifeld, V. (1996b) Effect of lipopolysaccharides on body temperature and hypothalamic PGE_2 response in developing rats. In: *Thermal Physiology*, Memphis (in press).

Klir, J.J., McClellan, J.L., Kozak, W., Szelenyi, Z., Wong, G.H. and Kluger, M.J. (1995) Systemic but not central administration of tumor necrosis factor-α attenuates LPS-induced fever in rats. *Am. J. Physiol.*, 268: R480–R486.

Kluger, M.J. (1986) Is fever beneficial? *Yale J. Biol. Med.*, 59: 89–95.

Kluger, M.J. (1991) Fever: Role of pyrogens and cryogens. *Physiol. Rev.*, 71: 93–127.

Kozak, W., Conn, C.A. and Kluger, M.J. (1994) Lipopolysaccharide induces fever and depresses locomotor activity in unrestrained mice. *Am. J. Physiol.*, 266: R125–R135.

Kozak, W., Conn, C.A., Klir, J.J., Wong, G.H.W. and Kluger, M.J. (1995) TNF soluble receptor and antiserum against TNF enhance lipopolysaccharide fever in mice. *Am. J. Physiol.*, 269: R23–R29.

Krueger, J.M., Kapas, L., Opp, M.R. and Obal, F. Jr. (1992) Prostaglandins E_2 and D_2 have little effect on rabbit sleep. *Physiol. Behav.*, 51: 481–485.

Lipton, J.M. and Ticknor, C.B. (1979) Influence of sex and age on febrile responses to peripheral and central administration of pyrogens in the rabbit. *J. Physiol.*, 295: 263–272.

Lopez-Valpuesta, F.J. and Myers, R.D. (1995) Cytokines and thermoregulation: interleukin-9 injected in preoptic area fails to evoke fever in rats. *Brain Res. Bull.*, 36: 181–184.

Macari, M., Furlan, R.L., Gregorut, E.P., Secato, E.R. and Guerreiro, J.R. (1993) Effects of endotoxin, interleukin-1 β and prostaglandin injections on fever response in broilers. *Br. Poult. Sci.*, 34: 1035–1042.

Milton, A.S. (1989) Thermoregulatory actions of eicosanoids in the central nervous system with particular regard to the pathogenesis of fever. *Ann. New York Acad. Sci.*, 539: 392–410.

Minano, F.J., Sancibrian, M., Vizcaino, M., Paez, X., Davatelis, T., Fahey, T., Sherry, B., Cerami, A. and Myers, R.D. (1990) Macrophage inflammatory protein-1: unique action on hypothalamus to evoke fever. *Brain Res. Bull.*, 24: 849–852.

Molenaar, G., Berkenbosh, F., van Dam, A.M., Lugard, C.M.J.E. (1990) Distribution of interleukin 1 β immunoreactivity within the porcine hypothalmus. *Brain Res.*, 33: 248–255.

Morimoto, A., Murakami, N., Sakata, Y., Watanabe, T. and Yamaguchi, K. (1990) Functional and structural differences in febrile mechanism between rabbits and rats. *J. Physiol. (Lond.)*, 427: 227–239.

Morimoto, A., Long, N.C., Nakamori, T. and Murakami, N. (1991) The effect of prostaglandin E_2 on the body temperature of restrained rats. *Physiol. Behav.*, 50: 249–253.

Murphy, S. and Pearce, B. (1988) Eicosanoids in the CNS: sources and effects. *Prostaglandins Leukotrienes Essent. Fatty Acids*, 31: 165–170.

Murphy, S., Pearce, B., Jeremy, J. and Dandoma, P. (1988) Astrocytes as eicosanoid-producing cells. *Glia*, 1: 241–245.

Nakamori, T., Morimoto, A., Yamaguchi, K., Watanabe, T. and Murakami, N. (1994) Interleukin-1 β production in the rabbit brain during endotoxin-induced fever. *J. Physiol. (Lond.)*, 476: 177–186.

Nam, M.J., Thore, C. and Busija, D. (1995) Protein kinases and prostaglandin production in ovine astroglia. *Prostaglandins*, 50: 33–45.

Navarra, P., Pozzoli, G., Becherucci, C., Preziosi, P., Grossman, A.B. and Parente, L. (1993) Prostaglandin E_2 and bacterial lipopolysaccharide stimulate bioactive interleukin-1 release from hypothalamic explants. *Neuroendocrinology*, 57: 257–261.

Norman, D.C., Grahn, D. and Yoshikava, T.T. (1985) Fever and aging. *J. Am. Geriatr. Soc.*, 33: 859–863.

O'Rourke, S.T. and Rudy, T.A. (1984) Intracerebroventricular and preoptic injections of leukotrienes C_4, D_4 and E_4 in the rat: lack of febrile effect. *Brain Res.*, 295: 283–288.

Parrott, R.F., Vellucci, S.V., Forsling, M.L. and Goode, J.A. (1995) Hyperthermic and endocrine effects of intravenous prostaglandin administration in the pig. *Domest. Anim. Endocrinol.*, 12: 197–205.

Romero, S.D., Chyatte, D., Byer, D.E., Romero, J.C. and Yaksh, T.L. (1984) Measurement of prostaglandins in the cerebrospinal fluid in cat, dog, and man. *J. Neurochem.*, 43: 1642–1649.

Roth, J., Conn, C.A., Kluger, M.J. and Zeisberger, E. (1993) Kinetics of systemic and intrahypothalamic IL-6 and tumor necrosis factor during endotoxin fever in guinea pigs. *Am. J. Physiol.*, 262: R653–R658.

Rothwell, N.J. (1992) Eicosanoids, thermogenesis and thermoregulation. *Prostaglandins Leukotrienes Essent. Fatty Acids*, 46: 1–7.

Rothwell, N.J. (1994) CNS regulation of thermogenesis. *Crit. Rev. Neurobiol.*, 8: 1–10.

Rothwell, N.J., Hardwick, A.J. and Lindley, I. (1990) Central action of interleukin-8 in rat are independent of prostaglandins. *Horm. Metab. Res.*, 22: 595–596.

Ruwe, W.D., Naylor, A.M., Dinarello, C.A. and Veale, W.L. (1988) Characteristics of pyrogen fever are altered in the aged rabbits. *Exp. Gerontol.*, 23: 103–113.

Saper, C.B. and Breder, C.D. (1992) Endogenous pyrogens in the CNS: role in the febrile response. *Prog. Brain Res.*, 93: 419–428.

Scarpace, P.J., Borst, S.E. and Bender, B.S. (1992) The association of *E. coli* peritonitis with an impaired and delayed fever response in senescent rats. *J. Gerontol.*, 47: B142–B145.

Seydel, U., Brandenburg, K. and Reitschel, E.T. (1994) A case for an endotoxic conformation. *Prog. Clin. Biol. Res.*, 388: 17–30.

Simpson, C.W., Ruwe, W.D. and Myers, R.D. (1994) Prostaglandins and hypothalamic neurotransmitter receptors involved in hyperthermia: a critical evaluation. *Neurosci. Biobehav. Rev.*, 18: 1–20.

Sirco, S.I., Bishai, I. and Coceani, F. (1989) Prostaglandin formation in the hypothalamus *in vivo*: effect of pyrogens. *Am. J. Physiol.*, 256: R616–R624.

Spangelo, B.L. and Gorospe, W.C. (1995) Role of cytokines in the neuroendocrine-immune system axis. *Front. Neuroendocrinol.*, 16: 1–22.

Spangelo, B.L., Judd, A.M., MacLeod, R.M., Goodman, D.W. and Isakson, P.C. (1990) Endotoxin-induced release of interleukin-6 from rat medial basal hypothalmi. *Endocrinology*, 127: 1779–1785.

Spatz, M., Stanimirovic, D.B., Uematsu, S. and McCarron, R.M. (1994) Vasoactive peptides and prostaglandin D_2 in human cerebrovascular endothelium. *J. Auton. Nerv. Syst.*, 49 Suppl.: S123–S127.

Splawinski, J.A., Gorka, Z., Zachy, E. and Wojtaszek, B. (1978) Hyperthermic effects of arachidonic acid, prostaglandin E_2 and $F_{2\alpha}$ in rats. *Pflüg. Arch.*, 341: 15–21.

Stitt, J.T. (1991) Differential sensitivity in the sites of fever production by prostaglandin E_1 within the hypothalamus of the rat. *J. Physiol.*, 432: 99–110.

Strijbos, P.J., Hardwick, A.J., Relton, J.K., Carey, F. and Rothwell, N.J. (1992) Inhibition of central actions of cytokines on fever and thermogenesis by lipocortin-1 involves CRF. *Am. J. Physiol.*, 263: E632–E636.

Strijbos, P.J., Horan, M.A., Carey, F. and Rothwell, N.J. (1993) Impaired febrile responses of aging mice are mediated by endogenous lipocortin-1 (annexin-1). *Am. J. Physiol.*, 265: E289–E297.

Takahata, R., Matsumura, H., Kantha, S.S., Kubo, E., Kawase, K., Sakai, T. and Hayaishi, O. (1993) Intravenous administration of inorganic selenium compounds, inhibitors of prostaglandin D synthase, inhibits sleep in freely moving rats. *Brain Res.*, 623: 65–71.

Takao, T., Culp, S.G. and De Souza, E.B. (1993) Reciprocal modulation of interleukin-1β (IL-1β and IL-1 receptors by lipopolysaccharide (endotoxin) treatment in the mouse brain-endocrine-immune axis. *Endocrinology*, 132: 1497–1504.

Teisner, B. and Haahr, S. (1974): Poikilothermia and susceptibility of suckling mice to Coxackie B1 virus. *Nature*, 247: 568.

Ueno, R., Narumiya, S., Ogorochi, T., Nakayama, T., Ishikava, Y. and Hayaishi, O. (1982) Role of prostaglandin D_2 in the hypothermia of rats caused by bacterial lipopolysaccharide. *Proc. Natl. Acad. Sci. USA*, 79: 6093–6097.

Ueno, R., Osama, H., Urade, Y. and Hayaishi, O. (1985) Changes of enzymes involved in prostaglandin metabolism and prostaglandin binding proteins in rat brain during development and aging. *J. Neurochem.*, 45: 483–489.

Wahl, M. and Schilling, L. (1993) Regulation of cerebral blood flow. *Acta Neurochir. Suppl. Wien*, 59: 3–10.

Watanabe, T., Clark, W.G., Ceriani, G. and Lipton, J.M. (1994) Elevation of plasma ACTH concentration in rabbits made febrile by systemic injection of bacterial endotoxin. *Brain Res.*, 652: 201–206.

Watanabe, Y., Tokumoto, H., Yamashita, A., Narumiya, S., Mizuno, N. and Hayaishi, O. (1985) Specific bindings of prostaglandin D_2, E_2, and $F_{2\alpha}$ in postmortem human brain. *Brain Res.*, 342: 110–116.

Weidenfeld, J., Amir, I. and Shohami, E. (1993) Role of glucocorticoids in the regulation of brain prostaglandin biosynthesis under basal conditions and in response to endotoxin. *Endocrinology*, 132: 941–945.

Zampronio, A.R., Souza, G.E.P., Silva, C.A., Cunha, F.Q. and Ferreira, S.H. (1994) Interleukin-8 induces fever by a prostaglandin-independent mechanism. *Am. J. Physiol.*, 266: R1670–R1674.

Zampronio, A.R., Silva, C.A., Cunha, F.Q., Ferreira, S.H., Pela, I.R. and Souza, G.E.P. (1995) Indomethacin blocks the febrile response induced by interleukin-8 in rabbits. *Am. J. Physiol.*, 269: R1469–R1474.

H.S. Sharma and J. Westman (Eds.)
Progress in Brain Research, Vol 115

CHAPTER 10

Biogenic amines and thermoregulatory changes

Eugen Zeisberger*

Physiologisches Institut, Klinikum der Justus-Liebig-Universität Giessen, Aulweg 129, 35392 Giessen, Germany

Introduction

Organisms produce heat by metabolic processes that are dependent on ambient temperature. Homeothermic organisms gained certain independence from changes in ambient temperature, because they are not only able to detect environmental changes, but developed appropriate mechanisms to maintain their core temperature stable (Hensel et al., 1973; Ruben, 1995). The homeostatic mechanisms are coordinated by the central nervous system. In homeotherms, the limbic system and hypothalamus in particular are the parts of the brain involved in the control of homeostatic systems. Although there has been great progress in knowledge about the organization of these brain parts and their function (Nieuwenhuys, 1985; Shepherd, 1988), the roles of neurotransmitters participating in thermoregulation and thermal adaptation have not been elucidated sufficiently, and the experimental evidence is largely controversial. In the past 20 years there were several reviews collecting this evidence (Hellon, 1975; Bligh, 1979; Clark and Clark, 1980; Dascombe, 1985; Brück and Zeisberger, 1990; Nagai, 1991) and ascribing the diversity either to methodology or to interspecies differences. In two previous reviews (Brück and Zeisberger, 1990; Zeisberger and Roth, 1996), we tried to find a more natural explanation for this diversity. Animals differ in their size and therefore develop different thermoregulatory or thermoadaptive mechanisms and strategies, that can be activated subsequently, depending on time factors, and governed by the rules of economy. The purpose of the present paper is to review the possible roles of biogenic amines in thermoregulatory reactions to hot environment. Only an overview of the most important aspects of this topic can be given here. As examples for small and large organisms, only the changes found in guinea pigs or rats, and in humans will be analyzed. Thus the bibliography cannot be complete and for the most part reviews are referred to instead of the original literature. In this review the general principles of the organization of the thermoregulatory system will be described first, followed by thermoregulatory reactions to hot environment and the probable roles of biogenic amines in these responses.

Organization of the thermoregulatory system

The hypothalamus is the highest center of the autonomic system and is concerned with complex responses, which can be described as regulatory strategies subserving the homeostatic functions such as energy balance (including control of food intake, of cell metabolism, of body nutrient stores), the closely connected heat balance (thermogenesis, heat loss), water balance (thirst, water

*Corresponding author. Tel: +49 641 9947230; fax: +49 641 9947239; e-mail: eugen.zeisberger@physiologie.med.uni-giessen.de

intake, extracellular fluid volume, water excretion and sweating), the control of the balanced immune system, and of the balanced and timely coordinated development and reproduction. The evidence is growing that multisensor neurons (Hori et al., 1988; Boulant and Silva, 1989) sensitive to different local stimuli (temperature, osmolality, metabolic substances, hormones, cytokines) are integrated in the hypothalamus with many different neurotransmitter systems carrying information from peripheral sensory systems and instructions from higher parts of the CNS. The signals derived from this integration are differentiated in neurons producing releasing hormones and enhanced in cells of the endocrine system (Gale, 1973; Marques et al., 1981; Slaunwhite, 1988). They influence, via the autonomic nervous system or directly via circulation, the target cells, not only in the periphery of the body, but also within the CNS (Zeisberger, 1990).

The properties of the thermoregulatory system, which were intensively studied in the past 30 years (for reviews cf. Hammel, 1965, 1968; Benzinger, 1969; Hardy, 1972; Bligh, 1973; Hensel, 1973; Wyndham, 1973; Cabanac, 1975; Simon et al., 1986; Brück and Zeisberger, 1990; Jessen, 1990; Werner, 1990; Gagge and Gonzalez, 1996), can be summarized in the simplest way as follows. The thermoregulatory system is organized hierarchically, the highest controller being localized in the hypothalamus. The central controller receives information on the temperature from the body surface and from different parts of body core. Body surface temperature is measured by cutaneous thermal sensors (Pierau, 1996), core temperature by central sensors and thermosensitive structures within the preoptic area in limbic septum, anterior hypothalamus, brain stem, spinal cord and possibly some other places (Jessen, 1990; Boulant, 1996). Although two types of sensors, warm and cold sensitive structures have been found in the skin and in body core, it seems that in afferent nerve fibres from the skin, the information from cold sensitive structures dominates, and on the other hand, among the thermosensitive structures of the body core, only few are cold sensitive.

In cybernetic considerations two signal inputs into the hypothalamic controller were considered (for reviews cf. Brück and Zeisberger, 1978; Brück and Zeisberger, 1990; Jessen, 1990; Werner, 1990; Boulant, 1996): (1) The composite skin temperature signal (from cutaneous cold receptors) combined with input from central cold sensitive structures, and (2) the composite core temperature signal (from the large majority of warm sensitive central structures) combined with input from cutaneous warm sensors. These inputs are coupled with effectors in such a way that the composite skin temperature signal from cold sensors activates the mechanisms for conservation and production of the heat, and the composite core temperature signal from warm sensors activates the heat loss mechanisms (Fig. 1).

As known from various experimental approaches, the cold input may inhibit the heat defence branch and vice versa (cf. Bligh, 1972 for review and references). Therefore, inhibitory neurones have been proposed, in the central controller, interconnecting the two parallel branches for cold and heat defence. By this way the activation of the cold defence can be evoked only after overcoming the inhibition from central warm sensors, and vice versa the heat defence can begin after surpassing the input from cold sensors. Thus the activation of thermoregulatory responses starts at certain combinations of central and peripheral temperatures = threshold temperatures.

In an attempt to imitate the hypothalamic integration of thermal signals, some authors relate thermoregulatory responses to mean body temperature (T_b), which is a species-specific combination of a representative central temperature and the mean peripheral temperature. The weighting factors determining T_b seem to vary with body size ranging from 0.4:1 to 1:1 (central/mean peripheral temperature) in small animals like rats or guinea pigs, 3:1 in rabbits, 4:1 in dogs and from 8:2 to 9:1 in humans (Colin et al., 1971; Cabanac, 1975). This indicates that the relatively large surface area in a small animal represents an important thermoregulatory input, whose importance diminishes in large organisms. Whereas the cold defence effectors are present in the inner parts of

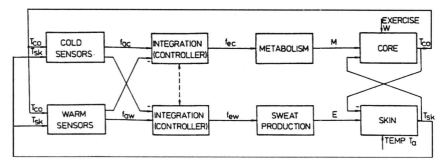

Fig. 1. Simple model of cold and warm defence (vasomotor effector assumed to be either at minimum or maximum). Tco = core temperature; Tsk = skin temperature; fa = (integrative) afferent frequency; fe = (integrative) efferent frequency; index c = cold; index w = warm; M = metabolic heat production; E = evaporative heat loss; Ta = air temperature; W = work load [from Werner (1996), reprinted with kind permission of Oxford University Press, New York, USA].

the body (core), the warm defence mechanisms are primarily active via the body surface. Therefore, it seems, that the thermoregulatory tasks in organisms varying in body size are different. While, small animals have problems how to produce enough heat to compensate their high heat loss, the large organisms must solve the problem of how to dissipate the heat produced by metabolism via the relatively small surface area.

The way of integration of thermal signals from cold and warm sensors in the hypothalamic controller led to speculation that the set point of the thermoregulatory system may thus be created (cf. Bligh, 1979 for review and references). This simple concept of the thermoregulatory system caused many researchers, including us, to construct similarly simple neuronal connectivity models (see Fig. 2, as an example).

Such models had the advantage of being a convenient didactic aid in explaining to students how the controller might be constructed, but also the disadvantage of a strong oversimplification leading to the belief that the system could be easily manipulated if the few specific inputs were represented by certain transmitters. The model shown in Fig. 1 also proposed a hard-wired circuitry which would result in a stable thermoregulatory set-point. Since it was known that between thermoregulatory threshold temperatures for the onset of heat production and dissipation, a zone

rather than a point existed, additional modulatory inputs into the controller were inferred. Examples of these are represented in the model shown in Fig. 2 by areas rich in catecholaminergic neurons (SC) and of serotonergic neurons (NR) in the lower brain stem, that send ascending fibres to the hypothalamic controller modifying the integration of thermal inputs, and descending fibres to the spinal cord modifying the output signals to thermoregulatory effectors. Our group in Giessen investigated the effects of these inputs on changes of the respective thermoregulatory thresholds in small animals and in humans (cf. Brück and Zeisberger, 1978, 1990; Brück and Hinckel, 1990; Zeisberger and Roth, 1996 for reviews and references). These modulatory inputs receive information from thermal sensors which is integrated with nonthermal inputs. It was proposed that such integration of thermal and nonthermal inputs takes place at all levels of hierarchy in the thermoregulatory system, and that it is necessary for creation of efferent signals with the spatial and temporal characteristics (Gordon and Heath, 1986). Thus, there exist multiple modulatory inputs that are not all monoaminergic. They all may participate in changes of thermoregulatory thresholds documented experimentally during thermal adaptation, fever, or under the influence of different other stressors (cf. Zeisberger and Roth, 1996 for review).

162

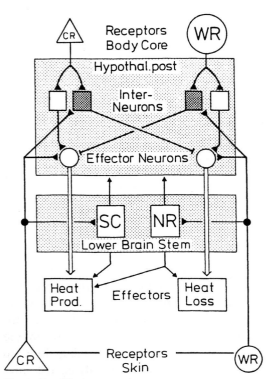

Fig. 2. Simplified model of neuronal connectivities related to temperature control. Heat loss mechanisms are driven prevailingly by the input from central warm sensors (WR in body core), supported by the input from peripheral warm sensors (WR skin) and inhibited by the central interneurons transmitting the composite signal from cold sensors. Heat production mechanisms are driven by the input from peripheral cold sensors (CR skin), supported by the input from central cold sensitive structures (CR in body core), opposed by the central interneurons transmitting the composite signal from warm sensors. Both the integration of thermal inputs into the hypothalamic controller and the outgoing signals to thermoregulatory effectors can be modified by ascending or descending nerve fibres from modulatory catecholaminergic (SC = subcoeruleus region) or serotonergic (NR = raphé nuclei) neurons in the lower brain stem, that also receive thermal inputs [from Brück (1987), reprinted with kind permission of Springer-Verlag, Berlin/Heidelberg, Germany].

Peripheral transmitters

Biogenic amines, mainly catecholamines — noradrenaline (NA), adrenaline (A), dopamine (DA) — and serotonin (5-hydroxytryptamine, 5-HT), have been thought to play an important role in thermoregulation. This belief was based on the fact that increased levels of NA and A were found in circulation, or excreted in urine, during different thermal loads. It is worth noting that NA and A found in peripheral blood or in urine originate mostly from sympathetic nerve endings or from the adrenal medulla. They represent a spillover of mediators released in sympathetic postganglionic neurons by impulses from the CNS evoked by a wide variety of stimuli. With the exception of skeletal musculature, which is controlled by the somatomotor nervous system, all of the so-called thermoregulatory effectors are activated by sympathetic nerves of the autonomic nervous system (Fig. 3).

In fact, the thermoregulatory system has no specific effector organs of its own, but shares them with other homeostatic systems. Even the nonshivering thermogenesis in brown adipose tissue and sweat secretion, which seem to serve exclusively the thermoregulation, may have a metabolic function, or subserve the system controlling the water balance as well. Therefore, the release of transmitters activating the thermoregulatory effectors need not in all cases represent the thermoregulatory reaction. Nevertheless, from Fig. 3, it can be concluded that two neurotransmitters are important for the control of thermoregulatory effectors, namely acetylcholine (ACh) and NA. The somatomotor nervous system controls via release of ACh in the neuromuscular junctions the tension in the skeletal musculature and the heat production by shivering (cf. Kleinebeckel and Klussmann, 1990 for review). By means of other stimulatory patterns the same system mediates voluntary movements and behavioral responses (cf. Cabanac, 1996b; Satinoff, 1996 for reviews). The ACh receptors in mammalian skeletal muscle are of nicotinic type, i.e. the actions of ACh can be mimicked by nicotine and blocked by curare. Somewhat different ACh receptors, but also of the nicotinic type, mediate the transmission from preganglionic to postganglionic neurons in the autonomic nerve system. The nicotinic receptors for ACh have been found also in different parts of the CNS. About four subtypes of nicotinic receptors have been described. All

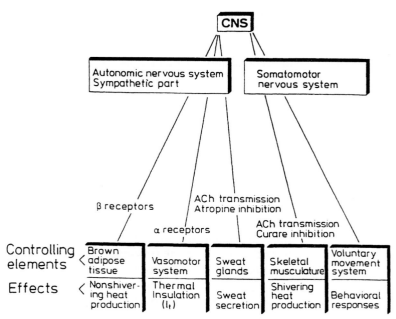

Fig. 3. Diagram of the neural control of the thermoregulatory controlling elements (effectors) and their effects (actions) [from Brück (1987), reprinted with kind permission of Springer-Verlag, Berlin/Heidelberg, Germany].

are closely connected to ion channels in the cell membrane (cf. McCarthy et al., 1986 for review on ultrastructure of the receptors). However, ACh released from postganglionic parasympathetic endings and from postganglionic sympathetic fibres to sweat glands stimulates the smooth muscle and the glands via ACh receptors of muscarinic type, i.e. the actions of ACh can be mimicked by muscarine and blocked by the drug atropine. Muscarinic receptors are very different from nicotinic receptors. Five subtypes have been cloned, that are all coupled via G proteins to adenylate cyclase or phospholipase C (Venter et al., 1989). Thus sweat secretion is stimulated from sympathetic ganglia by postganglionic cholinergic neurons via muscarinic receptors. ACh is very rapidly inactivated enzymatically in all types of synapses. Therefore, there is no measurable spillover of ACh into the blood. The other sympathetically-induced effects such as piloerection, vasomotor reactions and nonshivering thermogenesis (for reviews cf. Jansky, 1973; Nicholls and Locke, 1984; Himms-Hagen, 1990; Cannon et al.,

1994; Jansky, 1995) are all mediated by NA released from postganglionic sympathetic endings or by A secreted by the adrenal medulla and transported to the effectors via the blood flow. Both NA and A act on α- and β-receptors, with NA having a greater affinity for α- and A for β-receptors. Both types of receptors are linked to G proteins and there are multiple subtypes of each (Hille, 1992; Summers and McMartin, 1993; Ruffolo and Hieble, 1994). NA is removed from synapses by an active re-uptake mechanism. However, it is released not only at endings close to receptors, but at all varicosities of the active fibre and therefore its spillover into the blood is substantial. It is slowly metabolized to biologically inactive products by oxidation and methylation. The findings of increased circulating levels of NA and A during acute or chronic exposure to cold are therefore not surprising.

Central transmitters

Biogenic amines have also been shown to be

produced and released in the CNS where they act on specific receptors. The first proposals that monoamines such as catecholamines and 5-HT might modify the set point of the thermoregulatory system appeared in the late fifties (Brodie and Shore, 1957; Euler, 1961). In an attempt to prove this hypothesis, Feldberg and Myers (1963) injected these amines into cerebral ventricles and into the hypothalamus, and found that NA decreased, and 5-HT increased, body temperature in the cat. On the basis of these experiments, the authors postulated that the control of body temperature depends on the balance between the release of catecholamines and 5-HT in the rostral hypothalamus. This so-called new theory of thermoregulation stimulated many similar experiments in other mammals which, however, led to conflicting results. Some species reacted similarly to the cat, others reacted in just the opposite way, i.e. NA increased, and 5-HT decreased body temperature (for refs. see Hellon, 1975; Bligh, 1979; Lomax and Schönbaum, 1979; Clark and Clark, 1980; Myers, 1980; Blatteis, 1981). According to the thermoregulatory effect of the respective amine, different authors tried to attribute certain mediators to distinct elements in the simplified neuronal models (cf. Bligh, 1979), and failed to develop universally valid concepts. In our earlier review (Brück and Zeisberger, 1990), we tried to analyze the neuroanatomical and thermophysiological evidence in order to find out, what kind of signals the monoaminergic systems transmit, and how are they integrated into the thermoregulatory system. We came to the conclusion that these systems receive information from several sensory systems and that they seem to create additional modulatory signals, which may interfere with processing of specific thermal information at several sites. Theoretically, the central monoamines may participate in the control of thermal input, in the central integration of thermal signals, and in modification of output signals to thermoregulatory effectors. Best documented is their modulatory action on thermosensitive and thermointegrative hypothalamic neurons. There, the monoamines 5-HT and NA act as antagonists,

which enhance or diminish the effects of thermal afferents mediated by other transmitters. Moreover, the antagonistic monoaminergic systems are interconnected and can influence each other at the level of the lower brain stem. The activity in central monoaminergic systems can also be modified by neurohumoral feedback mechanisms from the periphery. By means of these interrelations the vegetative responses of the organism can be corrected and optimized. These interrelations can also explain some cross-adaptive changes in the thermoregulatory thresholds evoked by nonthermal factors such as food intake and exercise. In a recent review (Zeisberger and Roth, 1996), we tried to include the increasing knowledge on different neurochemical transmitter systems in the hypothalamus and expanded the concepts by integrating the peripheral–central interactions between autonomic nervous, neuroendocrine and neuroimmune systems (Fig. 4).

We came to the conclusion that these interactions help to keep the balance in different vegetative functions, and to restore it, when it was suddenly altered by a stressful cognitive or noncognitive event. In this respect these interactions also play a central role in all adaptive processes. Although it seems that a specific behavioral response can be initiated by a stressful event, it is not clear how these events are further differentiated and how the response is sustained during a continuing stress. It seems that complex interactions between the signal substances, and sometimes even their sequential action, are required to evoke a specific behavioral response, and that not only the signal substances released from nerve endings, but also chemical signals from the blood and surrounding extracellular fluid participate in this process. There is also increasing evidence that different hypothalamic homeostatic systems are interconnected and use common modulatory signal substances. Therefore, a change in the thermoregulatory system, i.e. a change in a system controlling the energy balance, is accompanied by changes in other vegetative functions involved in the control of the immune system or of water balance. In different species, the thermoregulatory and thermoadaptive strategies may be different. Obviously, the strategy chosen by the animals depends on different factors, such as the availability of energy and water, the season and other environmental factors, the individual or the inherited experience. The adaptive process involves learning and is dependent on interactions of the whole organism. For more information and references see Zeisberger and Roth (1996).

Thermoregulatory responses to changes in ambient temperature

Homeotherms generally resist cold better than heat. They can tolerate with little harm a 15°C decrease in body temperature, whereas 5–6°C hyperthermia can be lethal. To keep the temperature in the body core constant, the heat production must be balanced by heat loss. Muscular exercise increases metabolic rate above resting levels and thus increases the rate at which heat must be dissipated. The body can also gain heat from the environment by sun radiation, or when the ambient temperature is higher than the skin by convection and conduction, and this also increases the amount of heat that the body must dissipate. Environmental heat stress and muscular exercise therefore interact synergistically and may strain physiological systems to their limits.

Structural modifications

The thermoneutral zone varies from species to species according to morphology and fur thickness. It is very narrow in unclothed humans, but its span is much broader in clothed humans and a wide variety of animals, depending on size and the insulative values of the clothing or pelt (cf. Hensel et al., 1973; Gagge and Gonzalez, 1996 for reviews and references). The thermal resistance of the pelage in mammals and the plumage in birds can be increased within certain limits by raising hair and feathers due to involuntary tensing of smooth muscles (arrectores pilorum) connected to the hair follicles (piloerection). The additional insulation layers such as pelt in animals and clothing in humans are useful in the cold, but in the warm environment they generally impair the mechanisms for heat dissipation. Therefore, some animals developed genetically fixed adaptations allowing them to change the winter fur for another with lower resistance value in summer. Since pelt may protect the animal from heating up by sun radiation, some animals, such as the camel, have pelt with a high resistance value on the back, but with low resistance value on the abdominal site of the body, which is not exposed to sun radiation. Some mammals, especially those living or diving in cold water, developed additional thermal insulation in the form of a subcutaneous fat layer, that can substantially enlarge the buffer zone between the environment and the core of the body. As already mentioned, animals of small size have a large surface/volume ratio and have no problems in dissipating heat as long as the ambient temperature does not exceed the temperature of the body core. Nevertheless, many animals developed specialized structures with a 7–10 times higher surface/volume ratio than that of the body (rat tail, bat wing, rabbit ear, dog tongue, human fingers) to allow rapid loss of heat produced by motor activity and exercise. Animals of cold climates tend to have smaller surface areas than animals of the same species of hot climates. For example, polar animals tend to be larger, heavier and have relatively short limbs or appendages, whereas tropic animals are tall and slim with long and thin extremities.

Behavior

Behavioral responses are most economical, and the animals use them preferentially both in the cold (Satinoff, 1996) and hot environments (Cabanac, 1996a). Exposure to a hot environment sets in motion a series of thermoregulatory reactions preventing the life threatening hyperthermia. They can include the following responses: expanded posture, increasing the relative surface of the organism, search for shadow, hiding in burrows, reduced activity, reduced food intake, but increased water intake, cooling by spreading saliva or water on the skin, bathing in water or in

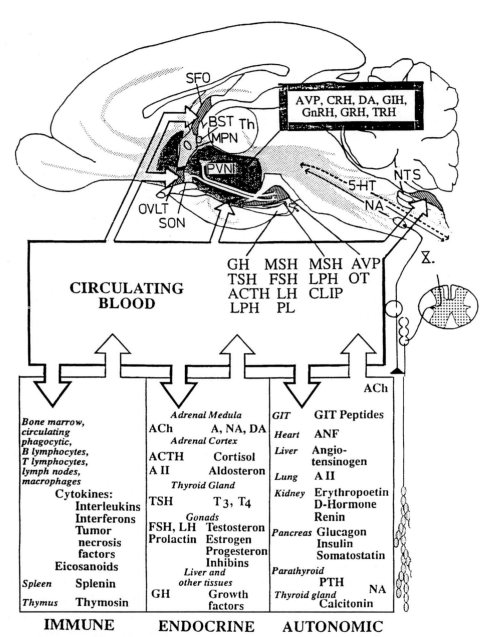

GH MSH MSH AVP
TSH FSH LPH OT
ACTH LH CLIP
LPH PL

**CIRCULATING
BLOOD**

Bone marrow, circulating phagocytic, B lymphocytes, T lymphocytes, lymph nodes, macrophages	*Adrenal Medula*	
	ACh	A, NA, DA
	Adrenal Cortex	
	ACTH	Cortisol
	A II	Aldosteron
	Thyroid Gland	
Cytokines:	TSH	T$_3$, T$_4$
Interleukins	*Gonads*	
Interferons	FSH, LH	Testosteron
Tumor	Prolactin	Estrogen
necrosis		Progesteron
factors		Inhibins
Eicosanoids	*Liver and other tissues*	
Spleen Splenin	GH	Growth
Thymus Thymosin		factors

GIT	GIT Peptides
Heart	ANF
Liver	Angiotensinogen
Lung	A II
Kidney	Erythropoetin
	D-Hormone
	Renin
Pancreas	Glucagon
	Insulin
	Somatostatin
Parathyroid	PTH
	NA
Thyroid gland	Calcitonin

ACh

IMMUNE   **ENDOCRINE**   **AUTONOMIC**

Fig. 4. Schematic representation of interactions between central and peripheral signal substances. In addition to somatic nerves, the CNS influences the peripheral tissues by means of signal substances released from autonomic nerves and from neuroendocrine system. In turn, the peripheral signal substances released from autonomic, endocrine and immune systems influence the CNS together with metabolic substrates and products in addition to signals from sensory systems. Explanations: On the parasagittal section of the guinea pig's brain (top) the bright shaded areas represent the multiple neurotransmitter systems of the medial forebrain bundle (among them also the ascending NA and 5-HT afferents to the hypothalamus). The dark shaded areas represent the integrative hypothalamic and limbic areas where neuroendocrine cells are distributed sending their axons not only to the median eminence and neurohypophysis, but also to different hypothalamic and extrahypothalamic sites such as the limbic septum,

mud, postponing the activity from the daytime to the night, migration into regions with cooler climate, and also more sophisticated human inventions such as dressing, ventilation and air conditioning in buildings. Along with behavioral responses, and not separable from them, are activated autonomic responses. They include metabolic, cardiovascular and evaporative adjustments.

Production and dissipation of heat

Heat production in homeotherms is clearly related to body size (cf. Hensel et al., 1973; Gagge and Gonzalez, 1996 for references). From a comparative point of view, the smallest mammal, the Etruscan shrew, needs about 175 times more oxygen per gram body weight and per unit of time than an elephant to keep its body temperature within the normal range. The high rate of metabolism of smaller species is only possible because the proportion of internal organs, compared with their total body weight, is much higher, than in larger animals, and because they can shiver with higher frequency (Kleinebeckel and Klussmann, 1990). Only small mammals up to 10 kg body weight have the additional ability for nonshivering thermogenesis (NST), and beyond this limit the contribution of NST to the total metabolic rate increases linearly with the reduction in body weight, being maximal in the smallest

mammals (Heldmaier, 1971). In hot environments, small homeothermic vertebrates reduce their activity. Some species developed the ability to enter regulated torpor, called estivation, in dry environments, especially when food and water are scarce. In the state of estivation the physiological functions are restricted, and metabolism is reduced below the basal value in the active state. Some species, for instance bats, often enter torpor even when energy supplies and body weight are adequate. Thus estivation may involve the integration of multiple physiological functions including energy conservation, biological rhythms and temperature regulation (cf. Ridesel and Folk, 1996 for review and references).

Circulatory adjustments

All homeotherms must balance any heat gain by subsequent heat dissipation through the skin and respiratory tract. The surface temperatures of the body are lower than the internal temperature, establishing thus the radial gradient necessary for the heat flux. Additionally, due to the countercurrent blood flow in central arteries and veins, the surface temperatures decrease along the longitudinal axes of the extremities. The axial gradient for the heat flux thus progressively decreases which diminishes also the radial gradient along the extremity. In this way excessive extremity heat loss is prevented in the cold. In hot environment,

---

amygdala or lower brain stem. The arrows protruding from the medial panel into the densely shaded brain areas indicate the special neurohemal exchange sites in some circumventricular organs, such as the subfornical organ (SFO) situated above the medial preoptic nucleus (MPN) near to bed nucleus of the stria terminalis (BST) rostral to thalamus (Th), the organum vasculosum of the lamina terminalis (OVLT), the median eminence and the posterior lobe of pituitary, or the area postrema in the lower brain stem near to the nucleus of the solitary tract (NTS). Abbreviations of hypothalamic releasing hormones listed in a frame in the brain section are: AVP = arginine vasopressin; CRH = corticotropin releasing hormone; DA = dopamine; GIH = growth hormone-inhibiting hormone; GnRH = gonadotropin releasing hormone; GRH = growth hormone-releasing hormone; TRH = thyrotropin releasing hormone. Abbreviations of hormones released from anterior, intermediate and posterior lobes of pituitary into the circulating blood are: GH = growth hormone; TSH = thyroid stimulating hormone; ACTH = adrenocorticotropic hormone; LPH = lipotropin; MSH = melanocyte stimulating hormone; FSH = follicle stimulating hormone; LH = luteinizing hormone; PL = prolactin; CLIP = corticotropin-like intermediate lobe peptide; AVP = arginine vasopressin; OT = oxytocin. Not explained abbreviations of peripheral hormones and mediators of autonomic system are: A II = angiotensin II; T3 = triiodothyronine; T4 = thyroxine; GIT = gastrointestinal tract; ANF = atrial natriuretic factor; PTH = parathyroid hormone [from Zeisberger and Roth (1996), reprinted with kind permission of Oxford University Press, New York, USA].

however, the blood delivered to the end of extremities by central arteries, returns to the body core via superficial veins. Thus the countercurrent heat exchange in central arteries and veins is interrupted, the surface temperature is nearly as high as core temperature, and more heat can be dissipated from the extremities to the environment. Moreover, the speed of the blood flow through the extremities and the skin can be modified by reflex activity. There are two distinct regions characterized according to the control: acral (or apical) and nonacral sites (Johnson et al., 1986). Acral sites include skin regions with high surface/volume areas such as the tips of extremities, nose, ears, tongue and lips, also called heat exchangers. Along with an abundance of arterioles, significant numbers of arteriovenous anastomoses (AVAs) were described in acral sites. These are shunt vessels between arterioles and venules. By means of opening the AVAs the blood flow, and therefore heat flux, through the acral sites can be substantially accelerated. The nonacral sites, such as the torso, forearms, upper arms and legs are characterized by a lack of AVAs.

The skin blood flow is primarily controlled by adrenergic vasoconstrictor nervous activity (Johnson et al., 1986; Johnson and Proppe, 1996), mediated by both α_1- and α_2-adrenergic receptors. The contribution of β-adrenergic receptor activity is limited. Vasodilation at normal core temperature levels seems to be the passive result of removing the cold-induced sympathetic vasoconstrictor α-adrenoreceptor drive (Grayson, 1990). Anaesthesia also removes the vasoconstrictor tone leading to peripheral vasodilation (Sessler, 1994). At high ambient temperatures during heat stress leading to hyperthermia, active cutaneous vasodilation has been described. The mechanisms for this additional dilatation are complex and not yet satisfactorily explained. It is induced by increase in sympathetic vasodilator activity which most likely involves the release of co-transmitters from cholinergic nerves (Kellogg et al., 1994). Therefore, the active cutaneous vasodilation has been linked to the sudomotor control of sweating, involving the formation or release of vasodilating peptides such as bradykinin, vasoactive intestinal peptide (VIP), calcitonin gene-related peptide (CGRP) and substance P. However, the possibility of the existence of separate vasodilator nerves releasing a non-adrenergic, noncholinergic and non-VIP mediator has not been ruled out. Many different candidates for the active vasodilator mediator, including also nitric oxide, were proposed, but the issue lacks clear resolution (cf. Johnson and Proppe, 1996 for review and references). Active vasodilation in dog tongue has been evoked through direct stimulation of sympathetic or parasympathetic nerves, which seems to include the AVAs vasodilation (Pleschka, 1984; Pleschka et al., 1987). In humans the acral blood flow and also the AVAs seem to be exclusively under adrenergic control (Hales et al., 1978). However, heat is an excellent and potent vasodilator per se (Grayson, 1990). Local heat, applied anywhere on the body, produces a localized vasodilation. Mechanisms for direct effects of elevated temperature of the skin may include altered adrenoceptor and adrenergic nerve function, but are, at least partially, independent of neural control (Johnson and Proppe, 1996).

At greater levels of heat stress, the degree to which the skin vasodilates, creates an enormous demand for blood flow. The delivery of blood flow is brought about by elevated cardiac output and redistribution of blood flow from splanchnic, renal and possibly skeletal muscle tissues to the skin. Adrenergic vasoconstrictor mechanisms, renin and angiotensin secretion are largely responsible for blood flow redistribution. The responses in cardiac output to elevated body temperature vary among species. In humans, a doubling of cardiac output has been described in resting, hyperthermic individuals (Brengelmann, 1983; Rowell, 1983) but some other species meet the demands for increased blood flow to the skin strictly by redistribution from other tissues without any change in cardiac output (Johnson and Proppe, 1996). The increase in cardiac output in humans is largely driven by increased heart rate, as stroke volume changes little.

Evaporation

Due to the high heat of vaporization of water (2.4 kJ/g), the evaporation from the surface of the skin and from the mucous membranes of the respiratory tract is a very effective means of heat loss. Evaporation from the skin is called sweating, the evaporation from the respiratory tract, combined with increase of the ventilation volume is generally called panting. The ventilation volume is typically increased by an increase in respiratory frequency (polypnoe, panting) accompanied by a reduction in volume of the individual breaths. There are large differences between species concerning the two mechanisms of evaporative heat loss. Panting is the prominent mechanism in birds, which lack sweat glands, and for most mammals with no or weak sweat secretion (mouse, rat, guinea pig, rabbit, cat, dog, sheep, pig, cow and others).

Panting

Panting in the furred mammal and feathered bird is the most efficient and direct route for dissipating metabolic body heat by evaporating water. Even neglecting the wastage of sweat dripping off the body surface, sweating in thermally insulated animals is less efficient in removing core heat from the body. The development and effectiveness of polypnoe vary within wide limits in individual species. In many species, respiratory frequency is increased proportionally to the increase in core temperature (sheep, pig, birds), while others pant as soon as the external temperature goes up (rabbit, dog, cat, cow). Some animals develop polypnoe with closed mouths (rat, guinea pig, rabbit, sheep), others pant with their mouth open, their tongues hanging out, and with copious secretion of saliva (dogs and cats), which is more effective. Some animals such as rabbits and sheep proceed to open-mouth panting when their core temperatures exceed 40°C. Panting is controlled by a motor nerve system from respiratory centers in medulla oblongata, which are modified by mod-ulatory inputs from the hypothalamus (cf. Hensel et al., 1973 for review and references).

Sweating

The postganglionic sympathetic fibers innervating sweat glands are nonmyelinated C fibers. They are primarily cholinergic in humans, but adrenergic in most other species (Robertshaw, 1975). The sweating in humans may also be facilitated by circulating catecholamines, in particular epinephrine, via α- and β-adrenergic receptors associated with eccrine sweat glands (Sato et al., 1989a, 1989b). The increase in body temperature from the sweating threshold induces the increase in thermoregulatory sweating. As sweating increases, there is initially a recruitment of sweat glands and than an increased sweat secretion per gland. Therefore, sweating is dependent both upon the density of sweat glands and the amount of sweat per gland. Different skin regions have different sweating responses for a given core temperature. In humans, the back and chest have the greatest sweating rates, while limbs have relatively low sweating rates. The sweating response may be enhanced by local heating of the skin. The mechanism of this effect is not entirely clear, but it seems that several factors are involved. Among them, the greater neurotransmitter release per nerve impulse arriving at the sweat gland and the increased responsiveness to a given amount of neurotransmitter substance have been discussed (cf. Sawka et al., 1996 for review and references). However, it should be kept in mind, that only some, prevailingly large mammalian species are equipped with sweat glands.

Probable roles of biogenic amines in thermoregulatory responses to hot environment

It is difficult to make a generalized statement concerning the role of biogenic amines in defence against overheating in respect to large differences between different species in the strategies they use to protect themselves from overheating, and in their abilities to dissipate heat. Looking at catecholamine levels found in the blood plasma or excreted in urine during acute or prolonged exposures to hot environment, everybody is confronted with the diversity of findings. But it should not be forgotten that the levels of catecholamines in blood plasma or urine represent an overall spillover of transmitters released at different prevailingly peripheral sites. This may be interpreted as an indicator of the activity in the sympathoadrenomedullar (SAM) system. It can be subdivided into sympathetic and adrenal outflow. The sympathetic output represents the regulatory signals sent by the CNS to the peripheral organs. The adrenal output results from activation of neuroendocrine HPA-axis and represents a nonspecific response of the CNS to the activation of different sensory systems by new, or highly loading stimuli, called stressors. Moreover, the sympathetic output is regionally differentiated as was demonstrated experimentally. Local heating of the hypothalamus (Iriki et al., 1971), spinal cord (Walther et al., 1970), and skin (Riedel et al., 1972) in anesthetized rabbits all evoked a decrease of sympathetic activity in cutaneous nerves (withdrawal of sympathetic vasoconstriction) and a simultaneous increase of sympathetic activity in splanchnic nerves (increasing of the vasoconstrictor tone). Both responses serve the redistribution of cardiac output to increase the blood flow in the skin and reduce it in splanchnic and muscle beds, so that the blood pressure can be minimally disturbed (cf. Johnson and Proppe, 1996 for review and references). Similar progressive increases in splanchnic nerve activity were also demonstrated in anesthetized rats by whole-body hyperthermia at core temperatures from 37°C to 41°C (Gisolfi et al., 1991). Decreased blood flow to the small intestine by 30–45% were also demonstrated in unanesthetized baboons, sheep and rats. These decreases could be prevented by blockade of α-adrenergic receptors (Proppe, 1980). The renal blood flow is also partly mediated by adrenergic α-receptors, supported by activation of the renin-angiotensin-aldosteron system which seems to be controlled by β-receptors (cf. Johnson and Proppe, 1996 for references). The control of the heat-induced redistribution of the blood flow is complex and achieved by an interaction of local regulatory substances, arterial baroreceptors, atrial stretch receptors, peripheral chemoreceptors and central nervous modulators. Among them is NA released from sympathetic nerves, and A released from adrenal medulla, as well as AVP released from the posterior lobe of pituitary and also hormones released by activation of the renin-angiotensin-aldosteron system, which all support the actions of catecholamines. The AII receptors in the CNS appear to play an important role for these responses. Intracerebroventricular application of a specific AII antagonist abolishes the increase in sympathetic nerve activity to the splanchnic region in response to heat challenge. Interestingly, the increase in AVP observed after heat stress is also reversed after central AII blockade (Kregel et al., 1994).

Thus during the blood flow redistribution, a decrease in sympathetic tone in one vascular bed can be compensated for by increases in others. If these changes were balanced, nothing should change in the total SAM output. However, in some species, these changes are not balanced, especially in large animals and in humans, where the cardiac output increases in addition to blood redistribution. Therefore, in these species the SAM output is regularly increased by a component necessary for driving the increase in heart rate. Correspondingly, increased levels of NA were reported in these species. Moreover, this sympathetic output may be supported by NA and A released from adrenal medulla in response to different thermal and nonthermal stressors. It seems, however, that the specific heat-stress response is activated at very high temperatures. Thus in the anesthetized rat the circulating catecholamines do not increase until the internal temperature exceeds 41°C (Gisolfi et al., 1991). In anesthetized cancer patients subject to therapeutic hyperthermia, plasma A concentration did not increase until internal temperature exceeded 39.5°C (Kim et al., 1979). However, in conscious individuals, the adrenal secretion may be activated at lower body temperatures by a combination of different stressors. Thus in dogs, the circulating catecholamines did not increase, when they were exposed to 35°C ambient temperature, but circulating levels of A and NA were elevated five- and threefold, respectively, after 3 h at 41°C. In humans, exercise in warm environment elicited elevations in plasma NA that were greater than the sum of the values observed during passive heating or exercise in a thermoneutral environment (cf. Francesconi, 1996 for review and references). Elevated plasma concentrations of NA and A have been found in hyperthermic animals and humans (cf. Gisolfi et al., 1991 for references) and in heat stroke patients (cf. Hales et al., 1996 for review).

In this review, I have tried to demonstrate that differences in release of monoamines found in different mammalian species can be expected, and are therefore not very surprising. Small species like the rat or the guinea pig are confronted with the problem of how to produce enough heat to survive in a cold environment rather than how to dissipate it in a hot environment. Therefore, small animals in a cold environment increase their food intake and metabolic rate and develop an additional thermogenic capacity in the form of nonshivering thermogenesis in brown adipose tissue, which is controlled by the activity of the SAM system (cf. Horwitz, 1996; Himms-Hagen, 1996 for reviews and references). The metabolic rate, the basic values of which are 5–10 times higher in small mammals than in humans, can in small species increase up to 10 times in the cold in comparison to at most, a threefold increase due to shivering in human adults (cf. Roberts, 1996 for review). The maximal SAM activity in small species can thus be expected during cold exposure in a cold-adapted state. In hot environments these animals first reduce their metabolic rate, activity and food consumption, which is achieved by the reduction of activity in the SAM system. Since they are protected by their fur against sun radiation, and avoid the direct confrontation behaviorally, they generally need to dissipate only the strongly reduced metabolic heat by convecting it to the skin. This is an easy task due to the large surface/volume ratio of the small animals. They increase the blood flow to the skin via the redistribution of the resting sympathetic activity, open the special heat exchangers in the ears or tail, and pant. Thus minimal activity in the SAM system can be expected under these conditions, unless it is increased additionally by exercise or some other stressors.

Exactly this has been found in our experimental investigations. In guinea pigs the amounts of NA and its main metabolite MHPG (3-methoxy-4-hydroxyphenylglycol) excreted in urine were increased 6.5 times and 4.3 times, respectively, in animals adapted to 5°C for 3 weeks in comparison to controls adapted to 22°C. In warm-adapted guinea pigs (28°C) the excreted amounts of NA and MHPG were reduced to 63% resp. 67% of levels found in controls adapted to 22°C (Roth et al., 1987). The blood plasma levels of NA and DHPG (dihydroxyphenylglycol) were also found to increase in cold-adapted guinea pigs, 5.7-fold and 2.3-fold, respectively, in comparison to controls adapted to 22°C (Roth et al., 1988; Zeisberger and Roth, 1989). Similar changes have also been found in non-hibernating golden hamsters during thermal adaptation (Roth et al., 1990).

However, in mammals of large body size, like humans, the situation is very different. There is still a relatively high NA excretion in a newborn baby, that can produce heat by NST in BAT, which is, however, less than 0.3 of that found in the newborn guinea pig (both related to the excreted amount of creatinine). In adult humans, who have lost the ability to produce heat by means of NST, the activity of the SAM system is lower and the excretion of NA decreases to about 25% of that found in the newborn baby (Zeisberger and Roth, 1988). Even the exposure to cold does not increase the catecholamine excretion much in adult humans, because they produce heat by shivering. Some increase occurs, however, which is due to circulatory efforts, peripheral vasoconstriction, and due to release of catecholamines from adrenals during thermal and emotional stress. Also exposure to hot environment increases the release of catecholamines in humans due to circulatory efforts connected with redistribution of the blood flow and the increase in cardiac output. The increased catecholamine levels found experimentally, support sweating in humans and control it in other large sweating species (Robertshaw, 1975). Further increase in catecholamine release may be caused by exercise, extreme heat stress and other combinations of different stressors. Also patients with heat stroke regularly have increased catecholamine levels in blood plasma (Hales et al., 1996).

Since peripheral–central interconnections seem to exist between the catecholamine levels (Brück and Zeisberger, 1978; Zeisberger and Roth, 1988; Brück and Zeisberger, 1990; Zeisberger, 1990), the balance between modulatory NA and 5-HT brain stem systems, ascending to the hypothalamus, can be changed, and thus the thermoregulatory system and other hypothalamic functions may be influenced. We reviewed these possibilities recently (Zeisberger and Roth, 1996) and therefore, in this context, I would like to add only one additional piece of experimental evidence supporting this concept. From different experiments in which we microinjected or microinfused monoamines into the thermointegrative area of the hypothalamus or selectively blocked aminergic receptors in this area, we concluded that in the guinea pig the hypothalamic release of NA due to activation of brain stem afferents may increase body temperature, whereas the blockade of hypothalamic adrenergic receptors or a neurochemical lesion induced by microinjected 6-hydroxydopamine (6-OHDA) reduced body temperature. As a functional antagonist of NA, 5-HT also decreased body temperature. Since intrahypothalamically administered neurotoxins might have destroyed not only the terminals of specific aminergic afferents, but also modified the function of thermointegrative neurons in this area,

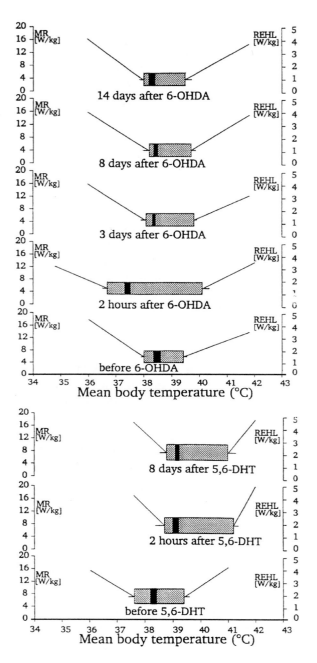

Fig. 5. A comparison of changes in thermoregulatory threshold temperatures for heat production (left borders of the shaded bars) and for heat loss (right borders of the shaded bars) before and at different time intervals after the neurotoxin lesions in the lower brain stem in guinea pigs. The dark areas within the shaded interthreshold zones indicate the initial mean body temperature of the guinea pigs before the start of cooling or heating tests. The lines indicate the slopes of the responses to cooling or heating. The effects of 6-OHDA lesion are shown on the top, those of 5,6-DHT lesion below [from Jöckel and Zeisberger (1994), reprinted with kind permission of Birkhäuser Verlag AG, Basel, Switzerland].

the conclusions were verified in another series of experiments. In these experiments the neurotoxins were injected into the areas in the lower brain stem from which the ascending catecholaminergic or serotonergic pathways originate, far away from the thermointegrative hypothalamic neurons. The results of the series are summarized in Fig. 5.

The upper part of the diagram depicts the responses of animals to experimental cooling and heating before, and at different time intervals after the lesion of catecholaminergic pathways by means of 6-OHDA (lower to upper). The shaded bars represent the width of the interthreshold zone between the threshold for heat production (left borders, TbSh = shivering threshold) and heat dissipation (right borders, TbREHL = threshold for respiratory evaporative heat loss). The dark areas within the shaded bars indicate the initial mean body temperature of the guinea pigs, before the start of cooling or heating tests. The lines ascending from the borders, denoting the thermoregulatory thresholds, indicate the slopes of the responses to cooling or heating. The lower part of the diagram depicts the responses, before and after the lesions of serotonergic pathways by means of 5,6-DHT (5,6 dihydroxy-tryptamine, from below to top). These results support the view that, in the guinea pig, catecholaminergic and serotonergic afferents to the hypothalamus have antagonistic, modulatory roles in the control of heat production. Activation of catecholaminergic afferents increases the TbSh and elevates body temperature. Therefore, the destruction of this system leads to a decrease of TbSh and body temperature. This decrease is transient, because it can be compensated by reduced activity in antagonistic, serotonergic afferents. The onset of heat loss is turned down merely by the activity of serotonergic afferents. Their destruction thus increases the TbREHL, a change which cannot be compensated. Although only thermoregulatory effects were described here, the specific neurochemical lesions acutely influenced the cardiovascular system, respiration, metabolic rate, food and water intake as well (see Jöckel and Zeisberger, 1994 for more details).

The monoaminergic modulatory systems seem to participate also in a number of other neurovegetative systems and hypothalamic functions including the stress-induced release of hormones and the neuroendocrine control of the immune system. They represent important modulatory signals needed for integration of hypothalamic systems, but they do not seem to transmit specific thermal signals. The complexity of the hypothalamic circuitry, schematically depicted in Fig. 4, exceeds our contemporary possibilities for experimental investigation and will for a long time remain a challenge for integrative physiologists.

Summary

This review recapitulates the general principles of the organization of the thermoregulatory system, describes the thermoregulatory reactions of small and large mammals to hot environment and analyzes the probable roles of biogenic amines in these responses. Catecholamines found in peripheral blood plasma or excreted in urine represent a spillover of mediators released partly from sympathetic nerve endings and partly from the adrenal medulla. Since the thermoregulatory efforts differ between small and large mammals in cold and hot environments, the peripheral release of catecholamines is also different in these animals. The levels of these signal substances in the blood, as well as their peripheral metabolic and functional effects, serve as feedback signals for the hypothalamic integrative circuitry. The roles of antagonistic modulatory monoaminergic systems, ascending from the lower brain stem to the hypothalamus, in these integrations were discussed only partly, because this was a topic of another recent review (Zeisberger and Roth, 1996).

References

Benzinger, T.H. (1969) Heat regulation: homeostasis of central temperature in man. *Physiol. Rev.*, 49: 671–759.

Blatteis, C.M. (1981) Functional anatomy of the hypothalamus from the point of view of temperature regulation. In: Z. Szelenyi and M. Szekely (Eds.), *Advances in Physiological Sciences, Volume 32, Contributions to Thermal Physiology*, Pergamon Press, Hungary, pp. 3–12.

Bligh, J. (1972) Neuronal models of mammalian temperature

regulation. In: J. Bligh and R.E. Moore (Eds.), *Essays on Temperature Regulation*, North-Holland, Amsterdam, pp. 105–120.

Bligh, J. (1973) *Temperature Regulation in Mammals and other Vertebrates*, North-Holland, Amsterdam, 436 pp.

Bligh, J. (1979) The central neurology of mammalian thermoregulation. *Neuroscience*, 4: 1213–1236.

Boulant, J.A. (1996) Hypothalamic neurons regulating body temperature. In: M.J. Fregly and C.M. Blatteis (Eds.), *Handbook of Physiology, Section 4: Environmental Physiology*, Volume I, Oxford University Press, New York, pp. 105–126.

Boulant, J.A. and Silva, N.L. (1989) Multisensory hypothalamic neurons may explain interactions among regulatory systems. *News Physiol. Sci.*, 4: 245–248.

Brengelmann, G.L. (1983) Circulatory adjustments to exercise and heat stress. *Annu. Rev. Physiol.*, 45: 191–212.

Brodie, B.B. and Shore, P.A. (1957) A concept of the role of serotonin and norepinephrine as chemical mediators in the brain. *Ann. New York Acad. Sci.*, 66: 631–642.

Brück, K. (1987) Significance of brain stem neuronal connectivities for thermoregulation and thermal adaptation. In: B. Scharrer, H.-W. Korf and H.-G. Hartwig (Eds.), *Functional Morphology of Neuroendocrine Systems*, Springer, Berlin, pp. 51–64.

Brück, K. and Hinckel, P. (1990) Thermoafferent networks and their adaptive modifications. In: E. Schönbaum and P. Lomax (Eds.), *Thermoregulation: Physiology and Biochemistry*, Pergamon Press, New York, pp. 129–152.

Brück, K. and Zeisberger, E. (1978) Significance and possible central mechanisms of thermoregulatory threshold deviations in thermal adaptation. In: L.C.H. Wang and J.W. Hudson (Eds.), *Strategies in Cold: Natural Torpidity and Thermogenesis*, Academic Press, New York, pp. 655–694.

Brück, K. and Zeisberger, E. (1990) Adaptive changes in thermoregulation and their neuropharmacological basis. In: E. Schönbaum and P. Lomax (Eds.) *Thermoregulation: Physiology and Biochemistry*, Pergamon Press, New York, pp. 255–307.

Cabanac, M. (1975) Temperature regulation. *Annu. Rev. Physiol.*, 37: 415–439.

Cabanac, M. (1996a) Heat stress and behavior. In: M.J. Fregly and C.M. Blatteis (Eds.), *Handbook of Physiology, Section 4: Environmental Physiology*, Volume I, Oxford Universitiy Press, New York, pp. 261–283.

Cabanac, M. (1996b) The place of behavior in physiology. In: M.J. Fregly and C.M. Blatteis (Eds.), *Handbook of Physiology, Section 4: Environmental Physiology*, Volume II, Oxford University Press, New York, pp. 1523–1536.

Cannon, B., Bengtsson, T., Dicker, A., Jacobsson, A., Kuusela, P., Thonberg, H., Tvrdik, P., Zhao, J. and Nedergaard, J. (1994) The role of adrenergic stimulation in regulation of heat production and recruitment of adipose tissue. In: E. Zeisberger, E. Schönbaum and P. Lomax (Eds.), *Thermal Balance in Health and Disease*, Birkhäuser, Basel, pp. 87–102.

Clark, W.G. and Clark, Y.L. (1980) Changes in body temperature after administration of adrenergic and serotonergic agents and related drugs including antidepressants. *Neurosci. Biobehav. Rev.*, 4: 281–375.

Colin, J., Timbal, J., Houdas, Y., Boutelier, C. and Guieu, J.D. (1971) Computation of mean body temperature from rectal and skin temperature. *J. Appl. Physiol.*, 31: 484–489.

Dascombe, M.J. (1985) The pharmacology of fever. *Prog. Neurobiol.*, 25: 327–373.

Euler, C.V. (1961) Physiology and pharmacology of temperature regulation. *Pharmacol. Rev.*, 13: 361–368.

Feldberg, W. and Myers, R.D. (1963) A new concept of temperature regulation by amines in the hypothalamus. *Nature*, 200: 1325.

Francesconi, R.P. (1996) Endocrinological and metabolic responses to acute and chronic heat exposures. In: M.J. Fregly and C.M. Blatteis (Eds.), *Handbook of Physiology, Section 4: Environmental Physiology*, Volume I, Oxford Universitiy Press, New York, pp. 245–260.

Gagge, A.P. and Gonzalez, R.R. (1996) Mechanisms of heat exchange: Biophysics and physiology. In: M.J. Fregly and C.M. Blatteis (Eds.), *Handbook of Physiology, Section 4, Environmental Physiology*, Volume I, Oxford University Press, New York, pp. 45–84.

Gale, C.C. (1973) Neuroendocrine aspects of thermoregulation. *Annu. Rev. Physiol.*, 35: 391–430.

Gisolfi, C.V., Matthes, R.D., Kregel, K.C. and Oppliger, R. (1991) Splanchnic sympathetic nerve activity and circulating catecholamines in the hyperthermic rat. *J. Appl. Physiol.*, 70: 1821–1826.

Gordon, C.J. and Heath, J.E. (1986) Integration and central processing in temperature regulation. *Annu. Rev. Physiol.*, 48: 595–612.

Grayson, J. (1990) Responses of the microcirculation to hot and cold environments. In: E. Schönbaum and P. Lomax (Eds.), *Thermoregulation Physiology and Biochemistry*, Pergamon Press, New York, pp. 221–234.

Hales, J.R.S., Iriki, M., Tsuchiya, K. and Kozawa, E. (1978) Thermally-induced cutaneous sympathetic activity related to blood flow through capillaries and arteriovenous anastomoses. *Pflüg. Arch. Eur. J. Physiol.*, 375: 17–24.

Hales, J.R.S., Hubbard, R.W. and Gaffin, S.L. (1996) Limitation of heat tolerance. In: M.J. Fregly and C.M. Blatteis (Eds.), *Handbook of Physiology, Section 4: Environmental Physiology*, Volume I, Oxford University Press, New York, pp. 285–355.

Hammel, H.T. (1965) Neurons and temperature regulation. In: W.S. Yammamoto and J.R. Brobeck (Eds.), *Physiological Controls and Regulations*, Saunders, Philadelphia, pp. 71–79.

Hammel, H.T. (1968) Regulation of internal body temperature. *Annu. Rev. Physiol.*, 30: 641–710.

Hardy, J.D. (1972) Models of temperature regulation-a review. In: J. Bligh and R.E. Moore (Eds.), *Essays on Temperature Regulation*, North-Holland, Amsterdam, pp. 163–186.

Heldmaier, G. (1971) Zitterfreie Wärmebildung und Körpergröße bei Säugetieren. *Z. Vergl. Physiol.*, 73: 222–248.

Hellon, R.F. (1975) Monoamines, pyrogens and cations: Their actions on central control of body temperature. *Pharmacol. Rev.*, 26: 289–321.

Hensel, H. (1973) Neural processes in thermoregulation. *Physiol. Rev.*, 53: 948–1017.

Hensel, H., Brück, K. and Raths, P. (1973) Homeothermic organisms. In: H. Precht, J. Christophersen, H. Hensel and W. Larcher (Eds.), *Temperature and Life*, Springer, Berlin, pp. 503–779.

Hille, B. (1992) G protein-coupled mechanisms and nervous signaling. *Neuron*, 9: 187–195.

Himms-Hagen, J. (1990) Brown adipose tissue thermogenesis: role in thermoregulation, energy regulation and obesity. In: E. Schönbaum and P. Lomax (Eds.), *Thermoregulation: Physiology and Biochemistry*, Pergamon Press, New York, pp. 327–414.

Himms-Hagen, J. (1996) Neural and hormonal responses to prolonged cold exposure. In: M.J. Fregly and C.M. Blatteis (Eds.), *Handbook of Physiology, Section 4: Environmental Physiology*, Volume I, Oxford University Press, New York, pp. 439–480.

Hori, T., Nakashima, T., Koga, H., Kiyohara, T. and Inoue, T. (1988) Convergence of thermal, osmotic and cardiovascular signals on preoptic and anterior hypothalamic neurons in the rat. *Brain Res. Bull.*, 20: 879–885.

Horwitz, B.A. (1996) Homeostatic responses to acute cold exposure: thermogenic responses in birds and mammals. In: M.J. Fregly and C.M. Blatteis (Eds.), *Handbook of Physiology, Section 4, Environmental Physiology*, Volume I, Oxford University Press, New York, pp. 359–377.

Iriki, M., Riedel, W. and Simon, E. (1971) Regional differentiation of sympathetic activity during hypothalamic heating and cooling in anesthetized rabbits. *Pflüg. Arch. Eur. J. Physiol.*, 328: 320–331.

Jansky, L. (1973) Non-shivering thermogenesis and its thermoregulatory significance. *Biol. Rev.*, 48: 85–132.

Jansky, L. (1995) Humoral thermogenesis and its role in maintaining energy balance. *Physiol. Rev.*, 75: 237–259.

Jessen, C. (1990) Thermal afferents in the control of body temperature. In: E. Schönbaum and P. Lomax (Eds.), *Thermoregulation. Physiology and Biochemistry*, Pergamon Press, New York, pp. 153–183.

Johnson, J.M. and Proppe, D.W. (1996) Cardiovascular adjustments to heat stress. In: M.J. Fregly and C.M. Blatteis (Eds.), *Handbook of Physiology, Section 4: Environmental Physiology*, Volume I, Oxford Universitiy Press, New York, pp. 215–243.

Johnson, J.M., Brengelmann, G.L., Hales, J.R.S., Vanhoutte, P.M. and Wenger, C.B. (1986) Regulation of the cutaneous circulation. *Fed. Proc.*, 45: 2841–2850.

Jöckel, J. and Zeisberger, E. (1994) Thermoregulatory changes after neurochemical lesions of catecholaminergic and serotonergic neurons in the lower brain stem of the guinea pig. In: E. Zeisberger, E. Schönbaum and P. Lomax (Eds.), *Thermal Balance in Health and Diesease. Advances in Pharmacological Sciences*, Birkhäuser, Basel, pp. 73–78.

Kellogg, D.L. Jr., Pérgola, P.E., Piest, K.L., Kosiba, C., Crandall, C.G. and Johnson, J.M. (1994) Cutaneous active vasodilation in humans is mediated by cholinergic nerve cotransmission. *FASEB J.*, 8: A263.

Kim, Y.D., Lake, C.R., Lees, D.E., Schutte, W.H., Bull, J.M., Weise, V. and Kopin, I.J. (1979) Hemodynamic and plasma catecholamine responses to hyperthermic cancer therapy in humans. *Am. J. Physiol.*, 237: H570–H574.

Kleinebeckel, D. and Klussmann, F.W. (1990) Shivering. In: E. Schönbaum and P. Lomax (Eds.), *Thermoregulation Physiology and Biochemistry*, Pergamon Press, New York, pp. 235–253.

Kregel, K.C., Stauss, H. and Unger, T. (1994) Modulation of autonomic nervous system adjustments to heat stress by central ANG II receptor antagonism. *Am. J. Physiol.*, 266: R1985–R1991.

Lomax, P. and Schönbaum, E. (1979) *Body Temperature: Regulation, Drug Effects and Therapeutic Implications*, Modern Pharmacology-Toxicology 16, Dekker, New York.

Marques, P.R., Illner, P., Williams, D.D., Green, W.L., Kendall, J.W., Davis, S.L., Johnson, D.G. and Gale, C.C. (1981) Hypothalamic control of endocrine thermogenesis. *Am. J. Physiol.*, 241: E420–E427.

McCarthy, M.P., Earnest, J.P., Young, E.F., Choe, S. and Stroud, R.M. (1986) The molecular neurobiology of the acetylcholine receptor. *Annu. Rev. Neurosci.*, 9: 383–413.

Myers, R.D. (1980) Hypothalmic control of thermoregulation. Neurochemical mechanisms. In: P.J. Morgane and J. Panksepp (Eds.), *Handbook of the Hypothalamus*, Volume 3, Dekker, New York, pp. 83–210.

Nagai, M. (1991) Participation of monoaminergic systems in body temperature regulation. In: M. Yoshikawa, M. Uono, H. Tanabe and S. Ishikawa (Eds.), *New Trends in Autonomic Nervous System Research*, Elsevier, Amsterdam, pp. 71–74.

Nicholls, D.G. and Locke, R.M. (1984) Thermogenic mechanisms in brown fat. *Physiol. Rev.*, 64: 1–64.

Nieuwenhuys, R. (1985) *Chemoarchitecture of the Brain*, Springer, Berlin, 246 pp.

Pierau, F.-K. (1996) Peripheral thermosensors. In: M.J. Fregly and C.M. Blatteis (Eds.), *Handbook of Physiology, Section 4: Environmental Physiology*, Volume I, Oxford University Press, New York, pp. 85–104.

Pleschka, K. (1984) Control of tongue blood flow in regulation of heat loss in mammals. *Rev. Physiol. Biochem. Pharmacol.*, 100: 75–120.

Pleschka, K., Sugahara, M., Hashimoto, M., Sommerlad, U., Lürkens, I. and Ernst, C. (1987) Local circulatory control in thermal stress. In: Dejours (Ed.), *Comparative Physiology of Environmental Adaptation*, Vol. 2, Karger, Basel, pp. 107–122.

Proppe, D.W. (1980) α-Adrenergic control of intestinal circulation in heat-stressed baboons. *J. Appl. Physiol.*, 48: 759–764.

Riedel, W., Iriki, M. and Simon, E. (1972) Regional differentiation of sympathetic activity during peripheral heating and cooling in anesthetized rabbits. *Pflüg. Arch. Eur. J. Physiol.*, 332: 239–247.

Ridesel, M.L. and Folk, G.E., Jr. (1996) Estivation. In: M.J. Fregly and C.M. Blatteis (Eds.), *Handbook of Physiology, Section 4, Environmental Physiology*, Volume I, Oxford University Press, New York, pp. 279–283.

Roberts, J.C. (1996) Thermogenic responses to prolonged cold exposure: birds and mammals. In: M.J. Fregly and C.M. Blatteis (Eds.), *Handbook of Physiology, Section 4, Environmental Physiology*, Volume I, Oxford University Press, New York, pp. 399–418.

Robertshaw, D. (1975) Catecholamines and control of sweat glands. In: R.O. Greep and E.B. Astwood (Eds.), *Handbook of Physiology, Endocrinology*, Section 7, Vol. 4, Am. Physiol. Soc., Bethesda, MD, pp. 591–603.

Roth, J., Zeisberger, E. and Schwandt, H.J. (1987) Changes in peripheral metabolism of catecholamines in guinea-pig during thermal adaptation. *J. Therm. Biol.*, 12: 39–44.

Roth, J., Zeisberger, E. and Schwandt, H.J. (1988) Influence of increased catecholamine levels in blood plasma during cold-adaptation and intramuscular infusion on thresholds of thermoregulatory reactions in guinea-pigs. *J. Comp. Physiol. B*, 157: 855–863.

Roth, J., Merker, G., Nürnberger, F., Pauly, B. and Zeisberger, E. (1990) Changes in physiological and neuroendocrine properties during thermal adaptation of golden hamsters (*Mesocricetus auratus*). *J. Comp. Physiol. B*, 160: 153–159.

Rowell, L.B. (1983) Cardiovascular adjustments to thermal stress. In: J.T. Shepherd and F.M. Abboud (Eds.), *Handbook of Physiology, Peripheral Circulation and Organ Blood Flow*, Section 2, Vol. 3, Am. Physiol. Soc., Bethesda, MD, pp. 967–1024.

Ruben, J. (1995) The evolution of endothermy in mammals and birds: from physiology to fossils. *Annu. Rev. Physiol.*, 57: 69–95.

Ruffolo, R.R. Jr. and Hieble, J.P. (1994) alpha-Adrenoceptors. *Pharmacol. Ther.*, 61: 1–64.

Satinoff, E. (1996) Behavioral thermoregulation in the cold. In: M.J. Fregly and C.M. Blatteis (Eds.), *Handbook of Physiology, Section 4, Environmental Physiology*, Volume I, Oxford University Press, New York, pp. 481–505.

Sato, K., Kang, W.H., Saga, K. and Sato, K.T. (1989a) Biology of sweat glands and their disorders. I. Normal sweat gland function. *J. Am. Acad. Dermatol.*, 20: 537–563.

Sato, K., Kang, W.H., Saga, K. and Sato, K.T. (1989b) Biology of sweat glands and their disorders. II. Disorders of sweat gland function. *J. Am. Acad. Dermatol.*, 20: 713–726.

Sawka, M.N., Wenger, C.B. and Pandolf, K.B. (1996) Thermoregulatory responses to acute exercise-heat stress and heat acclimation. In: M.J. Fregly and C.M. Blatteis (Eds.), *Handbook of Physiology, Section 4: Environmental Physiology*, Volume I, Oxford University Press, New York, pp. 157–185.

Sessler, D.I. (1994) Thermoregulation and heat balance: general anesthesia. In: E. Zeisberger, E. Schönbaum and P. Lomax (Eds.), *Thermal Balance in Health and Disease*, Birkhäuser, Basel, pp. 251–265.

Shepherd, G.M. (1988) *Neurobiology*, Oxford University Press, New York, 689 pp.

Simon, E., Pierau, F.K. and Taylor, D.C.M. (1986) Central and peripheral thermal control of effectors in homeothermic temperature regulation. *Physiol. Rev.*, 66: 235–300.

Slaunwhite, W.R., Jr. (1988) *Fundamentals of Endocrinology*, Marcel Dekker, New York, 422 pp.

Summers, R.J. and McMartin, L.R. (1993) Adrenoceptors and their second messenger systems. *J. Neurochem.*, 60: 10–23.

Venter, J.C., Fraser, C.M., Kerlavage, A.R. and Buck, M.A. (1989) Molecular biology of adrenergic and muscarinic cholinergic receptors. A perspective. *Biochem. Pharmacol.*, 38: 1197–1208.

Walther, O.-E., Iriki, M. and Simon, E. (1970) Antagonistic changes of blood flow and sympathetic activity in different vascular beds following central thermal stimulation. II. Cutaneous and visceral sympathetic activity during spinal cord heating and cooling in anesthetized rabbits and cats. *Pflüg. Arch. Eur. J. Physiol.*, 319: 162–184.

Werner, J. (1990) Functional mechanisms of temperature regulation, adaptation and fever: complementary system theoretical and experimental evidence. In: E. Schönbaum and P. Lomax (Eds.), *Thermoregulation. Physiology and Biochemistry*, Pergamon Press, New York, pp. 185–208.

Werner, J. (1996) Modeling homeostatic responses to heat and cold. In: M.J. Fregly and C.M. Blatteis (Eds.), *Handbook of Physiology, Section 4: Environmental Physiology*, Volume I, Oxford University Press, New York, pp. 613–626.

Wyndham, C.H. (1973) The physiology of exercise under heat stress. *Annu. Rev. Physiol.*, 35: 193–220.

Zeisberger, E. (1990) Central modulators of thermoregulation. *J. Basic Clin. Physiol. Pharmacol.*, 1: 277–289.

Zeisberger, E. and Roth, J. (1988) Role of catecholamines in thermoregulation of cold-adapted and newborn guinea pigs. In: W. Künzel and A. Jensen (Eds.), *The Endocrine Control of the Fetus*, Springer, Berlin, pp. 288–299.

Zeisberger, E. and Roth, J. (1989) Changes in peripheral and central release of hormones during thermal adaptation in the guinea pig. In: A. Malan and B. Canguilhem (Eds.), *Living in the cold. II*, John Libbey Eurotext, Paris, pp. 435–444.

Zeisberger, E. and Roth, J. (1996) Central regulation of adaptive responses to heat and cold. In: M.J. Fregly and C.M. Blatteis (Eds.), *Handbook of Physiology, Section 4: Environmental Physiology*, Volume I, Oxford University Press, New York, pp. 579–595.

H.S. Sharma and J. Westman (Eds.)
Progress in Brain Research, Vol 115

CHAPTER 11

Immunological and neuroendocrine modulation of fever in stress

Joachim Roth*

Physiologisches Institut, Klinikum der Justus-Liebig-Universität Giessen, Aulweg 129, 35392 Giessen, Germany

Introduction

Fever is one of the most common components of the array of host defence responses in an infected organism. The febrile increase of body temperature creates an internal hot environment within the infected host, in which the brain has to function and which is even generated by signals from the brain. Fever is not the result of an inability to regulate body temperature, which might occur in an external hot environment leading to a passive rise of core temperature termed hyperthermia. The febrile organism regulates body temperature at a higher level meaning that the increased thermoregulatory set-point is actively defended by adequate effector mechanisms. The febrile shift of regulated body temperature to a higher value is controlled by the brain, predominantly by the anterior part of the hypothalamus. There is agreement that fever, like other components of the acute phase response, is beneficial for the infected host because the higher body temperature helps to accelerate and facilitate the activation of the immune defence (Kluger, 1991, 1994) and restricts a wide range of gram-negative bacteria from synthesizing their protective lipopolysac-

charides and thereby enabling serum complement to perforate and kill the invading pathogens (Green and Vermeulen, 1994). On the other hand, an excessive and dangerous rise of body temperature during fever is prevented by control mechanisms, the so-called endogenous antipyretic systems (Zeisberger and Merker, 1992). These antipyretic systems include pathways and signal substances, which act in part within, and in part outside, the central nervous system. The antipyretic pathways are already activated during the time course of the febrile response (Zeisberger et al., 1986, 1994), so that magnitude and duration of fever are controlled and limited by a number of feed-back mechanisms. The signal molecules involved in endogenous antipyretic pathways include neuropeptides and hormones, which are released in increased amounts under a variety of stressful conditions. Therefore, it is not surprising that different kinds of stress alter the febrile response of the infected host. On the other hand, under certain experimental conditions, psychological stress itself is capable of evoking a rise of body temperature, which seems to fulfil several criteria of a fever (Kluger, 1991, 1994).

In the first part of this paper, the current opinions on the mediators and mechanisms involved in the generation of fever are summarized emphasizing the different hypotheses on the

---

*Corresponding author. Tel: +49 641 9947248; fax: +49 641 9947239; e-mail: eugen.zeisberger@physiologie.med.uni-giessen.de

transfer of febrile signals from the periphery of the body into the brain. In a second part the different endogenous antipyretic systems are introduced and the modulation of the activity of the immune system and the changes of the febrile response under the influence of different stressors are analyzed. Finally, it is discussed if the stress-induced rise of core temperature, which is accompanied by the release of soluble immune mediators and possibly stimulated by some stress hormones, represents a condition of fever under nonpathological conditions.

Generation of fever

In most cases confrontation of the infected host with invading microorganisms starts somewhere in the periphery of the body. Here, microbial products such as lipopolysaccharide (LPS) from gram-negative bacteria or muramyl-dipeptide (MDP) predominantly produced by gram-positive bacteria stimulate macrophages, monocytes and other cells to synthesize and release cytokines, the so-called endogenous pyrogens. Cytokines usually act locally subserving specific immunological tasks. In situations when released in increased amounts they spill over into the systemic circulation like hormones and may also affect other organ systems including the brain. As a consequence of the peripheral cytokine induction, several brain-controlled functions are modified resulting in generation of fever, suppression of food intake (anorexia), psychological changes collectively termed 'sickness behavior' or in the activation of the hypothalamic-pituitary-adrenal (HPA) axis (Kent et al., 1992; Rothwell and Hopkins, 1995). Most of these listed functions are controlled by and within the hypothalamus. An explanation why these functions are modified after peripheral injection of LPS was given by the discovery of increased amounts of the pyrogenic cytokines interleukin-6 (IL-6) and tumor necrosis factor α (TNFα) not only in the systemic circulation but also in hypothalamic push–pull perfusates during the time course of LPS-induced fever in guinea pigs and rats (Klir et al., 1993;

Roth et al., 1993). After peripheral injection of LPS, increased amounts of IL-6 and TNFα in plasma and in perfusates of the anterior hypothalamus precede the onset of the febrile response (Jansky et al., 1995). Both of these cytokines are capable of inducing a fever when administered into the anterior hypothalamus (Blatteis et al., 1990; Klir et al., 1993; Roth et al., 1994a) and are able to stimulate hypothalamic CRH-secreting neurons and thereby the HPA-axis (Sharp et al., 1989; Navarra et al., 1991). After peripheral injection of a fever-inducing dose of LPS, we like others (for review see: Kluger, 1991) failed to detect a substantial increase of IL-1 in plasma or perfusates of the anterior hypothalamus. In spite of this fact, localized actions of IL-1, which is regarded as the most important endogenous pyrogen (Dinarello et al., 1988), seem to be critical for the generation of fever. Systemic administration of an IL-1 receptor antagonist has been shown to inhibit LPS-fever and to attenuate circulating IL-6 (Luheshi et al., 1996). Even more important for the development of a febrile response seems to be the production and action of IL-1 within the brain. Peripherally administered LPS induces the expression of IL-1 (and other cytokines) in several brain areas including the anterior hypothalamus (Gatti and Bartfai, 1993; Laye et al., 1994; Nakamori et al., 1994). Interestingly, fever and rise of hypothalamic IL-6 could be blocked in rats by microinjection of anti-rat IL-1β antibodies into the anterior hypothalamus prior to peripheral injection of LPS (Klir et al., 1994). As a neurophysiological correlate of the fever induction by actions of cytokines within the anterior hypothalamus it has been shown *in vitro* that TNFα, IL-1 and IL-6 are able to induce hypothalamic neuronal activity changes that are consistent with fever production, i.e. inhibition of warm-sensitive neurons and excitation of cold-sensitive neurons (Hori et al., 1991; Shibata and Blatteis, 1991; Xin and Blatteis, 1992). The integration of these modified neuronal signals shifts the thermoregulatory set-point to a higher level. The organism feels cold and activates a variety of heat generating and heat conserving reflexes until the new set-point is reached and maintained. The appearance and actions of cytokines within the hypothalamus thus provide a reasonable explanation for the modification of brain-controlled temperature regulation (and other functions) during peripheral infection or inflammation.

Are these bioactive cytokines, measurable within the hypothalamus during fever, transported from the blood into the brain (Gutierres et al., 1993; Banks et al., 1994) or are they produced locally in response to some signal in the fever pathway? The following three arguments support the hypothesis that the detection of cytokine-activities within the hypothalamus during LPS-induced fever results rather from a local intrahypothalamic production than from a transport via blood to brain.

(1) The kinetics of systemic and intrahypothalamic TNFα and IL-6 are completely different. Peak-activity of TNFα in the systemic circulation can be detected soon after peripheral injection of LPS followed by a rapid decline and disappearance. In the hypothalamus, however, the highest activity of TNFα was measured at the peak of fever. Systemic activity of IL-6 rises and declines parallel with the febrile changes of body temperature, while hypothalamic IL-6 shows peak-activity in the early stage of the febrile response, which declines rather slowly.

(2) Attempts failed to detect radioactive labelled cytokines or human recombinant cytokines in hypothalamic push–pull perfusates after their intra-arterial injection or infusion.

(3) Intrahypothalamic microinjection of anti-rat IL-1β antibodies (see above) blocked the LPS-induced rise of IL-6 in the anterior hypothalamus, while systemic levels of IL-6 remained unchanged.

Although there is evidence that production of cytokines in the CNS is finally responsible for the modulation of brain-controlled functions during infection, there is still the open question of how the signals from peripherally released endogenous pyrogens enter the brain. Currently two hypotheses exist of how peripherally released cytokines might transfer signals into the brain. By the so-called neurohormonal hypothesis it is proposed that circulating endogenous pyrogens (cytokines) enter the perivascular clefts in one of the circumventricular organs in the brain, namely the organum vasculosum laminae terminalis (OVLT). This hypothesis is based on the fact that electrolytic lesions of the OVLT (Blatteis et al., 1983) or disruption of the OVLT from the hypothalamic thermoregulatory centers (Hashimoto et al., 1994) cause a suppression of fever. As a possible mechanism for the induction of fever via the OVLT it has been proposed that cytokines entering the perivascular space of the OVLT influence brain functions by prostaglandin-dependent mechanisms, since IL-1 and other cytokines can stimulate the synthesis and release of prostaglandins within brain tissue. Prostaglandins released within the OVLT by blood-borne cytokines may then diffuse to adjacent brain areas or activate neuronal pathways to the hypothalamus, finally resulting in an intrahypothalamic release of locally produced cytokines (see above).

The alternative hypothesis for explaining the influence of peripherally released endogenous pyrogens on brain-controlled functions suggests an activation of neuronal pathways of communication between the immune system and the brain (Dantzer, 1994; Watkins et al., 1995b). In particular, the afferent fibers of the vagus nerve seem to mediate a wide range of illness responses due to intraperitoneal administration of LPS or cytokines. Subdiaphragmatic vagotomy has been shown to block the modifications of several brain-controlled functions due to intraperitoneal injections of exogenous (bacterial) or endogenous pyrogens including fever (Watkins et al., 1995a) and the induction of IL-1β in the brain (Laye et al., 1995). According to our own recent experiments, vagal afferent fibers seem, indeed, to play a crucial role in the transduction of immune signals from the abdominal cavity to the brain, because fevers induced by intraperitoneal injections of cytokine-inducing bacterial products were

TABLE 1

Mean fever-indices (the integrated febrile responses, the areas between the temperature curves of normothermic and febrile animals, for 8 h after pyrogen application expressed in °C·h) in vagotomized and sham-operated guinea pigs in response to intraperitoneal or intramuscular injections of the bacterial pyrogens LPS and MDP (see Zeisberger et al., 1996; Goldbach et al., 1997). Fever is suppressed in vagotomized guinea pigs only if the pyrogen is administered into abdominal cavity

Treatment	Pyrogen	Route of injection	Mean fever index (°C·h)
Vagotomy	LPS	Intraperitoneal	1.39
Sham. op	LPS	Intraperitoneal	5.58
Vagotomy	LPS	Intramuscular	7.07
Sham. op	LPS	Intramuscular	6.44
Vagotomy	MDP	Intraperitoneal	3.93
Sham. op	MDP	Intraperitoneal	5.87
Vagotomy	MDP	Intramuscular	6.78
Sham. op	MDP	Intramuscular	6.89

suppressed by subdiaphragmatic vagotomy in guinea pigs. Vagotomized guinea pigs could, however, develop normal fevers when the pyrogens were administered intramuscularly (Table 1).

We therefore conclude that the vagus nerve does not represent the only afferent pathway for signals from the immune system to the brain. Possibly other sensory afferent nerves are involved besides the vagus nerve. There is, however, one more argument that favors a role of circulating cytokines as important signals for modifying temperature regulation and other brain-controlled functions. In two studies (Roth et al., 1993, 1994b) we observed an excellent correlation between circulating cytokines (IL-6, TNFα) and the magnitude of the febrile response. This correlation remains manifest even under the experimental condition of the development of LPS-tolerance, when systemic production of cytokines and fever are attenuated progressively and in parallel. These results together with the observations made in vagotomized animals therefore support the view that there are different communication pathways between the immune system and the brain, which may act independently of each other or in a coordinated manner to induce fever, sickness behavior and all the other modulations of brain-controlled functions, which are observed during peripheral infection or inflammation.

Endogenous antipyresis

Body temperature only rarely exceeds 41°C during fever. It has therefore been proposed that the febrile rise in temperature must be controlled, limited and sometimes even prevented by the action of endogenous antipyretic substances liberated within the brain or systemically during fever. For any substance to be categorized as an endogenous antipyretic, several criteria should be fulfilled, corresponding to the criteria for endogenous pyrogens (Kasting, 1989; Kluger, 1991). These criteria include that the administration of the putative antipyretic substance at its site of action or the stimulation of endogenous release of the substance result in an attenuation of fever. Further, the blockade of the biological action or inhibition of the production of the substance should have some fever-enhancing effects. In this chapter, the experimental evidence for the roles of several molecules as endogenous antipyretics is summarized.

Arginine-vasopressin (AVP)

In 1979 the first report on the role of AVP as an endogenous antipyretic substance was published based on the observation that perfusion of the ventral septal area in the limbic system with AVP resulted in a suppression of fever (Cooper et al., 1979). Since then many studies on the antipyretic properties of AVP have been performed and reviewed (Cooper, 1987, 1995; Zeisberger, 1990; Pittman et al., 1993).

The antipyretically effective site for AVP is located in a small area of the brain, the ventral septum of the limbic system. Antipyresis induced by AVP is thus not due to an inhibitory effect of this cytokine on the immune system, but is rather caused by neuronal mechanisms (Zeisberger and Merker, 1992). Vasopressinergic projections from cell bodies of the hypothalamic paraventricular nucleus (PVN) and the septum have been demonstrated by immunocytochemical methods (Staiger and Nürnberger, 1989) and the release of AVP within the septum increases during fever (Landgraf et al., 1990). The released AVP seems to stimulate neurons within the septum via V_1 receptors (Poulin et al., 1988; Raggenbass et al., 1988). This excitation is then transmitted back to the hypothalamus via septofugal fibers which have also been demonstrated (Staiger and Wouterlood, 1990). In the hypothalamus the signals of these septofugal fibers may cancel the neuronal changes which have been induced by cytokines (see above). The activation of vasopressinergic projections from the hypothalamic paraventricular nucleus (PVN) to the limbic septum during fever and in response to several stressful stimuli can be demonstrated by immunohistochemical methods (Merker et al., 1989) and by measurement of intraseptal and systemic releases of AVP (Landgraf et al., 1990; Roth and Zeisberger, 1992; Roth et al., 1992). All these stressful situations are accompanied by reduced febrile responses. This is shown in Fig. 1, which summarizes the results from several of our studies on the role of AVP as an endogenous antipyretic substance.

The second column shown in Fig. 1 demonstrates the antipyretic effect of intraseptal microinfusions of AVP, which result in an attenuation of fever by about 80%. The next four columns represent stressful conditions, which are all accompanied by an activation of the antipyretic vasopressinergic pathways and a reduced febrile response, such as the last day of pregnancy, a moderate dehydration, cold adaptation or immobilization. The specific property of AVP to act as an antipyretic in the septum is demonstrated by the last two columns of Fig. 1. Electrical stimulation of the hypothalamic PVN results in an attenuation of fever by 60%, an effect which can be antagonized by intraseptal administration of a vasopressinergic V_1-receptor antagonist (for further details see Naylor et al., 1988; Unger et al., 1991; Bock et al., 1994).

Adrenocorticotrophic hormone (ACTH) and α-melanocyte stimulating hormone (α-MSH)

Antipyretic properties of ACTH and α-MSH can be demonstrated not only after their central (intraseptal), but also in response to their peripheral (intravenous) administration (Glyn and Lipton, 1981; Shih and Lipton, 1985). The property of ACTH and α-MSH to stimulate release of glucocorticoids from the adrenal glands is not the only mechanism of how these peptides exert their peripheral effect, since antipyresis can also be induced by ACTH in adrenalectomized animals (Zimmer and Lipton, 1981). In particular, α-MSH has pronounced immunosuppressive properties and antagonizes several effects of IL-1 on the immune system (Cannon et al., 1986). In contrast to AVP, the neuropeptides ACTH and α-MSH can thus be regarded as antipyretic substances, which exert their effects not exclusively by neuronal mechanisms, but also by an inhibitory influence on some components of the immune system.

γ-Melanocyte stimulating hormone (γ-MSH)

In contrast to α-MSH, which can be regarded as a natural metabolite of ACTH, γ-MSH is a direct derivative of the pro-opiomelanocortin. Antipyre-

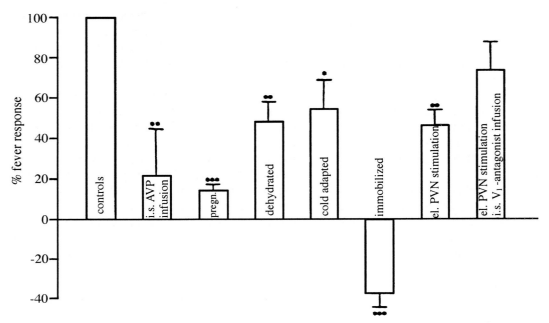

Fig. 1. Comparison of the mean fever indices (integrated thermal responses, see legend to Table 1) measured in several groups of guinea pigs as controls or under the influence of different stimuli. To compare data from several series of experiments, the control fever index was always defined as 100% fever response (i.s. = intraseptal; pregn. = pregnant; el. = electrical; PVN = paraventricular nucleus; *P < 0.05; **P < 0.01; ***P < 0.001; from Roth and Zeisberger, 1992; for further details, see Zeisberger, 1990; Roth et al., 1992).

sis is induced not only by microinfusion of γ-MSH into the limbic septum, but also in response to systemic (intra-arterial) infusion of this peptide (Bock et al., 1994). The suppression of fever by systemic administration of γ-MSH seems not to be due to an inhibitory influence on release of pyrogenic cytokines. LPS-induced increases in circulating levels of IL-6 and TNFα are not altered during the infusion of γ-MSH. The antipyretic effect of peripherally administered γ-MSH seems rather due to some feedback action on the central nervous system, finally leading to an activation of vasopressinergic pathways (Gruber and Callahan, 1989).

Glucocorticoids and lipocortin-1

Anti-inflammatory and immunomodulatory actions of glucocorticoids have been known for decades (Claman, 1993). Also the febrile response to injections of pyrogens is modulated by glucocorticoids. LPS-induced fever is greater in adrenalectomized than in sham-operated rats, and replacement of corticosterone by releasing-pellets attenuated the febrile and cytokine responses to endotoxin in the adrenalectomized animals (Coelho et al., 1992; Morrow et al., 1993). When the normal levels of cortisol are increased by systemic infusions in humans, fever and production of pyrogenic cytokines in response to LPS are attenuated (Barber et al., 1993). In recent experiments in our laboratory (prepared for publication) we increased circulating levels of cortisol in guinea pigs for several weeks to values, which are observed under conditions of stress, by implanting cortisol releasing-pellets and observed a significant suppression of the second phase of LPS-induced fever.

There is experimental evidence that the antipyretic effects of glucocorticoids are mediated by lipocortin-1, a glucocorticoid-inducible protein, which is a potent inhibitor of phospholipase A_2. In rats, administration of lipocortin-1 results in a suppression of fevers induced by several pyrogenic cytokines (Carey et al., 1990; Strijbos et al., 1992).

Most of the endogenous antipyretic substances listed above are released in increased amounts under stressful conditions. From Fig. 1 it becomes obvious that immobilization stress not only resulted in an attenuation of LPS-induced fever, but rather in a hypothermic response. This hypothermia after injection of LPS cannot simply be explained by the activation of vasopressinergic pathways, because in dehydrated or cold-adapted guinea pigs a higher release of AVP is observed than under conditions of immobilization stress, and still a fever develops. Therefore, we analysed the LPS-induced production of endogenous pyrogens and several stress hormones in freely moving and immobilized guinea pigs.

Suppression of fever by immobilization stress

About 30 years ago, it was reported that rabbits restrained in a position with extended legs were unable to develop a fever in response to bacterial endotoxin, but became rather hypothermic (Sheagren and Wolff, 1966). Serum collected from these animals could, however, induce a fever in recipient rabbits. The authors concluded that a production of endogenous pyrogen occurred in absence of a febrile response in immobilized animals but failed to provide a reasonable explanation for the suppression of fever by the immobilization stress.

The phenomenon of complete fever suppression can also be demonstrated in immobilized guinea pigs as shown in Fig. 2.

Immobilization of guinea pigs in a stretched position results in a complete abrogation of LPS-induced fever, and the animals even develop a hypothermia of about 1°C below their normal abdominal temperature. Figures 3 and 4 show the results of the analysis of several classic stress-hormones and the pyrogenic cytokines TNFα and

IL-6 before and after injection of LPS in freely moving and immobilized guinea pigs.

Fig. 3 summarizes the circulating levels of the stress-hormones noradrenaline (NA), AVP and cortisol 60 min before and at selected times after injection of LPS. By immobilization, for all of the three hormones, levels in blood plasma are significantly increased 60 min prior to injection of LPS. The injection of LPS per se induces a stimulation of release of NA, AVP and cortisol, which again finally leads to higher levels in immobilized than in freely moving guinea pigs. For AVP, an antipyretic action was confirmed in the septum of the limbic system; and in addition to the higher circulating levels of AVP, increased amounts of this peptide can also be detected in septal push–pull perfusates of immobilized guinea pigs. The anti-inflammatory and immunomodulatory actions of cortisol have been mentioned above. An innervation of lymphatic tissue and organs of immunological importance by the sympathetic nervous system has been demonstrated (Madden and Felten, 1995). The sympathetic influence on the immune system seems to be inhibitory (Katafuchi et al., 1993). Increased levels of NA and cortisol in immobilized animals may therefore contribute to an inhibition of some components of the immune system.

The circulating activities of TNFα (peak in the early phase of fever) and IL-6 (peak at the maximum of fever) were attenuated in immobilized guinea pigs to about one-third of the values measured in freely moving animals. Stress also downregulates LPS-induced expression of proinflammatory cytokines in the brain (Goujon et al., 1995). The results shown in Fig. 4 confirm the older observation mentioned above, that in plasma of immobilized rabbits some amount of endogenous pyrogen is still produced in spite of the absence of fever (Sheagren and Wolff, 1966). All results documented in Figs. 3 and 4 confirm that not only pyrogenic immune signals are attenuated by immobilization stress and contribute to the suppression of fever. In addition, also antipyretic vasopressinergic pathways acting within the brain of immobilized animals are already activated be-

184

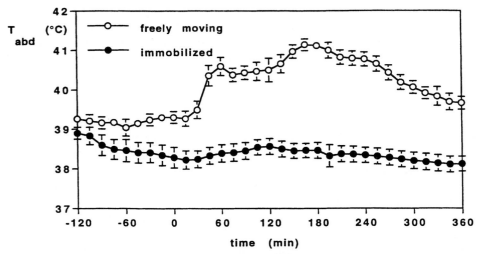

Fig. 2. Thermal response to intramuscular injections of 20 μg/kg LPS in freely moving (open cicles) and immobilized (filled cicles) guinea pigs. LPS was injected at time 0. Abdominal temperature was recorded by use of battery-operated biotelemetry transmitters implanted intraperitoneally (from Zeisberger and Roth, 1996).

fore injection of LPS so that the remaining pyrogenic signals fail to evoke a febrile response. Finally immobilization in a stretched position prevents animals from curling up in the cold and thereby from reducing heat loss. This effect is, however, not considered as the most important contribution for the hypothermic response in immobilized animals, because the complete suppression of fever can also be observed in a warm environment, which is accompanied by activated heat loss mechanisms.

It has to be mentioned that the hypothermic response to immobilization in rabbits and guinea pigs is not observed in all species of experimental animals. It is known that the expression of behavioral and neurochemical responses evoked by stressors depends on recent individual experience, a phenomenon called habituation or tolerance (Zeisberger and Roth, 1996). Also genetic factors determine the expression of responses to stressors, thus leading to striking differences between the reactions of different species to the same stressor. For example, the restrained rat visually increases motor activity, becomes aggressive and develops a hyperthermia; but under conditions of restraint stress the rat is also unable to develop a fever in response to injections of different pyrogens, which rather evoke a hypothermic response (Long et al., 1991a,b).

Despite the general observation that different kinds of stress cause an activation of endogenous antipyretic pathways (Fig. 1) and a reduction in release of endogenous pyrogens finally leading to an attenuation or even suppression of fever, under certain experimental conditions, stressors are able to cause a rise of body temperature without an external infectious or inflammatory stimulus. What are the reasons for this stress-induced rise of body temperature?

Evidence for stress-induced rise of body temperature as a nonpathological fever

Exposure of rats for a certain time to the novel environment of a so-called 'open field' (a large illuminated chamber) results in a rise of abdominal temperature (Kluger, 1991; Morrow et al., 1993). A similar observation is made when the cages of guinea pigs or rats are changed as shown in Fig. 5.

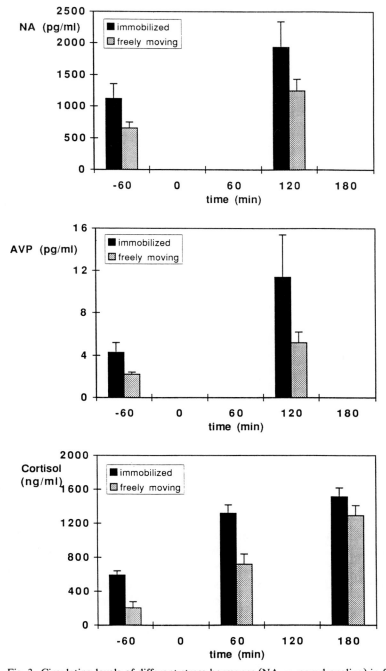

Fig. 3. Circulating levels of different stress hormones (NA = noradrenaline) in freely moving and immobilized guinea pigs 60 min before and at selected times after intramuscular injection of 20 μg/kg LPS at time 0. NA was analyzed by means of HPLC with electrochemical detection, AVP and cortisol by specific radioimmunoassays.

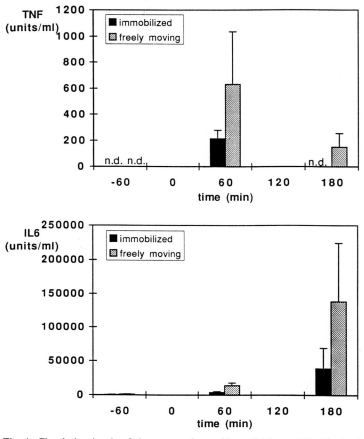

Fig. 4. Circulating levels of the pyrogenic cytokines TNFα and IL-6 in freely moving and immobilized guinea pigs 60 min before and at selected times after intramuscular injection of 20 μg/kg LPS at time 0. TNFα- and IL-6-activities were measured by specific bioassays.

Abdominal temperature of guinea pigs increases by about 0.5°C by such an exposure to a novel environment. In rats the rise in core temperature by about 1.3°C is even more pronounced. This stress-induced rise of body temperature can, in part, be blocked by pretreatment with antipyretic drugs like sodium salicylate or indomethacin (Singer et al., 1986; Kluger, 1991). This observation and the following listed findings support the hypothesis that the rise of body core temperature during stress is a fever. The stress-induced increase of abdominal temperature is adjusted by adequate thermoregulatory effector mechanisms and thus different from a passive hyperthermia (Briese and Cabanac, 1991). Stress elicits some components of the acute-phase response in rabbits (Morimoto et al., 1987). Exposure to physical or psychological stressors elevates circulating IL-6, a pyrogenic cytokine (LeMay et al., 1990; Zhou et al., 1993). A possible explanation for the the induction of cytokines in stressful situations was given recently by studies using an isolated perfused rat liver (Liao et al., 1995a,b). At low doses, stress-hormones like corticosterone or epinephrine induced the production of cytokines by the Kupfer cells of the perfused liver. Thus it may be possible that the elevation of circulating stress-hormones, due to the exposure

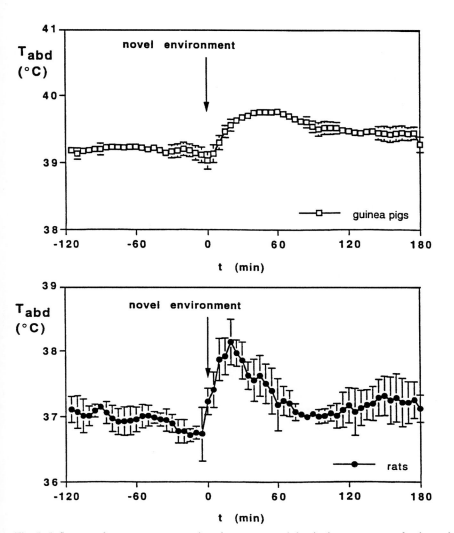

Fig. 5. Influence of exposure to a novel environment on abdominal temperature of guinea pigs (upper part) and rats (lower part). Abdominal temperature was recorded by use of battery-operated biotelemetry transmitters implanted intraperitoneally.

to a novel environment, evokes a systemic release of cytokines and thereby a fever. Interestingly, high doses of corticosterone which attenuate LPS-induced fever, have also a suppressive effect on LPS-induced production of cytokines by the isolated perfused liver. If the levels of stress-hormones are rising above a certain level or increase for a longer period of time, their antipyretic properties will counteract release of cytokines and attenuate the fever in response to exogenous pyrogens like LPS.

Final conclusions

Various stressors, several of which have been mentioned in this paper, activate different sensory systems and central nervous pathways. Acutely, they may evoke some common responses, leading to an activation of the sympathico-adrenal system and the HPA-axis. Under conditions of an activated immune system, sympathetic nerve fibers to lymphoid tissue or spleen as well

188

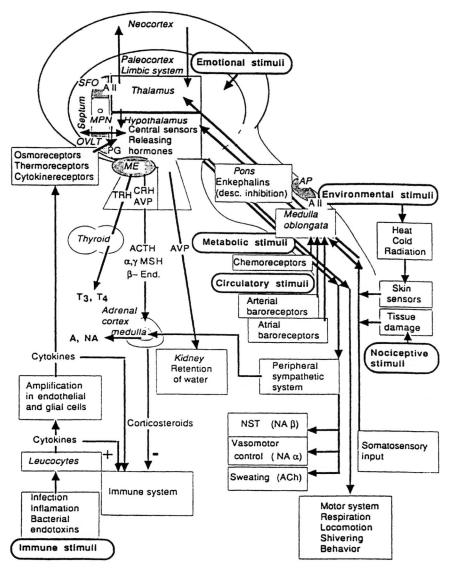

Fig. 6. Schematic illustration of the convergence of signals evoked by different external and internal stimuli (denoted by bold type) into the hypothalamus and of the hypothalamic outputs to peripheral organs mediated by motor nerves, peripheral vegetative nerves and the endocrine system [from Zeisberger et al. (1994), reprinted with kind permission of John Libbey Eurotext, Paris, France].

as a stimulation of the HPA-axis represent the most important negative-feedback loops, which may help in that the potentially dangerous machinery of the immune system is restricted in its activity to limited time periods and finally turned off again. An attempt to demonstrate and sum-

marize the different external and internal stimuli (stressors) which may interfere with the homeostasis of the organism is shown in Fig. 6 (see Zeisberger et al., 1994; Zeisberger and Roth, 1996).

Environmental, nociceptive, metabolic, circulatory and immune stimuli act on different peripheral and internal sensors, whose signals are conveyed by afferent pathways to the central nervous system, where their integration and modulation occur. The hypothalamus represents the most important integrative center, which contains multisensor neurons sensitive to different stimuli like temperature, osmolality, metabolic substances, hormones and cytokines. The signals produced by the integration of this information are differentiated in neurons producing releasing hormones and potentiated in cells of the endocrine system. The resulting efferent endocrine or neural signals alter peripheral functions or systemic metabolism to counteract the disturbance from the original stressor. All the external and internal stimuli shown in Fig. 6 are able to activate the sympathico-adrenal- and the HPA-systems. Fever is induced by actions of mediators of the immune system on the central nervous system either by neurohormonal or by neuronal mechanisms. Soon after its induction it is suppressed again by different antipyretic mechanisms which are predominantly activated together with the HPA-axis. This activation can be regarded as a negative feedback mechanism in the complex neuroendocrine reflexes finally serving to reestablish the normal state of activity in the immune system. If the HPA-axis is activated by stressors of non-immune origin, the febrile response can be attenuated in magnitude and duration or even suppressed.

In the introduction it has been pointed out that the febrile rise of body temperature is beneficial. The brain which is used to work at about 2°C lower temperatures than observed under conditions of fever has developed several mechanisms to take care that the internal hot environment created by signals from the immune system is limited in magnitude and duration. Thereby an excessive rise of body temperature which may harm cells generally, and nerve cells particularly, is prevented. Another question is if a febrile rise of body temperature is also beneficial under conditions of an external hot environment or generally under conditions of demands on heat de-fence. In this case two concurrent disturbances that impose a load on the thermoregulatory system, but evoke opposite thermoeffector responses have to be counteracted by the organism. Under such conditions of combined stressors a change from beneficial to detrimental effects of fever may occur. This is indicated by a higher mortality of experimental animals in situations in which disturbances like an injection of a pyrogen, hot environment and severe dehydration are combined (Blatteis et al., 1994). Since only a few studies have been performed on the activity of the immune system during experimental infections combined with stressors like heat exposure, long-term exercise or severe dehydration, final conclusions about the beneficial effects of fever under such conditions cannot yet be drawn. However, this interesting question merits further studies.

References

Banks, W.A., Kastin, A.J. and Gutierrez, E.G. (1994) Penetration of interleukin-6 across the murine blood–brain-barrier. *Neurosci. Lett.*, 179: 53–56.

Barber, A.E., Coyle, S.M., Marano, M.A., Fischer, E., Calvano, S.E., Fong, Y., Moldawer, L.L. and Lowry, S.F. (1993) Glucocorticoid therapy alters hormonal and cytokine responses to endotoxin in man. *J. Immunol.*, 150: 1999–2006.

Blatteis, C.M., Bealer, S.L., Hunter, W.S., Llanos, Q.J., Ahokas, R.A. and Mashburn, T.A.J. (1983) Suppression of fever after lesions of the anteroventral third ventricle in guinea pigs. *Brain Res. Bull.*, 11: 519–526.

Blatteis, C.M., Quan, N., Xin, L. and Ungar, A.L. (1990) Neuromodulation of acute phase responses to interleukin-6 in guinea pigs. *Brain Res. Bull.*, 25: 895–901.

Blatteis, C.M., Ungar, A.L. and Howell, R.B. (1994) Thermoregulatory responses of rabbits to combined heat exposure, pyrogen and dehydration. In: A.S. Milton (Ed.), *Temperature Regulation: Recent Physiological and Pharmacological Advances*, Birkhäuser, Basel, pp. 71–74.

Bock, M., Roth, J., Kluger, M.J. and Zeisberger, E. (1994) Antipyresis caused by stimulation of vasopressinergic neurons and intraseptal or systemic infusions of γ-MSH. *Am. J. Physiol.*, 266: R614–R621.

Briese, E. and Cabanac, M. (1991) Stress hyperthermia: physiological arguments that it is a fever. *Physiol. Behav.*, 49: 1153–1157.

Cannon, J.G., Tatro, J.G., Reichlin, S. and Dinarello, C.A. (1986) Alpha-melanocyte stimulating hormone inhibits immunostimulatory and inflammatory actions of interleukin-1. *J. Immunol.*, 137: 2232–2236.

Carey, F., Forder, R., Edge, M.D., Greene, A.R., Horan, M.A., Strijbos, P.J.L.M. and Rothwell, N.J. (1990) Lipocortin 1 fragment modifies pyrogenic actions of cytokines in rats. *Am. J. Physiol.*, 259: R266–R269.

Claman, H.N. (1993) Corticosteroids as immunomodulators. *Ann. New York Acad. Sci.*, 685: 288–292.

Coelho, M.M., Souza, G.E.P. and Pela, I.R. (1992) Endotoxin-induced fever is modulated by endogenous glucocorticoids in rats. *Am. J. Physiol.*, 263: R423–R427.

Cooper, K.E. (1987) The neurobiology of fever: thoughts on recent developments. *Annu. Rev. Neurosci.*, 10: 297–324.

Cooper, K.E. (1995) *Fever and Antipyresis — The Role of the Nervous System*, Cambridge University Press, Cambridge, 182 pp.

Cooper, K.E., Kasting, N.W., Lederis, K. and Veale, W.L. (1979) Evidence supporting a role for endogenous vasopressin in natural suppression of fever in the sheep. *J. Physiol. (Lond.)*, 295: 33–45.

Dantzer, R. (1994) How do cytokines say hello to the brain? Neural versus humoral mediation. *Eur. Cytokine Netw.*, 5: 271–273.

Dinarello, C.A., Cannon, J.G. and Wolff, S.M. (1988) New concepts on the pathogenesis of fever. *Rev. Infect. Dis.*, 10: 168–189.

Gatti, S. and Bartfai, T. (1993) Induction of tumor necrosis factor-α mRNA in the brain after peripheral endotoxin treatment: comparison with interleukin-1 family and interleukin-6. *Brain Res.*, 624: 291–294.

Glyn, J.R. and Lipton, J.M. (1981) Hypothermic and antipyretic effects of centrally administered ACTH (1-24) and α-melanotropin. *Peptides*, 2: 177–187.

Goldbach, J.M., Roth, J. and Zeisberger, E. (1997) Fever suppression by subdiaphragmatic vagotomy in guinea pigs depends on the route of pyrogen administration. *Am. J. Physiol.*, 272: R675–R681.

Green, M.H. and Vermeulen, C.W. (1994) Fever and the control of gram-negative bacteria. *Res. Microbiol.*, 145: 269–272.

Gruber, K.A. and Callahan, M.F. (1989) ACTH-(4-10) through γ-MSH: evidence for a new class of central autonomic nervous system-regulating peptides. *Am. J. Physiol.*, 257: R681–R694.

Gutierres, E.G., Banks, W.A. and Kastin, A.J. (1993) Murine tumor necrosis factor alpha is transported from blood to brain in the mouse. *J. Neuroimmunol.*, 47: 169–176.

Goujon, E., Parnet, P., Laye, S., Combe, C., Kelley, K.W. and Dantzer, R. (1995) Stress downregulates lipopolysaccharide-induced expression of proinflammatory cytokines in the spleen, pituitary, and brain of mice. *Brain Behav. Immun.*, 9: 292–302.

Hashimoto, M., Ueno, T. and Iriki, M. (1994) What role does the organum vasculosum laminae terminalis play in fever in rabbits? *Pflüg. Arch.*, 429: 50–57.

Hori, T., Nakashima, T., Take, S., Kaizuka, Y., Mori, T. and Katafuchi, T. (1991) Immune cytokines and regulation of body temperature, food intake and cellular immunity. *Brain Res. Bull.*, 27: 309–313.

Jansky, L., Vybiral, S., Pospisilova, D., Roth, J., Dornand, J., Zeisberger, E. and Kaminkova, J. (1995) Production of systemic and hypothalamic cytokines during the early phase of endotoxin fever. *Neuroendocrinology*, 62: 55–61.

Kasting, N.W. (1989) Criteria for establishing a physiological role for brain peptides. A case in point: the role of vasopressin in thermoregulation during fever and antipyresis. *Brain Res. Rev.*, 14: 143–153.

Katafuchi, T., Take, S. and Hori, T. (1993) Roles of the sympathetic nervous system in the suppression of cytotoxicity of spleenic natural killer cells in the rat. *J. Physiol. (Lond.)*, 465: 343–357.

Kent, S., Bluthe, R.M., Kelley, K.W. and Dantzer, R. (1992) Sickness behavior as a new target for drug development. *Trends Pharmacol. Sci.*, 13: 24–28.

Klir, J.J., McClellan, J.L. and Kluger, M.J. (1994) Interleukin-1β causes the increase in anterior hypothalamic interleukin-6 during LPS-induced fever in rats. *Am. J. Physiol.*, 266: R1845–R1848.

Klir, J.J., Roth, J., Szelenyi, Z., McClellan, J.L. and Kluger, M.J. (1993) Role of hypothalamic interleukin-6 and tumor necrosis factor-α in LPS-fever in rat. *Am. J. Physiol.*, 265: R512–R517.

Kluger, M.J. (1991) Fever: role of pyrogens and cryogens. *Physiol. Rev.*, 71: 93–127.

Kluger, M.J. (1994) Fever and antipyresis. In: E. Zeisberger, E. Schönbaum and P. Lomax (Eds.), *Thermal Balance in Health and Disease: Recent Basic Research and Clinical Progress*, Birkhäuser, Basel, pp. 343–352.

Landgraf, R., Malkinson, T.J., Veale, W.L., Lederis, K. and Pittman, Q.J. (1990) Vasopressin and oxitocin in rat brain in response to prostaglandin fever. *Am. J. Physiol.*, 259: R1056–R1062.

Laye, S., Parnet, P., Goujon, E. and Dantzer, R. (1994) Peripheral administration of lipopolysaccharide induces the expression of cytokine transcripts in the brain and pituitary of mice. *Mol. Brain Res.*, 27: 157–162.

Laye, S., Bluthe, R.M., Kent, S., Combe, C., Medina, C., Parnet, P., Kelley, K. and Dantzer, R. (1995) Subdiaphragmatic vagotomy blocks induction of IL-1β mRNA in mice brain in response to peripheral LPS. *Am. J. Physiol.*, 268: R1327–R1331.

LeMay, L.G., Vander, A.J. and Kluger, M.J. (1990) The effects of psychological stress on plasma interleukin-6 activity in rats. *Physiol. Behav.*, 47: 957–961.

Liao, J., Keiser, J.A., Scales, W.S., Kunkel, S.L. and Kluger, M.J. (1995a) Role of corticosterone in TNF and IL-6 production in isolated perfused rat liver. *Am. J. Physiol.*, 268: R699–R706.

Liao, J., Keiser, J.A., Scales, W.E., Kunkel, S.L. and Kluger, M.J. (1995b) Role of epinephrine in TNF and IL-6 production from isolated perfused rat liver. *Am. J. Physiol.*, 268: R896–R901.

Long, N.C., Morimoto, A., Nakamori, T. and Murakami, N. (1991a) The effect of physical restraint on IL-1β- and LPS-induced fever. *Physiol. Behav.*, 50: 625–628.

Long, N.C., Morimoto, A., Nakamori, T., Yamashiro, O. and Murakami, N. (1991b) Intraperitoneal injections of prostaglandin E2 attenuate hyperthermia induced by restraint or interleukin-1 in rats. *J. Physiol. (Lond.)*, 444: 363–373.

Luheshi, G., Miller, A.J., Brouwner, S., Dascombe, M.J., Rothwell, N.J. and Hopkins, S.J. (1996) Interleukin-1 receptor antagonist inhibits endotoxin fever and systemic interleukin-6 induction in the rat. *Am. J. Physiol.*, 270: E91–E95.

Madden, K.S. and Felten, D.L. (1995) Experimental basis for neural-immune interactions. *Physiol. Rev.*, 75: 77–106.

Merker, G., Roth, J. and Zeisberger, E. (1989) Thermoadaptive influence on reactivity pattern of vasopressinergic neurons in the guinea pig. *Experientia*, 45: 722–726.

Morimoto, A., Watanabe, T., Myogin, T. and Murakami, N. (1987) Restraint induced stress elicits acute-phase response in rabbits. *Pflüg Arth.*, 410: 554–556.

Morrow, L.E., McClellan, J.L., Conn, C.A. and Kluger, M.J. (1993) Glucocorticoids alter fever and IL-6 responses to psychological stress and to lipopolysaccharide. *Am. J. Physiol.*, 264: R1010–R1016.

Nakamori, T., Morimoto, A., Yamaguchi, K., Watanabe, T. and Murakami, N. (1994) Interleukin-1β production in the rabbit brain during endotoxin-induced fever. *J. Physiol. (Lond.)*, 476: 177–186.

Navarra, P., Tsagarakis, S., Faria, M.S., Rees, L.H., Besser, G.M. and Grossman, A.B. (1991) Interleukins-1 and -6 stimulate the release of corticotropin-releasing hormone-41 from rat hypothalamus *in vitro* via the eicosanoid cyclooxygenase pathway. *Endocrinology*, 128: 37–44.

Naylor, A.M., Pittman, Q.J. and Veale, W.L. (1988) Stimulation of vasopressin release in the ventral septum of the rat brain suppresses prostaglandin E fever. *J. Physiol. (Lond.)*, 399: 177–189.

Pittman, Q.J., Poulin, P. and Wilkinson, M.F. (1993) Role of neurohypophysial hormones in temperature regulation. *Ann. New York Acad. Sci.*, 689: 375–381.

Poulin, P., Lederis, K. and Pittman, Q.J. (1988) Subcellular localization and characterization of vasopressin binding sites in the ventral septal area, lateral septum and hippocampus of the rat brain. *J. Neurochem.*, 50: 889–898.

Raggenbass, M. Dubois-Dauphin, M., Tribollet, E. and Dreifuss, J.J. (1988) Direct excitatory action of vasopressin in the lateral septum of the rat brain. *Brain Res.*, 459: 60–69.

Roth, J. and Zeisberger, E. (1992) Evidence for antipyretic vasopressinergic pathways and their modulation by noradenergic afferents. *Physiol. Res.*, 41: 49–55.

Roth, J., Schulze, K., Simon, E. and Zeisberger, E. (1992) Alteration of endotoxin fever and release of arginine vasopressin by dehydration in the guinea pig. *Neuroendocrinology*, 56: 680–686.

Roth, J., Conn, C.A., Kluger, M.J. and Zeisberger, E. (1993) Kinetics of systemic and intrahypothalamic IL-6 and tumor necrosis factor during endotoxin fever in guinea pigs. *Am. J. Physiol.*, 265: R653–R658.

Roth, J., Bock, M., McClellan, J.L., Kluger, M.J. and Zeisberger, E. (1994a) Fever induction by a cytokine network in guinea pigs: the roles of tumor necrosis factor and interleukin-6. In: A.S. Milton (Ed.), *Temperature Regulation: Recent Physiological and Pharmacological Advances*, Birkhäuser, Basel, pp. 11–16.

Roth, J., McClellan, J.L., Kluger, M.J. and Zeisberger, E. (1994b) Attenuation of fever and release of cytokines after repeated injections of lipopolysaccharide in guinea pigs. *J. Physiol. (Lond.)*, 477: 177–185.

Rothwell, N.J. and Hopkins, S.J. (1995) Cytokines and the nervous system II: actions and mechanisms of action. *Trends Neurosci.*, 18: 130–136.

Sharp, B.M., Matta, S.G., Peterson, P.K., Newton, R., Chao, C. and McAllen, K. (1989) Tumor necrosis factor-α is a potent ACTH secretagogue: comparison to interleukin-1β. *Endocrinology*, 124: 3131–3133.

Sheagren, J.N. and Wolff, S.M. (1966) Demonstration of endogenous pyrogen in afebrile rabbits. *Nature*, 210: 539–541.

Shibata, M. and Blatteis, C.A. (1991) Differential effects of cytokines on thermosensitive neurons in guinea pig preoptic area slices. *Am. J. Physiol.*, 261: R1996–R1103.

Shih, S.T. and Lipton, J.M. (1985) Intravenous α-MSH reduces fever in the squirrel monkey. *Peptides*, 6: 685–687.

Singer, R., Harker, C.T., Vander, A.J. and Kluger, M.J. (1986) Hyperthermia induced by open-field stress is blocked by salicylate. *Physiol. Behav.*, 36: 1179–1182.

Staiger, J.F. and Nürnberger, F. (1989) Pattern of afferents to the lateral septum in the guinea pig. *Cell Tissue Res.*, 257: 471–490.

Staiger, J.F. and Wouterlood, F.G. (1990) Efferent projections from the lateral septal nucleus to the anterior hypothalamus in the rat: a study combining Phaseolus vulgaris-leucoagglutinin tracing with vasopressin immunocytochemistry. *Cell Tissue Res.*, 261: 17–23.

Strijbos, P.J., Hardwick, A.J., Relton, J.K., Carey, F. and Rothwell, N.J. (1992) Inhibition of central actions of cytokines on fever and thermogenesis by lipocortin-1 involves CRF. *Am. J. Physiol.*, 263: E632–E636.

Unger, M., Merker, G., Roth, J. and Zeisberger, E. (1991) Influence of noradrenergic input into the hypothalamic paraventricular nucleus on fever in the guinea pig. *Pflüg. Arch.*, 419: 394–400.

Watkins, L.R., Goehler, L.E., Relton, J.K., Tartaglia, N., Silbert, L., Martin, D. and Maier, S.F. (1995a) Blockade of interleukin-1 induced hyperthermia by subdiaphragmatic vagotomy: evidence for vagal mediation of immune-brain communication. *Neurosci. Lett.*, 183: 27–31.

Watkins, L.R., Maier, S.F. and Goehler, L.E. (1995b) Cytokine-to-brain communication: a review and analysis of alternative mechanisms. *Life Sci.*, 57: 1011–1026.

Xin, L. and Blatteis, C.M. (1992) Hypothalamic neuronal responses to interleukin-6 in tissue slices: effects of indomethacin and naloxone. *Brain Res. Bull.*, 29: 27–35.

Zeisberger, E. (1990) The role of septal peptides in thermoregulation and fever. In: J. Bligh and K. Voigt (Eds.), *Thermoreception and Temperature Regulation*, Springer, Berlin, pp. 273–283.

Zeisberger, E. and Merker, G. (1992) The role of OVLT in fever and antipyresis. In: A. Ermisch, R. Landgraf and H.J. Rühle (Eds.), *Circumventricular Organs and Brain Fluid Environment, Progress in Brain Research*, Vol. 91, Elsevier, Amsterdam, pp. 403–408.

Zeisberger, E. and Roth, J. (1996) Central regulation of adaptive responses to heat and cold. In: M.J. Fregly and C.M. Blatteis (Eds.), *Handbook of Physiology, Section 4: Environmental Physiology*, Oxford University Press, New York, pp. 579–595.

Zeisberger, E., Merker, G., Blähser, S. and Krannig, M. (1986) Role of vasopressin in fever regulation. In: K.E. Cooper, P. Lomax, E. Schönbaum and W.L. Veale (Eds.), *Homeostasis and Thermal Stress: Experimental and Therapeutic Advances*, Karger, Basel, pp. 62–65.

Zeisberger, E., Roth, J. and Kluger, M.J. (1994) Interactions between the immune system and the hypothalamic neuroendocrine system during fever and endogenous antipyresis. In: K. Pleschka and R. Gerstberger (Eds.), *Integrative and Cellular Aspects od Autonomic Functions: Temperature and Osmoregulation*, John Libbey Eurotext, Paris, pp. 181–190.

Zeisberger, E., Goldbach, J.M. and Roth, J. (1996) Fever suppression by subdiaphragmatic vagotomy in guinea pigs depends on the route of pyrogen administration. *Pflüg. Arch.*, 431 (suppl., abstract) R51.

Zhou, D., Kusnecov, A.W., Shurin, M.R., DePaoli, M. and Rabin, B.S. (1993) Exposure to physical and psychological stressors elevates plasma interleukin-6: relationship to the activation of hypothalamic-pituitary-adrenal axis. *Endocrinology*, 133: 2523–2530.

Zimmer, J.A. and Lipton, J.M. (1981) Central and peripheral injections of ACTH (1-24) reduce fever in adrenalectomized rabbits. *Peptides*, 2: 413–417.

H.S. Sharma and J. Westman (Eds.)
Progress in Brain Research, Vol 115

CHAPTER 12

The effects of drugs on thermoregulation during exposure to hot environments

Peter Lomax[1]* and Eduard Schönbaum[2]

[1]*School of Medicine, University of California, Los Angeles, CA 90024, USA*
[2]*Department of Medical Pharmacology, LACDR, Leiden State University, Leiden, The Netherlands*

Introduction

During exposure to high ambient temperatures, the thermoregulatory centres in the brain and spinal cord activate appropriate physiological and behavioural responses so as to maintain the core temperature at the normal level of 37°C in the face of the external heat load. Should the latter be of a degree such as to overwhelm the regulatory system the internal body temperature rises and clinical heat stroke[†] may ensue. A large number of the fatal cases seen today involve military personnel undergoing training for deployment in tropical regions, or athletes training for various events. Indeed heat stroke is a leading cause of death, second only to head and spinal injuries, amongst American athletes (Knochel, 1975). The life threatening rise in internal temperature during severe physical exertion at a high ambient temperature (and frequently excessive humidity) is considered a distinct syndrome — 'stress-induced heat stroke' as opposed to 'classical heat stroke' (for detailed clinical descriptions see

Knochel, 1985). The main clinical characteristics of each type of heat stroke are listed in Table 1.

In addition to the hot environment, other factors have been implicated in the pathogenesis of classical heat stroke. Notable among these is the concomitant use of prescription drugs or exposure to exogenous chemicals (see review by Clark and Lipton, 1984) many of which are commonly used in agriculture and industry. Over the past few decades the inappropriate use of drugs and hormones has become a major problem in the case of professional athletes attempting to improve body function and competitive performance; and the practice persists in spite of the institution of strict and expensive drug testing programs.

In order to study the mechanism(s) by which such compounds may contribute to the development of heat stroke it is necessary briefly to review the physiology of normal temperature regulation.

Temperature regulation

Although there is evidence for secondary centres in the spinal cord, the major control of body temperature is exercised by neurones located in the rostral hypothalamus in the preoptic/anterior hypothalamic nuclear complex. Various models have been proposed to describe this central neu-

---

*Corresponding author. Present address: 25 Avenue du Soleil d'Or, 06230 Villefranche-sur-Mer, France.
[†]There appears to be a lack of consensus as to whether the term should be 'heat stroke', 'heat-stroke' or 'heatstroke'. The first form is consistent with the style of related disorders, e.g. 'heat cramps', 'heat exhaustion'.

TABLE 1

Comparison of the major clinical characteristics of classical and stress-induced heat stroke

Classical heat stroke	Stress-induced heat stroke
Older individuals	Young individuals
Frequently associated with chronic illness, alcoholism, heart disease, obesity	Subjects generally healthy and athletic
Precipitated by exposure to a hot, humid climate over several days	Rapid onset during severe exercise in hot, humid conditions
Commonly associated with medications that impair peripheral heat loss mechanisms	May be associated with substance abuse or environmental toxins

ronal system that is able to maintain the internal body temperature, in particular that of the brain stem, within a quite narrow range in the face of considerable changes in the external thermal environment. Hardy (1961) developed the hypothesis of proportional regulation based on engineering control theory. Several authors have since expanded on this model which seems to be consistent with most physiological observations in homeothermic species, including humans (see review by Hammel, 1968).

The regulated temperature is assumed to be that of the hypothalamus. The frequency and magnitude of the action potentials of the thermosensitive neurones vary with temperature (with a $Q_{10} > 2$ for warm-sensitive cells). These parameters are compared to those generated by an adjacent group of reference neurones. This latter group receives input from thermosensitive receptors in the skin and body core, and from proprioceptors in the muscles, which modulate the neuronal firing rates. Thus, the reference level (referred to as the *set point*) continually changes in response to fluctuations in the internal and external environment. This is a dynamic system which 'anticipates' the impact of environmental changes and responds appropriately so as to obviate any variation in the internal temperature within a narrow range of about $\pm 0.5-0.9°C$ (Cox et al.,

1975). Figure 1 depicts the thermoregulatory pathways within the model.

As an example of the response of this system let us consider exposure of an animal to a hot environment. The elevated external temperature activates warm receptors in the skin from which signals are relayed through the spinal ascending pathways to the rostral hypothalamic thermoregulatory centres. This afferent input results in a lowering of the set point (T_{set}) which is now below the actual hypothalamic temperature (T_{hyp}). The resulting offset activates heat loss mechanisms (vasodilatation in the skin, sweating, heat loss behaviour) so as to prevent any rise in core temperature (T_b) that might result from the external heat load. The system appears to have a hysteresis (determined from behavioural studies in rats) of no more than $0.3°C$ (Cox et al., 1976). Thus, no significant change in core temperature will occur unless the external heat stress is such as to overload the capacity of the system to dispel heat.

It should be noted that the physiological effectors have only a limited ability to maintain thermostasis within the normal environmental conditions under which the animal has evolved or become acclimated. This is particularly the case in the human species which depends pre-eminently on appropriate behaviour, such as manipulation of the environment, appropriate apparel,

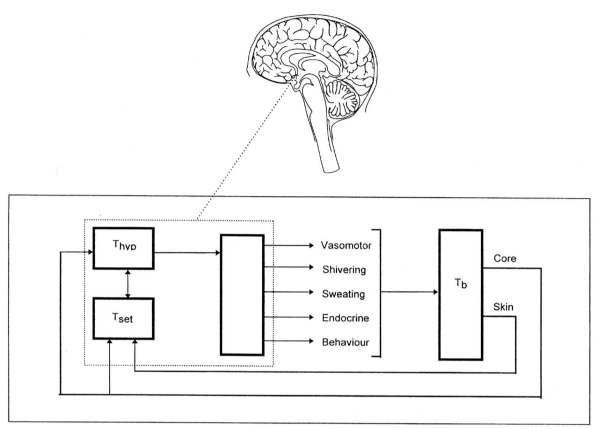

Fig. 1. Schematic diagram of the neuronal model of temperature regulation based on engineering theory of a variable set point. The primary control centres are located in the rostral hypothalamus seen in the sagittal section of the human brain. Thermoreceptors in the skin and body core relay to the rostral hypothalamus to modulate the firing rate of neurones (T_{set}) determining the set point. The rate is compared to that of central thermosensitive neurones (T_{hyp}). The values are integrated and if there is any offset, appropriate efferent systems are activated that regulate heat loss and heat production. Thus, body temperature (T_b) undergoes little significant change in the face of changes in the environmental temperature.

etc., in order to function under widely ranging climatic conditions on earth and in space. Not infrequently the appropriate behavioural response may be subjugated by the desire to succeed in competitive situations (e.g., in marathon runners). Such suppression of appropriate thermoregulatory behaviour can be a decisive factor in the pathogenesis of stress-induced heat stroke.

For more detailed discussion of the physiological control of body temperature, see reviews in Schönbaum and Lomax (1990a,b).

Modification of thermoregulation by drugs and environmental toxins

The sites and mechanisms of action of exogenous substances which interfere with normal temperature regulation have been studied extensively in animals (see Schönbaum and Lomax, 1979) but far less completely in human subjects.

In the case of thermoregulatory disorders during exposure to hot environments rather more attention has been focused on humans, largely as a result of the efforts undertaken by the Ministry of Health in Saudi Arabia to establish emergency treatment centres for pilgrims taking part in the Hajj to Medina and Mecca each year. Amongst the ∼ 2 000 000 pilgrims, heat-related illness is a common occurrence (see Khogali and Hales, 1983), especially in those years when the event falls in the hotter summer months. Substance abuse is rare during the Hajj but many pilgrims are using prescription drugs for various conditions (cardiovascular, metabolic, neurological, etc.) and these may substantially impair the central thermoregulatory and/or peripheral effector systems (Lomax, 1983).

The focus of the present volume is primarily on brain function during heat exposure. It needs to be remembered, however, that few, if any, central activities take place without input or feed back from the periphery. Also, effector systems that modulate body temperature have other primary physiological functions. For example, a major route for loss of heat in humans is via radiation from the skin by control of cutaneous blood flow. During exercise the vasomotor centres divert blood to the working muscles and reduce skin blood flow. In canines evaporation from the tongue during panting is a primary method of heat loss and inadequate water intake leads to serious hyperthermia. As a corollary, any drugs which modify these peripheral systems (such as peripherally acting antihypertensive agents) may seriously impair regulation of temperature during exposure to a hot environment.

These considerations dictate that one cannot restrict the discussion only to compounds with a direct action on the central nervous system when reviewing adverse effects during heat exposure.

Broadly, drugs may adversely affect thermoregulation in two ways — by changing the set point or by modifying peripheral effector systems. In the case of heat stroke interference with heat loss pathways mediating vasodilatation and sweating is of primary importance. Vasoconstrictors and anticholinergic drugs, respectively could suppress these functions. One needs to be aware, however, of anomalous reactions; usually these are due to

secondary effects of the compound in question. It should be recalled also that appropriate behaviour is the predominant protective measure during exposure to severe heat stress and can be impaired non-specifically by a variety of centrally active drugs.

Behavioural paradigms provide a relatively easy method to detect shifts in the thermoregulatory set point so long as the test compound does not impair the ability of the subject to respond to the test situation (Cox et al., 1976). Moreover, in humans, subjective feelings are sufficient to confirm a shift. For example, at the onset of fever the set point is raised when the core temperature is still at the normal level. But the subject feels 'cold' until the core temperature rises to the new level.

Apart from specific effects on the thermoregulatory system, drugs may cause life threatening changes in body temperature by modifying endogenous heat production. The most dramatic syndrome is the development of life threatening malignant hyperpyrexia in genetically predisposed individuals during general anaesthesia. These patients appear to have a defect in calcium transport by the sarcoplasmic reticulum (Denborough, 1980). The muscles become rigid and generate a great amount of heat. Excess muscular heat production may occur also following absorption of compounds that cause uncoupling of oxidative metabolism, that increase muscle tone, or that induce agitation, hyperactivity or seizures. With the exception of malignant hyperpyrexia these conditions do not usually endanger life under normal ambient temperatures. However, when combined with conditions of high environmental temperature and/or humidity they may prove fatal.

Specific drugs and toxins

Clark and Lipton (1984), in a review of drugs that may be implicated in the pathogenesis of heat stroke, divided them into two broad groups — those that impair heat loss and those that increase heat production. Many of the drugs discussed are, however, not really relevant to the development of exercise or stress-induced heat stroke; drugs which induce profound CNS depression, for example, would constrain most activities likely to cause stress, most notably in the case of athletes. A more useful approach for the present purposes is to select the compounds which are most likely to be applicable to the population under consideration. This population is not restricted to young people exercising while participating in various team games or individual sports. The upsurge in popularity of recreational exercise (walking, jogging, or running over various terrains, cycling, etc.) has occurred in countries world-wide, in regions of normally high ambient temperatures and in all age groups. More fit and healthy people nowadays are retiring from full employment for various reasons (largely because of economic cutbacks) so there is an increasing number of older individuals who have the time, and feel the need, to pursue these pastimes. Because of this widely expanded range of ages the repertoire of relevant drugs, particularly prescription drugs, has increased accordingly.

For the purpose of our discussion the compounds can be classified into three main groups: drugs taken for medical reasons (prescription and non-prescription); substance abuse; chemical environmental contaminants.

Drugs used for psychiatric disorders

The introduction of the antipsychotic or neuroleptic phenothiazines by Laborit et al. (1952) revolutionised the practice of psychiatry and almost emptied mental institutions around the globe. Today there are hundreds of thousands of patients under treatment with this class of drugs.

The occurrence of pyrexia during therapy with these neuroleptics was noted early (Garmany et al., 1954) and Bark (1982) has reviewed the literature on their role in the pathogenesis of heat stroke. The latter reported that the predominant number of casualties occurred in males of 20–50 years and the phenothiazines with a relatively higher anticholinergic potency had a greater propensity to precipitate heat stroke. Since sweating is suppressed by this class of drugs, it is likely that exertional stress underlay the onset of heat stroke in these patients. Although a raised ambient temperature is normally the principal precipitating factor in most cases, heat stroke following exertion at normal room temperatures in an adolescent undergoing therapy with chlorpromazine has been observed (Greenblatt and Greenblatt, 1973). Compared to atropine (which rarely triggers heat stroke in normal doses) the phenothiazines have a fairly weak peripheral cholinergic blocking action and it would seem unlikely that sweating would be suppressed sufficiently to account for the disruption in core temperature.

It has been demonstrated (Borbély and Loepfe-Hinkkanen, 1979) that the change in core temperature of animals treated with chlorpromazine is a function of the ambient conditions to which the subject is acclimated. At low ambient temperatures the drug induces hypothermia while a similar dose leads to hyperthermia at ambient temperatures above the thermoneutral range for the species. These effects are mediated at sites outside the CNS since the quaternary analogue N-methylchlorpromazine, which does not traverse the blood/brain barrier, leads to a fall in temperature in the rat at ambient temperatures below 18°C (Kirkpatrick and Lomax, 1971). Both compounds induce cutaneous vasodilatation in man, probably due to blockade of cholinergic transmission in the paravertebral autonomic ganglia. Injection of chlorpromazine or its quaternary analogue directly into the rostral hypothalamic thermoregulatory centres of the rat induces a rise in temperature (Kirkpatrick and Lomax, 1971) which most likely reflects a drug-induced elevation of the set point (Polk and Lipton, 1975).

One can conclude that these neuroleptics cause increased blood flow in the skin and so bolster radiant heat loss in a cold environment. Conversely, when the external temperature is above skin temperature heat will be absorbed and body temperature will rise. If, in addition, the set point is elevated by the drug the homeostatic mechanisms will not correct the rise in core temperature and irreversible heat stroke may ensue.

It was probably Delay et al. (1960) who first drew attention to the syndrome which subsequently has been labelled the 'neuroleptic malignant syndrome'. This can occur during treatment with several of the neuroleptics (see Clark and Lipton, 1984). Patients develop hyperpyrexia under normothermic (temperate) environmental circumstances. In 45 reported cases, 40 were 10–49 years of age and 28 were males. The clinical picture is characterised by psychomotor disorders, such as akinesia and stupor or hypertonus and dyskinesia, usually with concomitant respiratory discomfort. Mortality exceeds 20% and seems to be due to failure of organ systems rather than to the hyperthermia per se, although one cannot discount the possibility of the onset of disseminated intravascular coagulation (DIC) (a common terminal stage in severe heat stroke) in which hepatic and renal failure are conspicuous.

This syndrome may develop within a few days of the initiation of therapy. The precipitous rise in core temperature derives from heat production in the skeletal muscles (as in malignant hyperpyrexia) which demonstrate increased tone ascribed to the effect of the drug on the extrapyramidal system. There are no predictive criteria for this condition, but it should be considered in all patients who present with fever when being treated with these drugs.

Another widely prescribed group of drugs in the management of psychiatric disorders is the tricyclic antidepressants. Their effects on body temperature have been reviewed by Garattini and Jore (1979). Normally a fall in core temperature is seen which is a function of the antipsychotic potency of the drug. The tricyclic group manifests interactions with other neuropharmacological drugs which modify body temperature, such as reserpine, amphetamine, noradrenergic and cholinomimetic drugs. This interaction is used as a model for screening potential antidepressants (Garattini and Jore, 1979; Loskota and Schönbaum, 1979). Clinical heat illness, including heat stroke, has been reported with a combination of tranylcypromine (a monoamine oxidase inhibitor), propranolol and a benzodiazepine (King et al., 1979).

Amphetamine and its congeners

Amphetamine and derivatives, such as 3,4-methylene-dioxymethamphetamine (MDMA) or 'ecstasy', remain among the major drugs of abuse even though reports of their toxicity surfaced some 60 years ago (Anderson and Scott, 1936). It was another 24 years before Jordan and Hampson (1960) reported the association of these compounds with hyperpyrexia. On reviewing the literature Sellers et al. (1979) found a mortality rate of 69% in cases of amphetamine toxicity presenting with hyperpyrexia. Concern about the use of MDMA has recently resurfaced because of its use in association with the night-long dance sessions called 'raves' which involve prolonged physical exertion. Death consequent to ingestion of the drug prior to such exercise has been reported (Coore, 1996) in which a rectal temperature of 40.3°C was recorded. There are no supportable indications for the clinical use of these drugs today.

The amphetamines readily enter the brain after oral consumption where they excite the reticular activating system of the mid-brain, the thalamus and the cerebral cortex. This leads to intensified alertness accompanied by tremor, agitation and increased motor activity in addition to the elevation of mood, and, frequently, euphoria. The neuropharmacological effects are manifest primarily by release of noradrenaline from noradrenergic neurones in the CNS. It has generally been considered that the rise in body temperature is a result of augmented heat production in the muscles, although normally prescribed oral doses have little or no effect on temperature except during exposure to elevated ambient temperatures. However, enhanced noradrenergic neuronal activity in the rostral hypothalamus stabilises membrane potentials and could raise the thermoregulatory set point (see Cox and Lomax, 1977).

Drugs that modify cholinergic transmission

Because of its suppression of sweating the cholinergic blocking drug atropine is frequently cited as a classic example of a drug that precipitates stress-induced heat stroke. In human experimental studies healthy volunteers, administered greater than the normal therapeutic dose of atropine while exposed to high environmental temperatures, have failed to demonstrate that the core temperature rises to hazardous levels other than in infants and small children in whom even moderate doses can induce 'atropine fever'. Atropine may exert a central action on thermoregulation, particularly at high doses. In rats and other species, direct injection of atropine into the rostral hypothalamus leads to a rise in core temperature (Kirkpatrick and Lomax, 1971). At the same central site, injection of cholinomimetics or cholinesterase inhibitors causes hypothermia in animals due to a lowering of the set point (Cox et al., 1975). Such observations really have little relevance to stress-induced heat stroke since the use of atropine and related drugs is confined mainly to hospital treatment.

Of greater import to the present discussion is the group of compounds classified as organophosphates. These are constituents of many pesticides used in agriculture and domestic gardening and are the basis of a number of toxic nerve gases developed for military use. They are extremely potent, largely irreversible, inhibitors of the enzyme acetylcholinesterase and their clinical effects are characterised by hyperactivity of cholinergic systems throughout the body, including the CNS. In Japan alone (population approx. 100 000 000), ~ 20 000 deaths due to organophosphate insecticides were reported by the Ministry of Health and Welfare between 1954 and 1969. In cases of occupational poisoning, adsorption takes place largely through the skin and respiratory tract.

Depending on the ambient temperature, core temperature will rise or fall following toxic doses of these compounds. Moderate to severe fever was noted in 30% of the cases reviewed by Namba et al. (1971). The increased cholinergic activity leads to excess sweating but no clear relationship between its magnitude and the degree of change in temperature has been established. In animals, direct cholinergic stimulation of the rostral hypothalamic thermoregulatory centres causes a lowering of the set point and hypothermia (Cox et al., 1975). The clinical syndrome of cholinesterase suppression is characterised by serious metabolic disruption of which the high fever is but one aspect. Death is usually ascribed to cardiac failure. Cordner et al. (1986) described an unusual incident of poisoning with pilocarpine eye drops which appeared to have been added to the food of three hospital patients, of whom two died. High fever was noted in each instance.

Marihuana

Marihuana is listed as a restricted drug in many countries in Europe and North America, each practising its own degree of tolerance for those who use it habitually. Characteristic physiological or psychological responses to administration of the raw drug or its active ingredient, Δ^9-tetrahydrocannabinol (THC), even in excessively high doses, are difficult to demonstrate convincingly in animal or human experiments. A fall in body temperature of around 3°C occurs in rats following injection of THC (10 mg·kg^{-1} i.p.). A second dose 48 h later is without effect (Lomax, 1971). Jones et al. (1980) studied the effects of smoking marihuana cigarettes on groups of volunteers exposed to an ambient temperature of 23.5 or 40.6°C. The drug had no significant effect on tympanic membrane temperature at 23.5°C. At 40.6°C there was a rise in core temperature of ≈ 0.8°C (Fig. 2). During the period when the temperature was increasing sweating was suppressed and the subjects reported feeling 'less hot'. Such observations are consistent with a drug-induced rise in the set point which could herald the possibility of the onset of heat stroke if the individual were to be concurrently carrying out severe muscular exercise.

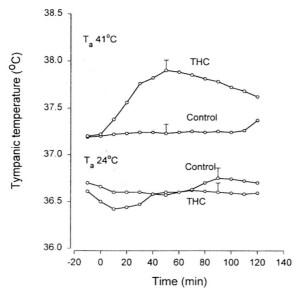

Fig. 2. The effect of smoling a placebo cigarette or a marihuana cigarette containing THC (18 mg) on core temperature (recorded at the tympanic membrane) in groups of six adults at environmental temperatures of 24°C or 41°C. Vertical bars represent ± 1 S.E.M. Data from Jones et al. (1980), courtesy of Karger, Basel.

Cocaine

Abuse of cocaine in its several forms, by all strata of society, continues to increase. Young athletes, amateur and professional, are amongst the most prevalent of identified users, especially of 'crack'. Since around 1984 scattered clinical reports of cocaine mortality have appeared in which terminal hyperpyrexia ($> 42°C$) and DIC have been prominent (for references see Lomax and Daniel, 1990a). Many of these cases have arisen during the course of participation in sports events, and in conditions of high ambient temperature and humidity.

Estimates of the recreational dose of cocaine cover a remarkably wide range. 'Mainliners' inject 10–20 mg intravenously (≈ 0.14–0.28 mg $\cdot$ kg^{-1}). The fatal dose in man is about 2.3 mg $\cdot$ kg^{-1} i.v. (160 mg total dose). Blood levels at necropsy ranged from 0.9–21 mg $\cdot$ kg^{-1} (mean 6.2 mg $\cdot$ kg^{-1}) (Mittleman and Welti, 1984).

In squirrel and Rhesus monkeys, intravenous injection of cocaine (0.1–5.0 mg $\cdot$ kg^{-1}) leads to significant increases in heart and respiratory rates and core temperature in a thermoneutral environment (around 24°C) (Wilson et al., 1976; Gonzalez and Byrd, 1977). Hyperthermia (up to 3.0°C) following cocaine injection has been noted in dogs, rabbits and guinea pigs, all at normal laboratory temperatures (Clark and Lipton, 1986).

Effects of cocaine in the rat

The Sprague–Dawley rat is an effective animal model for the study of stress induced heat stroke due to the ease with which it can be trained to exercise on a treadmill. Administration of cocaine (10–40 mg $\cdot$ kg^{-1}) to rats at rest at an ambient temperature (T_a) of 22°C leads to a dose-dependent fall in core temperature (T_c). When the animals were exposed to T_a 35°C, the T_c increased, as a function of the dose, over the same range (Lomax and Daniel, 1989). Repeated injections of cocaine at 1, 3, 8, 15, and 23 days did not modify the magnitude of the temperature change, compared to that following the first injection, i.e. neither tolerance nor potentiation occurred (Lomax and Daniel, 1990b). In rats trained to exercise on a treadmill, moderate running for 60

TABLE 2

Mean core temperature recorded in rats 60 min after the start of moderate exercise

Treatment (dose)	Number of animals	Core temperature (mean ± S.E.M.)
0.9% NaCl (0.1 ml $\cdot$ 100 g^{-1})	6	39.08 ± 0.07
Cocaine (10 mg $\cdot$ kg^{-1})	6	39.0 ± 0.17
Cocaine (20 mg $\cdot$ kg^{-1})	10	39.06 ± 0.11
Cocaine (30 mg $\cdot$ kg^{-1})	6	39.87 ± 0.28*

*Significantly different from 0.9% NaCl ($P < 0.05$; Students t-test).

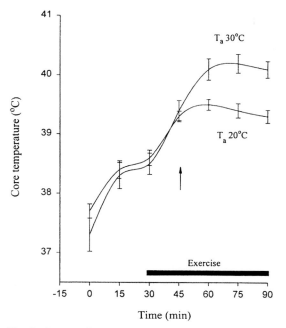

Fig. 3. Groups of rats were trained to exercise at a moderate rate on a treadmill for at least 60 min and core temperature was recorded. The ambient temperature (T_a) was set at 20°C or 30°C. Cocaine (20 mg·kg^{-1} i.p.) was injected at time indicated by the arrow. Vertical bars represent ±1 S.E.M. From 60 to 90 min the core temperature was significantly higher at T_a 30°C than at T_a 20°C ($P < 0.04$).

stroke. Indeed, rats will not survive in this experimental paradigm unless they are actively cooled.

Training the rats to exercise voluntarily on the treadmill occupies approximately 2 months and once proficient they were used for up to 24 months. This was justified since, as discussed above, it had been demonstrated that repeated testing revealed no evidence of tolerance to the effects of cocaine. However, it was noted anecdotally that in animals just recently trained the increase in T_c after 60 min running appeared to be less than that in rats that had been in the laboratory for 12 months or more. This observation prompted a study (Lomax and Daniel, 1990c) to compare 'young' and 'old' animals. The T_c stabilised at a higher level during exercise in old ($\approx$ 52 weeks old) than in young ($\approx$ 20 weeks old) rats both at 25°C and 30°C. Following administration of cocaine (20 mg·kg^{-1} i.p.) the older animals exhibited a greater temperature increase at both T_as after running for 60 min. The plateau was reached over a similar period of time ($\approx$ 30 min after the start of running) in both groups and, noting that the initial T_c was lower in the old group, the rate of rise was greater in the old rats. Older animals were heavier than the younger ones (355 g compared to 299 g) and so were working at a higher rate but the ratio was only 1.18:1.00 whereas the ratio of the rate of rise was 2:1. When the belt speed was reduced from 0.22 m·s^{-1} to 0.18 m·s^{-1} (1.22:1.00) the rate of rise was not significantly changed, i.e. the variance in weight does not account for the difference in the final plateau temperature. The rise in temperature during exercise reflects an elevation of the set point triggered by signals from the muscle proprioceptors. This upward setting is enhanced at higher T_as by input from cutaneous thermoreceptors (Jessen, 1990). Why the set point should increase more in older individuals is unclear, although it is conceivable that age-related changes in central neurotransmitter systems, particularly in catecholaminergic neurones, may be responsible. Certainly, these data indicate that the elderly may have a greater chance of developing stress-induced heat stroke in hot environ-

min at T_a 22°C led to a rise in T_c. Cocaine (10 or 20 mg·kg^{-1}) did not modify the rise in T_c compared to the same volume of 0.9% NaCl; on increasing the dose of cocaine to 30 mg·kg^{-1} the rise in T_c was significantly greater (Lomax and Daniel, 1990a) (Table 2). When rats acclimated to T_a 20°C were placed in the treadmill chamber heated to 30°C, the resting T_c increased by $\approx$ 0.6°C over a 30-min period. The animals were then exercised for 60 min by which time the T_c had increased by 1.05 ± 0.16°C to $\approx$ 39.6°C. Cocaine (20 mg·kg^{-1} i.p.), a dose that was ineffective at T_a 22°C, augmented the exercise-induced hyperthermia and the terminal T_c was over 40°C (Lomax and Daniel, 1993). Figure 3 summarises the conclusion relevant to the present discussion, viz, cocaine can induce significant hyperthermia during exercise at a high ambient temperature and this could progress to heat

ments and may be exposed to an increased tendency to cocaine toxicity under such conditions.

The central effects of cocaine appear to be mediated at multiple sites in the brain. Unlike other local anaesthetics in clinical use cocaine blocks the reuptake of catecholamines into the presynaptic terminal of noradrenergic and dopaminergic neurones. This is the basis of its powerful vasoconstrictor action when injected into the tissues which reduces surgical bleeding and prolongs the duration of local anaesthesia. Accumulation of dopamine in the synaptic cleft, due to a similar blockade of reuptake, may be the cause of the behavioural responses to the drug (see Fisher et al., 1987). Pretreatment with the dopamine D_1 antagonist, SCH 23390 protects rats from the lethal effects of cocaine but does not reduce the incidence of seizures (Witkin et al., 1989). The effects of SCH 23390 on the thermal responses to cocaine have been investigated by Lomax and Daniel (1991a, 1991b, 1993). Injection of SCH 23390 (1 mg $\cdot$ kg^{-1} i.p.) into the rat at T_a 22°C had no effect on T_c over the first 60 min; thereafter, however, the temperature steadily declined over the following 60 min and remained below that of the control animals for several hours. The hypothermic response to cocaine (20 mg $\cdot$ kg^{-1} i.p.) was considerably augmented in animals pretreated with SCH 23390 (1 mg $\cdot$ kg^{-1} i.p.) and the T_c remained low for up to 120 h. The rise in T_c induced by cocaine (20 mg $\cdot$ kg^{-1} i.p.) at T_a 30°C was abolished by injection of SCH 23390 15 min prior to cocaine, indeed the pre-treated rats developed significant hypothermia within 15 min, although SCH 23390 alone had no effect on T_c over 90 min at the high environmental temperature.

SCH 23390, even at low doses (0.1, 0.3 or 1.0 mg $\cdot$ kg^{-1} i.p.), suppresses spontaneous motor activity so that the rats would exercise on the treadmill only for 30–45 min after injection. Pre-treatment with the antagonist did not affect the rise in core temperature induced by cocaine at T_a 30°C (Lomax and Daniel, 1993).

If the thermoregulatory effects of cocaine are indeed mediated by central dopaminergic systems these findings are consistent with earlier conclu-

sions, using selective agonists and antagonists (Chipkin, 1988; Sánchez, 1989; Vasse et al., 1990), that D_1 receptor activation leads to a rise in T_c and D_2 activation causes a fall. When both receptor subtypes are triggered, the direction of the temperature change in the rat would seem to be a function of T_a and the consequent state of the thermoregulatory system in response to the input from peripheral thermosensors. At a T_a above the thermoneutral zone, the hyperthermic response is dominant but when the D_1 receptors are blocked hypothermia, mediated by the D_2 receptors, occurs. There is a relatively high density of D_1 compared to D_2 receptors in the CNS ($\approx$ 3–5:1 depending on the species), in addition to a probably distinct D_3 species in the limbic system. The majority of identified drug effects are manifest at the D_2 receptor with the D_1 being something of a mystery protein. One suggestion is that the D_1 receptor modulates the response of the D_2 receptor by expression of a signal protein. This could occur over an extended time frame that would account for the delayed onset and prolonged effect on T_c.

As noted above, in many cases of cocaine toxicity occurring in hot environments, stress-related heat stroke is the terminal event. The mortality rate in all forms of heat stroke is very high, exceeding 80% unless expeditious and skilled emergency treatment is available. The most urgent component of this is to lower the body temperature. In patients presenting with hyperthermia secondary to cocaine toxicity dopamine D_1 antagonists are unlikely to prove to be useful adjuvants to body cooling by physical methods.

Conclusion

When exposed to a hot environment a healthy individual, in whom the thermoregulatory system is unimpaired, would not be expected to develop a dangerous rise in deep body temperature (exceeding 2–3°C). Addition of another factor, viz, increased heat production as a result of muscular exercise, may overload the capacity of the heat loss mechanisms so that the body temperature rises and exertional heat stroke may develop. As we have seen, certain drugs can interfere with the central controlling system to alter the set point or impair the effector systems. Generally the subject and, in many cases, medical advisors seem to be unaware of these drug side effects. This is particularly the case with cocaine overdose where the terminal syndrome (DIC) is identical to that in severe heat stroke. The immediate emergency treatment of such patients must be directed towards lowering the core temperature. Clearly, education is required since the morbidity and mortality rates are extremely high in those cases in which drugs are implicated in the aetiology of exertional heat stroke.

References

Anderson, E.W. and Scott, W.C. (1936) Cardiovascular effects of benzedrine. *Lancet*, ii: 1461–1462.

Bark, N.M. (1982) Heatstroke in psychiatric patients: two patients and a review. *J. Clin. Psychiatry*, 43: 377–380.

Borbély, A.A. and Loepfe-Hinkkanen, M. (1979) Phenothiazines. In: E. Schönbaum and P. Lomax (Eds.), *Body Temperature: Regulation, Drug Effects and Therapeutic Implications*, Dekker, New York, pp. 403–426.

Chipkin, R.E. (1988) Effects of D1 and D2 antagonists on basal and apomorphine decreased body temperature in mice and rats. *Pharmacol. Biochem. Behav.*, 30: 683–686.

Clark, W.G. and Lipton, J.M. (1984) Drug related heatstroke. *Pharmacol. Ther.*, 26: 345–388.

Clark, W.G. and Lipton, J.M. (1986) Changes in body temperature after administration of adrenergic and serotonergic agents and related drugs including antidepressants: II. *Neurosci. Behav. Rev.*, 10: 153–220.

Coore, J.R. (1996) A fatal trip with ecstasy: a case of 3,4-methylene-dioxymethamphetamine/3,4-methylenedioxyamphetamine toxicity. *J. R. Soc. Med.*, 89: 51P–52P.

Cordner, S.M., Fysh, R.R., Gordon, H. and Whitaker, S.J. (1986) Deaths of two hospital inpatients poisoned by pilocarpine. *Br. Med. J.*, 293: 1285–1287.

Cox, B., Ary, M. and Lomax, P. (1976) Dopaminergic involvement in withdrawal hypothermia and thermoregulatory behavior in morphine dependent rats. *Pharmacol. Biochem. Behav.*, 4: 259–262.

Cox, B. and Lomax, P. (1977) Pharmacologic control of temperature regulation. *Annu. Rev. Pharmacol.*, 17: 341–353.

Cox, B., Green, M.D. and Lomax, P. (1975) Behavioral thermoregulation in the study of drugs affecting body temperature. *Pharmacol. Biochem. Behav.*, 3: 1051–1054.

Delay, J., Pichot, P., Lempériere, T., Elissalde, B. and Peigne, F. (1960) Un neuroleptique majeur non-phénothiazinique

et non-réserpinique, l'halopéridol dans le traitement des psychoses. *Ann. Médico-Psychologiques*, 118: 145–152.

Denborough, M.A. (1980) The pathophysiology of malignant hyperpyrexia. *Pharmacol. Ther.*, 9: 357–365.

Fisher, S., Raskin, A. and Uhlenhuth, E.H. (Eds.) (1987) *Cocaine and Biobehavioral Aspects*, Oxford University Press, New York.

Garattini, S. and Jore, A. (1979) Tricyclic antidepressant drugs. In: P. Lomax and E. Schönbaum (Eds.), *Body Temperature: Regulation, Drug Effects and Therapeutic Implications*, Dekker, New York, pp. 439–459.

Garmany, G., May, A.R. and Folkson, A. (1954) The use and action of chlorpromazine in psychoneuroses. *Br. Med. J.*, ii: 429–431.

Greenblatt, D.J. and Greenblatt, G.R. (1973) Chlorpromazine and hyperpyrexia: a reminder that this drug affects the mechanisms which regulate body temperature. *Clin. Pediatr.*, 12: 504–505.

Gonzalez, F.A. and Byrd, L.D. (1977) Physiological effects of cocaine in the squirrel monkey. *Life Sci.*, 21: 1417–1424.

Hammel, H.T. (1968) The regulation of internal body temperature. *Annu. Rev. Physiol.*, 30: 641–710.

Hardy, J.D. (1961) Physiology of temperature regulation. *Physiol. Rev.*, 41: 521–606.

Jessen, C. (1990) Thermal afferents in the control of body temperature. In: E. Schönbaum and P. Lomax (Eds.) *Thermoregulation: Physiology and Biochemistry*, Pergamon Press, New York, pp. 153–183.

Jones, R.T., Maddock, R., Farrel, T.R. and Herning, R. (1980) Marijuana and human thermoregulation in a hot environment. In: B. Cox, P. Lomax, A.S. Milton and E. Schönbaum (Eds.), *Thermoregulatory Mechanisms and their Therapeutic Implications*, Karger, Basel, pp. 62–64.

Jordan, S.C. and Hampson, F. (1960) Amphetamine poisoning associated with hyperpyrexia. *Br. Med. J.*, ii: 844.

Khogali, M. and Hales, J.R.S. (1983) *Heat Stroke and Temperature Regulation*, Academic Press, Australia.

King, I., Barnett, P.S. and Kew, M.C. (1979) Drug-induced hyperpyrexia. *S. Afr. Med. J.*, 56: 190–191.

Kirkpatrick, W.E. and Lomax, P. (1971) Temperature changes induced by chlorpromazine and *N*-methyl chlorpromazine in the rat. *Neuropharmacology*, 10: 61–66.

Knochel, J.P. (1975) Dog days and siriasis. How to kill a football player. *J. Am. Med. Assoc.*, 233: 513–515.

Knochel, J.P. (1985) Disorders due to heat and cold. In: J.B. Wyngaarden and L.H. Smith (Eds.), *Cecil Textbook of Medicine*, Saunders, Philadelphia, pp. 2304–2307.

Laborit, H., Huguenard, P. and Alluaume, R. (1952) Un nouveau stabilisateur végétatif, le 4560 RP. *Presse Medical.*, 60: 206–208.

Lomax, P. (1971) Animal pharmacology of marihuana. *Proc. West. Pharmacol. Soc.*, 14: 10–13.

Lomax, P. (1983) Drug-induced changes in the thermoregulatory system. In: M. Khogali and J.R.S. Hales (Eds.), *Heat*

204

Stroke and Temperature Regulation, Academic Press, Australia, pp. 197–211.

Lomax, P. and Daniel, K.A. (1989) Body temperature changes induced by cocaine in the rat. In: J.B. Mercer (Ed.), *Proceedings of the International Symposium on Thermal Physiology*, Excerpta Medica, Amsterdam, pp. 265–271.

Lomax, P. and Daniel, K.A. (1990a) Cocaine and body temperature in the rat: effect of exercise. *Pharmacol. Biochem. Behav.*, 36: 889–892.

Lomax, P. and Daniel, K.A. (1990b) Cocaine and body temperature in the rat: effects of ambient temperature. *Pharmacology*, 40: 103–109.

Lomax, P. and Daniel, K.A. (1990c) Cocaine and body temperature in the rat: effects of exercise and age. *Pharmacology*, 41: 309–315.

Lomax, P. and Daniel, K.A. (1991a) Cocaine and body temperature in the rat: effect of dopamine D_1 antagonists. *Proc. West. Pharmacol. Soc.*, 34: 5–9.

Lomax, P. and Daniel, K.A. (1991b) Dopamine antagonists and cocaine induced temperature changes. In: P. Lomax and E. Schönbaum (Eds.), *Thermoregulation: The Pathophysiological Basis of Clinical Disorders*, Karger, Basel, pp. 114–118.

Lomax, P. and Daniel, K.A. (1993) Cocaine and body temperature: effects of exercise at high ambient temperature. *Pharmacology*, 46: 164–172.

Loskota, W.J. and Schönbaum, E. (1979) Reserpine. In: P. Lomax and E. Schönbaum (Eds.), *Body Temperature: Regulation, Drug Effects and Therapeutic Implications*, Dekker, New York, pp. 427–437.

Mittleman, R.E. and Welti, C.V. (1984) Death caused by recreational cocaine use. *J. Am. Med. Assoc.*, 252: 1889–1893.

Namba, T., Nolte, C.T., Jackrel, J. and Grob, D. (1971) Poisoning due to organophosphate insecticides. *Am. J. Med.*, 50: 475–492.

Polk, D.L. and Lipton, J.M. (1975) Effects of sodium salicylate, aminopyrine and chlorpromazine on behavioral temperature regulation. *Pharmacol. Biochem. Behav.*, 3: 167–172.

Sánchez, C. (1989) The effects of dopamine D-1 and D-2 receptors on body temperature in male mice. *Eur. J. Pharmacol.*, 171: 201–206.

Schönbaum, E. and Lomax, P. (1979) *Body Temperature: Regulation, Drug Effects and Therapeutic Implications*, Dekker, New York.

Schönbaum, E. and Lomax, P. (1990a) *Thermoregulation: Physiology and Biochemistry*, Pergamon Press, Oxford.

Schönbaum, E. and Lomax, P. (1990b) *Thermoregulation: Pathology, Pharmacology and Therapy*, Pergamon Press, Oxford.

Sellers, E.M., Martin, P.R., Roy, M.L. and Sellers, E.A. (1979) Amphetamines. In: P. Lomax and E. Schönbaum (Eds.), *Body Temperature: Regulation, Drug Effects and Therapeutic Implications*, Dekker, New York, pp. 461–498.

Vasse, M., Chagrauoi, A., Henry, J-P. and Protais, P. (1990) The rise in body temperature induced by stimulation of dopamine D_1 receptors is increased in acutely reserpinized mice. *Eur. J. Pharmacol.*, 181: 23–33.

Wilson, M.C., Bedford J.A., Buelke, J. and Kibbe, A.H. (1976) Acute pharmacological effects of intravenous cocaine in the Rhesus monkey. *Psychopharmacology*, 2: 251–261.

Witkin, J.M., Goldberg, S.R. and Katz, J.L. (1989) Lethal effects of cocaine are reduced by the dopamine-1 receptor antagonist SCH 23390 but not by haloperidol. *Life Sci.*, 44: 1285–1291.

SECTION III

Molecular aspects

H.S. Sharma and J. Westman (Eds.)
Progress in Brain Research, Vol 115

CHAPTER 13

Heat shock protein response in the central nervous system following hyperthermia

Jan Westman and Hari Shanker Sharma*

Laboratory of Neuroanatomy, Department of Anatomy, Biomedical Centre, Box 571, Uppsala University, S-751 23 Uppsala, Sweden

Introduction

When cells and tissues are exposed to various stressful stimuli they respond with a rapid production of a highly conserved set of proteins called heat shock proteins (HSP) (Lindquist, 1986; Lindquist and Craig, 1988; Kumar, 1992). The term 'heat shock protein' was derived from the fact that these proteins were initially discovered to be induced by hyperthermic conditions (Bardwell and Craig, 1984; Craig, 1985; Anathan et al., 1986; Welch, 1992). However rapid advancement of new knowledge in this field showed that these proteins can also be induced by a wide variety of non-thermal noxious stimuli such as exposure to heavy metals, oxidants; pathophysiological stressors like bacterial and viral infections, inflammation, ischemia, trauma; as well as under the influence of various hormones, neoplastic drugs, chemicals and growth factors (Table 1) (Sharma et al., 1992a; Ciocca et al., 1993; Blake et al., 1994; Marcuccilli and Miller, 1994; Sharma et al., 1995; Marcuccilli et al., 1996; Sharma and Westman, 1997).

Due to these ubiquitous characteristics of HSP response after various types of stress, some workers prefer 'stress proteins' rather than 'heat-shock' proteins (Gonzalez et al., 1989; Gower et al., 1989). However with the recent discovery of induction of many other proteins following stress such as glucose-regulated proteins (GRP), ubiquitin, α B-crystalline which are also very closely related with HSP family (Kato et al., 1993), the term 'stress protein' as a replacement of 'heat shock' proteins will lead to more confusion. Thus in spite of induction of HSP in cells by various thermal and non-thermal stimuli, the term 'heat shock proteins' is widely used in the current literature (Lindquist, 1986; Lindquist and Craig, 1988; Welch, 1992) and is also followed in this review.

The HSP response is a universal response of all prokaryotic and eukaryotic species following subjection to noxious stressful situations (Hightower, 1980; Anathan et al., 1986; Barbe et al., 1988; Kaufmann, 1992; Welch, 1992). HSPs are synthesised in four general molecular weight classes: 95–100 kDa, 80–90 kDa, 70–75 kDa and 20–30 kDa, with minor variations in molecular weight which are species-specific (Craig, 1985; Lindquist, 1986; Lindquist and Craig, 1988; Kaufmann, 1992; Welch, 1992). These members of the HSP family (Table 2) have several features in common such as, they are preferentially expressed following hy-

---

*Corresponding author. Tel: +46 18 4714433; fax: +46 18 243899; e-mail: Sharma@anatomi.uu.se

TABLE 1

Factors influencing synthesis of various heat shock proteins

Stimuli	Type of HSP synthesis
Stressors	HSP 100, HSP 90, HSP 70, HSP 60, HSP 27
Heat stress[a]	
Heat shock	
Immobilization[a]	
UV radiation	
Amino acid analogues	
Arsenite	
Various chemicals	
Drugs	
Physiological stimuli	HSP 90, HSP 70, HSP 60, HSP 27
Hormones	
Growth factors	
Cell cycle	
Immunomodulators	
Pathological conditions	HSP 90, HSP 70, HSP 72
Trauma[a]	
Ischemia	
Hypoxia	
Infarction	
Infections	
Glucose starvation	
Anoxia	

[a]Authors own investigations; compiled from various sources (Ciocca et al., 1993; Marcuccilli and Miller, 1994; Sharma et al., 1995; Marcuccilli et al., 1996; Sharma and Westman, 1997; Sharma et al., 1997a).

perthermia; they are found in all living cells; their amino acid sequences are highly conserved throughout evolution except for the small molecular weight of HSPs; and they have a specific DNA motif (heat shock element) in the promotor region of their genes which is activated by specific heat shock transcription factor known as heat shock factor (HSF) (Sarge et al., 1991, 1993; Sorger, 1991; Marcuccilli and Miller, 1994).

Induction of HSP after stress is mediated by the multigene family of HSF (Morimoto, 1993; Marcuccilli and Miller, 1994). Recent discovery of multiple HSF genes in chicken, mouse and human raises the interesting possibility and diversity

of its function which is not yet well known (Morimoto, 1993). It is speculated that each HSF is responsible for a particular cellular response to different stressors or they are involved in certain processes of cell development (Sarge et al., 1994), a feature which however requires further investigation.

Studies on HSP response in the CNS following various stressors are, however, still lacking. On the other hand HSP response in other organs has resulted in the generation of a wealth of current information. The functional significance and physiological implication of such findings are largely obscure (Marcuccilli and Miller, 1994). It appears that the cellular HSP response is of great pathophysiological importance and can be used as a marker of cell reaction in different pathological conditions.

One of the fundamental problems in understanding the pathophysiological significance of HSP in the CNS is that most of our knowledge concerning HSP response in hyperthermia is based on exposure of glial cells or nerve cells in culture (Lindquist, 1986; Kaufmann, 1992; Welch, 1992). Thus it is not clear whether induction of HSP is beneficial or harmful to the cells in *in vivo* situations. Moreover, the influence of neuroprotective drugs on expression of HSP response in these hyperthermic or similar stress experiments is completely lacking. Thus our understanding of HSP response in the pathophysiology of CNS injury is still rudimentary.

This review focuses on the pathological significance of HSP response in the CNS following heat stress in *in vivo* situations which has largely been ignored in the past. In addition, the current knowledge about HSP induction, function and its significance is also reviewed. Finally, based on our own investigation in heat stress, the pharmacological modification of HSP response in relation to cell injury which is a new emerging subject, is also discussed.

HSP in normal cells

Most of the HSP are constitutively expressed in

TABLE 2

Heat shock protein types, their intracellular localisation and possible function

HSP type	Similar names in literature	Localisation	Possible function
The small HSP family			
HSP 27	HSP 28	Nucleus[a] cytoplasm	Cell survival, maintenance, stress resistance
HSP 32	Heme oxygenase	Endoplasmic reticulum membrane	Heme degradation
Ubiquitin		Cytoplasm	Protein degradation
HSP 70 family			
HSC 70	HSP 73 HSC 73	Cytoplasm	Protein maturation Protein translocation
HSP 70[b]	HSP 72	Nucleus nucleolus	Unknown, inducible?
GRP 78	BiP	Endoplasmic reticulum	Secretory proteins
GRP 75		Mitochondria	Protein translocation
HSP 90 family			
HSP 90		Cytoplasm	Protein maturation
HSP 90 α (86 kDa)			
HSP 90 β (84 kDa)		Steroid receptors	Inactive receptor
GRP 94	ERp99 endoplasmin	Endoplasmic reticulum	Protein folding, secretory proteins
HSP 110	HSP 100	Nucleus, cytoplasm nucleolus[a]	Thermotolerance

Due to different gel systems used in various laboratories, the HSP nomenclature is often quite complicated and rather confusing. For instance, many laboratories prefer to use HSP 70 which is present in both cytoplasm and nucleus as HSP 73 and HSP 72 (for details see text).
HSP = heat shock protein; HSC = heat shock cognate; GRP = glucose related protein; BiP = binding protein (for details see text); compiled from various sources (Welch, 1992; Ciocca et al., 1993; Marcuccilli and Miller, 1994; Sharma et al., 1995; Marcuccilli et al., 1996; Sharma and Westman, 1997; Sharma et al., 1997a).
[a] Incorporated after stress only.
[b] Expression occurs after stress only.

normal cells (Welch, 1992; Ciocca et al., 1993; Marcuccilli and Miller, 1994). Their proposed function is to regulate cell growth, maintenance and development (Welch, 1992, Kaufmann, 1992). One of these protein is identified as heat shock cognate 70 (HSC 70) or constitutive isoform of HSP 70 (Sorger, 1991; Kaneko et al., 1993). Other members of HSP 70 kDa family can be inducible (Marcuccilli and Miller, 1994). However, they share more than 90% similarity with HSC 70 and are also regarded to have similar functional properties (Sarge et al., 1993). This is evident from the fact that inducible HSP 70 can prevent

protein denaturation and help in refolding of damaged proteins after stress (Sarge et al., 1994). Members of the other HSP 70 family are known to play important roles in protein folding and translocation within the endoplasmic reticulum and mitochondria (Welch, 1992). These observations strongly indicate that HSP plays an important role in maintaining the physiological activity of the cells in the CNS.

HSP induction and cellular protection

There is evidence which suggests that HSP induction is related to the protection of both neural and non-neural cells in the CNS. Thus microinjection of antibodies to HSP 70 and HSC 70 in rat embryo fibroblast cells (REF-52) resulted in lethality when subjected to a 45°C heat shock treatment (Riabowol et al., 1988). On the other hand, injection of antibodies directed against tubulin, actin, Fos, Ras, HSP 28 and the catalytic subunit of cAMP dependent protein kinase, did not influence the cell survival in identical conditions. These observations suggest that induction of HSP or HSC 70 is protective in nature.

Further evidence in this direction came from the observations of Uney et al. (1993) who transfected rat dorsal root ganglion (DRG) cells in culture with an EF-1α promoter-HSP 70 expression vector. When these transfected cells were heated to 46°C for 20 min, the survival of these cells was significantly greater than non-transfected DRG cells. In an earlier similar experiment, Johnston and Kucey (1988) transfected the Chinese hamster ovary cells with a plasmid containing gene for dihydrofolate reductase under the control of a 5′ amino acid control sequence containing three binding sites for HSF. In these transfected cells, thermotolerance following heat shock was significantly higher than in the control cells.

HSP as marker of cell injury

In the CNS, induction of HSP occurs under a wide variety of experimental conditions such as hyperthermia (Sprang and Brown, 1987; Sharma et al., 1992a), kainic acid administration (Planas et al., 1995), chemically induced-status epilepticus (Lowenstein et al., 1990), ischemia (Kato et al., 1993), brain or spinal cord injury (Brown et al., 1989; Gower et al., 1989; Sharma et al., 1995). In various animal models of middle cerebral artery occlusion or intracerebral injection of kainic acid, the HSP induction following 24 h after insult was closely related with the areas of brain damage. Based on these observations, Gonzalez and his colleagues (1989) suggested that HSP 70 can be used as a marker of cell injury. However, further

studies are needed in this direction to establish this finding.

HSP and acquired thermotolerance and cross tolerance

Another aspect of HSP induction is related with thermotolerance which has attracted great attention by many workers (Barbe et al., 1988; Johnston and Kucey, 1988; Landry et al., 1989; Li et al., 1992; Kato et al., 1994). Thus cells when pretreated with a mild hyperthermia resulted in HSP induction (Lindquist, 1986). When these cells are subjected to further severe heat stress, they are resistant to cell damage compared to the untreated controls (Lindquist and Craig, 1988). In the mechanism of thermotolerance, most emphasis is given on HSP 70 induction, compared to other forms of HSPs (Kaufmann, 1992; Welch, 1992; Marcuccilli and Miller, 1994). Thus involvement of other members of HSP in thermotolerance needs further investigation.

The phenomenon by which a mild heat stress is used to induce HSP which protects the cells from further damage caused by excitotoxicity or other stressors, is known as 'cross tolerance' (Sanchez et al., 1992). The potential therapeutic value of this 'cross tolerance' could be enormous. Thus, using this 'cross tolerance' phenomenon, it is possible to use pyretics to induce fever which can induce HSP response before patients undergo surgery in order to minimise cellular trauma. Likewise, use of drugs such as cocaine can also induce HSP in many tissues (Blake et al., 1994). It appears that prior induction of HSP in these patients is beneficial (Jurivich et al., 1992). However no direct evidence is available either to accept or reject this hypothesis.

Cross tolerance is a well-known phenomenon in the CNS. Thus when rats are pretreated for 15 min heat exposure in a chamber at 41°C and then subjected to retinal damage by excessive exposure to light 18 h after the heat treatment, none of these rats exhibited any retinal damage (Barbe et al., 1988). On the other hand, severe retinal damage occurred in all the rats which did not receive prior heat treatment when subjected to similar light exposure (Barbe et al., 1988). This protection of retina is well correlated with induction of HSP 64 because both cell protection and induction of HSP 64 were reduced 50 h after heat treatment.

Heat pretreatment of rat cortical cell culture also exhibited similar protection. Thus treatment of these cells to heat at 42.5°C for 20 min resulted in induction of HSP 72 kDa and HSP 90 kDa 3 h after exposure. These cells were resistant to glutamate toxicity at 3 h and 24 h after heat treatment. However this protection was lost 48 h after heat treatment (Rordorf et al., 1991). Neuroprotection in cerebellar granule cells following excitotoxicity also occurs after a mild heat pretreatment (Lowenstein et al., 1991).

HSP and ischemic cross tolerance

Apart from mild heat treatment, ischemic tolerance in animals subjected to a mild brief period of ischemic episode is also demonstrated (Kitagawa et al., 1990; Kumar, 1992). Thus Mongolian gerbils subjected to a brief ischemia of 2 min duration daily for 2 days survived 5 min bilateral carotid artery occlusion performed 1–4 days after the primary insult. These animals did not show any major cell damage or necrosis in the CA1 region of the hippocampus and exhibited a profound upregulation of HSP 70 in the pyramidal cells of the CA1 sector (Kitagawa et al., 1990; Kirino et al., 1991). These results suggest that even pretreatment with mild ischemia can attenuate the effect of severe ischemia-induced cell damage and this protection of the cells is related to the induction of HSP 70 response. This phenomenon indicates a role of HSP in the process of adaptation which however, requires further investigation.

Regional variation in HSP response

The studies reported above do not shed any light on the possible mechanisms of HSP induction in specific neural or non-neural cells under any particular stress situation. Thus it is not clear whether HSP induction will vary between neurons and glial cells under a particular situation of stress. There are a few experiments in this line which suggest that a certain set of neurons and glial cells are activated under a particular type of stress leaving other neurons and non-neuronal cells completely intact (Marcuccilli et al., 1996). There is evidence which suggests that different brain regions or different cell types will show different patterns of HSP induction under similar stress situations. The mechanisms of such a selective and specific response to HSP in the CNS under stressful situations are still unclear.

Hyperthermia induced by lysergic acid diethylamide (LSD) in rabbits resulted in induction of HSC 70 mRNA in the CA1 and CA4 regions of the hippocampus as well as in the Purkinje and granule cell layers 1 h after hyperthermia. At this time period, induction of HSP mRNA was absent in hippocampal neurons, however glial cells showed a profound increase in the HSP mRNA (Sprang and Brown, 1987). This observation is different from ischemia in which hippocampal CA1 pyramidal neurons showed marked upregulation of HSP 70 expression indicating that different cell types may express different forms of HSP and that all HSP induction is not protective in nature (Vass et al., 1988; Marcuccilli and Miller, 1994).

HSF and HSP induction

New experimental evidence suggests that induction of HSP 70 gene is mediated by a heat shock factor (HSF) (Welch, 1992; Morimoto, 1993; Marcuccilli and Miller, 1994). This HSF binds to heat-shock elements located in the promoters of heat shock genes as described above (Morimoto et al., 1992; Lis and Wu, 1993; Morimoto, 1993). These HSF are part of a multigene family and mammalian HSF1 and HSF2 is now cloned in mouse and human (Sarge et al., 1991; Schuetz et al., 1991). The main mediator of HSP expression appears to be HSF1. However HSF2 is known to be activated by hemin (Sarge et al., 1993; Sistone et al., 1994). Thus it seems quite likely that multiple forms of HSF are present in one species type which are activated by different ways under a similar stress situation. This possibility is related to the differential expression of some CNS cell types such as astrocytes or nerve cells to a particular stressor. Studies showing patterns of HSF expression in different neuronal and non-neuronal cell types in a particular stress situation may explain the selective vulnerability of cells in many pathological and neurodegenerative diseases of the CNS. However, this is a new and emerging discipline which requires further investigation.

Induction of HSP response by stress

Cells are able to detect adverse changes in their microenvironment and are capable with intracellular machinery to cope with various emergency situations (Selye, 1976; Welch, 1992; Hughes and Dragunow, 1995). These cells may use temporary or permanent changes in their gene expression depending on the magnitude and severity of the primary insult (Hughes and Dragunow, 1995). In addition, the cells are equipped with abnormal expression of HSP under adverse situations for their survival. The mechanisms by which the cells recognise adverse changes in their surroundings and subsequently increase their HSP response are however, still unclear.

One major triggering factor of the synthesis of HSP following stress or trauma appears to be intracellular accumulation of abnormally folded proteins (Hightower, 1980). It seems quite likely that upregulation of HSP is somehow involved in the recognition and removal of denatured proteins in traumatised or stressed cells. This idea gets further support from the experiments of various workers in bacterial cells, frog oocytes and chicken fibroblast cells (Kelley and Schlesinger, 1978; Anathan et al., 1986; Goff and Goldberg, 1987). Thus, feeding of amino acid analogues to bacteria resulted in production of abnormally folded proteins and also the induction of HSP response (Goff and Goldberg, 1987). These authors found an increased expression of bacterial

protease which suggests that an overload on the cellular proteolytic system seems to be one of the most important signals for HSP induction that is necessary for removal of these denatured proteins. Earlier observations in chicken embryo fibroblast cell described by Kelley and Schlesinger (1978) is in line with this observation. One of the landmark findings in the field is the study carried out by Anathan et al. (1986) who achieved an induction of HSP response by injecting a collection of denatured proteins into frog oocyte. These observations strongly support the idea that intracellular accumulation of abnormally folded proteins is one of the main triggering mechanisms of HSP induction (Welch, 1992).

Most of the HSP are constitutively expressed in the cells and are responsible for cell growth and differentiation. The degree of individual HSP expression depends on the metabolic activity of the cells (Kaufmann, 1992; Welch, 1992). Thus expression of HSP is very high in growing or secretory cells compared to quiescent cells. Expression of HSP is also increased in cells infected with virus, particularly with the lytic one in which synthesis of viral proteins is usually very high (Nevins, 1982). These observations suggest that HSP is essential for protein maturation. High expression of HSP in various conditions could be due to increased demand for protein synthesis by the cells. Thus, when cells are exposed to stress, their machinery of protein synthesis, secretory activity or the protein maturation systems are distorted resulting in accumulation of folded proteins which may result in induction of one or more types of HSP (Welch, 1992).

Alteration in cell physiology following induction of HSP response

Most studies are directed at understanding the molecular biology and biochemistry of HSP induction. A few studies examined the consequences of alterations in cell physiology following induction of HSP response. Yeasts and bacterial cells initiated the expression of HSP for a short period of time when their ambient temperature was increased from 20°C to 37°C. However, normal patterns of protein synthesis and other activities are resumed by these poikilothermic organisms even if there is a further increase in the ambient temperature. On the other hand, mammalian cells when exposed to high ambient temperatures are not capable of acclimation above 42°C like most homeothermic organisms. These cells continue to synthesise HSP at all temperatures up to the point of their cell death.

Induction of HSP in the mammalian cells following hyperthermia is also associated with many other biochemical changes. Thus there is a rapid decline in intracellular pH, decreased levels of ATP and an increase in cytosolic levels of calcium (Stevenson et al., 1981; Findly et al., 1983; Weitzel et al., 1985). However, these intracellular changes by themselves do not seem to contribute to the induction of HSP response (Drummond et al., 1986).

Morphological alterations in the intracellular compartment following heat shock

Heat shock induces profound morphological changes in the nucleus, nucleolus, intermediate filaments and mitochondria. Alteration in morphology of the cell nucleus in mammalian cells is a common finding following heat shock-induced hyperthermia. Thus perichromatin granules representing unprocessed forms of HSP mRNA accumulate in the nucleus indicating that RNA splicing is perturbed in hyperthermia. However expression of many inducible forms of HSP mRNA does not depend on splicing machinery of the proteins (Lindquist, 1986). Appearance of rodlike filaments sometimes occurs in the nucleus of many mammalian cells after heat treatment (Pekkald et al., 1984).

Disintegrated nucleolus is the other most important finding in hyperthermia. Nucleolus is responsible for the assembly of ribosomes and other ribonucleoprotein complexes. An aggregation of these proteins occurs in the nucleolus following hyperthermia which, however, is dependent on the degree of heat shock. These morphological changes in nucleolus correlates well with inhibi-

tion of ribosomal RNA processing and ribosome biogenesis following hyperthermia (Ellgaard and Clever, 1971).

Hyperthermia exerts a most pronounced effect on the cell cytoskeleton known as intermediate filaments. These intermediate filaments are distributed in the cell as a fine meshwork throughout the cytoplasm and extend toward the cell periphery. After heat treatment, these intermediate filaments quickly redistribute and form a tight 'cage' around the nucleus followed by a redistribution of mitochondria and polysomes around the cell nucleus (Thomas et al., 1982).

Electron microscopic observations following heat shock revealed swollen mitochondria. Their individual cristae appear quite prominent and the intracristal space is much expanded (Welch and Suhan, 1985). These alterations in mitochondria represent inhibition of mitochondrial function and probably reflect a lower level of ATP in the cells after stress (Findly et al., 1983).

Apart from changes in the nucleus, nucleolus and mitochondria, heat shock also affects the morphology of protein secretory machinery of the cells, and particularly the Golgi complex. Thus Golgi complex which is a well organised collection of membrane stacks in normal unstressed cells appears disintegrated and fragmented after heat shock treatment (Welch and Suhan, 1985). The biological significance of these phenomena is not at all clear and no attempts has been made to decipher the probable mechanisms of such intracellular events following hyperthermia.

Interestingly, all these morphological abnormalities are reversible if the heat treatment is not severe enough. However it is not yet clear whether induction of HSP is related with the recovery process or with the damage of the intracellular machinery.

HSP and other related families of stress proteins

In the last 35 years, many individual stress proteins and their corresponding genes in various organisms have been isolated and characterised. It was found that members of bacterial HSP exhibits 50% sequence identity with humans indicating that HSP is very well conserved throughout evolution (Craig, 1985).

Depending on the origin of induction, the stress proteins are often divided into HSP and glucose-regulated proteins (GRP). The HSP are often referred to proteins whose synthesis is increased following subjection of cells to heat shock and is found in different masses of 8, 28, 58, 72, 73, 90 and 110 kDa (Lindquist, 1986). On the other hand, GRP is referred to those proteins which were first found in cells starved of glucose and found in masses of 78, 94 and 110 kDa. It was found later that GRP is also upregulated following various other kinds of insults to cells such as alterations in calcium homeostasis, protein synthesis, or hypoxia (Welch, 1992).

As mentioned above, most of the HSPs are constitutively expressed in normal cells except HSP 72 which is expressed in cells solely after stress. Moreover, in some cell types depending on the stressors, a co-ordinated increase in the synthesis of both HSP and GRP is observed. It is interesting to note that both these families of stress proteins are structurally and functionally related (Lindquist, 1986; Welch, 1992).

HSP 8 kDa (Ubiquitin)

Increased synthesis of about 8-kDa protein occurs following heat shock treatment of chicken embryo fibroblasts or yeast. The cDNA encoding of this small polypeptide is identical to ubiquitin (Bond and Schlesinger, 1986). Ubiquitin is a highly conserved protein and plays an important role in chromatin structure and protein degradation. It appears that increased ubiquitin synthesis facilitates removal of denatured proteins.

HSP 28 kDa (α-crystalline)

In mammalian and avian cells, the low molecular mass of HSP 25–30 kDa is often identified as HSP 27 (Ciocca et al., 1993). However, some laboratories still prefer to call it HSP 24 or HSP 28 (Welch, 1992; Marcuccilli and Miller, 1994).

This protein is expressed at a very low level in normal cells but after heat stress, a 10- to 20-fold increase in its synthesis is observed. This low molecular mass of HSP exhibits sequence homology with α-crystallines (Arrigo et al., 1988).

Immunofluorescence studies revealed that most of the HSP 27 is present in the cytoplasm in close proximity with the Golgi complex which is redistributed into the cell nucleus following heat shock and slowly returns to the cytoplasm after recovery from thermal stress (Ciocca et al., 1993). It appears that this increase in the synthesis of HSP 27 is important for cells to survive following heat shock. This is evident from the fact that normal cells when transfected with their corresponding cDNA resulting in expression of high levels of HSP 27, exhibit higher thermotolerance compared to non-transfected cells (Landry et al., 1989).

HSP 27 is also related to the growth and secretory function of the cells and can be influenced by steroid receptors and calcium ionophores (Welch, 1992; Ciocca et al., 1993). Recently, this protein was found to have a very close homology with the heme oxygenase, an enzyme responsible for production of carbon monoxide (for details see Sharma, Alm and Westman in this volume). However further studies are needed to find out the detailed biological function of HSP 27 in health and disease.

HSP 60 kDa (molecular chaperons)

HSP 60 (also characterised as HSP 58) in mammalian cells is encoded by nuclear genes and synthesised in the cell cytoplasm and then finally transported into the mitochondria. The possible function of HSP 60 is to help the newly synthesised proteins to be correctly folded and assembled into their final mature structure (Ellis and Van der Vies, 1991). Due to this property of HSP 60 in facilitating proper assembly and protein folding the HSP 60 family is referred to as 'molecular chaperons' (Ellis and Van der Vies, 1991). Some evidence suggests that mitochondrial HSP 70 is a co-factor in this mechanism, however further studies are needed to confirm this finding (Mizzen et al., 1991).

HSP 70 kDa and related proteins

This family of HSP is one of the most widely studied proteins in the CNS of many species. The HSP 70 family and related proteins are constitutively expressed in the normal cell whereas, some members are of strictly inducible type (Craig, 1985; Welch, 1992). The HSP 70 is bound to nucleotides particularly ADP and ATP and is present in many other intracellular compartments (Welch, 1992). The two isoforms of HSP 70 found in both cytoplasm and nucleus are also known as HSP 73 and HSP 72, respectively. The HSP 73 is synthesised constitutively in all mammalian cells and is referred to as HSP 70 cognate which is nowadays called HSC 70 as mentioned above. On the other hand, the synthesis of HSP 72 is solely restricted to the cells subjected to stress. Therefore, HSP 72 is known as the inducible form of HSP 70. Interestingly, these two proteins exhibit more than 95% sequence homology and share similar biochemical properties (Lindquist, 1986; Welch, 1992).

The first biochemical role of HSP 70 came to light due to the fact that the HSP 70 family of proteins is present within the endoplasmic reticulum which is identical to GRP 78, previously known as binding protein (BiP). BiP interacts with the newly synthesised heavy and light chain immunoglobulins within the lumen of endoplasmic reticulum (Bole et al., 1986). These secretory proteins interact with BiP transiently before their final assembly, whereas structurally altered or mutant proteins form a relatively stable complex with BiP within the lumen of the endoplasmic reticulum. This suggests that BiP monitors the proper assembly of secretory proteins and functions like a quality control system within the endoplasmic reticulum (Welch, 1992).

The cytosolic forms of HSP 70 (HSP 72 and HSP 73) are also involved in protein maturation because HSP 70 directly interacts with the newly synthesised proteins for the post-translational translocation from the cytosol into the endoplasmic reticulum. These observations suggest that the HSP 70 family has a widespread interaction with the newly synthesised proteins which is necessary for cell function.

Most of the research in the field is confined to HSP 72 protein which is one of the best known inducible isoforms of the HSP 70 family. Bardwell and Craig (1984) first isolated the gene encoding HSP 70 in *Drosophila* which is about 50% homologous to the *Escherichia coli* 70-kDa HSP known as danK (Bardwell and Craig, 1984). Mutations in this gene result in the inability of the mutant bacteria to grow at high ambient temperatures and exhibit marked alterations in cell metabolism, impaired DNA and RNA synthesis and disturbances in cell division (Georgopoulos et al., 1990). These observations show that HSP 70 plays an important role in the function of eukaryotic cells.

A third major form of HSP 70 is referred as the glucose-regulated protein 78 (GRP 78) also known as BiP. This protein resides in the lumen of the endoplasmic reticulum. A fourth form of HSP 70 was suggested by Welch (1992) as GRP 75 which is often found in mitochondria and chloroplasts. However the mammalian genes encoding GRP 75 have not yet been identified.

HSP 90 kDa (GRP 94) family

HSP 90 is one of the most abundant proteins in mammalian cells, the synthesis of which increases profoundly after stress. This family of HSP appears in multiple isoforms however, two genes encoding this protein have been identified as α- and β-subtypes (Welch, 1992). The function of HSP 90 is not well known; however it appears that this protein interacts with various cellular proteins and the steroid receptor family. The steroid receptor family which consists of progesterone, testosterone and glucocorticoid are present in the cell in an inactive form complexed with many other cellular proteins. These steroid receptor proteins are in close contact with HSP 90 and also HSP 70; however, the binding of HSP

70 with steroid receptor complex is still uncertain (Catelli et al., 1985).

When steroid hormone enters into the cell it binds to its receptor and activates its target genes to induce transcription. There are reasons to believe that HSP 90 binds to the steroid receptor in the absence of the hormone in order to prevent its interaction with DNA (Welch, 1992). Alternatively, HSP 90 binds directly with the DNA binding domain of the receptor (Pratt et al., 1989). There is some evidence that HSP 90 is associated with the phosphorylation of heme-regulated eukaryotic initiation factor (EIF) $2a$ kinase, a protein which is activated by a brief but severe exposure of cells to heat stress, and inhibits short-term protein synthesis (Welch, 1992). However, additional studies are needed to establish this interaction.

GRP 94

GRP 94 exhibits marked sequence homology with HSP 90 (Mazzarella and Green, 1987). However, HSP 90 is mainly a cytosolic protein, whereas the GRP 94 resides primarily within the endoplasmic reticulum and on the plasma membrane (Lewis et al., 1985). This protein exhibits calcium binding properties very similar to that of HSP 90. It seems quite likely that this protein plays an important role in cell secretion because GRP 94 is highly abundant in cells with secretory activity (Booth and Koch, 1989).

HSP 110 kDa

This family of HSP 110 protein was first described by Subjeck et al. (1983). However its structure and function is still unknown. The HSP 110 is constitutively expressed in mammalian cells and located within the cytoplasm, nucleus and nucleolus. The HSP 110 levels are increased in the nucleolus in the region of ribosomal RNA transcription after heat stress (Subjeck et al., 1983). In yeast, the mammalian HSP 110 is homologous to HSP 104 which seems to be involved in thermal tolerance. This is apparent from the fact that HSP 104 mutated genes are unable to survive with the second heat shock treatment (Subjeck et al., 1983; Welch, 1992). However, further studies are needed to understand the involvement of HSP 110 in thermal tolerance.

HSP and cellular stress

In spite of voluminous literature in the field of HSP and cellular stress, the mechanisms and functional significance behind its upregulation in the CNS in stressful situations are still speculative (Welch, 1992; Sharma et al., 1992a, 1995; Sharma and Westman, 1997). There is evidence that many stressors like elevated temperature, amino acid analogues and heavy metals are known protein denaturants. Thus it seems likely that increased expression of various HSPs which are linked with proteins are essential for cells to cope with the adverse situation. It is also likely that the cells responding to severe stress by expressing upregulation of HSP serve as a marker of cellular stress only. At the moment, we have no further experimental evidence either to support or reject any one of the above hypothesis.

HSP and immune response

There is strong evidence which suggests that HSP response is related to various aspects of immune response (Kaufmann, 1991). Fever is one example in which enhanced activity of endogenous pyrogens such as interleukins, tumor necrosis factors and interferons occur and is quite similar to that of elevated temperatures (Polla, 1988). Thus in both febrile response and elevated temperatures, enhanced white blood cell function is seen. There are some suggestions that the enhanced activity of white blood cells in fever and hyperthermia is related to the activation of cellular HSP expression. It may be that various lymphokines can influence the expression and/or phosphorylation of several HSP in different white blood cells (Peluso et al., 1978). However, apart from its role in facilitating protein maturation, whether HSP directly influences the immune reaction is still unclear.

Available evidence shows that the HSP 70 family is involved in some aspect of class II histocompatibility-mediated antigen presentation (Van Buskirk et al., 1989). This indicates that one or more genes encoding HSP 70-related proteins are present within the major histocompatibility locus (Gunther, 1991).

The other interesting aspect of HSP is their role as targets for the immune response following bacterial, viral or parasitic infections. Thus after invasion into the warm blooded host, these microbes express enhanced HSP activity which represents the immunodominant targets for both T- and B-cell responses (Winfield and Jarjour, 1991). Some autoimmune diseases may arise due to the activation of T- and B-cells which are specific for foreign HSP but they can also recognise the closely related HSP of the host. Thus antibodies to self HSP have been found in various autoimmune disorders like rheumatoid arthritis, systemic lupus, ankylosing spondylitis, Reiter's syndrome and Crohn's diseases (Winfield and Jarjour, 1991). However, it remains to be determined whether these autoantibodies are directly involved in the progression or persistence of such diseases.

Thus, it appears that HSP expression in cells can occur in a wide variety of conditions, but the functional significance of such response is not well understood. Further studies using pharmacotherapy and modification of the HSP response in a particular condition will throw some light on the possible significance of HSP expression.

HSP in hyperthermia

Upregulation of HSP in the CNS following systemic hyperthermia has not been well studied in the past. On the other hand expression of HSP in various cell lines, slices and cultures has been described. A few reports suggest that induction of HSP mRNA in the hippocampal pyramidal neurons occurs after heat shock at 42°C (Parude et al., 1992). In this case, glia of corpus callosum or CA-4 region of the hippocampus exhibited about a 20-fold higher level of HSP-70 than neurons of Ammon's horn (Parude et al., 1992). However, these findings are not consistent. Thus, other workers did not observe HSP 70 induction in hippocampal pyramidal neurons after heat shock (Sprang and Brown, 1987; McCabe and Simon, 1993). In contrast these authors reported a marked induction of HSP response in glial cells indicating that pyramidal neurons are less sensitive to heat than glial cells. This difference in ability to induce HSP in neurons versus glial cells has been suggested to be due to differences in the response of HSF in neurons compared to glial cells (Marcuccilli et al., 1996). However, the details are unclear and the subject appears controversial.

In other experiments, HSP 72 expression was found in rat brain including neurons, 24 h after whole body heating at 41.5°C for 15 min (Li et al., 1992). Similarly laser beam induced brain damage was associated with an increase in HSP 72 mRNA in the regions of intact microcirculation. The HSP 72 protein was localised in the perifocal zone of the lesion site 24 h after the insult. In these experiments, expression of c-*fos* mRNA and Fos protein of the proto-oncogene transcription factor occurred throughout the damaged hemisphere 2–3 h after the insult, (Linsberg et al., 1996).

Following hyperthermia in rabbits, although the constitutive expression of HSP 90 is high in cerebellum and cerebral hemispheres, increased expression of this protein in the brain stem was not detected (Manzerra and Brown, 1992a, 1992b; Manzerra et al., 1993). On the other hand, increased expression of HSP 70 was noted which showed a close parallelism with HSC 70 expression in these experiments.

These observations show that expression of HSP in the CNS following systemic hyperthermia is still not understood. Thus further research is highly warranted in order to understand the functional significance of HSP expression in the CNS in health and disease.

The concept of stress

Stress is originally defined as a non-specific re-

TABLE 3

A brief survey of alterations in gene expression during various kinds of stressors

Stressors	IEG type	Regional expression
Seizures (electrical/chemical)	c-fos, c-fos mRNA in nuclei of neurons, jun-B, zif 268, jun-D mRNA	Dentate gyrus pyriform, cingulate cortex, other cortical regions, hippocampus and limbic system
Kindling	Fos, Fos-B, c-jun, Jun-B, Jun-D, Krox-24, c-fos, c-jun	Amygdala, hippocampus
Focal brain injury and spreading depression	c-fos, c-fos mRNA, Fras, jun-B, c-jun, krox-24	Injured hempsphere, underlying subcortical regions
Spinal cord injury[a]	c-fos	Spinal sensory and motor neurons in the vicinity of lesion
Nerve transection	c-jun, jun-B, jun-D mRNA and protein	Axotomised neurons
Long-term potentiation and memory formation	c-fos mRNA, Fos-B, c-jun, jun-B, zif-268	Hippocampus, visual motor, olfactory cortex depending on training
Immobilisation	c-fos, c-jun, jun-B, jun-D, zif-268, fra-1	Paraventricular nucleus, amygdaloid nucleus
Handling, injection of saline, sensory stimulation (noxious, non-noxious, olfactory and visual)	c-fos, c-jun, zif-268, krox-24	PVN, amygdala, hippocampus, neocortex, spinal cord dorsal horn superficial layers I-III, thalamic region depending on the area involved
Sleep deprivation	fos protein/mRNA, NGFI-A mRNA, jun-B	Dorsal raphé, reticular formation, pontine region
Hypertension, stimulation of aortic depressor nerve, circulating angiotensin	fos protein, c-fos, NGF-1-A mRNA	area postrema, reticular formation, medullar, nucleus ambiguus, LC, supraoptic nucleus, inferior olive, hypothalamus, amygdala

IEG, immediate early genes; LC, locus coeruleus; NGF, nerve growth factor; PVN, paraventricular nucleus; Zif, zink finger.
Modified after Hughes and Dragunow (1995).
[a]Authors own investigation.

sponse of the organism following altered situation (Selye, 1976). However recent evidence suggests that various neuronal populations are selectively activated by different stressors (Hughes and Dragunow, 1995). Thus, c-fos, a marker of neuronal activation, and other immediate early genes are upregulated in specific brain regions following immobilisation, running and other kinds of stressors (Table 3). In most of these cases, HSP response is also activated as discussed above (Sharma et al., 1992a, 1995; Welch, 1992). Thus it appears that stressors can induce expression of immediate early genes in specific brain regions and this selectivity may be related to HSP induction.

Problems of heat stress

Heat is one of the best known stressors to mankind. The problems of heat stress and heat stroke is known since Biblical times (Judith 8: 2–3). Heat injury is the most severe illness caused by high ambient temperature to the human population and is the third largest killer in the World after cardiovascular and traumatic injuries to the CNS (Ellis, 1972; Sminia et al., 1994). However studies regarding the effects of heat on the CNS have been largely ignored in the past. The possible mechanisms behind brain damage caused by heat exposure are still poorly understood (Sharma, 1982; Sharma and Dey, 1986, 1987; Sharma and Cervós-Navarro, 1990a–c; Sharma et al., 1991a–c, 1992a–c, 1994, 1996a, 1997a–c; Sharma, Westman and Nyberg, this volume). Thus efforts should be made to understand the molecular mechanisms of brain damage following heat exposure in order to develop suitable therapeutic strategies.

Our investigation on HSP expression in the CNS following systemic hyperthermia

In the following section we describe HSP expression in the CNS following systemic hyperthermia using our rat model. In addition an attempt has been made to understand the functional significance of HSP reaction in the CNS with regard to cell injury using a pharmacological approach.

Pathophysiology of the HSP response and cell injury

The cellular HSP response in the CNS is of great pathophysiological importance (Sharma et al., 1992a; Marcuccilli and Miller, 1994; Sharma et al., 1995; Sharma and Westman, 1997). This is because of the fact that induction of HSP response occurs in both neural and non-neural cells in a large variety of brain pathologies such as ischemia, epileptic seizures, trauma neuroblastoma, multiple sclerosis or following administration of cocaine, L-glutamine or kainic acid (Fornace et al., 1989; Blake et al., 1990, 1994; Kaneko et al., 1993; Liu et al., 1993; Schreiber et al., 1993; Udelsman et al., 1993, 1994; Wang et al., 1993; D'Souza et al., 1994; Gao et al., 1994; Katayama et al., 1994; Kato et al., 1994; LeJohn et al., 1994). This HSP response may represent cell reaction in different pathological conditions (Sloviter and

Lowenstein, 1992; Welch, 1992; Tanon et al., 1993) or could be a result of some kind of defence mechanism of the traumatised cells (Lindquist, 1986; Kaufmann, 1992; Kumar, 1992; Suga and Nowak, 1992; Welch, 1992; Kato et al., 1993). It is still not certain whether the induction of HSP response is neuroprotective because in severe ischemia, some neurons are lethally injured without any preceding evidence of HSP-70 induction (Liu et al., 1993; Kato et al., 1994). Thus the pathophysiological significance of HSP response is still controversial.

Mechanisms of HSP induction in brain pathology

The mechanisms behind the induction of HSP response in brain pathology are not well understood. Previously, it has been shown that the HSP response can be induced in virtually all cell types in response to various stressors, chemicals, neurotransmitters and hormones or growth factors (Table 1) (Welch, 1992; Ciocca et al., 1993). Thus, ACTH and catecholamines have the capacity to induce the HSP response in adrenal glands and in aorta of rats (Blake et al., 1990, 1991, 1993, 1994; Udelsman et al., 1993, 1994). These chemicals are capable of inducing the stress response probably by influencing the signal transduction mechanisms via protein kinase C and calcium (Morimoto et al., 1992; Welch, 1992).

Since the signal transduction can be mediated by various neurochemicals via protein kinase C and ion channels (Brown et al., 1989; Blake et al., 1994), it appears that other neurochemicals may be involved in this response as well. One way of increasing the knowledge about the induction of HSP response in brain pathology is to use various pharmacological agents which have the capacity to influence neurochemical metabolism, edema and cell injury or the stress response itself.

HSP response in the CNS following heat stress

We undertook a series of investigations to expand our knowledge regarding induction of HSP response in the CNS following systemic heat stress. To that end, we exposed rats to 4 h heat stress at

38°C and examined the upregulation of HSP 72 kDa, the inducible isoform of the HSP 70 family. We employed an immunohistochemical approach to investigate the expression of the HSP (72 kDa) using light microscopy in various regions of the brain and spinal cord (Table 4) in heat stress (Sharma et al., 1992a). Electron microscopy was used to define the subcellular localisation of HSP immunoreactivity seen by light microscopy.

It appears that heat stress induces a cascade of

TABLE 4

Upregulation of HSP 72 (kDa) in the CNS of heat stress

CNS region	Control (n = 5)	Heat stress conscious (n = 6)	Heat stress anaesthetised (n = 4)
Cerebral cortex			
Cingulate anterior	−	+ + +	−
Cingulate posterior	−	+ + +	−
Frontal	− / + ?	+	− / + ?
Parietal	−	+ + +	−
Occipital	−	+ + +	− / + ?
Temporal	− / +	+ + +	−
Pyriform	−	+ +	− / +
Cerebellum			
Vermis	−	+ + +	−
Cortex	− / +	+ + +	− / + ?
Hippocampus			
CA1	−	+	−
CA2	−	+ +	−
CA3	− / + ?	+ +	− / +
CA4	−	+ + +	+
Dentate gyrus	−	+ +	− / +
Hilus	−	+ +	−
Caudate nucleus	−	+ +	−
Amygdala	−	+ + +	+
Colliculus			
Colliculi superior	−	+ +	−
Colliculi inferior	−	+ + +	− / +
Thalamus			
Massa internedia	−	+ + +	+
Dorsal thalamic nuclei	− / +	+ +	−
Ventral thalamic nuclei	−	+ + +	−
Lateral thalamic nuclei	−	+ + +	− / +
Hypothalamus			
Preoptic anterior	−	+ +	+
Posterior hypothalamic nuclei	−	+ + +	+
Brain stem	− / +	+ + +	− / +
Reticular formation	−	+ + +	− / + ?
Medulla	−	+ + +	−
Pons	−	+ + +	− / + ?

(Continued)

TABLE 4 (*Continued*)

CNS region	Control (n = 5)	Heat stress conscious (n = 6)	Heat stress anaesthetised (n = 4)
Spinal cord			
Dorsal horn	−	+ +	− / +
Ventral horn	−	+ + +	−
Lateral horn	−	+ + +	−
White matter	−	+	−
Central canal	−	+ +	− / +

Rats were subjected to 4 h heat stress at 38°C in a biological oxygen demand incubator (n = 6). A separate group of rats (n = 4) were given urethane (1.5 g/kg, i.p.) and then subjected to 4 h heat stress. Rats kept at normal room temperature (21 ± 1°C) served as controls.

− = negative, + = mild, + + = moderate, + + + = profound immunostaining, ? = found in a few cases only. Evaluations were made by two independent observers in a blind fashion.

pathophysiological events leading to cell and tissue injury (Sharma et al., 1991a–c, 1992a–c, 1996a, 1997a–c). Neurons, glial cells and microvessels in the CNS are exposed to a wide range of adverse thermal sensations in their cellular and fluid microenvironment following systemic heat injury (Sharma and Cervós-Navarro, 1990a–c; Sharma et al., 1992a–c). Obviously, some of the cells cannot withstand these changes and will die as a result of secondary injuries. The cells located in different regions in the CNS following thermal injury are thus exposed to a number of stressful events, such as breakdown of the BBB permeability, vasogenic edema and microvascular flow disturbances (Sharma and Dey, 1986; 1987; Sharma and Cervós-Navarro, 1990a–c; Sharma et al., 1991a–c, 1992b; 1996a; 1997a–c). Thus it seems quite likely that cells and tissues that are sensitive to heat stress will respond with a rapid production of HSP that can be used as a marker of cell reaction or the degree of cell injury.

To test this hypothesis, we used tissue samples from various brain regions after heat stress and examined the state of HSP expression, BBB permeability, edema and cell changes. Furthermore, in order to find out a probable relationship between HSP expression and cell injury, we used a pharmacological approach (for details, see Table 5). Thus, in order to gain insight into the mecha-

nisms of HSP expression, we influenced the BBB permeability, edema and cell changes by drugs and compared the HSP expression in these stressed rats in identical brain samples. Our results are the first to show that breakdown of the BBB permeability and edema correlates well with the induction of HSP expression in the CNS in heat stress. Thus drugs which attenuated the BBB breakdown in heat stress also reduced the expression of HSP response. On the other hand drugs which failed to prevent the leakage of the BBB were unable to downregulate the HSP expression. These results strongly indicate a prominent role of BBB disruption, edema and cell injury in HSP induction, not reported earlier (see below).

Experimental protocol

The experiments were carried out on male Wistar rats weighing between 100 and 150 g housed at controlled room temperature (21 ± 1°C) with a 12 h light, 12 h dark schedule. Food and tap water were supplied *ad libitum* before the experiments.

Exposure to heat stress

Rats were exposed to heat in a biological oxygen demand (BOD) incubator maintained at 38°C for

TABLE 5

Pharmacological manipulations in heat stress and HSP 72 kDa expression in the CNS

Drugs	Dosage and route of administration	No. of injections, schedule	Source
p-Chlorophenylalanine	100 mg/kg/day, i.p.	3 days, 1 day before HS	Sigma, USA
Indomethacin	10 mg/kg, i.p.	1, 30 min before HS	Sigma, USA
Naloxone	10 mg/kg, i.p.	1, 30 min before HS	Sigma, USA
Nimodipine	2 μg/kg/min for 2 h	30 min before HS	Bayer, FRG
6-OHDA	75 μg in 10 μl saline	i.c.v. 15 days before	Sigma, USA
Urethane	1.5 g/kg, i.p.	1, 10 min before	Merck, FRG

The drugs were given as pretreatment and rats were subjected to a 4 h heat stress at 38°C in a biological oxygen demand incubator (for details see text). After heat exposure, animals were perfused *in situ* with formalin-based fixative and HSP upregulation was examined in various brain regions using standard immunohistochemical methods (Sharma et al., 1995). The drugs in powder form were dissolved in isotonic saline or artificial CSF and the pH was adjusted to 7.4 before administration. Dosage adjusted according to Sharma (1982); Sharma and Dey (1986, 1987).

4 h. The relative humidity of 45–50% and the wind velocity of 20–25 cm/s was kept constant (Sharma, 1982; Sharma and Dey, 1986, 1987; Sharma et al., 1991a–c, 1992b,c). This experimental procedure was approved by the ethical committee of Uppsala University, Uppsala, Sweden.

HSP immunostaining

The HSP-immunohistochemistry using antibodies directed against HSP-72 kDa (Amersham, UK) was used in the brain and spinal cord samples obtained from controls, and 4 h heat stressed rats (Table 4) with or without pretreatment with drugs (Table 5).

Perfusion and fixation

Immediately after heat exposure, the animals were anaesthetised with Equithesin (3 ml/kg, i.p.) and the chest was opened. The right auricle was cut rapidly and a 20-gauge butterfly cannula was inserted into the left ventricle of the heart. Animals were perfused with about 50 ml of a 0.1 M phosphate buffer (pH 7.4) at room temperature in order to wash out the remaining blood from the

microvessels. Immediately after washout, the animals were perfused with 100 ml of fixative containing 2.5% glutaraldehyde, 0.5% paraformaldehyde in 0.1 M sodium phosphate buffer (37°C, pH 7.4). Perfusion pressure was maintained throughout the procedure at 90 torr (Sharma et al., 1995). After perfusion, the animals were wrapped in an aluminium foil and kept overnight in a refrigerator at 4°C. On the next day, the various tissue samples from the brain and spinal cord were selected for HSP expression (Table 4).

Vibratome sectioning and incubation with HSP antiserum

The selected tissue pieces from various brain and spinal cord regions (Table 4) were dissected out and sectioned transversely (60 μm thick) on a Vibratome (Oxford Instruments, UK). The sections were then transferred to the primary antibody solution, consisting of a primary antibody (mouse anti-HSP antiserum, Amersham, UK) diluted 1:500 and normal swine serum diluted 1:30 in phosphate buffer saline (PBS) and incubated free floating under agitation for 36 h at room temperature. Following six 10 min rinses in phosphate buffer saline (PBS) and Tris–HCl (pH 7.6), the sections were transferred to the secondary antibody solution (swine anti mouse 1:30 in PBS) and incubated for 60 min at room temperature under agitation. Thereafter, the sections were incubated in the PAP complex solution (1:20 in PBS) under the same conditions, with intervening rinses in PBS.

Immunolabelling

Immunocomplexes were localised by incubating the sections for 6–7 min in a solution containing 75 mg of DAB and 30 μl of 30% H_2O_2/100 ml of Tris–HCl buffer. The reaction was terminated by transferring the sections to Tris–HCl buffer. The sections were washed in 0.15 M sodium cacodylate buffer and post-fixed for 20 min in 2% osmium tetraoxide (OsO_4) dissolved in cacodylate buffer. They were then dehydrated in a graded series of ethanol, embedded in epon between acetate foils and polymerised at 60°C for 48 h. To serve as controls, consecutive sections were incubated in parallel with those intended for HSP immunohistochemistry, the only difference in treatment being that the primary antiserum was omitted in the first incubation of the control sections. Sections obtained from control, 4 h heat stressed animals with or without drug treatment were processed in parallel (Sharma et al., 1995).

After embedding, the sections were examined in a light microscope for evaluation of the immunolabelling. For comparison, one section in each group was not osmicated in order to see the labelled neurons against a light background. The nonosmicated section was examined and photographed.

Electron microscopy

For ultrastructural investigation of labelled neurons, osmicated sections were used. The desired tissue sections were attached to an Epon block and parts of the sections containing labelled neurones were trimmed out. Ultrathin sections were cut using a diamond knife (LKB, Ultramicrotome, Sweden), collected on one hole grid and stained with uranyl acetate and lead citrate. Some of the sections were kept unstained. A Phillips 300 or Hitachi transmission electron microscope was used.

Since the penetration of the antibodies was limited, serial sections beginning from the surface of the Vibratome sections were followed in the electron microscope from a level of poor preservation and strong immunolabelling to a level at which the preservation was good and immunolabelling was still visible, although often fainter than in the ultrathin sections from the surface of the Vibratome sections. If the neurons had been cut so that the nucleolus was present within the limits of the Vibratome sections, the neuron was photographed in the nucleolar plane at a magnification of ×2800–4000 (Sharma et al., 1995).

Drug treatment

Animals were treated with either p-CPA, indomethacin, naloxone, nimodipine or 6-OHDA prior to heat stress according to the standard protocol (for details, see Table 6). All drug treatments except 6-OHDA were found to be neuroprotective in nature (Sharma and Cervós-Navarro, 1990a,c; Sharma et al., 1994, 1997) as described below.

Characteristics of the heat shock response

The CNS of rats subjected to heat stress showed profound cell injury, edema and breakdown of the BBB permeability (Sharma and Dey, 1986, 1987; Sharma and Cervós-Navarro, 1990a–c; Sharma et al., 1991a–c, 1992b,c, 1994, 1996a, 1997). The neuropil was greatly expanded and spongy in appearance (Sharma and Cervós-Navarro, 1990). The nerve cells had distorted cell bodies; some were slightly swollen and others had shrunk (Sharma et al., 1992b,c, 1994, 1997a–c). Pretreatment with the p-CPA (Sharma and Cervós-Navarro, 1990), indomethacin (Sharma et al., 1994), naloxone (Sharma et al., 1997b) and nimodipine (Sharma and Cervós-Navarro, 1990b) but not with 6-OHDA (Sharma, 1982; Sharma et

224

TABLE 6

Summary of drug treatments on HSP 72 kDa upregulation in the brain of 4 h heat stressed rats

Type of experiment	Upregulation of HSP in the CNS				
	Cerebral cortex	Hippocampus	Cerebellum	Thalamus	Hypothalamus
Control	−	−	−	−	− / + ?
4 h HS	+ + +	+ + +	+ + +	+ + +	+ + +
Urethane + HS	−	− / +	− / + ?	−	− / + ?
p-CPA + HS	− / +	+	+	− / +	−
Indomethacin + HS	−	+	−	+	+
Naloxone + HS	+	− / +	− / +	+	+
Nimodipine + HS	−	−	− / + ?	−	−
6-OHDA + HS	+ + +	+ + +	+ + +	+ + +	+ + +

− = negative, + = mild, + + = moderate, + + + = profound immunostaining, ? = found in few cases only. Evaluations were made by two independent observers in a blind fashion.

al., 1997a), markedly diminished the heat induced cell damage, edema and microvascular permeability disturbances. Thus, the nerve cell changes in drug treated heat stressed rats were much less pronounced than those seen in the untreated or 6-OHDA treated stressed rats.

A representative example of cell changes seen at light microscopy following 4 h heat stress in the occipital cortex and brain stem is shown in Fig. 1. Thus, many nerve cells are dark and distorted (Figs. 1a,c) and the neuropil looks spongy in appearance. On the other hand, pretreatment with p-CPA (Fig. 1b) or naloxone (Fig. 1c) significantly attenuated the nerve cell damage caused by heat exposure. Thus many nerve cells are normal in appearance and a distinct neuronal cytoplasm containing cell nucleus can easily be seen (Fig. 1). The neuropil is less edematous compared to the untreated stressed animal.

At electron microscopy, dark and distorted nerve cells with signs of membrane damage, edema, and vascular reactions are very common in many brain regions. One example of nerve cell damage in the occipital cortex and brain stem is shown in Figs. 2 and 3, respectively. In these brain regions, vascular reaction, as evident with partial or completely collapsed microvessels, perivascular edema, membrane disruption, vesicu-

lation of myelin, synaptic damage and abnormal cellular changes in the neuropil are quite prominent.

These cell changes were considerably reduced by pretreatment with p-CPA, indomethacin, naloxone and nimodipine (Sharma and Cervós-Navarro, 1990a,b; Sharma et al., 1994, 1997b). However, pretreatment with 6-OHDA did not reduce these cell changes in any parts of the brain after heat stress (Sharma, 1982; Sharma et al., 1997a).

HSP immunoreaction in heat stress

The CNS of normal rats did not show any evidence of HSP immunoreactivity (Fig. 4a and Fig. 5a; Table 4). However, after 4 h heat exposure, there was a marked increase in the immunostaining of HSP in neurons in several brain and spinal cord regions (Figs. 4b,c and Figs. 5b–h; Table 4). This immunolabelling of HSP was not seen in anaesthetised animals subjected to heat exposure (Fig. 6b; Table 4) indicating that stress associated with heat plays an important role in induction of the HSP response. These observations are in line with our hypothesis that passive heating alone is not responsible for cell damage in the CNS.

Neuroprotection

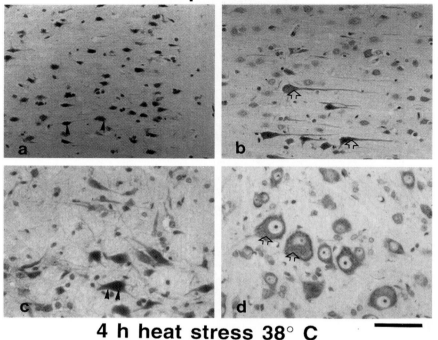

4 h heat stress 38° C

Fig. 1. Cell changes in the cingulate cortex (a) and brain stem (c) in 4 h heat stressed rats and their modification with p-CPA (b) and naloxone (d) pretreatment. In untreated rat, many dark and distorted nerve cells (arrow heads) can be seen. Pretreatment with drugs protected many nerve cells (blank arrows) after heat stress (bar a,b = 100 μm, c = 60 μm, d = 50 μm) (for details see text).

The HSP immunolabelling is seen in the nerve cells of various brain regions and in the spinal cord. A representative example of HSP immunostaining in the dorsal and ventral horn of the cervical spinal cord is shown in Fig. 7. It is interesting to note that marked upregulation of HSP can be seen in the spinal cord dorsal horn where the first central relay of thermoceptive pathways are situated. Immunostaining of HSP in the nerve cell nucleus and in the neuronal cytoplasm is quite frequent (Figs. 4b, 5b–h and 6a). In Epon-embedded vibratome sections, immunostaining of HSP as dark black reaction products in the nucleus is very common (Fig. 8a).

Ultrastructural investigation demonstrated dark reaction products of HSP in dendrites and cytoplasm of nerve cell bodies. One example of a few labelled dendrites from the dorsal horn of the spinal cord of one heat stressed animal is shown in Fig. 9. The immunolabelling seen as black dark particles is mainly attached to the surface of organelles including cytoskeleton and endoplasmic reticulum (Fig. 9).

This induction of HSP response in heat stress is no longer evident in rats pretreated with drugs which reduced the cell damage. Thus, upregulation of HSP following heat stress was not observed in rats pretreated with p-CPA (Fig. 6c), indomethacin, naloxone (results not shown) or nimodipine (Fig. 8b). On the other hand, pretreatment with 6-OHDA which did not reduce the cell changes, was unable to reduce the upregulation of HSP response after heat exposure (Fig. 6d). These observations strongly indicate that induction of HSP response is closely associated with the magnitude of cell injury.

nerve cell reaction and edema
occipital cerebral cortex

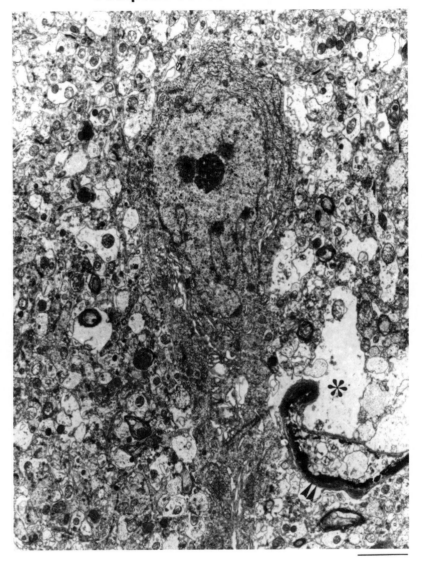

4 h heat stress 38° C

Fig. 2. Electron micrograph of one dark and distorted nerve cell in the occipital cortex of a 4 h heat stressed rat. The cytoplasm of the nerve cell is electron dense and dark in appearance. The nerve cell nucleus shows abnormally folded nuclear membrane and dense heterochromatin granules in the karyoplasm. One completely collapsed microvessel (arrow heads) alongwith signs of perivascular edema (*) can be seen. Other signs of membrane disruption and damage to neuropil are common (bar = 2 μm).

Brain stem

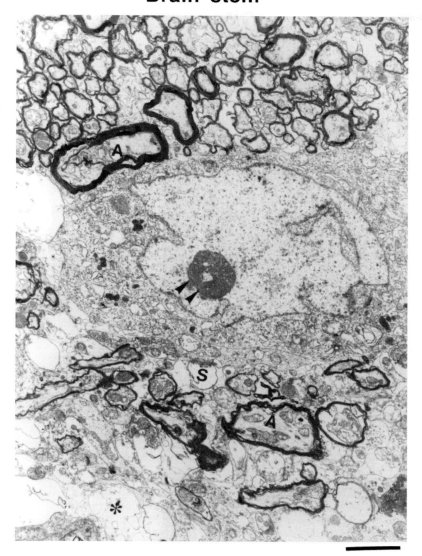

4 h heat stress 38° C

Fig. 3. Electron micrograph of one distorted nerve cell in the brain stem of a 4 h heat stressed rat. The cell nucleus shows abnormally folded nuclear membrane and an eccentric nucleolus (arrow heads). The cytoplasm contains many heterochromatin granules mainly concentrated around the nuclear membrane. Damage to many myelinated axons (A) and synapses (S) is clearly visible. Signs of edema (*) and membrane disruption are very common (bar = 2.5 μm).

Mechanisms of HSP response in heat stress

Our observations are the first to show that the immunoreactivity of HSP 72 kDa occurring in neurons following hyperthermic brain injury can be prevented by pretreatment of rats with drugs known to influence serotonin, prostaglandins and opioid neurotransmission, or by blocking the L-

228

HSP (72 kD) immunostaining

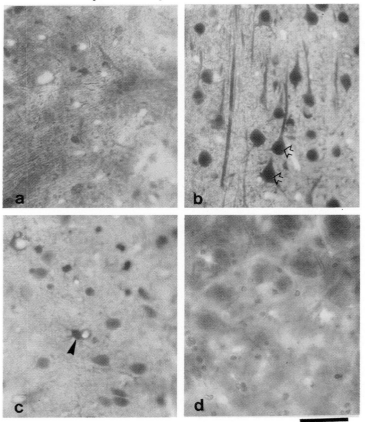

4 h heat stress 38° C

Fig. 4. A representative example of HSP 72 kD immunostaining in heat stress. (a) Positive control in the occipital cortex of one normal rat showing apparently no HSP immunostaining; (b) upregulation of HSP immunostaining in the occipital cortex of heat stressed rat can be seen in many nerve cells (blank arrows); (c) HSP positive nerve cells and one glia cell, probably astrocyte (arrow head) around one microvessel in the thalamus are visible; (d) negative control staining from the occipital cortex of one heat stressed rat. In this section, the primary antibody was omitted (bar = 80 μm).

type calcium channels, in the CNS. Interestingly, these drugs also significantly reduced the occurrence of cell injury, edema and the breakdown of the BBB permeability in heat stress (Sharma et al., 1997a–c). These results suggest that the cellular HSP response following thermal brain injury is reduced by drugs attenuating the secondary cell injury mechanisms in the CNS. These observations are in line with our hypothesis that reduc-

tion in cellular stress and/or injury will attenuate the HSP response (Sharma et al., 1992a, 1995; Sharma and Westman, 1997).

The HSP immunoreactivity was detected in neuronal cytoplasm attached to the surface of organelles including endoplasmic reticulum, in the nerve cell nucleus and in dendrites. To our knowledge, this study is the first to provide direct evidence of HSP immunoreactivity at the ultra-

HSP 72 kD immunostaining

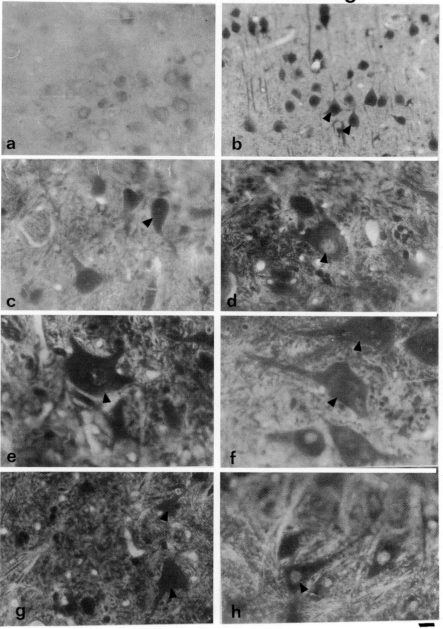

4 h heat stress 38 °C

Fig. 5. Upregulation of HSP in the CNS of a 4 h heat stressed rat. (a) Control, (b) anterior cingulate cortex, (c) cerebellar vermis, (d) thalamus, (e) medulla, (f) pons, (g) cervical spinal cord (C5), and (h) thoracic spinal cord (T4). Marked HSP immunostaining in nerve cells (arrows) is very common in many regions of the brain and spinal cord (bar a,b = 90 μm, c,d = 60 μm, e,f = 40 μm, g, h = 50 μm).

HSP 72 kD immunostaining
4 h heat stress 38 °C

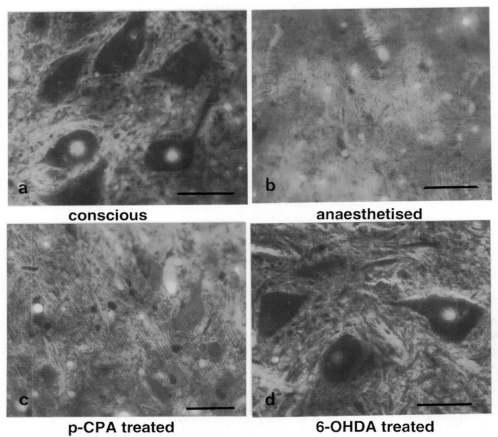

Fig. 6. HSP immunostaining in the spinal cord of 4 h heat stressed rats and its modification by anaesthesia and drugs. (a) Marked upregulation of HSP is seen in motoneurons of the rat spinal cord in the C5 segment. The immunostaining is clearly seen in the neuronal cytoplasm and in some cases within the nucleus; (b) subjection of urethane anaesthetised rats to similar heat stress did not result in the upregulation of HSP in the spinal cord; (c) depletion of serotonin synthesis by pretreatment with p-CPA prevented the HSP response in the conscious rats exposed to heat stress; (d) pretreatment with 6-OHDA, a catecholaminergic nerve toxin, did not prevent the induction of HSP response in motoneurons of the rat spinal cord after heat stress (for details see text; bar = 30 μm).

structural level in the CNS of hyperthermic rats confirming some recently reported biochemical studies suggesting HSP binding sites at membrane levels (Katayama et al., 1994; LeJohn et al., 1994; Sanchez et al., 1992). This immunolabelling was not evident in animals subjected to heat stress in drug pretreated rats. This indicates that the cells in these drug treated rats did not get

sufficient signals to induce upregulation of HSP response at the cellular level probably by modification of either the stress response itself or due to the altered neurochemistry of the nervous system before heat exposure.

The detailed mechanisms of induction of HSP response in the CNS following hyperthermic brain injury are unclear. However, it seems likely that

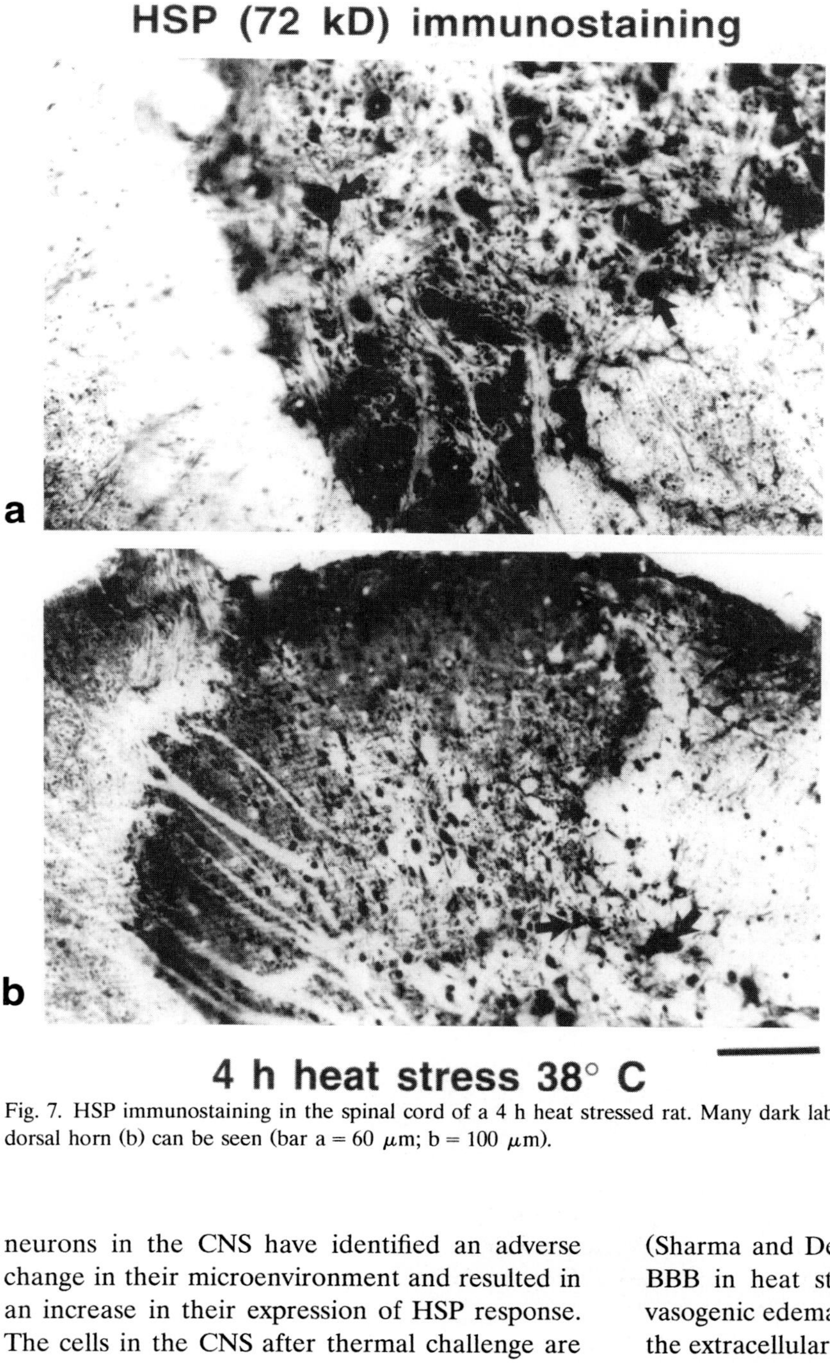

HSP (72 kD) immunostaining

4 h heat stress 38° C

Fig. 7. HSP immunostaining in the spinal cord of a 4 h heat stressed rat. Many dark labelled neurons in the ventral horn (a) and dorsal horn (b) can be seen (bar a = 60 μm; b = 100 μm).

neurons in the CNS have identified an adverse change in their microenvironment and resulted in an increase in their expression of HSP response. The cells in the CNS after thermal challenge are exposed to marked changes in their fluid microenvironment as evident from a breakdown of the BBB permeability in many brain regions (Sharma and Dey, 1986, 1987). Disruption of the BBB in heat stress is instrumental in inducing vasogenic edema and will alter the composition of the extracellular fluid micro-environment (Sharma and Cervós-Navarro, 1990a–c; Sharma et al., 1991a–c, 1992b,c, 1994, 1996a, 1997a–c). Furthermore, numerous compounds from damaged cells

232

will be added to the edema fluid (Sharma et al., 1995). As a result the ionic, chemical, immunologic and physiological microenvironment of nerve cells are markedly perturbed (Sharma et al., 1996a,b). This will result in disturbances in the regulatory functions of the nerve cells and will

lead to an abnormal increase in their HSP expression.

It may be that edema by itself or a component of the edema fluid trigger the cellular stress response (Sharma et al., 1995). This idea is in line with recent observations that various humoral

HSP (72 kD) immunostaining

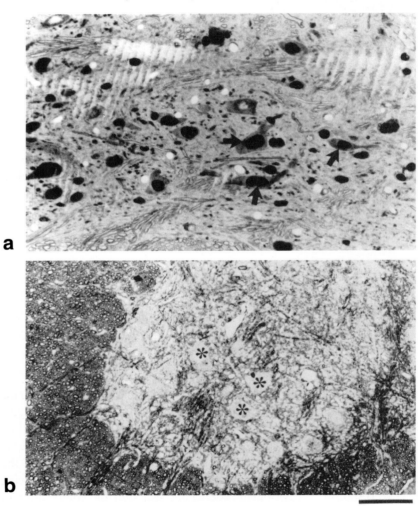

4 h heat stress 38° C

Fig. 8. Epon-embedded semi-thick section (1 μm) from the spinal cord of one untreated 4 h heat stressed rat (a), and one nimodipine pretreated stressed rat (b). Many HSP labelled neurons (arrow) can be seen in the untreated heat stressed rat whereas virtually no immunolabelled neurons are present (*) in the nimodipine treated rat (bar = 50 μm).

HSP (72 kD) immunostaining

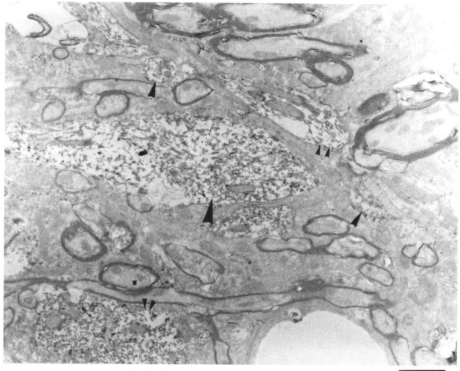

4 h heat stress 38° C

Fig. 9. Electron micrograph taken from the dorsal horn of the cervical spinal cord (C5) of a 4 h heat stressed rat showing HSP immunolabelling (arrow heads) at the ultrastructural level. HSP immunolabelling evident as black dark particles often attached to the endoplasmic reticulum in the dendrites of different diameters. This section is not contrasted with lead citrate or uranyl acetate (bar = 2.5 μm).

factors such as ACTH, catecholamines and cytokines have the capacity to induce HSP response in various neural or non-neural cells (Blake et al., 1994; D'Souza et al., 1994; Marcuccilli and Miller, 1994; Udelsman et al., 1994).

There are reasons to believe that various neurochemicals released after heat stress will influence the cellular machinery of the CNS to induce synthesis of protein kinase C and then act via opening of Ca^{2+} gated channels (Morimoto et al., 1992; Katayama et al., 1994; LeJohn et al., 1994; Marcuccilli and Miller, 1994; Udelsman et al., 1994). Our study further indicates that perhaps

serotonin, prostaglandins, and opioids may induce the HSP response probably via increasing the intracellular Ca^{2+} permeability through opening of calcium ion channels and stimulation of protein kinase C mechanisms (Ciocca et al., 1993; Blake et al., 1994; Marcuccilli et al., 1996; Sharma et al., 1997a; Sharma and Westman, 1997).

This is evident from the fact that pretreatment with serotonin synthesis inhibitor p-CPA, prostaglandin synthesis inhibitor, indomethacin or opioid receptor antagonist, naloxone prevented the induction of HSP response in the CNS of heat stressed animals. This observation clearly indicates that serotonin, prostaglandins and opioids are important in the pathophysiology of HSP response and cell injury in heat stress.

The possibility that these neurochemicals are capable of influencing signal transduction mechanisms through Ca^{2+} is in line with the results obtained using nimodipine, which is a potent inhibitor of Ca^{2+} channel (Sharma and Cervós-Navarro, 1990c). Since pretreatment with these drugs also prevented the BBB disruption and edema (Sharma et al., 1997a) it appears that alterations in fluid microenvironment of the CNS is an important factor responsible for induction of HSP expression.

We have shown previously that neurons of the CNS exhibit marked cell changes after heat stress (Sharma and Cervós-Navarro, 1990a–c; Sharma et al., 1991a–c, 1992b,c, 1994, 1997a–c). These nerve cell changes are present in regions with signs of edema and it is therefore on the basis of light and electron microscopy difficult to know if they represent true intravital changes or cellular artefacts in the edematous regions of the CNS. The present investigation confirms that the nerve cell changes in the CNS obviously represent true intravital stress phenomena since the HSP reaction is elicited. This concept is further strengthened by the fact that rats subjected to heat stress and pretreated with drugs exhibited a markedly reduced HSP response indicating a milder stress to these neurones. We believe that the neurons in the CNS must have been exposed to the same degree of thermal injury as in the group not given any drugs. Therefore, thermal injury in itself is not the inducer of the HSP response.

Serotonin, prostaglandins and opioids are thought to be the mediators of increased vascular permeability and formation of vasogenic edema. Thus, pretreatment with drugs modifying the metabolism of these neurochemicals will reduce the vascular permeability and edema in the CNS of heat stressed rats (Sharma et al., 1997a). The neurons in the CNS of these drug treated and heat stressed rats will therefore most probably be exposed to a milder change in their fluid microenvironment compared with the untreated heat stressed rats. This may be one of the most important reasons why the HSP response was so markedly reduced in the drug treated heat stressed rats. Alternatively, neurochemicals may have some direct inhibiting action on the HSP synthesis in the CNS.

Finally, microvascular flow reduction resulting in local ischemia may also be implicated in the production of the HSP response (Kawagoe et al., 1993; Liu et al., 1993; Kato et al., 1994). This is apparent from the fact that treatment of rats with drugs will reduce the ischemia caused by heat stress and other microvascular disturbances (Sharma and Cervós-Navarro, 1990a–c; Sharma et al., 1991a–c, 1992b,c, 1994, 1997a–c). However, this reduction in HSP response by drugs is not related to alterations in the hyperthermia, mean arterial blood pressure, blood gases or pH in heat stress (Table 7). This is evident from the fact that changes in these physiological variables following heat exposure were not significantly influenced by drug treatments (Table 7).

Conclusion

This study shows that HSP response is elicited in neurons in the CNS of rats subjected to 4 h heat stress. This HSP reaction does not occur if the rats are given a serotonin synthesis inhibitor, p-CPA; a prostaglandin synthesis inhibitor, indomethacin; an opioid receptor antagonist, naloxone; or a calcium channel blocker, nimodipine, before heat exposure. These drug treated rats subjected to a similar heat exposure exhibited less pronounced signs of BBB disruption, edema and cell changes in the regions exhibiting the HSP response. This indicates a milder stress to the cells after heat exposure in these drug treated rats. Thus, neurochemicals and calcium ions must somehow be involved in the process of inducing the HSP response in the CNS neurons in heat stress either by having some direct effect on cellular stress mechanisms or by its BBB disruption or edema inducing capacity.

TABLE 7

Mean arterial blood pressure and blood gases in rats subjected to heat stress and their modification with drugs

Type of experiment	n	Rectal T $\Delta°C$	MABP torr	P_aO_2 torr	P_aCO_2 torr	Arterial pH
Control	6	$+0.23 \pm 0.34$	108 ± 6	81.56 ± 0.23	33.58 ± 0.13	7.4 ± 0.04
HS 4 h	8	$+3.86 \pm 0.21**$	$75 \pm 3**$	82.48 ± 0.68	34.87 ± 0.33	7.3 ± 0.06
Urethane + HS	5	$+1.45 \pm 0.23^{a}**$	$90 \pm 6**$	81.67 ± 0.34	34.13 ± 0.11	7.4 ± 0.08
p-CPA + HS	6	$+3.18 \pm 0.18**$	$88 \pm 2**$	81.34 ± 0.44	33.87 ± 0.21	7.4 ± 0.02
Indomethacin + HS	5	$+3.04 \pm 0.21**$	$90 \pm 3**$	80.23 ± 0.32	32.34 ± 0.33	7.3 ± 0.05
Naloxone + HS	6	$+3.22 \pm 0.31**$	$89 \pm 4**$	81.43 ± 0.54	32.67 ± 0.56	7.3 ± 0.08
Nimodipine + HS	5	$+3.06 \pm 0.11**$	$82 \pm 6**$	81.01 ± 0.32	34.07 ± 0.23	7.4 ± 0.04
6-OHDA + HS	8	$+3.87 \pm 0.43**$	$76 \pm 4**$	82.45 ± 0.54	34.76 ± 0.32	7.3 ± 0.04

Values are mean $\pm$ standard deviation, Indom. = indomethacin, 6-OHDA = 6-hydroxydopamine, p-CPA = p-chlorophenylalanine,
[a] $P < 0.05$ compared to 4 h heat stress, ANOVA followed by Dunnett test.
** $P < 0.01$ compared to control.

Future direction

Further studies in our laboratory using other HSP families of 27 kDa, 60 kDa, 90 kDa and 110 kDa in the CNS of heat stressed rats are in progress to understand the possible significance of HSP expression in cell injury mechanisms. Expression of other molecular markers of cell injury such as c-*fos* and c-*jun*, growth factors and their receptors in relation to HSP upregulation and their modification with various pharmacological agents are needed for a better understanding of HSP induction in health and disease, which is currently under investigation in our laboratory.

Acknowledgements

Due to space limitations only key references are included. Financial support for this investigation was received from Swedish Medical Research Council project no. 2710; Göran Gustafsson Foundation, Stockholm, Sweden; Torsten and Ragner Söderberg Stiftelse, Sweden; Alexander von Humboldt Foundation, Bonn, Germany; The University Grants Commission, New Delhi, and The Indian Council of Medical Research, New Delhi, India. We are grateful to Kärstin Flink, Ingmarie Olsson, R. Esparza, Elisabeth Scherer, Franziska Drum, Katja Deparade, Hana Plückhan for technical assistance; Tord Löving for outstanding help in library work and Frank Bittkowski for photography. The secretarial assistance of Eva Lundberg, GunBritt Lind, Angela Ludwig, Katherin Kern, and Aruna Misra is highly appreciated.

References

Anathan, J., Goldberg, A.L. and Voellmy, R. (1986) Abnormal proteins serve as eukaryotic stress signals and trigger the activation of heat shock genes. Science Wash. DC, 232: 252–254.

Arrigo, A.P., Suhan, J.P. and Welch, W.J. (1988) Dynamic changes in the structure and intracellular locale of the mammalian low-molecular-weight heat shock protein. Mol. Cell. Biol., 8: 5059–5071.

Barbe, M.F., Tytell, M., Gower, D.J. and Welch, W.J. (1988) Hyperthermia protects against light damage in the rat retina. Science Wash. DC, 241: 1817–1820.

Bardwell, J.C. and Craig, E.A. (1984) Major heat shock gene of Drosophila and the heat inducible dnaK gene are homologous. Proc. Natl. Acad. Sci. USA, 81: 848–849.

Blake, M.J., Gershon, D., Fargnoli, J. and Holbrook, N.J. (1990) Discordant expression of heat shock protein mRNA

236

expression in tissues of heat-stressed rats. *J. Biol. Chem.,* 265: 15275–15279.

Blake, M.J., Udelsman, R., Feulner, G.J., Norton, D.D. and Holbrook, N.J. (1991) Stress-induced heat shock protein 70 expression in adrenal cortex: An adrenocorticotropic hormone sensitive, age-dependent response. *Proc. Natl. Acad. Sci. USA,* 88: 9873–9877.

Blake, M.J., Buckley, D.J. and Buckley, A.R. (1993) Dopaminergic regulation of heat shock protein-70 expression in adrenal gland and aorta. *Endocrinology,* 132: 1063–1070.

Blake, M.J., Buckley, A.R., Buckley, D.J., LaVoi, K.P., Bartlett T (1994) Neural and endocrine mechanisms of cocaine-induced 70-kD heat shock protein expression in aorta and adrenal gland. *J. Pharmacol. Exp. Ther.,* 268: 522–529.

Bole, D.G., Hendershot, L.M. and Kearney, J.F. (1986) Post-translational associations of immunoglobulin heavy chain binding protein with nascent heavy chains in non-secreting and secreting hybridomas. *J. Cell Biol.,* 102: 1558–1566.

Bond, U. and Schlesinger, M.J. (1986) Ubiquitin is a heat shock protein in chicken embryo firbroblasts. *Mol. Cell. Biol.,* 5: 949–956.

Booth, C. and Koch, G.L.E. (1989) Perturbation of cellular calcium induces secretion of luminal ER proteins. *Cell,* 59: 729–737.

Brown, I.R., Rish, S. and Ivy, G.O. (1989) Induction of a heat shock gene at the site of tissue injury in the rat brain. *Neuron,* 2: 1559–1564.

Catelli, M.G., Binart, N., Jong-Testas, I., Renoir, J.M., Baulieu, E. and Feramisco, J.R. (1985) The common 90 kD protein of '8S' steroid receptors is a heat shock protein. *EMBO J.,* 4: 3131–3137.

Ciocca, D.R., Oesterreich, S., Chamness, G.C., McGuire, W.L. and Fuqua, S.A.F (1993) Biological and clinical implications of heat shock protein 27000 (Hsp 27): a review. *J. Natl. Cancer Inst.,* 85: 1558–1570.

Craig, E.A. (1985) The heat shock response. *CRC Crit. Rev. Biochem.,* 18: 239–280.

D'Souza, S.D., Antel, J.P. and Freedman, M.S. (1994) Cytokine induction of heat shock protein expression in human oligodendrocytes: an interleukin-1-mediated mechanism. *J. Neuroimmunol.,* 50: 17–24.

Drummond, I.A., McClure, S.A., Poenie, M., Tsien, R.Y. and Steinhardt, R.A. (1986) Large changes in intracellular pH and calcium observed during heat shock are not responsible for the induction of heat shock proteins in Drosophila melanogaster. *Mol. Cell. Biol.,* 6: 1767–1775.

Ellgaard, E.G. and Clever, U. (1971) RNA metabolism during puff induction in *Drosophila melanogaster. Chromosome,* 36: 60–78.

Ellis, F.P. (1972) Mortality from heat illness and heat-aggravated illness in the United States. *Environ. Res.,* 5: 1–58.

Ellis, R.J. and Van der Vies, S.M. (1991) Molecular chaperones. *Annu. Rev. Biochem.,* 60: 321–347.

Fornace, A.J., Alamo, I., Hollander, M.C. and Lamoreaux, E.

(1989) Induction of heat shock protein transcripts and B2 transcripts by various stresses in chinese hamster cells. *Exp. Cell Res.,* 182: 61–74.

Findly, R.C., Gillies, R.J. and Shulman, R.G. (1983) *In vivo* phosphorous-31 nuclear magnetic resonance reveals lowered ATP during heat shock of tetrahymena. *Science Wash. DC,* 219: 1223–1225.

Gao, Y.L., Raine, C.S. and Brosnan, C.F. (1994) Humoral response to HSP 65 in multiple sclerosis and other neurologic conditions. *Neurology,* 44: 941–946.

Georgopoulos, C., Ang, D., Liberek, K., Zylicz M. (1990) Properties of the *Escherichia coli* heat shock proteins and their role in bacteriophage λ growth. In: R. Morimoto, A. Tissieres and C. Georgopoulos (Eds.), *Stress Proteins in Biology and Medicine,* Cold Spring Harbor, New York, pp. 191–222.

Goff, S.A., Goldberg, A.L. (1987) Production of abnormal proteins in *E. coli* stimulates transcription of ion and other heat shock genes. *Cell,* 41: 587–595.

Gonzalez, M.F., Shiraishi, K., Hisanga, K., Sagar, S.M., Mandabach, M. and Sharp, F.R. (1989) Heat shock proteins as markers of neural injury. *Mol. Brain Res.,* 6: 93–100.

Gower, D.J., Holiman, C., Lee, K.S. and Tytell, M. (1989) Spinal cord injury and the stress protein response. *J. Neurosurg.,* 70: 605–611.

Gunther, E. (1991) Heat shock genes and the major histocompatability complex. In: S.H.E. Kaufmann (Ed.), *Current Topics in Microbiology and Immunology,* Vol. 167, Springer, New York, pp. 57–70.

Hightower, L.E. (1980) Cultured animal cells exposed to amino acid anologues or puromycin rapidly synthesize several polypeptides. *J. Cell. Physiol.,* 102: 407–424.

Hughes, P. and Dragunow, M. (1995) Induction of immediate-early genes and the control of neurotransmitter-regulated gene expression within the nervous system. *Pharmacol. Rev.,* 47: 133–178.

Johnston, R.N. and Kucey, B.L. (1988) Competitive inhibition of hsp 70 gene expression causes thermosensitity. *Science,* 242: 1551–1554.

Jurivich, D.A., Sistonen, L., Kroes, R.A. and Morimoto, R.I. (1992) Effect of sodium salicylate on the human heat shock response. *Science,* 255: 1243–1245.

Kaneko, M., Abe, K. Kogure, K., Saito, H. and Matsuki, N. (1993) Correlation between electroconvulsive seizure and HSC 70 mRNA induction in mice brain. *Neurosci. Lett.,* 157: 195–198.

Katayama, S., Shuntoh, H., Matsuyama, S. and Tanaka, C. (1994) Effect of heat shock on intracellular calcium mobilization in neuroblastoma × glioma hybrid cells. *J. Neurochem.,* 62: 2292–2299.

Kato, S., Hiarno, A., Kato, M., Herz, F. and Ohama, E. (1993) Comparative study on the expression of stress-response protein (srp) 72, srp 27, αB-crystallin and ubiquitin in brain tumors. An immunohistochemical investigation. *Neuropathol. Appl. Neurobiol.,* 19: 436–442.

Kato, H., Liu, Y., Kogure, K. and Kato, K. (1994) Induction of 27-kDa heat shock protein following cerebral ischemia in a rat model of ischemic tolerance. *Brain Res.,* 634: 235–244.

Kawagoe, J.I, Abe, K., Aoki, M. and Kogure, K. (1993) Induction of HSP 90α heat shock mRNA after transient global ischemia in gerbil hippocampus. *Brain Res.,* 621: 121–125.

Kaufmann, S.H.E. (1991) Heat shock proteins and immune response. In: S.H.E. Kaufmann (Ed.), *Current Topics in Microbiology and Immunology,* Vol. 167, Springer, New York.

Kaufmann, S.H.E. (1992) Heat shock proteins in health and disease. *Int. J. Clin. Lab. Res.,* 21: 221–226.

Kelley, P.M. and Schlesinger, M.J. (1978) The effects of amino acid analogs and heat shock in gene expression in chicken embryo fibroblasts. *Cell,* 19: 1277–1286.

Kirino, T., Tsujita, Y. and Tamura, A. (1991) Induced tolerance to ischemia in gerbil hippocampal neurons. *J. Cereb. Blood Flow Metab.,* 11: 299–307.

Kitagawa, K., Matsumoto, M., Tagaya, M., Hata, R., Ueda, H., Niinobe, M., Handa, N., Fukunaga, R., Kimura, K., Mikoshiba, K. and Kamada, T. (1990) 'Ischemic tolerance' phenomenon found in the brain. *Brain Res.,* 528: 21–24.

Kumar, K. (1992) Heat schock proteins in brain ischemia: Role undefined as yet. *Metab. Brain Dis.,* 7: 115–123.

Landry, J., Chrétien, P., Lambert, H., Hickey, E. and Weber, L.A. (1989) Heat shock resistance conferred by expression of the human hsp 27 gene in rodent cells. *J. Cell Biol.,* 109: 7–15.

LeJohn, H.B., Cameron, L.E., Yang, B., MacBeath, G., Barker, D.S. and Williams, S.A. (1994) Cloning and analysis of a constituitive heat shock (cognate) protein 70 gene inducible by L-glutamine. *J. Biol. Chem.,* 269: 4513–4522.

Lewis, M.R., Mazzarella, R.A. and Green, M. (1985) Structure and assembly of the endoplasmic reticulum. *J. Biol. Chem.,* 260: 3050–3057.

Li, G.C., Li, L., Liu, R.Y., Rehman, M. and Lee, W.M.F. (1992) Heat shock protein hsp 70 protects cells from thermal stress even after deletion of its ATP-binding domain. *Proc. Natl. Acad. Sci. USA,* 89: 2036–2040.

Linsberg, P.J., Frerichs, K.U., Siren, A-L, Hallenbeck, J.M. and Nowak, T.S. Jr (1996) Heat-shock protein and c-*fos* expression in focal microvascular brain damage, *J. Cereb. Blood Flow Metab.,* 16: 82–91.

Liu, Y., Kato, H., Nakata, N. and Kogure, K. (1993) Temporal profile of heat shock protein 70 synthesis in ischemic tolerance induced by preconditioning ischemia in rat hippocampus. *Neuroscience,* 56: 921–927.

Lindquist, S. (1986) The heat-shock response. *Annu. Rev. Biochem.,* 55: 1151–1191.

Lindquist, S. and Craig, E.A. (1988) The heat-shock proteins. *Annu. Rev. Genet.,* 22: 631–677.

Lis, J. and Wu, C. (1993) Protein traffic on the heat shock promoter: parking, stalling, and trucking along. *Cell,* 74: 1–4.

Lowenstein, D.H., Simon, R.P. and Sharp, F.R. (1990) The pattern of 72 kDa heat shock protein-like immunoreactivity in the rat brain following flurothyl-induced status epilepticus. *Brain Res.,* 531: 173–182.

Lowenstein, D.H., Chan, P.H. and Miles, M.F. (1991) The stress protein response in cultured neurons: characterization and evidence for a protective role in excitotoxicity. *Neuron,* 7: 1053–1060.

Manzerra, P. and Brown, I.R. (1992a) Expression of heat shock genes (hsp 70) in rabbit spinal cord: localization of constitutive and hyperthermia inducible mRNA species. *J. Neurosci. Res.,* 31: 606–615.

Manzerra, P. and Brown, I.R. (1992b) Distribution of constitutive- and hyperthermia-inducible heat shock mRNA species (hsp 70) in the Purkinje layer of the rabbit cerebellum. *Neurochem. Res.,* 17: 559–564.

Manzerra, P., Rush, S.J. and Brown, I.R. (1993) Temporal and spatial distribution of heat shock mRNA and protein (hsp 70) in the rabbit cerebellum in response to hyperthermia. *J. Neurosci. Res.,* 36: 480–490.

Marcuccilli, C.J. and Miller, R.J. (1994) CNS stress response: too hot to handle. *Trends Neurosci.,* 17: 135–138.

Marcuccilli, C.J., Mathur, S.K., Morimoto, R.I. and Liller, R.J. (1996) Regulatory differences in the stress response of hippocampal neurons and glial cells after heat shock. *J. Neurosci.,* 16: 478–485.

Mazzarella, R.A. and Green, M. (1987) ERp 99, an abundant conserved glycoprotein of the endoplasmic reticulum is homologous to the 90 kDa heat shock protein (hs 90) and the glucose regulated protein (grp 94). *J. Biol. Chem.,* 262: 8875–8883.

McCabe, T. and Simon, R.P. (1993) Hyperthermia induces 72 kDa heat shock protein expression in rat brain in non-neural cells. *Neurosci. Lett.,* 159: 163–165.

Mizzen, L.A., Kabiling, A.N. and Welch, W.J. (1991) The two mammalian mitochondrial stress proteins, grp 75 and hsp 58, transiently interact with newly synthesized mitochondrial proteins. *Cell Regul.,* 2: 165–179.

Morimoto, R.I. (1993) Cells in stress: transcriptional activation of heat shock genes. *Science,* 259: 1409–1410.

Morimoto, R.I., Sarge, K.D. and Abravaya, K. (1992) Transcriptional regulation of heat shock genes. *J. Biol. Chem.,* 267: 21987–21990.

Nevins, J.R. (1982) Induction of the synthesis of a 70,000 dalton mammalian heat shock protein by the adenovirus EIA gene product. *Cell,* 29: 913–919.

Parude, S., Groshan, K., Raese, J.D. and Morrison-Bogorad, M. (1992) Hsp 70 mRNA induction is reduced in neurons of aged rat hippocampus after thermal stress. *Neurobiol. Aging,* 13: 661–672.

Pekkald, D., Heath, B. and Silver, J.C. (1984) Changes in chromatin and the phosphonylation of nuclear proteins during heat shock of *Achlya ambisexualis. Mol. Cell. Biol.,* 4: 1198–1205.

Peluso, R.W., Lamb, R.A. and Choppin, P.W. (1978) Infection with paramyxovirus stimulates synthesis of cellular polypeptides that are also stimulated in cells transformed by Rous

Sarcoma virus or deprived of glucose. *Proc. Natl. Acad. Sci. USA*, 75: 6120–6124.

Planas, A.M., Soriano, M.A., Ferrer, I. and Rodriguez, F.E. (1995) Kainic acid-induced heat shock protein-70 mRNA and protein expression is inhibited by MK-801 in certain rat brain regions. *Eur. J. Neurosci.*, 7: 293–304.

Polla, B.S. (1988) A role for heat shock proteins in inflammation? *Immunol. Today*, 9: 134–137.

Pratt, W.-B., Sanchez, Bresnick, E.H., Meshinchi, S., Scherrer, L.C., Dalman, F.C. and Welch, M.J. (1989) Interaction of the glucocorticoid receptor with the Mr 90,000 heat shock protein: an evolving model of ligand-mediated receptor transformation and translocation. *Cancer Res.*, 49 Suppl.: 2222s–2229s.

Riabowol, K., Mizzen, L.A. and Welch, W.J. (1988) Heat shock induced lethality in cells microinjected with antibodies specific for hsp 70. *Science Wash. DC*, 242: 433–436.

Rordorf, G., Koroshetz, W.J. and Bonventre, J.V. (1991) Heat shock protects cultured neurons from glutamate toxicity. *Neuron*, 7: 1043–1051.

Sanchez, Y., Taulien, J., Borkovich, K.A. and Lindquist, S. (1992) Hsp 104 is required for tolerance to many forms of stress. *EMBO J.*, 11: 2357–2364.

Sarge, K.D., Zimarino, V., Holm, K., Wu, C. and Morimoto, R.I. (1991) Cloning and characterisation of two mouse heat shock factors with distinct inducible and constitutive DNA-binding ability. *Genes Dev.*, 5: 1902–1011.

Sarge, K.D., Murphy, S.P. and Morimoto, R.I. (1993) Activation of heat shock gene transcription by heat shock factor 1 involves oligomerization, acquisition of DNA-binding activity, and nuclear localization and can occur in the absence of stress. *Mol. Cell. Biol.*, 13: 1392–1407.

Sarge, K.D., Park-Sarge, O.K., Kirby, J.D., Mayo, K.E. and Morimoto, R.I. (1994) Regulated expression of heat shock factor 2 in mouse testis: potential role as a regulator of *hsp* gene expression during spermatogenesis. *Biol. Reprod.*, 50: 1334–1343.

Schuetz, T.J., Gallo, G.J., Sheldon, L., Tempst, P. and Kingston, R.E. (1991) Isolation of a cDNA for HSF2: evidence for two heat shock factor genes in humans. *Proc. Natl. Acad. Sci. USA*, 88: 6911–6915.

Selye, H. (1976) *Stress in Health and Disease*, Butterworths, London.

Schreiber, S.S., Najm, I., Tocco, G. and Baudry, M. (1993) Co-expression of HSP 72 and c-*fos* in rat brain following kainic acid treatment. *Neuroreport*, 5: 269–272.

Sharma, H.S. (1982) *Blood-Brain Barrier in Stress*, Ph.D. thesis, Banaras Hindu University, Varanasi, India, pp. 1–85.

Sharma, H.S. and Cervós-Navarro, J. (1990a) Brain oedema and cellular changes induced by acute heat stress in young rats. *Acta Neurochir. (Wien)*, Suppl. 51: 383–386.

Sharma, H.S. and Cervós-Navarro, J. (1990b) Nimodipine improves cerebral blood flow and reduces brain edema, cellular damage and blood–brain barrier permeability following

heat stress in young rats. In: J. Krieglstein and H. Oberpichler (Eds.), *Pharmacology of Cerebral Ischemia*, 1990, CRC Press, Boca Raton, FL, pp. 303–310.

Sharma, H.S. and Cervós-Navarro, J. (1990c) Pathophysiology of blood–brain barrier in stress. *Clin. Neuropathol.*, 9: 111.

Sharma, H.S. and Dey, P.K. (1986) Probable involvement of 5-hydroxytryptamine in increased permeability of blood–brain barrier under heat stress. *Neuropharmacology*, 25: 161–167.

Sharma, H.S. and Dey, P.K. (1987) Influence of long-term acute heat exposure on regional blood–brain barrier permeability, cerebral blood flow and 5-HT level in conscious normotensive young rats. *Brain Res.*, 424: 153–162.

Sharma, H.S. and Westman, J. (1997) Prostaglandins modulate constitutive isoform of heat shock protein (72 kD) response following trauma to the rat spinal cord. *Acta Neurochir.*, Suppl. 71: 134–137.

Sharma, H.S., Zimmer, C. and Cervós-Navarro, J. (1991a) Neuropathological aspects of acute heat exposure in young rats. *Clin. Neuropathol.*, 10: 315.

Sharma, H.S., Cervós-Navarro, J. and Dey, P.K. (1991b) Acute heat exposure causes cellular alteration in cerebral cortex of young rats. *NeuroReport*, 2: 155–158.

Sharma, H.S., Cervós-Navarro, J. and Dey, P.K. (1991c) Rearing at high ambient temperature during later phase of the brain development enhances functional plasticity of the CNS and induces tolerance to heat stress. An experimental study in the conscious normotensive young rats. *Brain Dysfunct.*, 4: 104–124.

Sharma, H.S., Westman, J., Cervós-Navarro, J. and Gosztonyi, G. (1992a) Acute systemic heat exposure increases heat shock protein (HSP-70 kD) immunoreactivity in the brain and spinal cord of young rats. *Clin. Neuropathol.*, 11: 174–175.

Sharma, H.S., Zimmer, C., Westman, J. and Cervós-Navarro, J. (1992b) Acute systemic heat stress increases glial fibrillary acidic protein immunoreactivity in brain. An experimental study in the conscious normotensive young rats. *Neuroscience*, 48: 889–901.

Sharma, H.S., Kretzschmar, R., Cervós-Navarro, J., Ermisch, A., Rühle, H-J. and Dey, P.K. (1992c) Age-related pathophysiology of the blood-brain barrier in heat stress. *Prog. Brain Res.*, 189–196.

Sharma, H.S., Westman, J., Nyberg, F., Cervós-Navarro, J. and Dey, P.K. (1994) Role of serotonin and prostaglandins in brain edema induced by heat stress. An experimental study in the rat. *Acta Neurochir. (Wien)*, Suppl. 60: 65–70.

Sharma, H.S., Olsson, Y. and Westman, J. (1995) A serotonin synthesis inhibitor, p-chlorophenylalanine reduces heat shock protein response following trauma to the rat spinal cord. An immunohistochemical and ultrastructural study in the rat. *Neurosci. Res.*, 21: 241–249.

Sharma, H.S., Westman, J., Cervós-Navarro, J. and Nyberg, F. (1996a) A 5-HT$_2$ receptor mediated breakdown of the blood–brain barrier permeability and brain pathology in heat stress. An experimental study using cyproheptadine and ketanserin in young rats. In: P. Couraud and A. Scherman (Eds.), *Biology and Physiology of the Blood–Brain Barrier*, Plenum Press, New York, pp. 117–124.

Sharma, H.S., Westman, J., Cervós-Navarro, J., Dey, P.K. and Nyberg, F. (1996b) Probable involvement of serotonin in the increased permeability of the blood–brain barrier by forced swimming. An experimental study using Evans blue and ^{131}I-sodium tracers in the rat. *Behav. Brain Res.,* 72: 189–196.

Sharma, H.S., Westman, J., Cervós-Navarro, J., Dey, P.K. and Nyberg, F. (1997a) Blood–brain barrier in stress: a gateway to various brain diseases. In: R. de Kloet, D. Ben-Nathan and R. Levy (Eds.), *New Frontiers of Stress: Modulation of Brain Function*, Harwood, Amsterdam.

Sharma, H.S., Westman, J., Cervós-Navarro, J., Dey, P.K. and Nyberg, F. (1997b) Opioid receptor antagonists attenuate heat stress induced reduction in cerebral blood flow, increased blood–brain barrier permeability, vasogenic edema and cell changes in the rat. *Ann. New York Acad. Sci.,* 813: 559–571.

Sharma, H.S., Westman, J., Alm, P., Sjöquist, P.-Ö., Cervós-Navarro, J. and Nyberg, F. (1997c) Involvement of nitric oxide in the pathophysiology of acute heat stress in the rat. Influence of a new antioxidant compound 290/51. *Ann. New York Acad. Sci.*, 813: 581–590.

Sloviter, R.S. and Lowenstein, D.H. (1992) Heat shock protein expression in vulnerable cells of the rat hippocampus as an indicator of excitation-induced neuronal stress. *J. Neurosci.,* 12: 3004–3009.

Sminia, P., Van der Zee, J., Wondergem, J. and Haveman, J. (1994) Effect of hyperthermia on the central nervous system: a review. *Int. J. Hyperthermia*, 10: 1–30.

Sistone, L., Sarge, K.D. and Morimoto, R.I. (1994) Human heat shock factors 1 and 2 are diffrentially activated and can synergistically induce hsp 70 gene transcription. *Mol. Cell. Biol.,* 14: 2087–2099.

Sorger, P.K. (1991) Heat shock factor and heat shock response. *Cell,* 65: 363–366.

Sprang, G.K. and Brown, I.R. (1987) Selective induction of a heat shock gene in fibre tracts and cerebellar neurons of the rabbit brain detected by *in situ* hybridization. *Mol. Brain Res.,* 3: 89–93.

Stevenson, M.A., Calderwood, S.K. and Hahn, G.M. (1981) Rapid increases in inositol trisphosphate and intracellular Ca^{2+} after heat shock. *Biochem. Biophys. Res. Commun.,* 137: 826–833.

Subjeck, J.R., Shyy, T., Shen, J. and Johnsson, R.J. (1983) Association between mammalian 110,000 dalton heat shock proteins and nucleoli. *J. Cell. Biol.,* 97: 1389–1398.

Suga, S. and Nowak, T.S. (1992) Pharmacology of the postischemic stress response: effects of temperature on hsp 70 expression after transient ischemia and hypothermic action of NBQX in the gerbil. In: J. Krieglstein and H. Oberpichler-Schwenk (Eds.), *Pharmacology of Cerebral Ischemia,* 1992 edn. Wissenschaftliche, Stuttgart, pp. 279–286.

Tanon, H., Nockels, R.P., Pitts, L.H. and Noble, L.J. (1993) Immunolocalization of heat shock protein after fluid percussive brain injury and relationship to breakdown of the blood–brain barrier. *J. Cereb. Blood Flow Metab.,* 13: 116–124.

Thomas, G.P., Welch, W.J., Mathews, M.B. and Feramisco, J.R. (1982) Molecular and cellular effects of heat shock and related treatments of mammalian tissue culture cells. *Cold Spring Harbor Symp. Quant. Biol.,* 46: 985–996.

Udelsman, R., Blake, M.J., Stagg, C.A., Li, D., Putney, J. and Holbrook, N.J. (1993) Vascular heat shock protein expression in response to stress: Endocrine and autonomic regulation of the age-dependent response. *J. Clin. Invest.,* 91: 465–473.

Udelsman, R., Blake, M.J., Stagg, C.A. and Holbrook, N.J. (1994) Endocrine control of stress-induced heat shock protein 70 expression *in vivo. Surgery,* 115: 611–616.

Uney, J.B., Kew, J.N.C., Staley, K., Tyres, P. and Sofroniew, M.V. (1993) Transfection-mediated expression of human Hsp 70i protects rat dorsal root ganglion neurons and glia from severe heat stress. *FEBS Lett.,* 334: 313–316.

Van Buskirk, A., Crump, B.L., Margoliash, K. and Pierce, S.K. (1989) A peptide binding protein having a role in antigen presentation is a member of the hsp 70 heat shock family. *J. Exp. Med.,* 170: 1759–1809.

Vass, K., Welch, W.J. and Nowak, T.S. (1988) Localization of 70 kDa stress protein induction in gerbil brain after ischemia. *Acta Neuropathol.,* 77: 413–424.

Wang, S., Longo, F.M., Chen, J., Butman, M., Graham, S.H., Haglid, K.G. and Sharp, F.R. (1993) Induction of glucose regulated protein (grp 78) and inducible heat shock protein (hsp 70) mRNAs in rat brain after kainic acid seizures and focal ischemia. *Neurochem. Int.,* 23: 575–582.

Weitzel, G., Pilatus, G.U. and Rensing, L. (1985) Similar dose response of heat shock protein synthesis and intracellular pH changes in yeast. *Exp. Cell Res.,* 159: 252–256.

Welch, W.J. (1992) Mammalian stress response: cell physiology, structure/function of stress proteins, and implications for medicine and diseases. *Physiol. Rev,* 72: 1063–1081.

Welch, W.J. and Suhan, J.P. (1985) Morphological study of the mammalian stress response: characterization of changes in cytoplasmic organelles, cytoskeleton, and nucleoli and appearance of intranuclear actin filaments in rat fibroblasts after heat shock treatment. *J. Cell Biol.,* 101: 1198–1211.

Winfield, J.B. and Jarjour, W.N. (1991) Stress proteins, autoimmunity and autoimmune disease. In: S.H.E. Kaufmann (Ed.), *Current Topics in Microbiology and Immunology,* Vol. 167, Springer, New York, pp. 191–208.

H.S. Sharma and J. Westman (Eds.)
Progress in Brain Research, Vol 115
© 1998 Elsevier Science BV. All rights reserved.

CHAPTER 14

Glial reactions in the central nervous system following heat stress

Jorge Cervós-Navarro[1], Hari Shanker Sharma[1,2]*, Jan Westman[2],
Erik Bongcam-Rudloff[3]

[1]*Institute of Neuropathology, Free University Berlin, Klinikum Steglitz, Hindenburgdamm 30, D-12 203 Berlin, Germany*
[2]*Laboratory of Neuroanatomy, Department of Anatomy, Biomedical Centre, P.O. Box 571,
Uppsala University, S-751 23 Uppsala, Sweden*
[3]*Department of Cell Biology, The Wenner-Gren Institute, University of Stockholm, S-712 34 Stockholm, Sweden*

Introduction

In the central nervous system (CNS), most attention is usually paid to neurons in spite of the fact that nerve cells are outnumbered by their non-neural neighbours, the glial cells and the endothelial cells (Glees, 1955; Varon and Somjen, 1979; Orkand, 1983; Arenander and Vellis, 1984; Duffy, 1984; Fedoroff and Vernadakis, 1986; Barres, 1994; Kettenmann and Ransom, 1995). On the basis of light microscopy, the glial cells are classified as astrocytes, oligodendrocytes and microglia (Glees, 1955; Orkand, 1983; Duffy, 1984). Out of these, the astrocytes are one of the most widely studied glial cells in the CNS during health and disease using both *in vivo* and *in vitro* conditions (Bignami et al., 1980; Amaducci et al., 1981; Duffy, 1984; Eng, 1985; Fedoroff and Vernadakis, 1986; Althaus and Siefert, 1987; Eng et al., 1992; Brenner, 1994; Galea et al., 1995). Their name is derived from the characteristic star-like configurations formed by their well-developed processes

as seen in optical microscopy (Glees, 1955; Duffy, 1984; Fedoroff and Vernadakis, 1986). At the fine structural level, sheet-like expansions of the terminals of these cell processes which completely ensheath the blood vessels of the CNS are virtually in direct contact with the endothelial cells themselves (Ling and Leblond, 1973; Beck et al., 1986; Kimelberg and Ransom, 1986; Tao-Cheng and Brightman, 1988; Kettenmann and Ransom, 1995). Only the basal laminae intervenes within the narrow extracellular space that separates the endothelial cells from the astrocytic processes (Glees, 1955; Duffy, 1984; Fedoroff and Vernadakis, 1986).

Although normally quiescent, there is now abundant evidence indicating that the astrocytes are one of the most sensitive indicators of pathological brain injury (Bignami et al., 1980; Amaducci et al., 1981; Hertz, 1981; Arenander and Vellis, 1984; Barrett et al., 1984; Chiu and Goldmann, 1985; Bernstein and Goldberg, 1987; Isacson et al., 1987; Aquino et al., 1988; Cavicchioli et al., 1988; Goshgarian et al., 1989; Condorelli et al., 1990; Hozumi et al., 1990; Kimelberg and Kettenmann, 1990; Dusart et al., 1991; Eng et al., 1992; Sharma et al., 1992a; Ahlsen et al., 1993; Sharma et al., 1993; Eng and Ghirnikar, 1994;

---

* Corresponding author. Department of Anatomy, Laboratory of Neuroanatomy, Box 571, Biomedical Centre, Uppsala University, S-751 23 Uppsala, Sweden. Tel: +46 18 4714433; fax: +46 18 243899; e-mail: Sharma@anatomi.uu.se

Gomi et al., 1996). The astrocytes respond by dividing, swelling, extending cellular processes and change their morphological features resulting in an increased number of cytoplasmic organelles and filaments (Morrison et al., 1985; Kimelberg and Ransom, 1986; Mucke et al., 1991; Norton et al., 1992; Lu et al., 1993; Masood et al., 1993; McLendon and Bigner, 1994). These phenomena are collectively referred to as astrocytosis (Orkand, 1983; Arenander et al., 1988; Brenner, 1994a). Glial fibrillary acidic protein (GFAP) is a highly conserved intermediate filament protein found predominantly in astrocytes (Eng et al., 1971; Brenner, 1994a,b; Eng and Ghirnikar, 1994). It is also found in the peripheral nervous system (PNS) as well as non-neural tissues; however, it remains a specific marker for differentiated astrocytes in the CNS (Orkand, 1983; Duffy, 1984). It is the principal cytoskeletal protein in astrocytes and is thought to provide structural support for maintenance of cell shape (Glees, 1955; Duffy, 1984; Eng, 1985). The relatively slow metabolic turnover rate for GFAP is consistent with a possible structural role for glial filaments (Fedoroff and Vernadakis, 1986). Changes in the expression of GFAP by astrocytes is observed in the initial induction of GFAP expression during the development of immature neuroectodermal cells into astrocytes and during glial scar formation, a pathological process common to a large number of neurological disorders (Barrett et al., 1984; Chiu and Goldmann, 1985; Sharma et al., 1992a; Torres-Aleman et al., 1992; Morgan et al., 1993; Sharma et al., 1993; Brenner, 1994a,b). In many pathological conditions, increased GFAP immunoreactivity is usually associated with a breakdown of the BBB and vasogenic edema (Schmidt-Kastner et al., 1990; Eng et al., 1992; Sharma et al., 1992a,b,c, 1993). These observations suggest that breakdown of the BBB and edema could be one of the important endogenous signals for glial cell activation, a feature which requires additional investigation.

There is now enough experimental evidence that hyperthermia will cause brain injury and may lead to cellular damage via modification of the BBB through an altered chemical and metabolic fluid microenvironment (Sharma and Dey, 1986; Sharma and Cervós-Navarro, 1990a,b; for details see Sharma, Westman and Nyberg, in this volume). However, activation of glial cells following thermal brain injury is still poorly understood. Previously, our laboratory was the only one to demonstrate activation of GFAP following hyperthermic brain injury (Sharma et al., 1992a). To our knowledge, this is the first report which suggests that 4 h of thermal insult is sufficient to induce GFAP expression in the CNS. However, the detailed mechanisms and the functional significance of this finding are not well known.

This review focuses on glial reactions in the CNS following heat stress which is mainly based on our own investigations. In addition, recent developments in the molecular aspects of the GFAP function in health and diseases is also summarised. Finally, an attempt has been made to find out the possible role of the BBB breakdown as an endogenous signal responsible for GFAP expression in the CNS in our rat model using a pharmacological approach.

Glial cells are important constituents of brain function

In 1846, Rudolf Virchow observed a connective tissue in the brain which he named as neuroglia. At that time the function of neuroglia was not known. After about 150 years since this fundamental discovery, new research in the field suggests that the glial cells are one of the most important constituents of the CNS involved in many physiological as well as pathological reactions of the brain and spinal cord (Pfrieger and Barres, 1996). Thus, there is recent evidence that glial cells regulate the formation and function of synapses (Pfrieger and Barres, 1996), provide structural and trophic support, regulate neurotransmitter metabolism and are involved in information processing of the nervous system (see below).

The growing trend of recent literature suggests that the glial cells, particularly astrocytes play an important role in the maintenance of normal BBB function and the fluid microenvironment of the brain (Beck et al., 1986; Tao-Cheng and Brightman, 1988). Astrocytes were previously considered as static constructional elements of the brain. However, in the last few years a physiological role for astrocytes in ion regulation, neurotransmitter metabolism and production of neurotrophic factors has been established (Miller et al., 1986; Murphy and Pearce, 1987; Arenander et al., 1988; McMillan et al., 1994; Pfrieger and Barres, 1996). The astrocytes, thus situated in and around neurons and maintaining a close contact with the vasculature via their end-feet are implicated in neuronal guidance, induction of the BBB, trophic support of neurons and promotion of local neurite outgrowth (Pfrieger and Barres, 1996; Rubin and Sanes, 1996; Staddon and Rubin, 1996). More specifically, astrocytes are potential targets for chemical signals released from neurons and possess binding sites for neuroactive peptides, amino acids, amines and eicosanoids which are known to be released from neurons (Murphy and Pearce, 1987; Atwell, 1994; Smith, 1994; Chiu and Kriegler, 1994; Barres, 1996).

There is recent evidence indicating that glial cells are one of the most sensitive indicators of pathological brain injury as mentioned above. Glial reaction to injury is expressed in terms of increased GFAP immunoreactivity. Thus, noxious mechanical, metabolic, or chemical insults to the brain and vasogenic edema will result in reactive gliosis depending on the magnitude and severity of the stimuli (Schmidt-Kastner et al., 1990). Our earlier observation on chronic hypoxia revealed a marked increase of GFAP activity in selected areas of brain (Zimmer et al., 1991). However, there are several other reports showing an increase of GFAP expression in brain under various pathological conditions (Chiu and Goldmann, 1985; Eng and Ghirnikar, 1994). Interestingly, in many of the above pathological conditions showing an increased GFAP immunoreactivity, is usually associated with a breakdown of the BBB (Beck et al., 1986; Janzer and Raff, 1987; Lum and Malik, 1994). This indicates that astrocytes

play an important role in the CNS homeostasis in health and diseases, and thus could be activated markedly following an alteration in the brain micro-fluid environment, a hypothesis which will require additional investigation.

Glial cells influence neurochemical metabolism

Astrocytes are the potential target of many chemical substances that are released from neurons (Table 1). Thus astrocytes seem to participate actively in the fluid microenvironment of the brain (Maxwell et al., 1987; McCarthy et al., 1988; Juurlink and Devon, 1990). It is now established that glial cells apart from working as an electric insulation to the nerve cells, provide trophic support to neurons and influence their ability to regenerate after injury (Deitmer and Rose, 1996; Tsacopoulos and Magistretti, 1996). Recent evidence strongly supports the idea that astrocytes are actively involved in the information processing of the CNS (Walz, 1989; Kettenmann and Ransom, 1995). This is evident from the ability of astrocytes to control local ion and neurotransmitter metabolism as mentioned above (Murphy and Pearce, 1987; Landis, 1994; Pfrieger and Barres, 1996).

Work done in the past 13 years has identified synthesis of various neurotransmitters, neuropeptides, cytokines and growth factors in astrocytes both in cell culture as well in *in vivo* situations (Table 1). The functional significance of such findings is not well known. There are reports indicating that expression of neurochemical receptors and growth factors following brain injury is restricted to the affected astrocytes in the CNS which seems to be one of the major contributing factors in the development of brain pathology (Miller et al., 1986; for review, see McMillan et al., 1994).

Glial cells modulate synaptic function

There is new evidence which suggests that the glial cells are also involved in synaptogenesis (for review see Pfrieger and Barres, 1996). Previously, synaptogenesis was regarded as the sole function of neurons (Vaughn, 1989). However, new findings on neuronal–glial interaction suggest that glial cells can also regulate the function of synapses (Haydon and Drapeau, 1995; Pfrieger and Barres, 1996). Experimental evidence to support the view that glial cells are influencing synaptogenesis came from the meticulous experiments by Nakanishi et al. (1994). These authors demonstrated that the synchronisation of calcium oscillations among cultured neurons is enhanced in astrocyte-rich cultures. Further experiments to test glial influence on synaptogenesis were done in purified neurons that were cultured with or without neuroglia. The results show that sympathetic neurons which are mainly adrenergic exhibit cholinergic synapses if cultured in the presence of glial cells. However, in this experiment it is not certain whether glia cells promoted the formation of synapses or changed the neurotransmitter phenotype of sympathetic neurons from adrenergic to cholinergic type (Jones et al., 1995; Pfrieger and Barres, 1996).

Pfrieger and his group further confirmed the role of glia in synaptogenesis using retinal ganglion cells in culture. These authors studied the synapse formation in the retinal ganglion cells in culture in the complete absence of the glial cells. Their results show that without glial cells, the neurons displayed only a low level of spontaneous synaptic activity and formed only a few synapses. Addition of neuroglia to the culture significantly enhanced the synaptic activity and the number of synaptic connections. These observations strongly indicate that glial-derived signals are important in the formation of synapses and glial cells promote synapse formation (Pfrieger and Barres, 1996).

The dynamic association between synapses and glial cells as described above indicates a potential importance of neuroglia during the development and remodelling of synaptic connections. However, it remains to be seen whether glial cells can influence synaptic plasticity following injury and repair mechanisms in the CNS following ischemic, traumatic or hyperthermic insults, a subject which will require further investigation.

Astrocytes are heterogeneously distributed in the CNS

Astrocytic processes surround almost all neuronal and vascular elements in the CNS (Peters et al., 1991). However, the precise distribution of astrocytic processes and their function markedly vary in different regions of the brain. Thus the composition of astrocytic membrane over the cell surface is not uniform in gray and white matter. The astrocytic processes have a very high concentration of intramembrane structures known as 'assemblies' on the brain surface and on the vascular elements. On the other hand, very few assemblies are present involving synapses and almost no assemblies are present on the astrocytic processes covering the neuronal cell body (Landis and Reese, 1982). Thus, the astrocytes are polarised, because their membrane structure varies according to the type and nature of the adjacent cellular processes.

In addition to their differences in membrane structure, astrocytes are also functionally different in various regions of the CNS (Zimmer and Sunde, 1984; Maxwell et al., 1987; McCarthy et al., 1988; Petito et al., 1990). Thus morphologically identified polygonal astrocytes referred to as protoplasmic astrocytes found in gray matter will respond to cAMP, pituitary extracts and epidermal growth factors. On the other hand, astrocytes which look stellate in appearance and are known as fibrous astrocytes present in white matter, do not respond to these growth factors or cAMP (Ernsberger et al., 1990; Juurlink and Devon, 1990; Whitaker-Azmita et al., 1990; Landis, 1994). These observations strongly indicate that astrocytes are structurally and functionally different in different regions of the CNS and perform important functions to maintain homeostasis.

GFAP is a marker of glial cell reaction

There is now enough evidence in the literature which suggests that GFAP represents a good marker of glial cell activation (Brenner, 1994; Cervós-Navarro and Urich, 1995; Pfrieger and

Barres, 1996). Thus, in response to various kinds of noxious insults to the CNS caused by physical trauma, ischemia, anoxia, chemical induced neurotoxicity, viral diseases and/or genetic disorders, the astrocytes react by an increased synthesis of GFAP filaments (Lynch, 1976; Chiu and Goldmann, 1985; Graeber and Kreutzberg, 1986; Schiffer et al., 1986; Yu et al., 1989; Petito et al., 1990; Ahlsen et al., 1993; Le Prince et al., 1993; Masood et al., 1993; McLendon and Bigner, 1994; for review see Kettenmann and Ransom, 1995). This response is part of the phenomena known as 'astrogliosis' (Brenner, 1994; Eng and Ghirnikar, 1994). However, studies on gliosis in various animal models of brain injury, neurotoxic damage, genetic diseases and/or inflammatory demyelination show that reactive gliosis is not a stereotypic response but varies widely in duration, degree of hyperplasia, and expression of GFAP (reviewed by Norton et al., 1992). Based on these studies, it appears that there are different biological mechanisms for induction and maintenance of reactive gliosis, an issue which is still controversial.

Astrocytes with an increased amount of GFAP also appear in neoplastic and metabolic diseases affecting the CNS (Cervós-Navarro and Urich, 1995), in traumatic brain and spinal cord injuries (Amaducci et al., 1981; Aquino et al., 1988; Goshgarian et al., 1989; Dusart et al., 1991; Eng et al., 1992; Sharma et al., 1993), chronic hypoxia (Zimmer et al., 1991), brain demyelination (Bignami et al., 1980), multiple sclerosis (Raine and Bornstein, 1970; Gorny et al., 1990) and in degenerative diseases such as Alzheimer's disease, Creutzfeldt-Jakob disease, and in Huntington's disease (Cervós-Navarro and Urich, 1995). Upregulation of GFAP is present in the Rosenthal fibres in Alexander's disease (Tomokane et al., 1991). Elevated concentrations of GFAP are also found in acute myelitis (Kaiser and Lucking, 1993), dementia (Le Prince et al., 1993) and autism (Ahlsen et al., 1993). These observations suggests that reactive gliosis and brain damage is somehow related in various pathological conditions of the CNS. However, the functional significance of glial cell reaction and the endogenous signals responsible for gliosis are not well understood.

Molecular aspects of the GFAP gene

As mentioned above, the intermediate filament commonly referred to as GFAP, is the major cytoskeletal protein in astrocytes, where it is expressed in a cell specific manner. This quality has made GFAP a widely used marker of normal, pathological and neoplastic astrocytes (Duffy, 1984). Increased synthesis of GFAP is a part of the reactive response to almost any type of CNS injury. Due to this characteristic, GFAP is regarded as an important marker of glial cell injury in trauma, ischemia, hypoxia or many other neurodegenerative diseases of the CNS.

Due to the cell specific expression of the GFAP gene, the GFAP-promoter has been used to direct exogenous genes exclusively to the brain. However, very little is known about the biological function of GFAP protein and of the regulation of GFAP gene expression. The best known reaction of astrocytes is their response to different insults, a response commonly known as astrogliosis as mentioned above. Following injury astrocytes become 'activated' to accomplish metabolic and structural roles in the CNS. In affected areas, activated astrocytes express high amounts of GFAP and form glial scars. Astrogliosis is often characterised by hyperplasia, hypertrophy of nuclei, cell bodies, and cytoplasmic processes, and extensive synthesis of GFAP (Eng and Ghirnikar, 1994). However the details of this reaction are still not known.

The gene: cDNA

GFAP was first isolated in 1971 by Eng and his colleagues from glial scars (plaques) derived from a patient with multiple sclerosis, a demyelinating disease of the CNS (Eng et al., 1971). Since the subunit was found to be an acidic protein, it has been designated glial fibrillary acidic protein. About 13 years after this fundamental discovery of GFAP, a GFAP clone was isolated in 1984 from a mouse cDNA library (Lewis et al., 1984).

This cloning constituted the starting point for the molecular genetic studies of GFAP. With the help of this cDNA fragment the murine GFAP gene was isolated and sequenced (Balcarek and Cowan, 1985). A few years later, the human cD-NAs were isolated and characterised by several groups (Reeves et al., 1989, Brenner et al., 1990; Bongcam-Rudloff et al., 1991; Kumanishi et al., 1992). The GFAP gene has been isolated and characterised also in the rat by Feinstein et al. (1992) and in the goldfish by Cohen and Schwartz (1993).

Genomic clones and chromosome localisation

The entire mouse GFAP gene has been sequenced and it encompasses 9.8 kilobases including nine exons separated by introns ranging in size from 0.2 to 2.5 kb. A comparison of the murine GFAP DNA genomic sequence shows great homology with other isolated intermediate filament genes (Balcarek and Cowan, 1985). The entire human genomic GFAP gene has also been sequenced but the sequence has not been published (Brenner, 1994b). The mouse GFAP gene was mapped to the distal arm of chromosome 11 by Southern blot analysis of mouse-Chinese hamster cell hybrids (Bernier et al., 1988) and by studies of Eco R1 RFLP segregation of GFAP alleles in 75 backcross progenies between C57BL/6 mice and *Mus spretus*. The human GFAP gene was assigned to chromosome 17q21 by screening of a panel of rodent-human cell hybrids and by *in situ* hybridisation to metaphase chromosomes (Bongcam-Rudloff et al., 1991). These results were later corroborated by other investigators using hybridisation to fluorescent-sorted chromosomes (Kumanishi et al., 1992) and Southern blotting (Brownell et al., 1991). Interestingly, there seems to be a cluster of intermediate filament genes in this chromosomal region (Rosenberg et al., 1988). Rogaev et al. (1993) have mapped the causative genetic defect of familial keratosis palmaris et plantaris, a disease characterised by extreme keratinization and desquamation of the skin of the palmar and plantar sur-

faces of the hands and feet, to an 8 cM interval on 17q12-24 in or close to the acidic keratin (type I) gene cluster. Linkage analyses have also shown that the disease traits of epidermolytic hyperkeratosis are linked to the keratin gene clusters on chromosome 17 (Leigh and Lane, 1993).

GFAP expression during development

In the mouse, the regulation of GFAP expression seems to be related to astrocyte proliferation and astroglial cell differentiation. During mouse brain maturation, GFAP mRNA levels show a biphasic expression pattern. GFAP mRNA increases between birth and day 15 (period of astrocytic proliferation) and then decreases until day 55 (period of astrocytic morphological differentiation) (Riol et al., 1992). In the human CNS, GFAP can be visualised immunohistochemically 8–9 weeks postconceptionally in radial glia of the spinal cord (Voronina and Preobrazhensky, 1994). In the brain, immunoreactive astrocytes are found initially deep in the white matter, and positive cells are gradually extended into the superficial white matter. This process continues until birth (Takashima and Becker, 1983). In the adult, GFAP expression is restricted to protoplasmic astrocytes in the grey matter, fibrous astrocytes in the white matter as well as Bergmann glia and subependymal astrocytes bordering the cerebral ventricles (McLendon and Bigner, 1994). The highest density of GFAP positive cells is found in the glia limitans, which forms an outer barrier surrounding the whole CNS. The suprachiasmatic nucleus, the site of the biological pacemaker, has been shown to undergo circadian variations in the expression of GFAP in the Syrian hamster. In this species, a 24-h rhythm in the distribution of GFAP immunoreactivity occurs in the suprachiasmatic nucleus supporting the hypothesis of astrocyte participation in the clock function (Lavialle and Serviere, 1995). Despite all the extensive work in the field of astrocyte biology the precise function of the GFAP protein has not been clearly elucidated.

Alternative forms of GFAP mRNA

As mentioned above, GFAP found in the rat PNS is known as GFAP-beta (Galea et al., 1995). This alternate form of GFAP is primarily produced in rat Schwann cells and has been described by Feinstein et al. (1992). These authors show that the mRNA extends 11 nucleotides upstream of the start point of the GFAP mRNA as described in the human GFAP (Brenner et al., 1990; Bong-cam-Rudloff et al., 1991). Tryptic peptide mapping of GFAP protein prepared from cultured astrocytes and Schwann cells, revealed one major peptide fragment present in CNS GFAP but absent from PNS GFAP (Galea et al., 1995). However, these results are still controversial. Other putative types of alternate GFAPs are the subject of studies by other groups, but there are no conclusive data at this point. Recently, a GFAP variant lacking the first exon has been reported by Zelenika and co-workers (1995). From a mouse bone marrow cDNA library they isolated GFAP cDNAs which start in the 3' part of intron 1 and contain all the downstream GFAP exons. The new GFAP mRNAs, which they call GFAP gamma mRNAs, are already present in the brain at embryonic day 15 and in adult forebrain and cerebellum. Their presence in astrocytic cell lines suggests that astrocytes may be the site of *in vivo* expression of these mRNAs. Furthermore in human an analogous GFAP mRNA containing the 3' part of intron 1 and lacking the exon 1 is also present in adult brain (Zelenika et al., 1995). These results suggest a new regulation of the GFAP gene expression, which however requires further investigation.

Knockout mice

In order to further understand the biology of GFAP several groups have created GFAP-null mice (Pekny et al., 1995; McCall et al., 1996; Gomi et al., 1996; Liedtke et al., 1996). The results of those studies suggests that (a) GFAP is important for astrocyte–neuronal interactions, and that astrocyte processes play a vital role in modulating synaptic efficacy in the CNS (McCall et al., 1996); (b) mice devoid of GFAP display abnormal myelination; myelinating oligodendrocytes in adults, nonmyelinated axons in optic nerve, and reduced myelin thickness in spinal cord (Liedtke et al., 1996); (c) mutant mice had a poor vascularization of the white matter and the BBB was structurally and functionally damaged; (d) moreover in the study by Liedtke et al. (1996), mice deprived of GFAP showed hydrocephalus associated with white matter loss. These studies suggest that astrocytic proteins are important in maintaining normal physiological functions of the CNS.

GFAP and vimentin

In transfection experiments with a human GFAP cDNA clone we have studied the formation of GFAP fibrils by immunofluorescence analysis using confocal microscopy. Double immunofluorescence analysis showed that the initially punctate GFAP was distributed along the pre-existing vimentin fibrils, and that the GFAP fibrils were developed from these dots on the framework of vimentin fibrils (Fig. 1). This result, showing copolymerization, is strongly supported by data from other groups suggesting that in cells that synthesise both types of intermediate filaments, GFAP and vimentin subunits are co-assembled and integrated into the same intermediate filament structures (Sharp et al., 1982; Quinlan and Franke, 1983; Abd-el-Basset et al., 1992; Lu et al., 1993). This view is consistent with the finding that purified GFAP microinjected in cells expressing vimentin organises into proper intermediate filament structures. On the other hand, in vimentin-free cells, GFAP was only seen as a disorganised juxtanuclear structure (Wiegers et al., 1991). Furthermore in a study by Galou et al. (1996) the authors showed that in mice devoid of vimentin the GFAP network is disrupted in astrocytes that normally co-express vimentin and GFAP. It is important to note that during glial differentiation, GFAP expression is found later

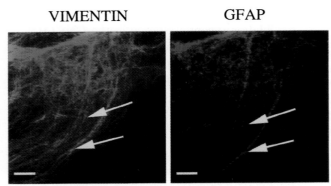

VIMENTIN GFAP

Fig. 1. Double fluorescence analysis of a GFAP-negative human glioma cell line transfected with a human GFAP cDNA. The newly synthesised GFAP is incorporated into the pre-existing vimentin network. Vimentin filament network visualised by indirect immunofluorescence for antivimentin antibodies and FITC labelled second antibodies. GFAP visualised by indirect immunofluorescence for anti-GFAP antibodies and Rhodamin labelled second antibodies (bar = 40 μm).

than the expression of vimentin in the same cells (Giordana, 1990; Stagaard Janas et al., 1991a,b). It has even been suggested that GFAP is expressed exclusively in vimentin positive normal or neoplastic cells (Abd-el-Basset et al., 1992).

Gene regulation

Recently, several studies have been done to understand the factors governing the mechanisms behind the transcription regulation of GFAP. These observations indicate that many factors including steroids, growth factors and cytokines are involved in the regulation of GFAP expression (for review see Laping et al., 1994b). Two regulatory elements have been identified to be essential for astrocytic specificity in human (Masood et al., 1993; Bongcam-Rudloff et al., unpublished observation), mouse (Miura et al., 1990; Sarkar and Cowan, 1991a,b; Sarid, 1991), and rat (Kaneko and Sueoka, 1993). A regions which spans -1612 to -1489 was also necessary to give a strong signal in GFAP-positive cells (Masood et al., 1993; Sarid, 1991). Furthermore the work of Nakatani et al. (1990) in the human and of Sarid (1991) in the mouse showed that *in vitro*, in a chloracetyl transferase-assay, the GFAP promoter had the strongest chloracetyl transferase-activity when 40 bases were present in the 5' end of the coding region. Some of these in

vitro studies have, however, given contradictory results (Laping et al., 1994a,b). *In vitro*, the cell-type specificity of GFAP appears to be determined by a combination of transcription factors that are not unique to the permissive cell type (Miura et al., 1990). However, the regulation of the GFAP gene is complex and it is not clear if only one or both regulatory regions contains the elements that restrict the expression to the astrocytes (for review see Brenner, 1994a). Therefore, the establishment of an *in vivo* transgenic model for studies of cis elements involved in GFAP expression is a matter of high priority.

Transgenic mice

The GFAP promoter has been used as a tool to direct exogenous genes to the glial cells in transgenic animals. In the human a 2.2-kb 5' fragment of the human GFAP gene ($-2163-+47$) confers astrocyte-specific expression in transgenic mice (Brenner et al., 1994). An *in vitro* study argues for the presence of an element in the first intron of the GFAP gene that suppresses expression in non-glial (HeLa) cells (Sarkar and Cowan, 1991b). Neither studies in our group (Bongcam-Rudloff et al., unpublished observation) in which we used a 1.8-kb 5' flanking region of the GFAP gene, nor other transgenic studies with the human promoter (Schonrich et al., 1991; Brenner et al., 1994), provide any evidence that intron sequences are required to suppress ectopic expression. The lack of detectable mRNA or lacZ staining in tissues outside of the central nervous system certainly indicates that the 1.8 kb 5′ flanking region confers a tightly controlled, tissue specific promoter activity. Other groups have instead used 2 kb of the murine GFAP 5′ flanking region promoter ligated to the prokaryotic Beta galactosidase gene to generate transgenic mice (Mucke et al., 1991; Jones et al., 1995; Galou et al., 1994; Verderber et al., 1995) and in all cases, x-gal staining showed a high degree of localisation of blue colour, due to galactosidase activity in glia cells in imprints from the brain tissues. In studies by Mucke et al. (1991) and others, these workers have inserted the exogenous genes into the first exon of the murine GFAP gene using the whole genomic sequence (Mucke et al., 1991; Rall et al., 1994; Toggas et al., 1994).

Glial cell reaction in hyperthermic brain injury

Activation of astrocytes following hyperthermic brain injury is a new subject which was not well studied in the past, as mentioned above. Previously, using routine light microscopy, a few sporadic observations of glial cell reaction in the CNS caused by local heating were described (for review see Sminia et al., 1994; Sharma, Westman and Nyberg, in this volume). A few studies describe glial cell changes at the ultrastructural level in cell culture following hyperthermia. However, these authors did not use any specific immunoreactive markers for glial cell activation. These *in vivo* and *in vitro* experiments are not comparable to each other because of the great variation in the magnitude and duration of heat exposure, survival periods and model used. Moreover, some authors using *in vivo* situation believe that the changes observed in glial cells are probably artefact (see review by Sminia et al., 1994 and in this volume). Thus, previous observations on glial cell injury in hyperthermia are mainly inconclusive and additional investigation

in this field is definitely needed to clarify this point.

Problems of heat stress and involvement of glial cells

Heat stress and associated hyperthermia is a common problem in many parts of the world (Austin and Berry, 1956; Gottschalk and Thomas, 1966; Shibolet et al., 1967a,b; Brahams, 1989; Gillett, 1989; Sterner, 1990). The problems of heat stress are usually associated with fever, radiotherapy for tumours, and exercise in hot environment (Sminia et al., 1994). In all these cases the body temperature rises (Field et al., 1944; Frankel et al., 1963; Burger and Fuhrman, 1969). Most of the attention in the field of thermal biology is placed on understanding the function of nerve cells, alterations in neurotransmitter metabolism and other immunological functions (Milton, 1993; Zeisburger et al., 1994; Blatteis, 1997). Interestingly, an involvement of glial cells in thermoregulatory mechanisms during health and diseases has still not been considered (Milton, 1993; Zeisburger et al., 1994; Blatteis, 1997). Since glial cells participate in the information processing of the CNS (Pfrieger and Barres, 1996), and possess receptors for various neurochemicals and endogenous pyrogens such as cytokines and prostaglandins, it seems quite likely that glial cells participate in thermoregulatory mechanisms in the CNS. It may be that hyperthermia-induced altered neurotransmitter metabolism or perturbed fluid microenvironment of the brain plays an important endogenous signal for glial cell activation, a hypothesis which requires detailed investigation.

Heat stress induces alteration in brain fluid microenvironment

Studies carried out by Sharma and his group in the past strongly indicate that heat stress has the capacity to influence fluid microenvironment of the brain (Sharma, 1982; Sharma and Dey, 1984, 1986, 1987; Sharma et al., 1986, 1991a,b; 1992a,b,c; 1994; 1996b; 1997a,b,c,d; Sharma and Cervós-Navarro, 1990a,b). This is evident from the fact that heat stress induces widespread breakdown of the BBB permeability to proteins (Sharma and Dey, 1986, 1987) and induces damage of nerve cells, glial cells and probably axons. This effect of heat stress on the BBB permeability is supposed to be influenced by various neurochemical mediators in the CNS (for review see Sharma, Westman and Nyberg, this volume).

Although, the probable mechanisms of hyperthermia-induced cell injury are still not known in complete detail, it seems quite likely that heat stress and associated hyperthermia will induce disturbances of the brain energy metabolism resulting in cellular energy failure (Siesjö, 1978). A failure of thermoregulatory mechanisms will lead to an increase in the whole body and brain temperature (Sharma et al., this volume). An increased brain temperature will mainly be responsible for alterations in the metabolism of various neurochemicals (Sharma and Dey, 1986, 1987; Sharma and Cervós-Navarro, 1990; Sharma et al., 1991, 1992, 1994, 1997a,b; Milton, 1993; Zeisburger et al., 1994; Blatteis, 1997) which in turn will influence the BBB permeability disturbances, cerebral blood flow and metabolism (Siesjö, 1978; Sharma and Dey, 1987; Sharma et al., 1991, 1992a,b,c), as well as inactivation of cellular enzyme proteins (Siesjö, 1978; Sharma et al., 1986, 1992b).

Alterations in neurochemical metabolism may disrupt the endothelial cell permeability probably via a receptor-mediated mechanism. A disruption of the BBB will expose the cellular compartments of the brain to various serum constituents including neurochemicals and immunologically active materials which were previously unable to enter into the CNS due to an intact BBB (Bradbury, 1992; Black, 1995; Sharma et al., 1996a,b). This increased microvascular permeability is likely to cause vasogenic edema and cellular reaction within the CNS (Sharma et al., this volume).

Thus various biochemical, immunological and pathophysiological reactions will be initiated after a breakdown of the BBB which may lead to alteration in the brain fluid microenvironment. Since a slight alteration in the composition of the extracellular fluid in which the neuron and glial cells bath will lead to abnormal brain function, it seems quite likely that a breakdown of the BBB along with an altered neurochemical metabolism and vasogenic edema may result in cell damage involving neuroglial cells as well.

Our own investigations on glial cell reaction in heat stress

In the following section, we describe our own investigations on heat stress induced glial cell reaction in various regions of the CNS in our rat model (see below). To examine the glial reaction in heat stress, we used GFAP and vimentin immunohistochemistry at the light microscopy level. These light microscopic observations were confirmed in selected regions using electron microscopy.

The rat model

We used an experimental model of heat stress originally described by Sharma and his group (Sharma, 1982; Sharma and Dey, 1984, 1986). This model consists of exposure of young animals to a 4-h heat exposure at 38°C. The relative humidity 50–55%, and wind velocity 20–25 cm/s were kept constant (Sharma and Dey, 1987, Sharma and Cervós-Navarro, 1990a,b; Sharma et al., 1991a,b).

Earlier, Sharma and his group demonstrated a marked increase in the BBB permeability to proteins, reduction in regional cerebral blood flow (CBF), elevation of plasma and brain serotonin levels, edema as well as cellular changes following heat stress. These changes were considerably reduced by pretreatment with various drugs modifying the function of serotonin, prostaglandins, opioids, histamine and calcium ion channels (for details see Sharma, Westman and Nyberg, this volume).

Since the glial cells are sensitive to various noxious insults to the brain and actively participate in the regulatory processes of the BBB, chemical and metabolic microenvironment, and contain receptors to various neurotransmitters as mentioned above (for details see Table 1), it appears that pharmacological modification of these neurotransmitters before heat stress may influence the glial cell response in heat stress as well.

TABLE 1

Increased expression of neurochemicals and their receptors by astrocytes

Neurochemicals	Normal conditions	CNS injury
Cytokines		
Interleukin 1	+ +	+ +
Interleukin 6	+ +	+ / − ?
Tumour necrosis factor a	+	+
Prostaglandins		
Prostacyclin	+	+ +
PGE2	+	+ +
Amines		
Serotonin	+ +	+ /?
Catecholamines	+	+
Histamine	+ /?	− /?
Growth factors		
Nerve growth factor	+ +	+
Ciliary neurotrophic factor	+	+
Brain-derived neurotrophic factor	+ +	+ / − ?
Neurotrophin-3	+	?
Glia cell line derived neurotrophic factor	+ +	+ / − ?
Transforming growth factor α	+	+
Transforming growth factor β	+	?
Insulin-like growth factor I	+ +	+
Basic fibroblast growth factor	+	+
Colony stimulating factor	+	?
Amino acid		
GABA	+ +	+ +
Glutamate	?	+ +
Taurine	+	+
Aspartate	+ +	+ / − ?
		(Continued)

TABLE 1   *(Continued)*

Neurochemicals	Normal conditions	CNS injury
Neuropeptides		
Enkephalins	+	+
Endothelins	+ +	+ +
Neuropeptide Y	+	?
Substance P	?	+
Somatostatin	+	?
Atrial natriuretic peptide	+ +	?
Angiotensinogen	+ +	+ +

Modified after Murphy and Pearce, 1987; McMillan et al., 1994; Sharma et al., 1992a,b, 1993. + = mild, + + = moderate, − = not detected, ? = uncertain.

The working hypothesis

Keeping the above information on the function of neuroglial cells in the CNS and its reaction in brain pathology, it appears that breakdown of the BBB permeability is instrumental in glial cell reaction in heat stress. Thus it would be interesting to see whether pharmacological manipulation of the BBB function in heat stress will also influence the glial reaction.

In order to understand the role played by the BBB disruption in glial cell activation, we pharmacologically attenuated the breakdown of the BBB permeability in heat stress by drugs known to influence the function of serotonin, prostaglandins, opioids and calcium channels and examined the GFAP immunoreactivity in the CNS using standard protocol (see below).

GFAP and vimentin immunostaining

The GFAP and vimentin immunostaining was examined in separate groups of control and heat stressed rats with or without pretreatment with various drugs (Table 2). For this purpose, the animals were perfused (under urethane anaesthesia, 1 g/kg, i.p.) transcardially with about 100 ml of a glutaraldehyde-based fixative (2.5% glutaraldehyde, 2% paraformaldehyde in 0.1 M phosphate buffer, pH 7.4 containing 2.5% picric acid) preceded by a brief saline rinse (0.9% NaCl, about 50 ml). The perfused animals were wrapped in an aluminium foil and kept in a refrigerator at 4°C overnight. Next day, the brain was removed and kept in the same fixative at 4°C for a minimum of 3–4 days. The desired portions of the brain were embedded in paraffin (Pellegrino et al., 1979). Multiple 3-μm-thick sections were cut and processed for GFAP and vimentin immunostaining using commercial protocol (Zimmer et al., 1991). In brief, for GFAP after deparaffinization, endogenous peroxidase was inhibited with 0.3% hydrogen peroxide with 1% non-immune horse serum in phosphate-buffered saline (PBS, pH 7.4) for 20 min and then for 8 h with monoclonal anti-GFAP serum (DAKO, Hamburg) diluted 1:500 in PBS or monoclonal anti-Vimentin (DAKO, Hamburg) diluted 1:100 in PBS, and thereafter the tissue sections were washed three time in PBS. After incubation with biotinylated horse anti-mouse immunoglobulin IgG at a 1:50-dilution and avidin-biotin complex (ABC; Vector, Burlingame) for 45 min, the brown reaction product was developed with 3,3′-tetra-aminobenzidine and hydrogen peroxide in 0.05 M Tris–HCl buffer (pH 7.4) for 4 min (Sharma et al., 1992a,b). The sections were counterstained with haemotoxylin–eosin. Some sections were incubated with preimmune horse serum at a 1:50 dilution as the primary antiserum. These control sections showed no immunoreactive product (Sharma et al., 1992a,b). The paraffin sections of the control and heat-stressed groups were processed simultaneously in parallel. The GFAP immunoreactivity in different brain regions was examined in a blind fashion by at least two independent observers.

Heat stress induces upregulation of GFAP

In normal animals, the GFAP-immunoreactivity was observed mainly in the perivascular glia limi-tans, subependymal fibre mesh around the ventricles, in the external glia limitans over the cerebral hemispheres and prominently in the radial Bergmann glia in cerebellum (Figs. 2 and 3) (Sharma et al., 1992a). Distinct GFAP-positive astrocytes were always seen in the corpus callosum and in some structures in the vicinity of the optic tracts (e.g. nucleus supraopticus) (Table 2).

Only a few positive astrocytes were found in the white matter as well as in the granular layer of the cerebellum (Figs. 3 and 4). In the hippocampus only the hilus of the dentate nucleus contained marked GFAP-stained astrocytes (Table 2), whereas other hippocampal structures like CA1 and CA2 sectors showed only very few stained astrocytes (Fig. 2). The glial cells of the cortex and brain stem stained weakly with GFAP (Figs. 2 and 3). Some GFAP-positive astrocytes were observed in the region of internal capsule. Further details are described in Table 2. The distribution of GFAP-immunoreactivity in normal rats was in accordance with our earlier observations and quite similar to the results described by other workers (Bignami et al., 1980; Hajos and Kalman, 1989; Kalman and Hajos, 1989; Zimmer et al., 1991; Sharma et al., 1992a).

The GFAP-immunoreactivity was remarkably increased in animals subjected to a 4-h heat stress at 38°C (Table 2) (Figs. 2–5). This staining was more intense in brain stem (pons, medulla), cerebellum, thalamus and hypothalamus, striatum and parts of the hippocampus (Fig. 2). The cortex showed an increase in GFAP immunoreactivity as compared with the controls in which no significant GFAP-positive astrocytes were seen (Figs. 2 and 4). In heat-stressed animals, immunostained astrocytes could be observed mostly in cortical layers III and IV (Table 2).

In heat-stressed animals, an increase in GFAP-positive astrocytes was noted in all parts of the hippocampus (Fig. 2). Thus, an increase in GFAP immunoreactivity following heat stress was observed in hippocampal areas like CA1 and CA2 sectors together with an obvious increase in the granular cell layer. The GFAP-positive astrocytes were often located around blood vessels and ex-

GFAP immunostaining

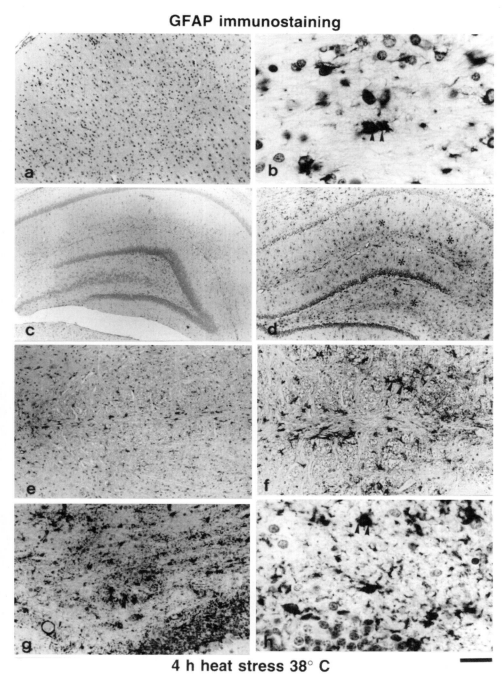

4 h heat stress 38° C

Fig. 2. Representative example of GFAP immunostaining (seen as dark black reaction product) in one control (a,c,e,g) and one 4 h heat stressed (b,d,f,h) rat. Only a few GFAP positive cells, if any, can be seen in the cortex (a), hippocampus (c), brain stem (e) and cerebellum (g). On the other hand, 4 h heat stress markedly increased the number of GFAP positive cells (arrow heads) in the cortex (b), hippocampus (*) (d), brain stem (f) and in cerebellum (h) (bar: a, c, d, e = 250 μm; b, h = 50 μm, f = 100 μm, g = 80 μm) (modified after Sharma et al., 1992).

TABLE 2

GFAP immunoreactivity in control and heat stressed rats

Region of brain[a]	GFAP immunoreactivity				
	Control	Heat stress (38°C)			
	$n = 5$	4 h $n = 5$	2 h $n = 3$	1 h $n = 3$	4 h[b] $n = 4$
Cerebral cortex					
Frontal	+	+ +	+	+	+
Parietal	+	+ +	+	+	+
Occipital	+ / −	+ +	+ / −	+ / −	+
Cingulate	+ +	+ + +	+ / −	−	−
Temporal	+ +	+ +	+ +	+ +	+
Pyriform	−	+ +	− / +	−	+ / − ?
Entorhinal	− / + ?	+ + +	+	+	+
Cerebellum					
Vermis	+	+ + + + +	+	+	+
Lateral cortex	+	+ + + +	+	−	+
Nucleus dentatus	+ +	+ + + + +	+ +	+	+ +
Nucleus emboliformis	+	+ + + + +	+	−	+
Nucleus fastigi	+	+ + + +	+	+	− / ?
Nucleus globus	− / ?	+ + +	− / ?	−	+
Inferior peduncle	+ / − ?	+ + + + +	+	−	+ / − ?
Paraflocculus	−	+ + + + +	−	+ +	+ +
Flocculus	−	+ + + +	+	+	+
Hippocampus					
CA1/2	−	+ +	−	+	+
CA3/4	+	+ + +	+	+	+
External fibre	+ +	+ + + +	+ / −	+	+
Dentate gyrus	+	+ + +	+ / −	+	+ / −
Striatum					
Caudate nucleus	+ + +	+ + + + +	+	+ +	+ + +
Globus pallidus	− / + ?	+ + +	+ +	+	+ + /?
Corpus callosum	+	+ + + +	+	−	+
Cingulum	+ +	+ + + +	+	−	+ +
Internal capsule	+ + +	+ + + +	+ +	+ +	+ + +
Thalamus					
Nucleus anterior	+	+ +	+	+	+ +
Nucleus posterior	+	+ + +	+	+	+ +
Nucleus dorsal	−	+ + + + +	−	−	+ / − ?
Nucleus medial	+ / − ?	+ + + +	− / ?	+	+ +
Nucleus ventral	− / +	+ + + + +	+ +	+	+ +
Nucleus lateral	+ +	+ + + + +	+	+	+ +
Substantia grisea	+ / −	+ + +	−	−	+
Substantia nigra	+	+ + +	+	−	+ +

(*Continued*)

TABLE 2   (*Continued*)

Region of brain[a]	GFAP immunoreactivity				
	Control $n = 5$	Heat stress (38°C)			
		4 h $n = 5$	2 h $n = 3$	1 h $n = 3$	4 h[b] $n = 4$
Hypothalamus					
Nucleus arcuates	+ +	+ + + + +	+	+	+ +
Nucleus anterior	+	+ + + +	+	+	+ +
Nucleus lateralis	+ / − ?	+ +	−	+ / − ?	+ / ?
Nucleus paraventricularis	+ +	+ + +	+	+	+ +
Nucleus posterior	+ +	+ + +	+	+	+ +
Nucleus venteromedialis	+	+ + +	+	+	+
Colliculi					
Superior	−	+	−	−	+ / ?
Inferior	−	+ +	−	−	−
Brain stem					
Nucleus ambiguus	−	+ + +	−	−	+
Nucleus cuneatus	− / + ?	+ +	−	+	+ / ?
Nucleus facialis	+ / −	+ + + +	−	−	+
Nucleus gracilis	−	+ + +	−	−	−
Nucleus hypoglossi	−	+ + +	−	−	−
Medial leminiscus	+ +	+ + + + +	+	+	+ + / ?
Nucleus occulomotor	−	+ + / ?	−	−	+
Nucleus pontis	+ +	+ + + + +	+ +	+	+
Nucleus raphe	+ +	+ + + + +	+ / ?	+	+ +
Nucleus superior olivary	+	+ + + +	+	+	+ / − ?
Nucleus trigeminalis	−	+ + +	−	−	+
Reticular formation	− / + ?	+ + + + +	+	−	−
Ventral tegmentum	−	+ + +	−	−	+
Corpus trapezoideum	+ / −	+ + + +	−	−	+
Tractus cerebellospinalis	− / +	+ + + +	−	+	+ + / ?
Tractus corticospinalis	+ +	+ + + + +	+	+	+ +
Tractus rubrospinalis	− / + ?	+ + +	−	+	+
Tractus tectospinalis	+	+ + +	+	−	+
Substantia gelatinosa	+ +	+ + + + +	+	+	+ +
Spinal cord					
Substantia gelatinosa	− / + ?	+ + + + +	+ +	+	+ +
Dorsal horn	+ / −	+ + + + +	+	+	+ +
Ventral horn	−	+ + + + +	+	+	+ +
Lateral horn	+	+ + + + +	+	+	+ +
Central canal	−	+ + + + +	+	+	+
White matter	+ +	+ + + + +	+ +	+ +	+ + +

Rats were subjected to acute heat exposure in a BOD incubator at 38°C (for details see text). The score of GFAP immunoreactivity was assigned arbitrarily by two independent workers in a blind fashion. The GFAP immunoreactivity on deparaffinised slides was developed using monoclonal anti GFAP sera and demonstrated using PAP technique. The slides from negative control (without primary antibody), control and heat stressed animals were processed simultaneously in parallel. Data modified after Sharma et al. (1992); − = negative, + = positive, ? = not seen in some cases; + = low, + + = mild, + + + = moderate, + + + + = high, + + + + + = very high.

[a]After Pellegrino et al. (1979).

[b]Urethane anaesthetised.

256

hibited intense binding of GFAP antibody as shown by a dark-brown reaction product (Fig 3).

An increase in GFAP-immunoreactive astrocytes was observed in various regions of the brain stem (Fig. 2), cerebellum (Fig. 4) and spinal cord (Fig. 5) in heat-stressed animals, as compared with normal animals. In cerebellum, strong GFAP positive astrocytes in the region of lateral cerebellar nuclei were seen (Fig. 4). Many GFAP-positive astrocytes were found in the molecular layer of the cerebellum of heat-stressed animals. The Bergmann glia of stressed animals showed a sig-

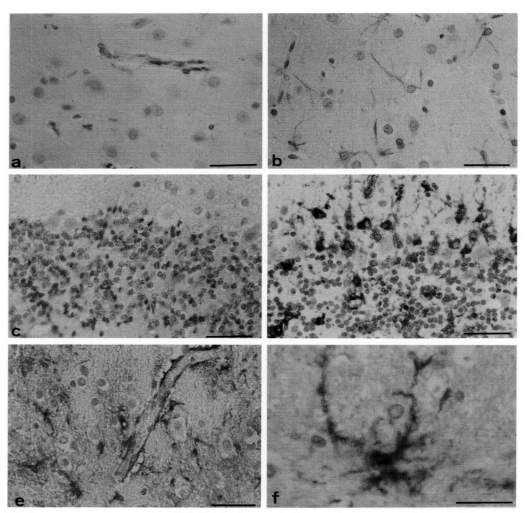

Fig. 3. A representative example of GFAP stained astrocytes from cerebral cortex, cerebellum and brain stem at high magnification of a control and a 4 h heat stressed animal. Only a very mild GFAP immunoreaction around a vessel in the cortex of a control animal (a) could be seen, whereas stronger GFAP stained cortical astrocytes are present in heat stressed animal (b). As compared to a normal animal (c), prominent GFAP positive astrocytes are seen around Bergmann glia in cerebellum after heat stress (d). In the brain stem reticular formation, strong GFAP stained astrocytes around an arteriole of heat stressed animal are apparent (e). In the same animal, a star-shaped astrocyte in the parietal cortex is clearly visible (f). (bars: a-e: 50 μm; f: 25 μm) (data from Sharma et al., 1992a).

GFAP immunostaining
cerebellum

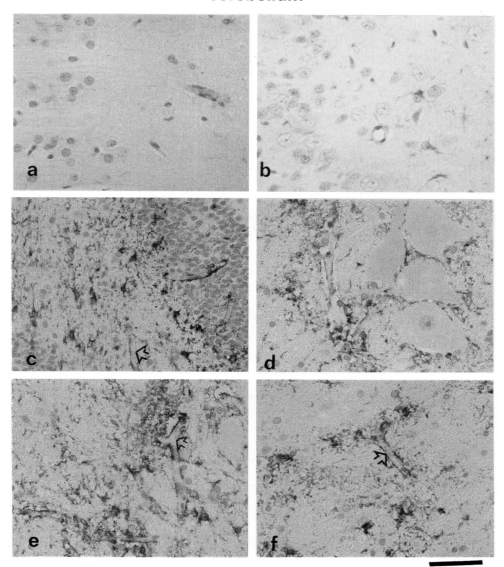

4 h heat stress 38°C

Fig. 4. A representative example of GFAP immunostaining in the cerebellum of a control (a, b) and a 4 h heat stressed rat (c–f). No significant GFAP staining in the cerebellum is evident in control (a, b), whereas a massive strong GFAP immunoreactivity was observed in many areas of cerebellum in heat stressed animal (c–f). Distinct GFAP expression in the region of lateral cerebellar nuclei (c) with some star-shaped GFAP positive astrocytes (d) is clearly visible. Mostly regressive changed astrocytes are located in the molecular (e) and in the granular layer (f) of the cerebellum. Staining of astrocytes around the blood vessels (blank arrow) is clearly apparent (bars: a, d = 80 μm, b = 30 μm, c = 100 μm, e,f = 50 μm).

GFAP immunostaining
spinal cord

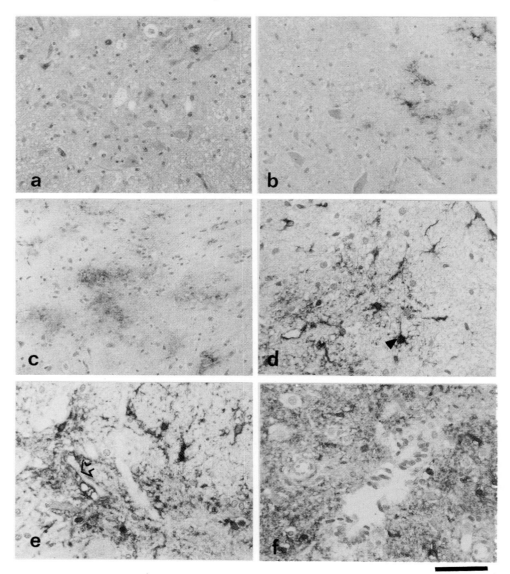

4 h heat stress 38°C

Fig. 5. A representative example of GFAP immunostaining in the spinal cord of a control (a–c) and a 4 h heat stressed rat (d–f). Very few GFAP positive cells if any can be seen in the spinal cord of control rat (a–c), whereas a marked increase in GFAP immunoreactivity was observed in different regions of the spinal cord of heat stressed rat (b–f). Distinct GFAP expression in the region of lateral gray matter (c) with some star-shaped GFAP positive astrocytes (filled arrow head) (d) is clearly visible. Regressive changed astrocytes are mainly located in the gray matter of ventral horn (e) and around the central canal (f) in the spinal cord. Intense immunostaining of astrocytes around the blood vessels (blank arrow) can easily be seen (bars: a–c = 150 μm, d,e = 80 μm, f = 60 μm).

nificant increase of GFAP immunoreactivity as compared with the controls. The GFAP immunoreactivity in granular layer astrocytes of stressed animals is quite apparent.

In brain stem a pronounced reactive gliosis was evident in stressed animals as compared with normal animals especially in the fasciculus solitarius, radial nucleus and tractus tectospinalis (Fig. 2). The raphe pontis and cross-sectioned pontine fiber-tracts showed strong GFAP-positive astrocytes following heat stress as compared with control (Fig. 2). Further details are described in Table 2.

In the spinal cord GFAP positive staining was located in both gray and white matter (Fig. 5). In general the intensity of GFAP immunostaining was mainly concentrated in the dorsal horn, ventral horn and around the central canal regions (Fig. 5). GFAP-stained cells are often found around the blood vessels in many parts of the brain (Fig. 3) indicating the importance of vascular glial interaction in the pathological mechanisms of heat stress.

On the other hand, subjection of conscious animals to heat stress either at shorter duration or anaesthetised rats for 4 h duration did not show any significant alteration in GFAP immunoreactivity as compared with the intact control group (Table 2). These observations suggest that duration of heat exposure and stress associated with heat are important factors in glial cell activation.

Heat stress induces upregulation of vimentin

Heat stress also upregulated vimentin expression in many parts of the brain. However, control animals did not show any vimentin immunoreactivity in any brain region examined. This observation is in line with previous works done by other workers (Pixley and De Vellis, 1984; Calvo et al., 1990). A marked increase in the immunoreactivity for vimentin expression was seen in the brain stem reticulum formation (Fig. 6), thalamus, cerebellum, corpus callosum and in some regions of the hippocampus. These observations indicate that heat stress induces selective upregulation of vimentin expression. Interestingly this increase in vimentin immunoreactivity was absent in either the anaesthetised animals exposed to 4 h heat stress or conscious animals exposed to 1 h or 2 h heat stress (results not shown). These observations are in line with the idea that increased vimentin expression is associated with glial cell pathology.

Heat stress induces ultrastructural changes in glial cells

The results obtained with GFAP immunostaining suggest that glial cells are activated in heat stress. To further confirm this, in a few heat stressed animals, we examined the glial cell reaction at the ultrastructural level using transmission electron microscopy (Sharma and Cervós-Navarro, 1990a,b; Sharma et al., 1991a). For this purpose, tissue pieces from the cerebral cortex, hippocampus, cerebellum and brain stem were embedded in epon and processed for standard transmission electron microscopy as described earlier (Sharma and Cervós-Navarro, 1990a,b).

Our results show that many damaged astrocytes and oligodendrocytes can be seen in various brain regions of the heat stressed rats (Figs. 7 and 8). A representative example of glial cell damage in the vicinity of a nerve cell (Fig. 8) and a microvessel (Fig. 7) in the cerebral cortex and thalamus can be seen, respectively. Cell swelling, edema and membrane disruption are quite prominent in the glia following heat stress. These ultrastructural observations are in line with our immunohistochemical studies and further confirm that the glial cells are one of the important potential targets of heat-induced brain damage, not reported earlier.

Pharmacological manipulation of GFAP activation in heat stress

Our results with various drug treatments and GFAP immunoreactivity in heat stress are shown in Table 3. The drugs used in this investigation

Vimentin immunostaining

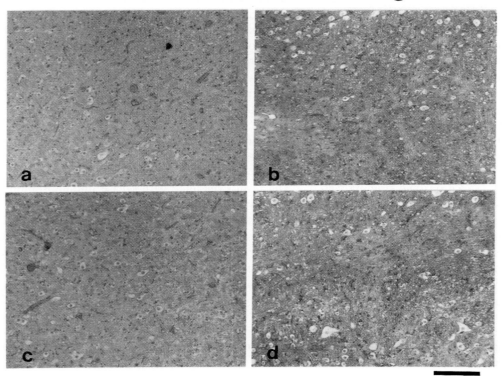

4 h heat stress 38° C

Fig. 6. Marked upregulation of vimentin immunostaining (seen as dark pink in colour) as a sign of strong gliosis in the brainstem raphe pontis (b) and cross-sectioned pontine fibre-tracts (d) of a 4 h heat stressed animal as compared to the normal rat (a, c) (bars: a–d: 250 μm).

are p-chlorophenylalanine (p-CPA), a serotonin synthesis inhibitor (Sharma and Cervós-Navarro, 1990a), indomethacin, a prostaglandin synthase inhibitor (Sharma et al., 1994), naloxone, an opioid receptor antagonist (Sharma et al., 1997b) or nimodipine, a calcium channel antagonist (Sharma and Cervós-Navarro, 1990b). Our results show that pretreatment with p-CPA, indomethacin, naloxone or nimodipine significantly reduced the GFAP positive cells in the CNS of heat-stressed rats (Table 3). The immunostaining of GFAP in these drug-treated stressed rats was very similar to that of the control group (Table 3). On the other hand, pretreatment with these drugs in normal animals however, did not influence the GFAP immunostaining (results not shown).

Heat stress alters fluid microenvironment of the brain

Changes in the fluid microenvironment of the brain in heat stress was examined by assessing the integrity of the BBB permeability. The BBB permeability was examined using Evans blue albumin extravasation in these rats (for details, see Sharma and Dey, 1986, 1987). In brief, a 2%

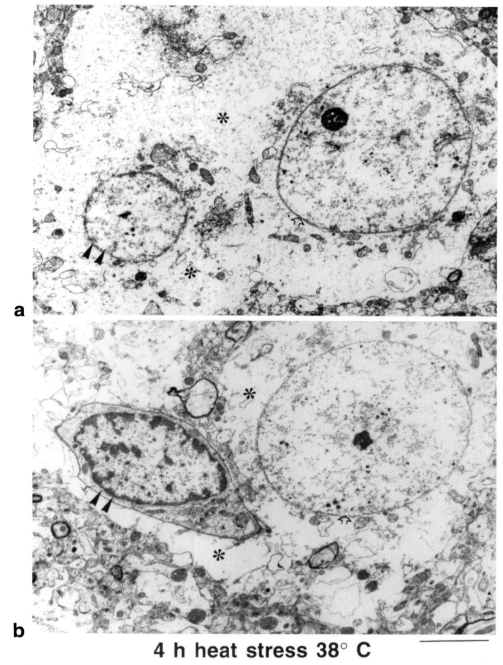

a

b

4 h heat stress 38° C

Fig. 7. High power electron micrograph showing swollen glial cell (arrow heads) around a nerve cell in the cerebral cortex (a) and thalamus (b) of a 4 h heat stressed rat. Membrane damage, vacuolation and edema (*) of the glial and nerve cell is quite distinct (bar = 300 nm).

vascular reaction and edema

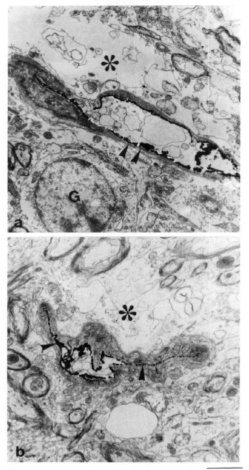

4 h heat stress 38° C

Fig. 8. Low power electron micrograph from the cerebral cortex (a) and brain stem (b) of a 4 h heat stressed rat. Signs of perivascular edema (*), vacuolation, membrane damage and myelin vesiculation are very common. Collapse of microvessels (filled arrow heads) and damage of one glial cell (G) is clearly visible (bar = 1.5 μm).

solution of Evans blue (0.3 ml/100 g body weight) was injected into the right femoral vein 3–5 min before perfusion (Sharma and Cervós-Navarro, 1990a). The intracerebrovascular dye was removed during saline infusion followed by perfusion with fixative solution. Before embedding the

brains for paraffin, the extravasation of Evans blue dye in the brain was visualised, using naked eye inspection (Table 4).

Subjection of conscious rats to 4-h heat stress resulted in a significant blue staining seen in many parts of the brain. However exposure of rats to a short duration of heat exposure or subjection of anaesthetised animals to 4 h heat stress did not result in blue staining of the brain except in non-barrier regions like the control group. These observations support the earlier observations of Sharma and Dey (1986) and further confirm that heat stress has the capacity to influence the brain fluid microenvironment depending on its magnitude and duration.

Investigations on BBB permeability in drug-treated rats suggest that pretreatment with p-CPA, indomethacin, naloxone or nimodipine significantly prevented the leakage of Evans blue in the brain after 4-h heat stress. These results further confirm our earlier observation that serotonin, prostaglandins, opioids and calcium channels are involved in the breakdown of the BBB permeability in heat stress (Sharma and Cervós-Navarro, 1990a,b; Sharma et al., 1994, 1997a,d).

Heat stress induces stress symptoms and alters physiological variables

In order to find a probable relationship with stress symptoms and the glial cell activation we observed the changes in body temperature, occurrences of salivation, behavioural prostration and gastric haemorrhages in the stomach (Sharma and Dey, 1986, 1987). In addition, the mean arterial blood pressure (MABP), arterial pH, P_aO_2 and P_aCO_2 were also examined (Table 5). Our results show that animals subjected to 4 h heat stress at 38°C exhibited marked hyperthermia (41.68 $\pm$ 0.36°C) compared to the control group (37.84 $\pm$ 0.28°C). Profuse salivation was noted in all animals, though the behavioural prostration was seen in more than 80% of the heat-stressed animals. At post-mortem examination, all the animals exhibited petechial haemorrhages in the gas-

TABLE 3

Effect of drugs on GFAP immunostaining in the CNS of 4-h heat-stressed rats

Region of the brain	GFAP immunostaining					
	Control $n = 5$	4 h HS $n = 6$	p-CPA $n = 6$	Indomethacin $n = 6$	Naloxone $n = 5$	Nimodipine $n = 6$
Cerebral cortex	+ / −	+ + +	+	+ / −	+	+
Hippocampus	+ / − ?	+ + + + +	+	+	+	+
Cerebellum	+ +	+ + + + +	+ +	+ +	+ + /?	+ + /?
Thalamus	+	+ + + + +	+	+	+	+ +
Hypothalamus	+ / −	+ + + +	+	+ +	+ +	+ +
Brain stem	+ +	+ + + + +	+ +	+ + /?	+ + /?	+ +
Spinal cord	+ / −	+ + + +	+ /?	+ /?	+	+ /?

− = negative, + = positive, ? = not seen in some cases; + = low, + + = mild, + + + = moderate, + + + + = high, + + + + + = very high.
Rats were subjected to acute heat exposure in a BOD incubator at 38°C (for details see text). The score of GFAP immunoreactivity was assigned arbitrarily by two independent workers in a blind fashion. The GFAP immunoreactivity on deparaffinised slides was developed using monoclonal anti GFAP sera and demonstrated using PAP technique. The slides from negative control (without primary antibody), control and heat stressed animals were processed simultaneously in parallel.
The drugs p-CPA (100 mg/kg/day, i.p. for 3 days, 1 day before heat stress), indomethacin (10 mg/kg, i.p., 30 min before heat stress), naloxone (10 mg/kg, i.p., 30 min before heat stress), nimodipine (2 μg/kg/min continuous infusion for 2 h before heat stress) were given in separate groups of rats according to the standard protocol (for details, see Sharma, Westman and Nyberg, this volume).

TABLE 4

Extravastion of Evans blue albumin in the CNS of 4-h heat-stressed rats and its modification with drugs

Region of the brain	Extravasation of Evans blue albumin					
	Control $n = 5$	4 h HS $n = 6$	p-CPA $n = 6$	Indomethacin $n = 6$	Naloxone $n = 5$	Nimodipine $n = 6$
Cerebral cortex	−	+ +	− / + ?	−	− / + ?	+ /?
Hippocampus	−	+ + +	−	−	−	−
Cerebellum	−	+ + +	−	− / + ?	−	−
Thalamus	−	+ + +	− / + ?	− / + ?	−	− / + ?
Hypothalamus	−	+ + +	−	−	−	−
Brain stem	−	+ + +	−	−	− / + ?	−
Spinal cord	−	+ +	−	−	−	− / + ?

The score of Evans blue extravasation was assigned arbitrarily by two independent workers in a blind fashion. The drugs p-CPA (100 mg/kg/day, i.p. for 3 days, 1 day before heat stress), indomethacin (10 mg/kg, i.p., 30 min before heat stress), naloxone (10 mg/kg, i.p., 30 min before heat stress), nimodipine (2 μg/kg/min continuous infusion for 2 h before heat stress) were given in separate groups of rats according to the standard protocol (for details see Sharma, Westman and Nyberg, this volume).
− = negative, + = positive; + + = mild, + + + = moderate, ? = uncertain some cases.

TABLE 5

Stress symptoms and physiological variables in control and heat-stressed animals

Type of experiment	Control $n = 6$	Heat stress at 38°C			
		4 h $n = 6$	2 h $n = 5$	1 h $n = 5$	4 h[a] $n = 5$
Stress symptoms					
Δ°C rectal temp.	+0.25 ± 0.01	+3.85 ± 0.06*	+1.25 ± 0.08*	+0.68 ± 0.04	+1.36 ± 0.16*
Salivation	Nil	+ + + +	+ +	+	+ +
Prostration	Nil	+ + +	Nil	Nil	Nil
Gastric ulcer	Nil	Many	Few	Nil	Few
Physiological variables					
MABP torr	110 ± 10	80 ± 8*	130 ± 10*	118 ± 12	98 ± 4
Arterial pH	7.37 ± 0.04	7.34 ± 0.08	7.36 ± 0.05	7.36 ± 0.04	7.35 ± 0.04
P_aO_2 torr	80.34 ± 0.64	82.56 ± 0.84*	81.56 ± 0.65	80.56 ± 0.89	81.34 ± 0.42
P_aCO_2 torr	34.33 ± 0.78	32.56 ± 0.89	33.73 ± 0.54	34.48 ± 0.81	34.24 ± 0.34

Animals were subjected to acute heat exposure in a BOD incubator at 38°C (for details see text). Data modified after Sharma et al. (1992). Values are mean ± S.D.
[a] Urethane anaesthetised.
*$P < 0.05$ Student's unpaired t-test, compared with control group.

tric mucosa. On the other hand, the animals with a shorter duration of heat exposure (1 h and 2 h) at 38°C or a similar duration of heat exposure (4 h) of anaesthetised rats showed only mild symptoms (Table 5). Subjection of animals to heat stress at 38°C for 4 h resulted in mild hypotension of about 20 ± 4 mmHg (Table 5). The P_aO_2 was significantly increased whereas, the P_aCO_2 values declined from the control value. The arterial pH was unaffected (Table 5).

Pretreatment with drugs however did not significantly attenuate the occurrence of stress symptoms and physiological variables (results not shown). These observations indicate that hyperthermia and other associated symptoms are not directly related to the magnitude of glial cell reaction or the BBB permeability disturbances.

Mechanisms of glial cell reaction in heat stress

Our results demonstrate a massive increase in the immunostaining of GFAP in selective brain regions in conscious young animals subjected to 4 h heat stress at 38°C. This observation strongly indicates that astrocytes are vulnerable in hyperthermic brain injury and further supports the idea that glial cells are involved in thermal information processing of the CNS.

This upregulation of GFAP immunoreactivity was not evident in animals subjected to a short duration (1 h and 2 h) of heat exposure indicating that the magnitude and severity of heat stress are important factors in eliciting astrocytic reaction in the CNS. Furthermore, subjection of urethane anaesthetised rats to 4 h heat exposure did not induce GFAP upregulation which is in line with the idea that stress caused by heat, rather than passive heating alone, is responsible for glial cell reaction.

Previously, activation of glial cell was thought to be a matter of late pathological outcome following traumatic, ischemic or hypoxic insult or in various neurodegenerative diseases of the CNS. Thus, increased GFAP immunostaining following trauma, stab wound, ischemia and hypoxia are described 48 h after the primary insult. An increase in GFAP-mRNA following ischemic insult to the brain was observed after 24 h by Cavicchioli et al. (1988). In contrast to these findings, our observations are the first to suggest that the expression of GFAP could be induced in the CNS even after a period of 4 h (the shortest survival period observed so far) following heat exposure. It appears that the severity and magnitude of noxious insult to the CNS, and alterations in the brain fluid microenvironment are important determining factors in precipitating glial cell reaction.

When the BBB is disrupted, numerous factors including many blood-born substances can activate the astrocytes (Arenander et al., 1988; Bologa et al., 1988; Gilad et al., 1990; Goldman and Abramson, 1990; Martin, 1992; Atwell, 1994; Chiu and Kriegler, 1994; Laping et al., 1994b; Barres, 1996; Deitmer and Rose, 1996). An increased BBB permeability following heat stress will thus lead to exposure of various neurotransmitters and ions to astrocytes (Sharma et al., 1997a,b,c,d). This could result in the alteration of the CNS microenvironment and swelling of astrocyte processes (Sharma et al., 1992a). This may alter the antigen reactivity causing an increase in antibody binding which would lead to an astrocytic reaction as reflected by in increase in immunocytochemical staining of GFAP (Sharma et al., 1992a,b, 1993). There are reports that neurochemicals may either directly or through second messengers like cAMP, exert their action on astrocytes resulting in a localised increase in GFAP immunoreactivity (Laping et al., 1994b; McMillan et al., 1994). However, in ischemia, a regional breakdown of the BBB and cellular damage are not apparently related to the increased GFAP immunostaining in the hippocampus (Schmidt-Kastner et al., 1990). This indicates a complex relationship between the time course and magnitude of the BBB opening, cell damage and astrocytic reaction.

That the breakdown of the BBB plays an essential role in GFAP activation is further shown by our observation that GFAP immunoreactivity was very similar to that of control animals in heat

stressed rats in which the BBB breakdown was prevented by pretreatment with various drugs (Table 4). Our results obtained with urethane anaesthetised animals in heat stress which did not exhibit either the breakdown of the BBB permeability or upregulation of GFAP are in line with this idea. These observations are the first direct evidence suggesting that alterations in the brain fluid microenvironment in the CNS plays an instrumental role in the glial cell reaction. Since these drug treatments in control rats did not elicit any major changes in the GFAP immunoreactivity of the CNS, a direct effect of these compounds on astrocytic activation seems most unlikely (Sharma et al., unpublished observations).

In rodent brain, the glial cells express the intermediate filament protein vimentin, during development before GFAP, and then either reduce or lose altogether this vimentin expression (Chiu and Goldmann, 1985). Increased expression of vimentin in adult brain following traumatic insults or ischemia is associated with glial cell pathology (Reifenberger et al., 1989). Thus, an increased expression of vimentin in young rats exposed to heat stress suggests that the glial cells are activated following heat injury and reflect the pathological alterations of astrocytes. This upregulation of vimentin immunostaining in heat stress also seems to be connected with the breakdown of the BBB and related disturbances in the brain fluid microenvironment (Sharma et al., 1992b).

The molecular mechanisms of increased GFAP immunostaining in heat stress are not well understood. In general, the response of astrocytes to a pathogenous noxa, consists of cell hyperplasia, hypertrophy and an increase in cell processes. The question whether hyperplasia takes place through mitoses is still under debate even though many mitoses are seen within a few days after injury within the wound. In long lasting brain injury as well as lengthy time after acute injury, the staining for GFAP well demonstrated the glial reaction, because the passage of astrocytes from the quiescent to the reactive state is accompanied by an increase of GFAP in relation to the development of processes: the filaments can migrate from the perinuclear position, giving rise to bundles converging on the cell processes. Our observation shows that an increased immunoreactivity of GFAP could be observed in early periods of survival following noxious heat stimulus depending on the severity and the magnitude of the primary insult to the CNS. Therefore, a mitotic activity does not seem to play a major role in the increase of GFAP immunostaining. Studies using double-labelling with GFAP antibodies and bromodeoxyuridine or tritiated thymidine to identify dividing astrocytes have shown that, at least in acute lesions, mitotic division (proliferation) of GFAP-expressing cells does not account for GFAP-positive cells that appear in the injury (Norton et al., 1992).

Since the turnover of GFAP in *in vivo* is slow and newly synthesised GFAP probably comprises only a small percentage of the existing pool, any change in the net accumulation would be detectable only after a long period of time. Increases in staining do not necessarily correlate with an increase in GFAP content or changes in its expression. Changes in antigen reactivity which might increase antibody binding or swelling of astrocyte processes, must be considered in such circumstances.

The term 'expression' should be used with some caution. In the lexicons of molecular biology, expression of a protein, beyond a basal level, connotes either an increase in the synthesis or, less frequently, a decrease of degradation of the protein in question. The immunoreaction is not quantitative and GFAP immunostaining intensity may not correlate with GFAP content (McLendon and Bigner, 1994). Cryogenic lesions in the rat brain reveal rapid increases in GFAP immunostaining without a detectable increase in GFAP content (Amaducci et al., 1981). Similarly, the early stages of experimental allergic encephalomyelitis reveal hypertrophy of astrocytic cell processes and intense GFAP immunoreactivity without an increase in GFAP content.

Thus, short-term changes may comprise biophysical and biochemical events such as transmembrane ion fluxes and post-translational modifications of pre-existing proteins. During the past decade, a wealth of data has been collected concerning short-term alterations that do not require de novo protein synthesis. The immediate early genes *fos*, *jun* and *Krox* belong to multigene families and constitute only a small part of the pool of rapidly inducible transcription factors (Bravo, 1990; Kiessling and Gass, 1994). They are thought to up- and down-regulate effector genes with preferential expression following various noxious stimuli in the CNS.

Astrogliosis is almost always associated with CNS damage. Thus, it may be difficult to discern whether astrocytes are the primary target of a disease process or are affected only secondarily. Very little is known about possible extracellular signals during regulating GFAP gene expression and the rapid GFAP synthesis during reactive astrogliosis. There are some indications of cAMP and protein kinase C involvement in this phenomena in cell culture studies (Condorelli et al., 1990).

Vasogenic edema was considered to be another important triggering mechanism of reactive astrocytosis for a long period of time (Schmidt-Kastner et al., 1990). Ultrastructural evidence suggests that enhanced exposure of epitopes may occur by disruption of the tight bundles of intermediate filaments secondary to edema. Swollen astrocytic processes filled with disrupted bundles of glial filaments and glycogen particles are well seen by electron microscopy in edematous brain tissue. The resulting edema allows the tight bundles of glial filaments to dissociate, resulting in more antigenic sites being available to GFAP antibodies (Eng et al., 1989). GFAP intermediate filament dissociation can also explain the rapid increase in GFAP staining following cryogenic lesions of the rat brain without an increase in GFAP content. Ultrastructural alterations in the astrocytes following heat exposure in this study further supports this contention.

The uneven regional distribution of GFAP immunostaining is markedly evident in heat stress. This uneven distribution of GFAP immunoreactivity in several brain areas following brain injury was observed previously. This indicates a heterogeneity in distinct subpopulations of astrocytes following injury (Miller et al., 1986). In chronic brain injury, the limbic cortex exhibits intensely stained evenly distributed astrocytes; the neocortex showed clearly stratified GFAP-staining with substantially less immunoreactivity occurring in the middle layers than in the areas close to the brain surface of the white matter; whereas, a regular staining pattern was observed in the hippocampus and the dentate gyrus. On the other hand, the striatum remained unstained in sharp contrast to the pallidum. In sham-operated animals, as well as in the contralateral side of the traumatic lesion in rats, the GFAP-stained astrocytes are present in the globus pallidus. Isacson et al. (1987) consistently found a larger area of GFAP-positive astrocytes in the traumatised hemisphere than those in the striatal and substantia nigra in control regions. Chronic hypoxia also revealed a marked increase in GFAP activity in specific brain regions (Zimmer et al., 1991). Thus, the remarkable consistency of GFAP-distribution reported from various laboratories working with different fixations and antisera suggests that this unevenness is neither accidental nor due to variations in staining methods (Kalman and Hajos, 1989). On the basis of these observations, Brenner (1994) suggested that the response of astrocytes can vary with the location within the CNS, which seems to be mediated or modified by interactions with the neighbouring non-neuroglial cells, such as nerve cells or endothelial cells.

The functional significance of such a selective increase in GFAP following heat stress is not known. It seems quite likely that local heterogeneity of astrocytes in terms of receptor bindings and sensitivity to neurochemical release from surrounding neurons may play an important role. The other possibility also exists that in heat stress, the regions involved in physiological mechanisms of thermal afferent sensation are more susceptible to hyperthermia-induced astrocytic reaction. The results obtained with GFAP immunostaining in the spinal cord are in line with this idea. Thus, the spinal cord dorsal horn exhibited a marked increase in GFAP-immunostaining in heat stress especially in the Rexe'd laminae I-II which is known to be involved in the pain and temperature pathways.

It may be that the increased expression of GFAP seems to be concomitant with the expression of heat shock proteins in glial cells. A robust glial heat shock response was demonstrated in in vitro studies (Nishimura et al., 1991). Also *in vivo* studies demonstrate a strikingly selective glial heat shock response (Marini et al., 1990). Accumulation of HSP 70 in astrocytic processes following hyperthermia is associated with accumulation of HSP in brain microvessels. This suggests that upregulation of HSP is involved in the changes of the BBB permeability. On the other hand, HSP presumably serve to protect cells after stress and promote cell recovery (Subjeck and Shyy, 1986). In this context, it is noteworthy that astrocytes synthesised significantly more HSP than neurons. However this aspect of cellular protection by HSP induction is still controversial (for details see Westman and Sharma in this volume).

Conclusion

Our results clearly demonstrate that the glial cells are one of the most important constituents of the CNS involved in the pathological mechanisms of hyperthermic brain injury. This activation of glial cells as evident from the marked increase in GFAP immunostaining depends on the magnitude and duration of heat exposure. Our observations further suggest that the glial cell activation is somehow related to alterations in the brain fluid microenvironment. Thus, a disruption of the BBB permeability reflecting a widespread alteration in the fluid microenvironment is found to be essential in precipitating glial cell reaction. This is further evident from the fact that pretreatment with drugs and anaesthesia which prevented the BBB disruption also prevented glial cell reaction. These observations are in line with our hypothesis that alteration in the brain fluid microenvironment plays an instrumental role in the pathophysiology of brain injury including neuroglial cell reaction.

Future direction

Our results provide strong experimental evidence that glial cells are involved in the pathological mechanisms of hyperthermic brain injury. Glial cells posses receptors to various neurochemicals and are involved in BBB function and synaptogenesis. Thus, it seems quite likely that glial cells are also involved in the physiological mechanisms of thermoregulation. However, this is a new subject which requires additional investigation.

The molecular mechanisms of GFAP upregulation in heat stress are still speculative. An increase in the number of astrocytes in a short survival period of 4 h is quite unlikely. Thus, an increase in the number of angiogenic site for binding of the GFAP antibodies, or a depolarisation of fibrillary acidic protein resulting in an increased exposure of antigenic sites, seems to be responsible for such an increased GFAP immunostaining in heat stress. A clear understanding of GFAP upregulation will emerge from studies using *in situ* hybridisation of specific GFAP mRNA with a cDNA probe in heat stress which is currently under investigation in our laboratory.

Acknowledgements

This study was supported by grants from the Swedish Medical Research Council Project 2710, Torsten and Ragner Söderberg Stiftelse, Sweden; Alexander von Humboldt Foundation, Bonn, Germany (HSS), University Grants Commission, New Delhi, India (HSS). The authors thank Professor P.K. Dey, Department of Physiology, Institute of Medical Sciences, Banaras Hindu University, Varanasi, India for extending laboratory facilities to HSS for animal experiments. The expert technical assistance of Kärstin Flink, Ingmarie Olsson, Katja Deparade, G. Kluge, R. Benz, R. Esparza and secretarial assistance of Angela Jan, Katherin Kern, and Aruna Misra are acknowledged with thanks.

References

Abd-el-Basset, E.M., Ahmed, I., Kalnins, V.I. and Fedoroff, S. (1992) Immuno-electron microscopical localization of vimentin and glial fibrillary acidic protein in mouse astrocytes and their precursor cells in culture. *Glia*, 6: 149–153.

Ahlsen, G., Rosengren, L. and Belfrange, M. (1993) GFAP in the cerebrospinal fluid of children with autism and other neuropsychiatric disorders. *Biol. Psychiatry*, 33: 734–743.

Althaus, H.H. and Siefert (1987) *Glial-neuronal Communication in Development and Regeneration*, Springer, Berlin.

Amaducci, L., Forno, K.I. and Eng, L.F. (1981) Glial fibrillary acid protein in cryogenic lesions of the rat brain. *Neurosci. Lett.*, 21: 27–32.

Arenander, A.T. and Vellis, J.D. (1984) Frontiers of glial physiology. In: *Neurobiology*, Vol. 53-91, Raven Press, New York.

Arenander, A.T., Lim, R., Varnum, B., Cole, R., Herschman, H.R. and de Villis, J. (1988) Astrocytes response to growth factors and hormones: early molecular events. In: P.J. Reier, R.P. Bunge and F.J. Seil (Eds.), *Current Issues in Neural Regeneration Research*, Alan R. Liss, New York, pp. 257–269.

Atwell, D. (1994) Glia and neurons in dialogue. *Nature*, 369: 707–708.

Austin, M.G. and Berry, J.W. (1956) Observation on one hundred cases of heatstroke. *J. Am. Med. Assoc.*, 161: 1525–1529.

Aquino, D.A., Chiu F.-C., Brosnan, C.F. and Norton, W.T. (1988) Glial fibrillary acidic protein increases in the spinal cord of Lewis rats with acute experimental autoimmune encephalomyelitis. *J. Neurochem.*, 51: 1085–1096.

Balcarek, J.M. and Cowan, N.J. (1985) Structure of the mouse glial fibrillary acidic protein gene: implications for the evolution of the intermediate filament multigene family. *Nucleic Acids Res.*, 13: 5527–43.

Barres, B.A. (1994) New roles for glia. *J. Neurosci.*, 11: 3685–3694.

Barres, B.A. (1996) Neuron-glial interaction. In: T.M. Jessel, L. Zipursky and M. Cowan (Eds.), *Neural Development*, Oxford University Press, Oxford.

Barrett, C.P., Donate, E.J. and Guth, L. (1984) Differences between adult and neonatal rats in their astroglial response to spinal injury. *Exp. Neurol.*, 84: 374–385.

Beck, D.W., Roberts, R.L. and Olson, J.J. (1986) Glial cells influence membrane-associated enzyme activity at the blood–brain barrier. *Brain. Res.*, 381: 131–137.

Bernstein, J.J. and Goldberg, W.J. (1987) Injury-related spinal cord astrocytes are immunoglobulin-positive (IgM and/or IgG) at different time periods in the regenerative process. *Brain Res.*, 426: 112–118.

Bignami, A., Dahl, D. and Rueger, D.C. (1980) Glial fibrillary acidic protein (GFAP) in normal neural cells and in pathological conditions. *Adv. Cell Neurobiol.*, 1: 285–319.

Black, K.L. (1995) Biochemical opening of the blood–brain barrier. *Adv. Drug Deliv. Rev.*, 15: 37–52.

Blatteis, C. (1997) Thermoregulation: Recent progress and new frontiers. *Ann. New York Acad. Sci.*, 813: 1–865.

Bologa, L., Cole, R., Chiappelli, F., Saneto, R.P. and De Villis, J. (1988) Expression of glial fibrillary acidic protein by differentiated astrocytes is regulated by serum antagonistic factors. *Brain Res.*, 457: 295–302.

Bongcam-Rudloff, E., Nister, M., Betsholtz, C., Wang, J.L., Stdenman, G., Huebner, K., Croce, C.M. and Westermark, B. (1991) Human glial fibrillary acidic protein: complementary DNA cloning, chromosome localization, and messenger RNA expression in human glioma cell lines of various phenotypes. *Cancer Res.*, 51: 1553–1560.

Bradbury, M.W.B. (1992) Physiology and pharmacology of the blood–brain barrier. *Handbook Exp. Pharmacol.*, 103: 1–450, Springer, Heidelberg.

Brahams, D. (1989) Heat stroke in training: a fatal case in Massachusetts. *Lancet*, ii: 1167.

Bravo, R. (1990) Growth factor responsive genes in fibroblasts. *Cell Growth Differ.*, 1: 305–309.

Bernier, L., Colman, D.R. and D'Eustachio, P. (1988) Chromosomal locations of genes encoding, 2′,3′ cyclic nucleotide, 3′-phosphodiesterase and glial fibrillary acidic protein in the mouse. *J. Neurosci. Res.*, 20: 497–504.

Brenner, M. (1994a) Glial fibrillary acidic protein (GFAP). *Brain Pathol.*, 4: 219–220.

Brenner, M. (1994b) Structure and transcriptional regulation of the GFAP gene. *Brain Pathol.*, 4: 245–257.

Brenner, M., Lampel, K., Nakatani, Y., Mill, J., Banner, C., Mearow, K., Dohadwala, M., Lipsky, R. and Freese, E. (1990) Characterization of human cDNA and genomic clones for glial fibrillary acidic protein. *Brain Res. Mol. Brain Res.*, 7: 277–286.

Brenner, M., Kisseberth, W.C., Su, Y., Besnard, F. and Messing, A. (1994) GFAP promoter directs astrocyte-specific expression in transgenic mice. *J. Neurosci.*, 14: 1030–1037.

Brownell, E., Lee, A.S., Pekar, S.K., Pravtcheva, D., Ruddle, F.H. and Bayney, R.M. (1991) Glial fibrillary acid protein, an astrocytic-specific marker, maps to human chromosome 17. *Genomics*, 10: 1087–1089.

Burger, F.J. and Fuhrman, F.A. (1969) Evidence of injury by heat in mammalian tissues. *Am. J. Physiol.*, 206: 1057–1061.

Calvo, J.L., Carbonell, A.L. and Boya, J. (1990) Coexpression of vimentin and glial fibrillary acidic protein in astrocytes of the adult rat optic nerve. *Brain Res.*, 532: 355–357.

Cavicchioli, L., Dickson, G., Prentice, H., Walsh, F.S., Vantini, G., Toffano, G. and Leon, A. (1988) Expression of the messenger RNA encoding the glial fibrillary acidic protein in rat basal forebrain following fimbria-fornix lesion. *Pharmacol. Res. Commun.*, 20: 609–610.

Cervós-Navarro, J. and Urich, H. (1995) *Metabolic and Degenerative Diseases of the Central Nervous System: Pathology, Biochemistry and Genetics*, Academic Press, New York, pp. 1–775.

Chiu, F.-C. and Goldmann, J.E. (1985) Regulation of glial fibrillary acidic protein (GFAP) expression in CNS development and in pathological states. *J. Neuroimmunol.*, 8: 283–292.

Chiu, S.Y. and Kriegler, S. (1994) Neurotransmitter-mediated signalling between axons and glial cells. *Glia*, 11: 191–200.

Cohen, I. and Schwartz, M. (1993) cDNA clones from fish optic nerve. *Comp. Biochem. Physiol. (b)*, 104: 439–447.

Condorelli, D.F., Dell'Albani, P., Kaczmarek, L., Messina, L., Spampinato, G., Avola, R., Messina, A. and Giuffrida Stella, A.M. (1990) Glial fibrillary acidic protein messenger RNA and glutamine synthetase activity after nervous system injury. *J. Neurosci. Res.*, 26: 251–257.

Deitmer, J.W. and Rose, C.R. (1996) pH regulation and proton signalling by glial cells. *Prog. Neurobiol.*, 48: 73–103.

Duffy, P.E. (1984) *Astrocytes, Normal, Reactive and Neoplastic*. Raven Press, New York.

Dusart, I., Marty, S. and Peschanski, M. (1991) Glial changes following an excitotoxic lesion in the CNS-II. Astrocytes. *Neuroscience*, 45: 541–549.

Eng, L.F., Vanderhaeghen, J.J., Bignami, A. and Gresti, B. (1971) An acidic protein isolated from fibrous astrocytes. *Brain Res.*, 28: 351–354.

Eng, L.F. (1985) Glial fibrillary acidic protein (GFAP):the major protein of glial intermediate filaments in differentiated astrocytes. *J. Neuroimmunol.*, 8: 203–214.

Eng, L.F. and Ghirnikar, R.S. (1994) GFAP and astrogliosis. *Brain Pathol.*, 4: 229–237.

Eng, L.F., D'Amelio, F.E. and Smith, M.E. (1989) Dissociation of GFAP intermediate filaments in EAE: observations in the lumbar spinal cord. *Glia*, 2: 308–317.

Eng, L.F., Yu, A.C.H. and Lee, Y.L. (1992) Astrocytic response to injury. In: *Neuronal–Astrocyte Interactions: Implications for Normal and Pathological CNS Function. Prog. Brain Res.*, 94: 353–365.

Ernsberger, P., Iacovitti, L. and Reis, D. (1990) Astrocytes cultured from specific brain regions differ in their expression of adrenergic binding sites. *Brain Res.*, 517: 202–208.

Fedoroff, S. and Vernadakis, A. (1986) *Astrocytes*, Vols. 1–3, Academic Press, Orlando.

Feinstein, D.L., Weinmaster, G.A. and Milner, R.J. (1992) Isolation of cDNA clones encoding rat glial fibrillary acidic protein: expression in astrocytes and in Schwann cells. *J. Neurosci. Res.*, 32: 1–14.

Field, J. (II), Fuhrman, F.A. and Martin, A.W. (1944) Effect of temperature on the oxygen consumption of the brain tissue. *J. Neurophysiol.*, 7: 117–126.

Frankel, H.M., Ellis (Jr), J.P. and Cain, S.M. (1963) Development of tissue hypoxia during progressive hyperthermia in dogs. *Am. J. Physiol.*, 205: 733–737.

Galea, E., Dupouey, P. and Feinstein, D.L. (1995) Glial fibrillary acidic protein mRNA isotypes: expression *in vitro* and *in vivo*. *J. Neurosci. Res*, 41: 452–461.

Galou, M., Colucci-Guyon, E., Ensergueix, D., Ridet, J.L., Gimenez, Y., Ribotta, M., Privat, A., Babinet, C. and Dupouey, P. (1996) Disrupted glial fibrillary acidic protein network in astrocytes from vimentin knockout mice. *J. Cell Biol.*, 133: 853–863.

Galou, M., Pournin, S., Ensergueix, D., Ridet, J.L., Tchelingerian, J.L., Lossouarn, L., Privat, A., Babinet, C. and Dupouey, P. (1994) Normal and pathological expression of GFAP promoter elements in transgenic mice. *Glia*, 12: 281–293.

Gilad, G.M., Shanker, G., Dahl, D. and Gilad, V.H. (1990) Dibutyryl cyclic AMP-induced changes in neuron-astroglia interactions and fibronectin immunocytochemistry in dissociated rat cerebellar cultures. *Brain Res.*, 508: 215–224.

Gillett, G. (1989) Another British soldier dies from heat illness. *Lancet*, ii: 1229.

Giordana, M.T. (1990) Neurocytogenesis and tumor development in the rat. *J. Neurosurg. Sci.*, 34: 167–170.

Glees, P. (1955) Neuroglia. *Morphology and Function.* Blackwell, Oxford.

Goldman, J.E. and Abramson, B. (1990) Cyclic AMP-induced shape changes of astrocytes are accompanied by rapid depolymerization of actin. *Brain Res.*, 528: 189–196.

Gomi, H.T.Y., Fujimoto, K., Ikeda, T., Katoh, A., Itoh, T. and Itohara, S. (1996) Mice devoid of the glial fibrillary acidic protein develop normally and are susceptible to scrapie prions. *Neuron*, 14: 29–41.

Gorny, M., Losy, J. and Wedner, M. (1990) Anti-GFAP antibodies in the cerebrospinal fluid of patients with multiple sclerosis and other neurologic diseases. *Neurol. Neurochir. Pol.*, 24: 17–22.

Goshgarian, H.G., Yu, X.-J. and Rafols, J.A. (1989) Neuronal and glial changes in the rat phrenic nucleus occurring within hours after spinal cord injury. *J. Comp. Neurol.*, 284: 519–533.

Gottschalk, P.G. and Thomas, J.E. (1966) Heat stroke. *Mayo Clin. Proc.*, 41: 470–482.

Graeber, M.B. and Kreutzberg, G.W. (1986) Astrocytes increase in glial fibrillary acidic protein during retrograde changes of facial motor neurones. *J. Neurocytol.*, 15: 363–373.

Hajos, F. and Kalman, M. (1989) Distribution of glial fibrillary acidic protein (GFAP)-immunoreactive astrocytes in the rat brain. II. Mesencephalon, rhombencephalon and spinal cord. *Exp. Brain Res.*, 78: 164–173.

Haydon, P.G. and Drapeau, P. (1995) From contact to connection: early events during synaptogenesis. *Trends Neurosci.*, 18: 196–201.

Hertz, L. (1981) Features of astrocytic function apparently involved in the response of central nervous tissue to ischemia-hypoxia. *J. Cereb. Blood Flow Metabol.*, 1: 143–153.

Hozumi, I., Aquino, D.A. and Norton, W.T. (1990) GFAP mRNA levels following stab wounds in rat brain. *Brain Res.*, 534: 291–294.

Isacson, O., Fischer, W. and Wictrorin, K. (1987) Astroglial response in the excitotoxically lesioned neostriatum and its projection areas in the rat. *Neuroscience*, 20: 1043–1056.

Janzer, R.C. and Raff, M.C. (1987) Astrocytes induce blood–brain barrier properties in endothelial cells. *Nature*, 325: 253–257.

Jones, B.W., Fetter, R.D., Tear, G. and Goodman, C.S. (1995) Glial cells missing: a genetic switch that controls glial versus neuronal fate. *Cell*, 82: 1013–1023.

Juurlink, B.H.J. and Devon, R.M. (1990) Macromolecular translocation — a possible function of astrocytes. *Brain Res.*, 533: 73–77.

Kaiser, R. and Lucking, C.H. (1993) GFAP-specific oligoclonal bands in the CSF of a patient with acute myelitis. *Acta Neurol. Scand.*, 88: 94–96.

Kalman, M. and Hajos, F. (1989) Distribution of glial fibrillary acidic protein (GFAP)-immunoreactive astrocytes in the rat brain. I. Forebrain. *Exp. Brain Res.*, 78: 147–163.

Kaneko, R. and Sueoka, N. (1993) Tissue-specific versus cell type-specific expression of the glial fibrillary acidic protein. *Proc. Natl. Acad. Sci. USA*, 90: 4698–4702.

Kettenmann, H. and Ransom, B.R. (1995) *Neuroglia*, Oxford University Press, New York.

Kiessling, M. and Gass, P. (1994) Immediate early gene expression in focal ischemia. *Brain Pathol.*, 4: 77–83.

Kimelberg, H.K. and Ransom, B.R. (1986) Physiological and pathological aspects of astrocytic swelling. In: S. Federoff and A. Vernadakis (Eds.) *Astrocytes*, Vol. 3. Cell Biology and Pathology of Astrocytes, Academic Press, Orlando, pp. 129–166.

Kimelberg, H.K. and Kettenmann, H. (1990) Swelling-induced changes in electrophysiological properties of cultured astrocytes and oligodendrocytes. *Brain Res.*, 529: 255–268.

Kumanishi, T., Usui, H., Ichikawa, T., Nishiyama, A., Katagiri, T., Abe, S., Yoshida, Y., Washiyama, K., Kuwano, R. and Sakimura, K. (1992) Human glial fibrillary acidic protein (GFAP): molecular cloning of the complete cDNA sequence and chromosomal localization (chromosome 17) of the GFAP gene. *Acta Neuropathol.*, 83: 569–578.

Landis, D.M.D. (1994) The early reactions of non-neural cells to brain injury. *Annu. Rev. Neurosci.*, 17: 133–151.

Landis, D.M.D. and Reese, T.S. (1982) Regional organisation of astrocytic membrane in cerebral cortex. *Neuroscience*, 7: 937–950.

Laping, N.J., Nichols, N.R., Day, J.R., Johnson, S.A. and Finch, C.E. (1994a) Transcriptional control of glial fibrillary acidic protein and glutamine synthetase *in vivo* shows opposite responses to corticosterone in the hippocampus. *Endocrinology*, 135: 1928–1933.

Laping, N.J., Teter, B., Nichols, N.R., Rozovsky, I. and Finch, C.E. (1994b) Glial fibrillary acidic protein: regulation by hormones, cytokines, and growth factors. *Brain Pathol.*, 4: 259–275.

Lavialle, M. and Serviere, J. (1995) Developmental study in the circadian clock of the golden hamster: a putative role of astrocytes. *Brain Res. Dev. Brain Res.*, 86: 275–282.

Le Prince, G., Delaere, P., Fages, C., Duyckaerts, C., Hauw, J.J. and Tardy, M. (1993) Alterations of GFAP mRNA level in the ageing brain and in senile dementia of the Alzheimer type. *Neurosci. Lett.*, 151: 71–73.

Leigh, I.M. and Lane, E.B. (1993) Mutation in the genes for epidermal keratins in epidermolysis bullosa and epidermolytic hyperkeratosis. *Arch. Dermatol.*, 129: 1571–1577.

Lewis, S.A., Balcarek, J.M., Krek, V., Shelanski, M. and Cowan, N.J. (1984) Sequence of a cDNA clone encoding mouse glial fibrillary acidic protein: structural conservation of intermediate filaments. *Proc. Natl. Acad. Sci. USA*, 81: 2743–2746.

Liedtke, W., Edelmann, W., Bieri, P.L., Chiu, F.-C, Cowan, N.J., Kucherlapati, R. and Raine, C.S. (1996) GFAP is necessary for the integrity of CNS white matter architecture and long-term maintenance of myelination. *Neuron*, 17: 607–615.

Ling, E.A. and Leblond, C.P. (1973) Investigation of glial cells in semithin sections. II. Variation with age in the numbers of the various glial cell types in rat cortex and corpus callosum. *J. Comp. Neurol.*, 149: 73–81.

Lu, X., Quinlan, R.A., Steel, J.B. and Lane, E.B. (1993) Network incorporation of intermediate filament molecules differs between preexisting and newly assembling filaments. *Exp. Cell Res.*, 208: 218–225.

Lum, H. and Malik, A.B. (1994) Regulation of vascular endothelial barrier function. *Am. J. Physiol.*, 267: 223–241.

Lynch, G. (1976) Normal and glial responses to the destruction of input: the 'deafferentiation syndrome'. In: P. Scheinberg (Ed.), *Cerebrovascular Diseases*, Raven Press, New York, pp. 209–227.

Marini, A.M., Kozuka, M., Lipsky, R.H. and Nowak Jr, T.S. (1990) 70-kilodalton heat shock protein induction in cerebellar astrocytes and cerebellar granule cells *in vitro*: Comparison with immunocytochemical localization after hyperthermia *in vivo*. *J. Neurochem.*, 54: 1509–1516.

Martin, D.L. (1992) Synthesis and release of neuroactive substances by glial cells. *Glia*, 5: 81–94.

McMillan, M.K., Thai, L., Hong, J.-S., O'Callaghan, J.P. and Pennypacker, K.R. (1994) Brain injury in a dish: a model for reactive gliosis. *Trends Neurosci.*, 17: 138–142.

Masood, K., Besnard, F., Su, Y. and Brenner, M. (1993) Analysis of a segment of the human glial fibrillary acidic protein gene that directs astrocyte-specific transcription. *J. Neurochem.*, 61: 160–166.

Maxwell, K., Berliner, J.A., Cancilla, P.A. (1987) Induction of γ-glutamyl transpeptidase in cultured cerebral endothelial cells by a product released by astrocytes. *Brain Res.*, 410: 309–314.

McCall, M.A., Gregg, R.G., Behringer, R.R., Brenner, M., Delaney, C.L., Galbreath, E.J., Zhang, C.L., Pearce, R.A., Chiu, S.Y. and Messing, A. (1996) Targeted deletion in astrocyte intermediate filament (GFAP) alters neuronal physiology. *Proc. Natl. Acad. Sci. USA*, 93: 6361–6366.

McCarthy, K., Salm, A. and Lerea, L. (1988) Astroglial receptors and their regulation of intermediate filament phosphorylation. In: H. Kimelberg (Ed.), *Glial Cell Receptors*, Raven Press, New York, pp. 1–18.

McLendon, R.E. and Bigner, D.D. (1994) Immunohistochemistry of the glial fibrillary protein: Basic and applied considerations. *Brain Pathol.*, 4: 221–228.

Miller, R.H., Abney, E.R., David, S., French-Constant, C., Lindsay, R., Patel, R., Stone, J. and Raff, M.C. (1986) Is reactive gliosis a property of a distinct subpopulation of astrocytes? *J. Neurosci.*, 6: 22–29.

Milton, A.S. (1993) *Physiology of Thermoregulation*, Birkhauser, Basel, pp. 1–405.

Miura, M., Tamura, T. and Mikoshiba, K. (1990) Cell-specific expression of the mouse glial fibrillary acidic protein gene: identification of the *cis*- and *trans*-acting promoter elements for astrocyte-specific expression. *J. Neurochem.*, 55: 1180–1188.

Morgan, T.E., Nichols, N.R., Pansinetti, G.M. and Finch, C.E. (1993) TGF-fl1 mRNA increases in macrophage/microglial cells of the hippocampus in response to deafferentiation and kainic acid-induced neurodegeneration. *Exp. Neurol.*, 120: 291–301.

Morrison, R.S., De Vellis, J., Lee, Y.L., Bradshaw, R.A. and Eng, L.F. (1985) Hormones and growth factors induce the synthesis of glial fibrillary acidic protein in rat brain astrocytes. *J. Neurosci. Res.*, 14: 167–176.

Mucke, L., Oldstone, M.B., Morris, J.C. and Nirenberg, M.I. (1991) Rapid activation of astrocyte-specific expression of GFAP-lacZ transgene by focal injury. *New Biol.*, 3: 465–474.

Murphy, S. and Pearce, B. (1987) Functional receptors for neurotransmitters on astroglial cells. *Neuroscience*, 22: 381–394.

Nakanishi, K., Okouchi, Y., Ueki, T., Asai, K., Isobe, I., Eksioglu, Y.Z., Kato, T., Hasegawa, Y. and Kuroda, Y. (1994) Astrocytic contribution to functioning synapse formation estimated by spontaneous neuronal intracellular Ca^{2+} oscillations. *Brain Res.*, 659: 169–178.

Nakatani, Y., Brenner, M. and Freese, E. (1990) An RNA polymerase II promoter containing sequences upstream and downstream from the RNA startpoint that direct initiation of transcription from the same site. *Proc. Natl. Acad. Sci. USA*, 87: 4289–4293.

Nishimura, R.N., Dwyer, B.E., Clegg, K., Cole, R. and de Vellis, J. (1991) Comparison of the heat shock response in cultured cortical neurons and astrocytes. *Mol. Brain Res.*, 9: 39–45.

Norton, W.T., Aquino, D.A., Hozumi, I., Chiu, F.C. and Brosnan, C.F. (1992) Quantitative aspects of reactive gliosis: a review. *Neurochem. Res.*, 17: 877–885.

Orkand, R.K. (1983) Glial cells. In: *Handbook of Physiology, The Nervous System*, Vol. I, pp. 855–875.

Pfrieger, F.W. and Barres, B.A. (1996) New views on synapse–glia interactions. *Curr. Opin. Neurobiol.*, 6: 615–621.

Pekny, M., Leveen, P., Pekna, M., Eliasson, C., Berthold, C.H., Westermark, B. and Betsholtz, C. (1995) Mice lacking glial fibrillary acidic protein display astrocytes devoid of intermediate filaments but develop and reproduce normally. *EMBO J.*, 14: 1590–1598.

Pellegrino, L.J., Pellegrino, A.S. and Cushman, A.J. (1979) *A Stereotaxic Atlas of the Rat Brain*, 2nd edn., Plenum Press, New York, pp. 1–122.

Peters, A., Palay, S.L. and Webster, H.F. (1991) *The Fine Structure of the Nervous System: The Neurons and Supporting Cells*, Oxford University Press, Oxford.

Petito, C.K., Morgello, S., Felix, J.C. and Lesser, M.L. (1990) The two patterns of reactive astrocytes in postischemic rat brain. *J. Cereb. Blood Flow Metabol.*, 10: 850–859.

Pixley, S.K. and De Vellis, J. (1984) Transition between radial glia and mature astrocytes studied with a monoclonal antibody vimentin. *Dev. Brain Res.*, 15: 201–209.

Quinlan, R.A. and Franke, W.W. (1983) Molecular interactions in intermediate-sized filaments revealed by chemical cross-linking. Heteropolymers of vimentin and glial filament protein in cultured human glioma cells. *Eur. J. Biochem.*, 132: 477–484.

Raine, C.S. and Bornstein, M.B. (1970) Experimental allergic encephalomyelitis — An ultrastructural study of experimental demyelination *in vitro*. *J. Neuropathol. Exp. Neurol.*, 29: 552–564.

Rall, G.F., Mucke, L., Nerenberg, M. and Oldstone, M.B. (1994) A transgenic mouse model to assess the interaction of cytotoxic T lymphocytes with virally infected, class I MHC-expressing astrocytes. *J. Neuroimmunol.*, 52: 61–68.

Reeves, S.A., Helman, L.J., Allison, A. and Israel, M.A. (1989) Molecular cloning and primary structure of human glial fibrillary acidic protein. *Proc. Natl. Acad. Sci. USA*, 86: 5178–5182.

Reifenberger, G., Bilzer, T., Seitz, R.J. and Wechsler, W. (1989) Expression of vimentin and glial fibrillary acidic protein in ethylnitrosourea-induced rat gliomas and glioma cell lines. *Acta Neuropathol.*, 78: 270–282.

Riol, H., Fages, C. and Tardy, M. (1992) Transcriptional regulation of glial fibrillary acidic protein (GFAP)-mRNA expression during postnatal development of mouse brain. *J. Neurosci. Res.*, 32: 79–85.

Rogaev, E., Rogaeva, E.K. and Ginter, E. (1993) Identification of the genetic locus for keratosis palmaris et plantaris on chromosome 17 near the RARA and keratin 1 genes. *Nat. Genet.*, 5.

Rosenberg, M., Raychaudhury, A., Shows, T.B., Lebeau, M.M., Fuchs, E. (1988) A group of type 1 keratin genes on human chromosome 17: Characterization and expression. *Mol. Cell Biol.*, 8: 722–736.

Rubin, L.L. and Sanes, J.R. (1996) Neuronal and glial cell biology. *Curr. Opin. Neurobiol.*, 6: 573–575.

Sarid, J. (1991) Identification of a *cis*-acting positive regulatory element of the glial fibrillary acidic protein gene. *J. Neurosci. Res.*, 28: 217–228.

Sarkar, S. and Cowan, N.J. (1991a) Intragenic sequences affect the expression of the gene encoding glial fibrillary acidic protein. *J. Neurochem.*, 57: 675–684.

Sarkar, S. and Cowan, N.J. (1991b) Regulation of expression of glial filament acidic protein. *J. Cell Sci.*, Suppl. 15: 97–102.

Schiffer, D., Giordana, M.T., Migheli, A., Giaccone, G., Pezzotta, S. and Mauro, A. (1986) Glial fibrillary acidic protein and vimentin in the experimental glial reaction of the rat brain. *Brain Res.*, 374: 110–118.

Schmidt-Kastner, R., Szymas, J. and Hossman, K.-A. (1990) Immunohistochemical study of glial reaction and serum protein extravasation in relation to neuronal damage in rat hippocampus after ischemia. *Neuroscience*, 38: 527–540.

Schonrich, G., Kalinke, U., Momburg, F., Malissen, M., Schmitt-Verhulst, A.M., Malissen, B., Hammerling, G.J. and Arnold, B. (1991) Down-regulation of T cell receptors on self-reactive T cells as a novel mechanism for extrathymic tolerance induction. *Cell*, 65: 293–304.

Sharma, H.S. (1982) *Blood-Brain Barrier in Stress*, Ph.D. thesis, Banaras Hindu University, Varanasi, India.

Sharma, H.S. and Dey, P.K. (1984) Role of 5-HT on increased permeability of blood–brain barrier under heat stress. *Indian J. Physiol. Pharmacol.*, 28: 259–267.

Sharma, H.S., Dey, P.K. and Ashok Kumar (1986) Role of circulating 5-HT and lung MAO activity in physiological processes of heat adaptation in conscious young rats. *Biomedicine*, 6: 31–40.

Sharma, H.S. and Dey, P.K. (1986) Probable involvement of 5-HT in increased blood–brain barrier permeability under heat stress in young rats. *Neuropharmacology*, 25: 161–167.

Sharma, H.S. and Dey, P.K. (1987) Influence of long-term acute heat exposure on regional blood–brain barrier permeability, cerebral blood flow and 5-HT level in conscious normotensive young rats. *Brain Res.*, 424: 153–162.

Sharma, H.S. and Cervós-Navarro, J. (1990a) Brain edema and cellular changes induced by acute heat stress in young rats. *Acta Neurochir. (Wien),*, Suppl. 51: 383–386.

Sharma, H.S. and Cervós-Navarro, J. (1990b) Nimodipine improves cerebral blood flow and reduces brain edema, cellular damage and blood–brain barrier permeability following heat stress in young rats. In: J. Krieglstein and H. Oberpichler (Eds.), *Pharmacology of Cerebral Ischemia, 1990*, CRC Press, Boca Raton, FL, pp. 303–310.

Sharma, H.S., Cervós-Navarro, J. and Dey, P.K. (1991a) Acute heat exposure causes cellular alteration in cerebral cortex of young rats. *NeuroReport*, 2: 151–154.

Sharma, H.S., Cervós-Navarro, J. and Dey, P.K. (1991b) Rearing at high ambient temperature during later phase of the brain development enhances functional plasticity of the CNS and induces tolerance to heat stress: An experimental study in the conscious normotensive young rats. *Brain Dysfunct.*, 4: 104–124.

Sharma, H.S., Zimmer, C., Westman, J. and Cervós-Navarro, J. (1992a) Acute systemic heat stress increases glial fibrillary acidic protein immunoreactivity in brain. An experimental study in the conscious normotensive young rats. *Neuroscience*, 48: 889–901.

Sharma, H.S., Kretzschmar, R., Cervós-Navarro, J., Ermisch, A., Rühle, H.-J. and Dey, P.K. (1992b) Age-related pathophysiology of the blood-brain barrier in heat stress. *Prog. Brain Res.*, 91: 189–196.

Sharma, H.S., Westman, J., Nyberg, F., Cervós-Navarro, J. and Dey, P.K. (1992c) Role of serotonin in heat adaptation an experimental study in the conscious young rat. *Endocrin. Regul.*, 26: 133–142.

Sharma, H.S., Olsson, Y. and Cervós-Navarro, J. (1993) p-Chlorophenylalanine, a serotonin synthesis inhibitor, reduces the response of glial fibrillary acidic protein induced by trauma to the spinal cord. *Acta Neuropathol. (Berlin)*, 86: 422–427.

Sharma, H.S., Westman, J., Nyberg, F., Cervós-Navarro, J. and Dey, P.K. (1994) Role of serotonin and prostaglandins in brain edema induced by heat stress. An experimental study in the rat. *Acta Neurochir.*, Suppl. 60: 65–70.

Sharma, H.S., Westman, J., Cervós-Navarro, J., Dey, P.K. and Nyberg, F. (1996a) Probable involvement of serotonin in the increased permeability of the blood–brain barrier by forced swimming. An experimental study using Evans blue and ^{131}I-sodium tracers in the rat. *Behav. Brain Res.*, 72: 189–196.

Sharma, H.S., Westman, J., Cervós-Navarro, J. and Nyberg, F. (1996b) A 5-HT$_2$ receptor mediated breakdown of the blood–brain barrier permeability and brain pathology in heat stress. An experimental study using cyproheptadine and ketanserin in young rats. In: P. Couraud and A. Scherman (Eds.), *Biology and Physiology of the Blood–Brain Barrier*, Plenum Press, New York, pp. 117–124.

Sharma, H.S., Westman, J. and Nyberg, F. (1998) Brain edema and cell changes following hyperthermic brain injury. In: H.S. Sharma and J. Westman (Eds.), *Brain Function in Hot Environment. Prog. Brain Res.*, Elsevier, Amsterdam, pp. 351–412.

Sharma, H.S., Westman, J., Cervós-Navarro, J., Dey, P.K. and Nyberg, F. (1997b) Opioid receptor antagonists attenuate heat stress induced reduction in cerebral blood flow, increased blood-brain barrier permeability, vasogenic edema and cell changes in the rat. *Ann. New York Acad. Sci.*, 813: 559–571.

Sharma, H.S., Westman, J., Alm, P., Sjöquist P-Ö, Cervós-Navarro, J. and Nyberg, F. (1997c) Involvement of nitric oxide in the pathophysiology of acute heat stress in the rat. influence of a new antioxidant compound H 290/51. *Ann. New York Acad. Sci.*, 813: 581–590.

Sharma, H.S., Westman, J., Cervós-Navarro, J., Dey, P.K. and Nyberg, F. (1997d) Blood–brain barrier in stress: a gateway to various brain diseases. In: R. de Kloet, D. Ben-Nathan and R. Levy (Eds.), *New Frontiers of Stress: Modulation of Brain Function*, Harwood, Amsterdam.

Sharp, G., Osborn, M. and Weber, K. (1982) Occurrence of two different intermediate filament proteins in the same filament in situ within a human glioma cell line. An immunoelectron microscopical study. *Exp. Cell Res.*, 141: 385–395.

Shibolet, S., Coll, R., Gilat, T. and Sohar, E. (1967a) Heatstroke: its clinical picture and mechanism in, 36 cases. *Q. J. Med.*, 36: 525–548.

Shibolet, S., Lancaster, M.C. and Danon, Y. (1967b) Heat stroke: a review. *Aviat. Space Environ. Med.*, 47: 280–301.

Siesjö, B.K. (1978) *Brain Energy Metabolism*, Wiley, Chichester, pp. 324–344.

Sminia, P., van der Zee, J., Wondergem, J. and Haveman, J. (1994) Effect of hyperthermia on the central nervous system: a review. *Int. J. Hypertherm.*, 10: 1–30.

Smith, S.J. (1994) Neuromodulatory astrocytes. *Curr. Biol.*, 4: 807–810.

Staddon, J.M. and Rubin, L.R. (1996) Cell adhesion, cell junctions and the blood-brain barrier. *Curr. Opin. Neurobiol.*, 6: 622–627.

Stagaard Janas, M., Nowakowski, R.S. and Mollgard, K. (1991a) Glial cell differentiation in neuron-free and neuron-rich regions. II. Early appearance of S-100 protein positive astrocytes in human fetal hippocampus. *Anat. Embryol.*, 184: 559–569.

Stagaard Janas, M., Nowakowski, R.S., Terkelsen, O.B. and Mollgard, K. (1991b) Glial cell differentiation in neuron-free and neuron-rich regions. I. Selective appearance of S-100 protein in radial glial cells of the hippocampal fimbria in human fetuses. *Anat. Embryol.*, 184: 549–558.

Sterner, S. (1990) Summer heat illness. *Postgrad. Med.*, 87: 67–73.

Subjeck, J.R. and Shyy, T.T. (1986) Stress protein of mammalian cells. *Am. J. Physiol.*, 250: (Cell. Physiol., 19) C1–C17.

Takashima, S. and Becker, L.E. (1983) Developmental changes of glial fibrillary acidic protein in cerebral white matter. *Arch. Neurol.*, 40: 14–18.

Tao-Cheng, J.-H. and Brightman, M.W. (1988) Development of membrane interactions between brain endothelial cells and astrocytes *in vitro*. *Int. J. Dev. Neurosci.*, 6: 25–37.

274

Toggas, S.M., Masliah, E., Rockenstein, E.M., Rall, G.F., Abraham, C.R. and Mucke, L. (1994) Central nervous system damage produced by expression of the HIV-1 coat protein gp120 in transgenic mice. *Nature*, 367: 188–193.

Tomokane, N., Iwaki, T., Tateishi, J., Iwaki, A. and Goldman J.E. (1991) Rosenthal fibers share epitopes with Beta-crystallin, GFAP, and ubiquitin, but not with vimentin. *Am. J. Pathol.*, 138: 875–885.

Torres-Aleman, I., Rejas, M.T., Pons, S. and Garcia-Segura, L.M. (1992) Estradiol promotes cell shape changes and glial fibrillary acidic protein redistribution in hypothalamic astrocytes *in vitro*: a neuronal-mediated effect. *Glia*, 6: 180–187.

Tsacopoulos, M. and Magistretti, P.J. (1996) Metabolic coupling between glia and neurons. *J. Neurosci.*, 16: 877–885.

Varon, S. and Somjen, G. (1979) Neuron–glial interactions. *Neurosci. Res. Prog. Bull.*, 17: 1–239.

Vaughn, J.E. (1989) Fine structure of synaptogenesis in the vertebrate central nervous system. *Synapse*, 3: 255–285.

Verderber, L., Johnson, W., Mucke, L. and Sarthy, V. (1995) Differential regulation of a glial fibrillary acidic protein-LacZ transgene in retinal astrocytes and Muller cells. *Invest. Ophthalmol. Vis. Sci.*, 36: 1137–1143.

Virchow, R. (1846) Uber das granulirte Aussehen der Wandungen der Gehirnventrikel. *Allg. Z. Psychiat.*, 3: 242–250.

Voronina, A.S. and Preobrazhensky, A.A. (1994) Developmental expression of glial fibrillary acidic protein gene in human embryos. *Neurosci. Lett.*, 174: 198–200.

Walz, W. (1989) Role of glial cells in the regulation of the brain ion microenvironment. *Prog. Neurobiol.*, 33: 309–333.

Westman, J. and Sharma, H.S. (1998) Heat shock protein response in the central nervous system in heat stress. In: H.S. Sharma and J. Westman (Eds.), *Brain Function in Hot Environment*, Elsevier, Amsterdam, this volume.

Whitaker-Azmita, P.A., Murphy, R. and Azmita, E.C. (1990) Stimulation of astroglial 5-HT1A receptors releases the serotonergic growth factor, protein S-100, and alters astroglial morphology. *Brain Res.*, 528: 155–158.

Wiegers, W., Honer, B. and Traub, P. (1991) Microinjection of intermediate filament proteins into living cells with and without preexisting intermediate filament network. *Cell Biol. Int. Rep.*, 15: 287–296.

Yu, A.C.H., Gregory, G.A. and Chan, P.H. (1989) Hypoxia-induced dysfunction and injury of astrocytes in primary cell cultures. *J. Cereb. Blood Flow Metabol.*, 9: 20–28.

Zelenika, D., Grima, B., Brenner, M. and Pessac, B. (1995) A novel glial fibrillary acidic protein mRNA lacking exon, 1. *Brain Res. Mol. Brain Res.*, 30: 251–258.

Zeisburger, E., Schönbaum, E. and Lomax, P. (1994) *Thermal Balance in Health and Diseases. Recent Basic Research and Clinical Progress*, Adv. Pharmacol. Sci., Birkhauser, Basel, pp. 1–485.

Zimmer, J. and Sunde, N. (1984) Neuropeptides and astroglia in intracerebral hippocampal transplants: an immunohistochemical study in the rat. *J. Comp. Neurol.*, 227: 331–347.

Zimmer, C., Sampaolo, S., Sharma, H.S. and Cervós-Navarro, J. (1991): Glial fibrillary acidic protein immunoreactivity in rat brain following chronic hypoxia. *Neuroscience*, 40: 353–361.

H.S. Sharma and J. Westman (Eds.)
Progress in Brain Research, Vol 115
© 1998 Elsevier Science BV. All rights reserved.

CHAPTER 15

Prostaglandin system in the brain: sites of biosynthesis and sites of action under normal and hyperthermic states

Kiyoshi Matsumura[1,2]*, Chunyu Cao[2], Yumiko Watanabe[1,2], Yasuyoshi Watanabe[1,2]

[1]*Subfemtomole Biorecognition Project, Japan Science and Technology Corporation*
[2]*Department of Neuroscience, Osaka Bioscience Institute, Furuedai 6-2-4, Suita, Osaka 565, Japan*

Introduction

Fever and hyperthermia are essentially distinct patho-physiological states, the former representing regulated elevation of the body temperature caused by immunological challenge and the latter representing its passive elevation caused by excessive heat load. In fact, inhibitors of prostaglandin (PG) synthesis, such as indomethacin, suppress fever but are not effective against hyperthermia. Febrile patients feel chilled whereas hyperthermic patients feel hot. In spite of these apparent distinctions, however, there is a common feature between fever and hyperthermia in that PG is involved in both. The involvement of PG in fever is well established and has been reviewed by Milton (1982). As for hyperthermia, Sharma et al. (1994) showed that in hyperthermic rats whose body temperature was raised to around 41°C by exposure to 38°C for 4 h, formation of edema, extravasation of plasma protein, and cellular damage took place in their brains. When the rats were pretreated with indomethacin, these pathological changes were greatly reduced. In addition, although body temperature was elevated by the

heat stress in both untreated and indomethacin-pretreated rats, the elevation was slightly but significantly smaller in the latter group. These results suggest that PGs are involved in the development of pathological changes associated with hyperthermia and that the hyperthermia itself might be partly mediated by PGs. PGs are also suspected to be the key molecules in other types of pathological conditions of the central nervous system. Release of PGs is dramatically increased by ischemia/reperfusion of the brain or by traumatic injury of the central nervous system (reviewed by Bazan et al., 1995), and treatment with a cyclooxygenase inhibitor, such as indomethacin, improves the neuronal injury (Sasaki et al., 1988; Sharma et al., 1993a,b, 1995). The onset and progression of Alzheimer's disease may also be slowed by the treatment with cyclooxygenase inhibitors (Rogers et al., 1993; Breitner et al., 1994). Thus, PGs are the key molecules involved in pathological changes in the central nervous system.

Since the first discovery of PG in the spermic fluid in 1930 (Kurzrok and Lieb, 1930), a huge number of studies have revealed the molecular nature of PGs, the enzymes involved in PG biosynthesis, and the receptors for PGs, not only in peripheral organs but also in the central ner-

---

*Corresponding author.

vous system (see reviews: Shimizu and Wolfe, 1990; Smith et al., 1991; Coleman et al., 1994). In contrast to the progress made in the molecular characterization, the physiological functions of PGs, especially those in the brain, largely remain to be elucidated. For further understanding of the functions of PGs in the brain under physiological as well as pathological states, such as hyperthermia, it is indispensable to clarify the localization of each molecule of the PG system in the brain. In this chapter, we review recent progress in research on the brain PG system with special attention paid to the *in vivo* location of enzymes involved in their biosynthesis and of their specific receptors under physiological as well as pathological conditions.

Enzymes involved in the biosynthesis of PGs

It is well established that PGs are biosynthesized from membrane phospholipids through three enzymatic steps (Smith et al., 1991). First, phospholipase A_2 (PLA_2) cleaves arachidonic acid from the membrane phospholipids. Arachidonic acid is then converted to PGH_2 by cyclooxygenase (COX). Although PGH_2 itself is biologically active in the blood vessel, all other active PGs are biosynthesized from PGH_2 by PG isomerases. In this enzymatic cascade, PLA_2 and COX are common to all PGs and are considered to play rate-limiting roles in the synthesis of PGs.

Phospholipase A_2

Three types of PLA_2s are well characterized in mammals. They are classified into cytosolic PLA_2 ($cPLA_2$) and secretory PLA_2 ($sPLA_2$). $sPLA_2$ is further divided into type I (pancreatic type) and type II (nonpancreatic type) (Glaser et al., 1993). In the brain, $cPLA_2$ and type-II $sPLA_2$ are either constitutively present or induced under some pathological conditions. Although several other proteins having PLA_2 activity have been found in the peripheral tissues or in cell lines derived from peripheral origins, their presence and significance in the brain remain to be elucidated.

$cPLA_2$

$cPLA_2$ is of high molecular weight (85 kDa for the human one), located in the cytoplasm, and activated by micromolar concentrations of Ca^{2+} (Clark et al., 1990, 1991; Yoshihara and Watanabe, 1990). Upon activation, $cPLA_2$ is translocated to the cell or nuclear membrane, where it exerts its enzymatic activity to release arachidonic acid from membrane phospholipids. Short-term regulation of $cPLA_2$ activity is thus accomplished by the intracellular Ca^{2+} level. Another mode of short-term regulation of $cPLA_2$ may be phosphorylation by mitogen-activated protein kinase (MAPK) and protein kinase C (PKC) (Exton, 1994). For the longer term, $cPLA_2$ can be induced by cytokine stimulation (Ozaki et al., 1994; Qvist et al., 1995) or as a consequence of brain ischemia (Bonventre and Koroshetz, 1993).

As for its localization in the brain, only limited information is available. Stephenson et al. (1994) showed by use of immunohistochemistry that $cPLA_2$-like immunoreactivity was located in the astrocytes of the gray matter in the human occipital cortex. No neuron was positively stained there. Since they only examined the occipital cortex, it is uncertain if this observation holds true for other brain regions as well. On the other hand, Owada et al. (1994) cloned cDNA for rat $cPLA_2$ and demonstrated using *in situ* hybridization that in normal rat brain, a faint but significant level of $cPLA_2$ mRNA was expressed in the neurons of the olfactory bulb, hippocampus, and cerebellum. After ischemic insult, expression of $cPLA_2$ mRNA was markedly enhanced in the hippocampal dentate granule cells (neurons) but not in those neurons of other brain regions. In the cell culture systems, both neuronal cells (Kim et al., 1995) and glial cells were reported to express $cPLA_2$ (Morii et al., 1994; Ozaki et al., 1994; Qvist et al., 1995).

Type-II $sPLA_2$

Type-II $sPLA_2$ is of low molecular weight (14 kDa), present in various types of cells, and is secreted in response to proinflammatory mediators such as interleukin-1 (see references in Glaser et al., 1993). In contrast to cPLA$_2$, type-II sPLA$_2$ requires millimolar concentrations of Ca^{2+} to be active. This means that type II sPLA$_2$ exerts its enzymatic activity only after having been secreted into the extracellular space. From the outside of the cells, this enzyme hydrolyzes membrane phospholipid to release arachidonic acid, which may either enter the cell again for further conversion to PGs or directly act on the cells from the outside. This enzyme is considered to play a significant role in the inflammation of the peripheral tissues.

In the brain, again only limited information is available on the location of this enzyme. Lauritzen et al. (1994) showed, using the *in situ* hybridization technique, that type-II sPLA$_2$ mRNA was not expressed in the normal brain. However, when rats were injected with LPS, the mRNA for this enzyme dramatically increased in the entire brain, with a particularly high level in the thalamus, caudate-putamen, hippocampus, and so on. In the same study, type-II sPLA$_2$ mRNA was also induced after global cerebral ischemia and reperfusion, but this induction was restricted to the hippocampus and cerebral cortex. Although the exact cell type was not identified, the mRNA-positive structures in the hippocampal layers seemed to well correspond to neuronal cells. On the other hand, Oka and Arita (1991) demonstrated that sPLA$_2$ is released from rat astrocyte cultures in response to inflammatory stimuli such as LPS and tumor necrosis factor.

Apparently, further studies are necessary to determine the location of cPLA$_2$ and sPLA$_2$ in the brain. Since both enzymes are induced by ischemia, their role in neuronal cell death associated with brain ischemia is suspected. In this context, they also could be involved in the pathological changes in the brain associated with hyperthermia.

Cyclooxygenase

The second enzyme involved in the synthesis of PGs is cyclooxygenase, which is also called prostaglandin endoperoxide synthase or PGH synthase (Smith et al., 1991). This enzyme catalyzes two chemical reactions that are from arachidonic acid to PGG$_2$ and then, from PGG$_2$ to PGH$_2$. Until recently, only one type of cyclooxygenase, constitutively expressed in various tissues, was recognized. In 1991, two research groups independently reported similar mRNA sequences that were immediately induced by stimuli such as a viral infection or phorbol ester treatment and whose deduced amino acid sequences were highly homologous to the previously determined sequence of cyclooxygenase (Kujubu et al., 1991; Xie et al., 1991). Soon thereafter, it was confirmed that the protein encoded by the mRNA sequence possessed enzymatic activity identical to that of cyclooxygenase (Fletcher et al., 1992). The former type of cyclooxygenase is now called cyclooxygenase-1 (COX-1), whereas the latter newly recognized one is called cyclooxygenase-2 (COX-2).

COX-1

COX-1 is constitutively expressed in various types of tissues, where it is considered to play physiological roles rather than pathological ones (Goppelt-Struebe, 1995). For example, COX-1 is present in the stomach mucosa and is responsible for mucosal protection.

Location of COX-1 in the brain

Before the discovery of COX-2, the location of COX-like immunoreactivity in the brain was investigated by two groups, one using monkeys (Tsubokura et al., 1991) and the other, sheep (Breder et al., 1992). Both groups used antibodies raised against cyclooxygenase from sheep seminal vesicle, which mainly consisted of COX-1. The former group showed in the monkey brain that both neuronal and glial cells contained COX-like immunoreactivity. On the other hand, the latter researchers demonstrated in sheep that almost all positive staining was neuronal. In both studies, neuronal staining was particularly prominent in the telencephalic regions including the cerebral cortex and hippocampus. It is also noteworthy in the latter study that COX-like immunoreactivity was present in the organum vasculosum laminae terminalis (OVLT), a circumventricular organ lacking the blood–brain barrier and supposedly being critical for the signaling of the brain by circulating cytokines. Unfortunately, however, neither of these studies examined the cross-reactivity of their antibodies to COX-2, probably because COX-2 had not been identified when these studies were carried out. Since COX-1 and COX-2 are highly homologous to each other, those antibodies might well have recognized both forms of COX. Thus, it is uncertain if the positively stained cells contained COX-1 or COX-2. In primary cultures of rat brain, however, Kawasaki et al. (1993) found that COX-1 mRNA and its protein were expressed in the neuronal cells but not in glial ones, although the expression was only transient. Location of COX-1 mRNA in the brain was reported by Li et al. (1993), who used an oligonucleotide antisense cDNA probe for their study. Positive signals were observed most prominently in the granular cell layer of the cerebellum followed by the pyramidal and granular cell layers of the hippocampus. As these regions contain a dense neuronal cell population, the majority of signals therefore seemed to be from neurons.

COX-2

Since the first two reports on COX-2 in 1991 (Kujubu et al., 1991; Xie et al., 1991), induction of COX-2 have been found in various types of cells with various types of stimulation (Goppelt-Struebe, 1995). One of the important findings among these studies is that inflammatory mediators, such as lipopolysaccharide (LPS), interleukin-1 (IL-1), and tumor necrosis factor (TNF), are potent stimuli for induction of COX-2 in various types of cells. In contrast, COX-1 was little affected by these stimuli. In addition, dexamethasone, a synthetic anti-inflammatory corticosteroid, was found to suppress COX-2 induction in some types of cells (Goppelt-Struebe, 1995). These results strongly suggest a significant role for COX-2 in the inflammatory response. The development of COX-2 specific inhibitors facilitated the elucidation of the role of COX-2 in

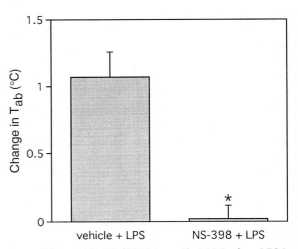

Fig. 1. Effect of NS-398 (COX-2-specific inhibitor) on LPS-induced fever. Adult male rats were pretreated with either NS-398 (3 mg/kg, i.p.) or its vehicle (400 μl of 50% DMSO) 1 h before LPS injection (100 μg/kg in 400 μl saline, i.p.). Abdominal temperature (T_{ab}) was monitored with a temperature transmitter implanted at least 1 week before the experiment. The values were obtained 2.5 h after the LPS treatment (the late rising phase of T_{ab}). Six to eight rats were used in each condition. *$P < 0.01$ vs. vehicle control.

the inflammatory process. One of the potent COX-2-specific inhibitors is NS-398 (Futaki et al., 1994), which inhibits COX-2 activity with an IC_{50} value of only a few μM, but does not affect COX-1 activity up to 100 μM. In contrast, indomethacin, a popular nonsteroidal anti-inflammatory drug (NSAID), inhibits both COX-1 and COX-2 equipotently. In an *in vivo* experimental model of inflammation, s.e., the carrageenan-air-pouch, NS-398 suppressed inflammation as well as PGE_2 production in the inflamed tissue (Futaki et al., 1993; Masferrer et al., 1994). These results suggested the possibility that COX-2 is also involved in fever. Indeed, oral administration of NS-398 suppressed fever in rats that had been injected with LPS intravenously (Futaki et al., 1993). We also confirmed the antipyretic action of NS-398 by using different timing and route of administration. When rats were pretreated with NS-398 (3 mg/kg, i.p.) 1 h prior to the LPS administration (100 μg/kg, i.p.), the subsequent fever was significantly suppressed (Fig. 1). Therefore, the location of COX-2, particularly that induced by pyrogens, in the brain would seem to be of importance in terms of the site of PGE_2 production during fever.

Location of COX-2 in the brain

The site of COX-2 mRNA in the brain was first reported in 1993 by Yamagata et al. (1993). They found that one of the genes induced in the rat brain by electrical convulsion coded for a protein nearly identical to that of murine COX-2. This group revealed using the *in situ* hybridization technique that COX-2 mRNA was constitutively expressed in the neurons of some discrete telencephalic regions including the cerebral cortex, hippocampus, and amygdala. Thus, the brain is an exceptional organ where COX-2 mRNA is constitutively expressed. The level of COX-2 mRNA in the neurons was, however, highly dependent on the neuronal activity; electrical convulsion or treatment with excitatory amino acid increased the amount of COX-2 mRNA, whereas an NMDA receptor antagonist decreased it. The increase in COX-2 mRNA was restricted in the telencephalic neurons after electrical activation. Neither neurons of other regions nor non-neuronal cells such as glia showed COX-2 mRNA signals. Distribution of COX-2-like immunoreactivity (COX-2-ir) in the rat brain was reported by Breder et al. (1995). Since COX-2 has a unique amino acid sequence near its carboxyl terminus, they were able to raise a specific antibody to COX-2 using this synthetic peptide region as an immunogen. The distribution of COX-2-ir was mostly in line with that of COX-2 mRNA in the telencephalic regions, although some differences were suggested in the hypothalamic and lower brain stem regions; however, the reasons for the differences are yet unknown.

Induction of COX-2 mRNA in the brain by pyrogens

In order to clarify the brain sites where COX-2 is induced by pyrogenic stimuli, we conducted a series of experiments using in situ hybridization techniques (Cao et al., 1995). Rats were either left untreated or injected with LPS (100 μg/kg in 400 μl saline, i.p.) or saline, and sacrificed at four time points after the injection. The time course of fever and the timing of sacrificing of the rats for *in situ* hybridization are shown in Fig. 2. Their brain sections were processed for *in situ* hybridization with a ^{35}S-labeled antisense cRNA probe for rat COX-2 or its sense cRNA probe as a negative control. Between the rats untreated and those injected with saline, no difference was observed in the distribution or intensity of COX-2 mRNA signals in the brain. In accordance with the results obtained by Yamagata et al. (1993), the brain sections from these rats showed constitutive expression of COX-2 mRNA in the neurons of discrete telencephalic regions (Fig. 3a for macroscopic view and Fig. 4A for light microscopic view). In addition, we found a low but significant level of COX-2 mRNA signal constitutively expressed in the OVLT (Fig. 4B), although the exact cell type still remains to be identified. One hour after the LPS injection (Fig. 3b), at which time the body temperature of the rats had not yet started to rise, the COX-2 mRNA signal in the telencephalic regions was slightly enhanced. At the same time, spot-like COX-2 mRNA signals appeared in both the telencephalic and non-telencepalic regions. This type of signal dramatically increased in number and intensity 2.5 h after the LPS injection (Fig. 3c), the time point corresponding to the late rising phase of fever. Similar signals were also observed in the brain surface. Microscopic observation revealed that the spot-like signals in the brain parenchyma were from the inner side of a certain type of blood vessel (Fig. 4C,D) and those in the brain surface were from yet identified cells in the leptomeninges (arachnoid membrane and pia matter; Fig. 4E). The induced COX-2 mRNA remained at a high level 4 h after the LPS injection (plateau phase of fever) (Fig. 3d). Seven hours after the LPS injection (falling phase of fever), the spot-like signals disappeared, and the signals from the telencephalic neurons returned to the preinjection level (Fig. 3e). Thus, in the brains of LPS-treated rats, COX-2 mRNA was induced in two distinct ways, i.e. a slight enhancement in the telencephalic neurons and a remarkable induction in the blood vessels and leptomeninges. Intraperitoneal injection of other pyrogenic cytokines, including interleukin-1β (Cao et al., 1996) and TNF-α (our unpublished observation), also resulted in a similar pattern of COX-2 mRNA induction in the blood vessels and leptomeninges. In contrast, interleukin-6, which was not pyrogenic when injected intraperitoneally, did not yield any COX-2 mRNA in these non-neuronal cells (our unpublished observation). Furthermore, detailed examination of the adjacent sections arranged in mirror image suggested that the vascular cells expressing COX-2 mRNA in response to IL-1β (Fig. 4 F1, G1) also expressed mRNAs for intercellular adhesion molecule-1 (ICAM-1; Fig. 4 F2) and IL-1 receptor type-1 (Fig. 4 G2) (Cao et al., 1996). Endothelial cells but not smooth muscle cells in the vessel were reported to express ICAM-1. Therefore, the COX-2 mRNA-positive cells in the blood vessels seem to be endothelial cells possessing the IL-1 type 1 receptor, suggesting that IL-1 in the blood acts on its receptor on

the endothelial cells and thereby induces COX-2.

How do these changes in COX-2 mRNA after a pyrogenic challenge relate to fever? In order to clarify their causal relation, we examined the possible correlation between fever and expression of COX-2 mRNA under several conditions in which either fever or COX-2 mRNA were experimentally manipulated. First, in rats that had been pretreated with the COX-2-specific inhibitor, intraperitoneal injection of LPS did not evoke fever (Fig. 1) but induced COX-2 mRNA in the blood vessels/leptomeninges and also slightly increased the level of neuronal COX-2 mRNA in the telencephalic regions (Cao et al., 1997). This result implies that the induction of COX-2 mRNA in both cellular groups were not the result of fever. Second, rats were made tolerant to LPS by repeated injections of LPS (400 μg/kg) every 3 or 4 days for a total of 10 times. In these rats, injection of LPS (100 μg/kg) induced neither fever nor COX-2 mRNA in the blood vessels/leptomeninges. On the other hand, COX-2 mRNA in the neurons was similar to that in the non-tolerant rats. When 10 rats were pretreated with LPS (100 μg/kg) at longer intervals (once a week) four times, the 5th injection of LPS resulted in various degrees of fever ranging from 0.2°C to 1.6°C among the 10 rats. In these rats, the magnitude of fever was well correlated with the level of COX-2 mRNA in the blood vessels/leptomeninges but not with that in the telencephalic neurons (Cao et al., 1997). These results suggest a close correlation between fever and vascular COX-2 mRNA. Thirdly, under urethane anesthesia, the basal level of neuronal COX-2 dramatically decreased and was only slightly enhanced by LPS. In contrast, under the same conditions, LPS induced both vascular COX-2 mRNA and fever (Cao et al., 1997). Taken together, these results support the idea that COX-2 mRNA in the blood vessels/leptomeninges is involved in fever.

Induction of COX-2 mRNA by LPS was also demonstrated by Breder and Saper (1996) in the mouse brain after systemic LPS treatment. The result was in line with ours in that non-neuronal cells were more sensitive to LPS than neuronal

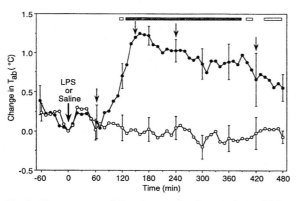

Fig. 2. Time courses of T_{ab} change after intraperitoneal injection of LPS (100 μg/kg) or its vehicle (400 μl of saline). Each value represents the mean $\pm$ S.E. of five rats. The change in T_{ab} was significantly different between LPS- and saline-injected rats in the time periods denoted by the dotted ($P < 0.01$) and open ($P < 0.05$) bars. The thick arrow indicates the time of injection; and the thin arrows, the time points at which the rats were sacrificed for the *in situ* hybridization study [from Cao et al. (1995), reprinted from *Brain Research* with kind permission of Elsevier Science B.V., Amsterdam, The Netherlands].

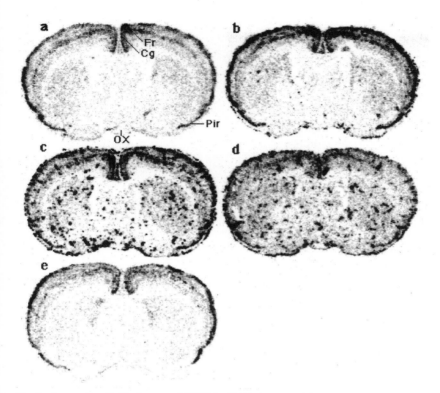

Fig. 3. Autoradiographic images of COX-2 mRNA in coronal brain sections of rats either untreated (a) or injected with LPS and sacrificed 1 h (b), 2.5 h (c), 4 h (d), or 7 h (e) after the LPS injection. Five rats were examined for each time point. Under ether anesthesia, the rats were perfused with saline followed by 4% paraformaldehyde. *In situ* hybridization was performed with a ^{35}S-labeled cRNA probe directed to 1 kb of rat COX-2 3′ cDNA sequence. The sections contain the optic chiasma (OX), rostral wall of the third ventricle, and preoptic area. Fr; frontal cortex, Cg; cingulate cortex, Pir; piriform cortex [from Cao et al. (1995), reprinted from *Brain Research* with kind permission of Elsevier Science B.V. Amsterdam, The Netherlands].

ones in expressing COX-2 mRNA. However, some discrepancies were noted on the types of cells responded to LPS. They demonstrated that choroid plexus and perivascular cells were positive for the mRNA while, in our case, induction of COX-2 mRNA in the choroid plexus was marginal and the COX-2 mRNA positive cells were likely to be the endothelial cells. These discrepancy may be, at least partly, explained by the differences of the animal species and of the dose of LPS.

COX-2 mRNA and its protein are also induced by transient focal ischemia in the rat brain (Planas et al., 1995). In this case, however, the majority of responsive cells were neurons. Thus, there seem to be two major sources of PGs in the brain. One source would be the non-parenchymal cells, including the cells in the leptomeninges and blood vessels (and possibly in the choroid plexus), where inflammatory stimuli, such as LPS and cytokines, induce COX-2 and subsequently enhance production of PGs. The second source would be the neuronal cells, where non-inflammatory stimuli, such as ischemia/reperfusion (Planas et al., 1995) and convulsion (Yamagata et al., 1993), induce COX-2 and enhance production of PGs. The pathophysiological roles of PGs in the latter case largely remain to be elucidated.

Enzymes downstream of COX

Biologically active PGs, i.e. PGE_2, PGD_2, $PGF_{2\alpha}$,

282

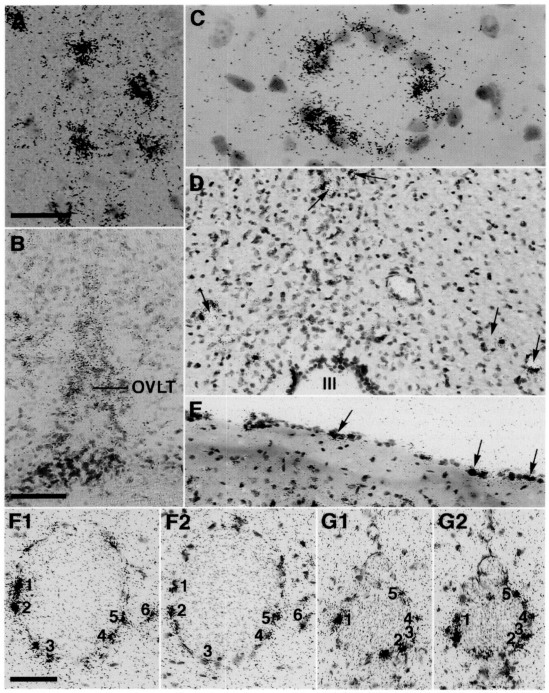

Fig. 4. Microautoradiographic view of COX-2 mRNA in the rat brain. (A) Under normal conditions, COX-2 mRNA signals (black dots) were present in the telencephalic neurons. (B) Under normal conditions, COX-2 mRNA signals were present in the organum

PGI$_2$, and thromboxane A$_2$, are isomerized from PGH$_2$ by enzymes specific for production of each PG. Up to the present, synthases for PGD$_2$, PGF$_{2\alpha}$, PGI$_2$, and thromboxane A$_2$ have been cloned and their molecular nature characterized (Watanabe et al., 1988; Yokoyama et al., 1991; Hara et al., 1994; Urade et al., 1995). Their brain location has, however, only been analyzed in detail for PGD$_2$ synthase. Among three distinct proteins possessing PGD$_2$ synthase activity, one form (glutathione-independent PGD synthase) is abundant in the brain (Urade et al., 1995). Immunoreactivity and mRNA for this type of PGD synthase were predominantly located in the leptomeninges and choroid plexus in the adult rat brain (Urade et al., 1987). Interestingly, PGD$_2$ synthase was found to be identical to one of the major constituent proteins in the cerebrospinal fluid (CSF) (Watanabe et al., 1994). This suggests that PGD synthase produced in the choroid plexus and leptomeninges is secreted into the CSF. PGD synthase in the CSF might be involved in the widespread control of brain function. Indeed, PGD$_2$ has a potent somnogenic action when applied to the ventral surface of the basal forebrain (Matsumura et al., 1994).

PGs

The existence of all biologically active PGs in the brain has been demonstrated in a large number of biochemical studies (Ogorochi et al., 1984). Their cellular localization is, however, poorly understood. This seems to be mainly due to the difficulty in the fixation of PGs in the tissue for histological study. There are two reports on the location of PGE$_2$-like immunoreactivity and one on that of PGF$_{2\alpha}$-like immunoreactivity. Fujimoto et al. (1992) reported that PGE$_2$ in the brain seems to be present in two components. PGE$_2$ in the first component could be extracted with ethanol, whereas the residual PGE$_2$ (second component) was extracted with HCl-acidified ethanol. The amount of PGE$_2$ in the first component was well affected by treatment with indomethacin or pentylenetetrasole, an convulsion inducer, which are known to decrease or increase PGE$_2$, respectively. On the other hand, PGE$_2$ in the second component did not change after either treatment. They reported that PGE$_2$-like immunoreactivity found in the histological study seemed to represent PGE$_2$ in the second component because the staining was resistant to ethanol, disappeared after treatment with ethanol plus HCl, and was not changed by indomethacin or pentylenetetrasole. In contrast, van Dam et al. (1993) reported that under normal conditions, no PGE$_2$-like immunoreactivity (PGE$_2$-ir) was present in the neurons and glial cells but faint staining was observed in the choroid plexus and microvasculature in the cortex. After administration of a large amount of lipopolysaccharide, PGE$_2$-ir was enhanced in the choroid plexus, microvessels, and paraventricular and supraoptic nuclei in the hypothalamus.

Ogawa et al. (1988) examined the localization of PGF$_{2\alpha}$-like immunoreactivity (PGF$_{2\alpha}$-ir) in the

---

vasculosum laminae terminalis (OVLT). Since the intensity of the signal in the OVLT is weaker than that of the telencephalic neurons, the signal in the OVLT region was not evident in the macroautoradiography (Fig. 2). (C) COX-2 mRNA signal appeared in the blood vessels 2.5 h after LPS injection (100 μg/kg, i.p.). Note that the signals are restricted to the inner side of the blood vessel. (D) Arrows indicate COX-2 mRNA-positive small blood vessels (arrows) in the rostro-medial part of the preoptic area 2.5 h after LPS injection. III, the third ventricle. (E) Arrows indicate COX-2 mRNA-positive cells in the leptomeninges 2.5 h after LPS injection. (F) Localization of COX-2 mRNA (F1) and ICAM-1 mRNA (F2) in the same blood vessel 4 h after intraperitoneal injection of recombinant human IL-1β (30 μg/kg). Two adjacent sections were arranged in a mirror image to obtain the same surface exposed to each cRNA probe. To facilitate the comparison of their location, one of the images was reversed in this figure. The corresponding numbers in the figures indicate that the signals seem to be from the same cells. G; Localization of COX-2 mRNA (G1) and IL-1 type-1 receptor mRNA (G2) in the same blood vessel 4 h after IL-1β. The details are the same as those in (F). Scale bars in A, B, and F1 represent 20 μm, 100 μm, and 50 μm, respectively. The scale bar in A is also for C, that in B is also for D and E, and that in F1 is also for F2, G1, and G2.

brains of rats that had been made anoxic for 30 s to 3 min and then reoxygenated for 5 min. Under normal conditions, only pial blood vessels were faintly positive for $PGF_{2\alpha}$-ir. Anoxia resulted in the occurrence of $PGF_{2\alpha}$-ir in the neurons of the hippocampus and cerebellum, the intensity being higher with longer anoxia. Interestingly, pretreatment with indomethacin suppressed the occurrence of $PGF_{2\alpha}$-ir in the neurons of anoxic rats.

Receptors for PGs

The variety of biological actions of PGs led to the notion that there should be specific receptors for each PG within the body. In the 1980s, receptors for PGE_2 (Malet et al., 1982; Ueno et al., 1985; Yumoto et al., 1986), PGD_2 (Shimizu et al., 1982; Ueno et al., 1985; Tokumoto et al., 1986) and $PGF_{2\alpha}$ (Malet et al., 1982) in the brain were demonstrated by analyzing the binding of radiolabeled PGs to the membrane fraction of the brain. These studies provided detailed information on their biochemical nature, i.e. dissociation constant, amount of receptor, ligand specificity, coupling to G proteins, and so on; however, little information was obtained on their localization in the brain. Since the first demonstration of the location of PGD_2 receptors in the rat brain (Yamashita et al., 1983), Watanabe and his colleagues have intensively studied the brain sites for receptors of PGE_2, $PGF_{2\alpha}$, and PGI_2 by the use of the *in vitro* receptor autoradiographic technique. Distinct localization of each PG receptor was demonstrated in adjacent monkey brain sections (Watanabe et al., 1989).

Molecular cloning of cDNAs for PG receptors first succeeded in 1991, revealing the structure of the human thromboxane A_2 receptor (Hirata et al., 1991). Based on the homology with the nucleotide sequence of TX receptor cDNA, cDNAs for all other PG receptors have been cloned and expressed in cultured cell lines for further characterization (Ushikubi et al., 1995). The receptor proteins are all coupled to G proteins and have seven transmembrane domains as a common feature of G-protein-coupled receptors. It is now possible to study the brain location of PG receptor mRNA by the use of the *in situ* hybridization technique. Comparison of the distribution of [^{3}H]PG binding sites with that of the mRNA for each PG receptor can provide new insight into the functions and modes of regulation of the receptors.

PGD_2 receptor

[^{3}H]PGD_2 bound to the membrane fraction of the brain with a relatively large K_d value (20–30 nM) and with a large B_{max} value (a few hundred fmol/mg protein) (Shimizu et al., 1982; Ueno et al., 1985; Tokumoto et al., 1986). The cloned cDNA for the PGD_2 receptor coded for a receptor protein to which [^{3}H]PGD_2 also bound with a large K_d value (40 nM), and stimulation of the receptor resulted in an enhanced production of cAMP (Hirata et al., 1994). There is, however, an apparent difference between the PGD_2 receptor in the membrane fraction of the brain and that expressed in the cloned cDNA sequence in a cell line. BW245C, one of the PGD_2 agonists, effectively displaced [^{3}H]PGD_2 bound to the cloned PGD_2 receptor but not that bound to the membrane fraction of the brain. Thus, the PGD_2 binding sites in the brain seem to represent a protein distinct from the cloned PGD_2 receptor.

Yamashita et al. (1983) demonstrated the distribution of PGD_2 binding sites in the rat brain by incubating frozen sections of the brain with [^{3}H]PGD_2. PGD_2 binding sites were found to be localized in discrete brain regions including olfactory bulb, nucleus accumbence, preoptic area, some diencephalic nuclei, amygdala, hippocampus, superior colliculus, central gray, cerebellum, and some areas of the cerebral cortex. More precisely, PGD_2 binding sites were localized in the Purkinje cell layer of swine brain (Watanabe et al., 1983) and some hypothalamic nuclei of monkey brain (Watanabe et al., 1989). In contrast, mRNA for the cloned PGD_2 receptor has not been detected in these brain regions. These results suggest the existence of multiple forms of PGD_2 receptors.

PGE₂ receptor

Based on differential sensitivity to various PGE_2 analogues, the PGE_2 receptor was classified into three subtypes, i.e. EP1, EP2, and EP3. Recently a 4th subtype, EP4, has been proposed (Coleman et al., 1994). Stimulation of EP1 increases intracellular Ca^{2+} concentration, whereas that of EP2 and EP4 increases cAMP. EP3 was considered to be coupled to Gi and to reduce cAMP when stimulated. Molecular cloning of the cDNAs for these receptors and their expression in cultured cell line, which cell did not express any of these PG receptors, has facilitated the characterization of their properties in a pure form (Sugimoto et al., 1992; Honda et al., 1993; Takeuchi et al., 1993; Watabe et al., 1993). It was further revealed that three isoforms of the EP3 receptor exist in the mouse, i.e. EP3α, EP3β, and EP3γ (Namba et al., 1993), two isoforms in rats i.e. rEP3A and rEP3B (Takeuchi et al., 1994), and four isoforms in the bovine, i.e. EP3A, EP3B, EP3C, and EP3D (Ushikubi et al., 1995). These isoforms only differ in the amino acid sequence near the C terminus in the cytoplasmic domain due to alternative splicing. Therefore, the isoforms have the same profile of binding to PGE_2 analogues but differ in their mode of coupling to G proteins. Northern blot analysis showed a detectable amount of EP3 in the mouse brain. It is, however, unclear which isoform of EP3 is predominant in the brain; because the isoforms are, in a large part, identical in both amino acid and nucleotide sequences, making it difficult to develop isoform-specific antibodies and oligonucleotide probes.

Distribution of PGE₂ binding sites in the brain

In 1988, the distribution of $[^3H]PGE_2$ binding sites, presumably PGE_2 receptors, was first demonstrated in the monkey diencephalon (Watanabe et al., 1988). The binding was high in the medial preoptic area, amygdala, and some hypothalamic and thalamic nuclei. This study was followed by more detailed analysis of $[^3H]PGE_2$ binding sites in the rat brain (Matsumura et al., 1990, 1992). As shown in Fig. 5, PGE_2 binding sites were located in a number of discrete brain regions, including some thalamic and hypothalamic nuclei, ventral hippocampus, central gray, superior colliculus, parabrachial nucleus, locus coeruleus, raphe nuclei, spinal trigeminal nuclei, and the nucleus tractus solitarius (NST). Although the results suggested a variety of PGE_2 functions in the brain, we were particularly interested in the finding that a dense distribution of PGE_2 binding sites was present in the anterior wall of the third ventricle (A3V; see Fig. 5A,K). PGE_2 binding sites there were distributed as if they surrounded the OVLT (Fig. 5K,I). This form of configuration was also observed in rabbits, guinea pigs (Matsumura et al., 1992), and monkeys (our unpublished observation).

Functions and properties of PGE₂ binding sites in the A3V region

What kind of physiological function do the PGE_2 binding sites have in the A3V region? PGE_2 had long been considered to be an endogenous mediator of fever. Since microinjection of PGE_2 into the preoptic/anterior hypothalamic area was most effective in evoking fever-like elevation in body temperature, it was presumed that the PGE_2 receptor is present in the preoptic area or its vicinity. Since the A3V and preoptic area are close to each other, we first speculated that A3V-PGE_2 binding sites may represent the main body of PGE_2 receptor sites involved in PGE_2-induced fever. To examine this possibility, we ablated the A3V region in rats by passing a high-frequency microwave current through an electrode positioned there. After recovery from the surgery (at least after two weeks), PGE_2 (10–100 ng in 1 μl saline) was microinjected into the preoptic area, which is located just caudal to the A3V region. In spite of the almost complete disappearance of the PGE_2 binding sites in the A3V region (Fig. 6), the febrile response to the microinjected PGE_2 occurred with no apparent difference from that observed in sham-operated rats (Fig. 7). These results imply that PGE_2 bind-

286

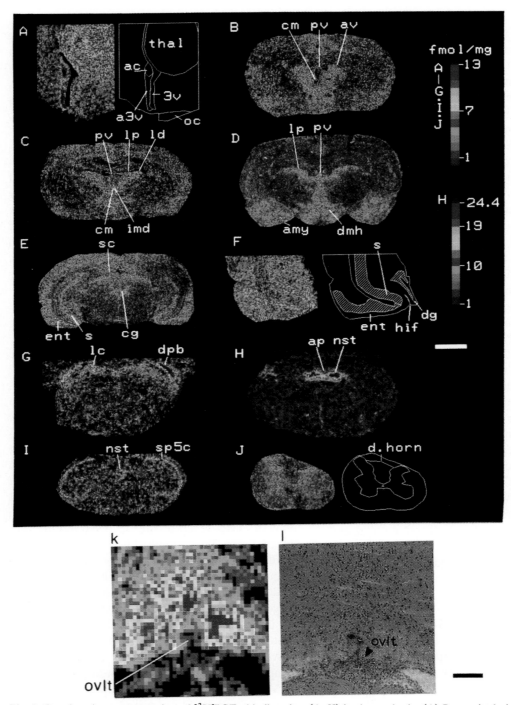

Fig. 5. Pseudo-color representation of [³H]PGE₂ binding sites (A–K) in the rat brain. (A) Parasagittal view of the preoptic area and hypothalamic region near the midline (left) and corresponding neuronal structures (right). (B–D) coronal sections containing the thalamus, and preoptic/hypothalamic region. (E) Coronal section containing midbrain and hippocampus. (F) Enlarged coronal view of the ventral hippocampus (left) and its neuronal organization (right). Striped area represents neuronal cell body-rich region.

ing sites in the A3V region are not essential to PGE$_2$-induced fever.

As mentioned above, there are four subtypes of the PGE$_2$ receptor. It is speculated that each subtype of this receptor plays a different role in the brain. In fact, Oka et al. (1994) microinjected subtype-specific agonists into the cerebral ventricle and demonstrated that the EP1 receptor might be involved in the febrile action of PGE$_2$ whereas EP3 is involved in the hyperalgesic action of it. So the question arose as to which subtype of PGE$_2$ receptor exists in the A3V region? This was examined by the displacement of [^{3}H]PGE$_2$ binding in the A3V region by subtype-specific receptor ligands, that is, 17-phenyl-trienor-PGE$_2$ (17-phenyl-PGE$_2$) for EP1, butaprost for EP2, and M & B 28767 for EP3. As shown in Fig. 8, M & B 28767 most effectively displaced [^{3}H]PGE$_2$ binding. This result implies that EP3 is predominant in the A3V region among the three PGE$_2$ receptor subtypes examined. The predominance of the EP3 subtype was also the case for all other brain regions possessing high levels of PGE$_2$ binding sites.

This result is in line with that of Northern blot analysis, i.e. mRNA for EP3 was detectable in the mouse brain (Sugimoto et al., 1992), whereas that for EP1 or EP2 was under the detection limit (Honda et al., 1993; Watabe et al., 1993). Sugimoto et al. (1994) conducted an *in situ* hybridization study for EP3 mRNA in mouse brain and found EP3 mRNA-positive cells to be neurons in

almost all cases. The distribution of EP3 mRNA-positive neurons in the mouse brain was similar to that of [^{3}H]PGE$_2$ binding sites in the rat brain. To avoid possible species difference, we conducted an *in situ* hybridization study for EP3 mRNA in rat brain and compared its distribution with that of PGE$_2$ binding sites. As shown in Fig. 9, EP3 mRNA was abundant in the thalamus, hypothalamus, midbrain, and lower brain stem. Importantly, this was also the case for the A3V region and neighboring preoptic nuclei. These results further indicate that PGE$_2$ receptors in the A3V region as well as in other brain regions are predominantly composed of the EP3 type.

However, a clear difference was noted between the distribution of PGE$_2$ binding sites and that of EP3 mRNA in some regions including the cerebral cortex, hippocampus, and the NST. Layers V and VI of the cerebral cortex and all neuronal layers in the hippocampus contained neurons possessing a high amount of EP3 mRNA, whereas PGE$_2$ binding in these regions was not distinguished. On the contrary, PGE$_2$ binding sites were abundant in the NST and spinal trigeminal nuclei, whereas no mRNA signal higher than the background level was detected there. These differences seem to be ascribable to the transport of EP3 protein to axons or dendrites after its synthesis in the cell soma. Indeed, we demonstrated that unilateral ablation of the vagus at a point between the nodose ganglion (a sensory ganglion in the vagal system) and brain reduced PGE$_2$ binding in

---

(G–J) Coronal sections of pons (G), medulla (H, I), and the cervical spinal cord (J). The white distance scale represents 3 mm for B–D and E and 1.5 mm for A and F–J. (K) Enlarged coronal image of the A3V region and corresponding Nissl-stained image. Note that the binding sites were densely distributed surrounding the OVLT. The distance scale (black) is for K and I and represents 200 μm. The rats were perfused with 20 mM phosphate-buffered saline under thiopental anesthesia. Their brains were frozen in dry-ice powder, and frozen sections of 10 μm thick were thaw mounted on glass slides. The sections were incubated with 20 nM [^{3}H]PGE$_2$ for 30 min at 4°C. Nonspecific binding was estimated in adjacent sections incubated with 20 nM [^{3}H]PGE$_2$ plus 100 μM unlabeled PGE$_2$. After removal of the unbound [^{3}H]PGE$_2$ by 4 × 30 s washing, the sections were dried and exposed to ^{3}H-sensitive films. After film development, the density of the autoradiographic images was quantitatively analyzed and pseudo-color coded. thal, thalamus; ac, anterior commissure; a3v, anterior wall of the 3rd ventricle; 3v, the 3rd ventricle; oc, optic chiasma; cm, central medial thalamic nucleus; pv, paraventricular thalamic nucleus; av, anteroventral thalamic nucleus; lp, lateroposterior thalamic nucleus; ld, laterodorsal thalamic nucleus; imd, intermediodorsal thalamic nucleus; amy, amygdala; dmh, dorsomedial hypothalamic area; sc, superior colliculus; ent, entorhinal cortex; s, subiculum; cg, central gray; dg, dentate gyrus; hif, hippocampal fissure; lc, locus coeruleus; dpb, dorsal parabrachial nucleus; ap, area postrema; nst, nucleus solitary tract; sp5c, spinal trigeminal nucleus (caudal part); d, dorsal horn of the spinal cord [modified from Matsumura et al. (1990, 1992), reprinted from *Brain Research* with kind permission of Elsevier Science B.V., Amsterdam, The Netherlands].

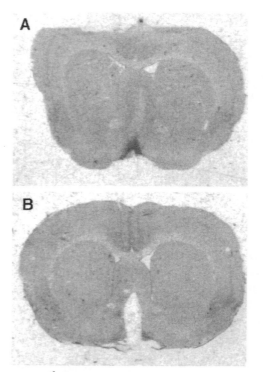

Fig. 6. [³H]PGE₂ binding in the anterior wall of the third ventricle (A3V) in the brain of a sham operated rat (A) and of a lesioned rat (B). Note that [³H]PGE₂ binding is almost completely absent in 'B'. The rats were anesthetized with pentobarbital and fixed in a stereotaxic frame. The lesion was made with an electrode to which microwave current was applied so that the temperature of the electrode tip became elevated to around 60°C. Autoradiography was done as described in the legend of Fig. 5.

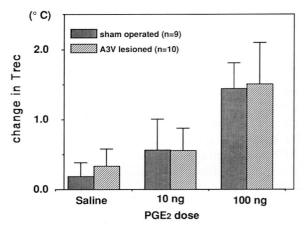

Fig. 7. Effect of A3V lesion on the febrile response to PGE₂ injected into the preoptic area. No apparent difference in the febrile response was noted between the two groups. The A3V region of each rat was ablated as described in the legend of Fig. 6. After a recovery period of at least 2 weeks, PGE₂ or saline was injected into the preoptic area. The maximum increases in the rectal temperature (T_{re}) were averaged from 9 or 10 rats.

the NST. Furthermore, the nodose ganglia and other sensory ones contained a high amount of EP3 mRNA (Fig. 9D,E). Thus, PGE₂ binding sites in the NST and spinal trigeminal nucleus seem to be transported from the corresponding sensory ganglia. This idea may also be applied to the inconsistency between distribution of PGE₂ binding sites and that of EP3 mRNA in the cerebral cortex and hippocampus, where EP3 protein may be transported from the cell soma to the dendrites and/or axons, resulting in a low and uniform appearance of the [³H]PGE₂ binding pattern.

Distribution of other PGE₂ receptor subtypes in the brain

At present, of the PGE₂ receptors, the EP1 receptor is then most likely one involved in the febrile action of PGE₂ in the brain. Where do they exist in the brain? Our trial to discriminate the EP1 subtype by looking at the displacement of [³H]PGE₂ binding by an EP1-specific receptor ligand failed, largely because the EP3 subtype-specific ligand displaced [³H]PGE₂ binding most effectively in all of the brain regions examined. Another critical point with this methodology involves the specificity of the ligands. Since the subtype-specific ligands used here more or less cross-reacted with other receptor subtypes at higher doses, detection of a small displacement of [³H]PGE₂ binding was difficult. An alternative approach would be *in situ* hybridization, which should discriminate the subtypes with higher specificity than could the ligand binding study. Batshake et al. (1995) performed *in situ* hybridization for mouse EP1 mRNA in the mouse

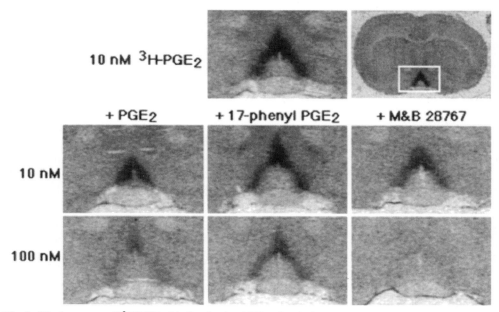

Fig. 8. Displacement of [³H]PGE₂ binding in the A3V region by its analogues.

brain. EP1 mRNA signals were detected in the paraventricular and supraoptic nuclei of the hypothalamus. No distinct signal was observed in the preoptic area or A3V region, presumed sites of the febrile action of PGE_2. This again raised a question as to whether the low expression level of EP1 mRNA in the preoptic area/A3V region could explain the potent febrile action of PGE_2 and an EP1-specific agonist. The correct answer to this question would be one of the following two: First, the low level of EP1 receptor is sufficient for the induction of fever. Second, there exists a yet unknown subtype of PGE_2 receptor to which 17-phenyl-PGE_2 can act as an agonist. Further studies are necessary to identify the exact sites of the febrile action of PGE_2.

As for EP2 and EP4 receptors, determination of their localization in the brain has not been reported in the brain. There is, however, evidence suggesting a possible role of EP2 in the brain. In primary cultures of cortical neurons, the addition of PGE_2 had a neuro-protective effect on glutamate-induced toxicity (Akaike et al., 1994). Using subtype specific receptor agonists, it was further

revealed that EP2 was responsible for the protective action because butaprost but neither 17-phenyl-PGE_2 nor M & B 25767 mimicked the action of PGE_2 (Akaike et al., 1994). It would be of interest to know if this is also the case in vivo. This finding also raises an essential question as to whether PGE_2 is protective or toxic to neurons because treatment with indomethacin, which inhibits PG biosynthesis, made the neuronal damage less under hyperthermic as well as traumatic conditions.

Another interesting finding in the PGE_2 receptor binding study was that the intermediate lobe (IML) of the pituitary gland has a high amount of PGE_2 binding sites (Matsumura et al., 1995). IML consists of melanotrophs, which secrete α-melanocyte stimulating hormone (α-MSH), a presumed endogenous antagonist of IL-1 and TNF. Displacement study and in situ hybridization study revealed that the PGE_2 receptors in the IML are of EP3 subtype. Application of PGE_2 (1–10 nM) on acutely isolated IML or primary cultures of the melanotrophs reduced intracellular Ca^{2+} ion concentration, suggesting that PGE_2 suppresses

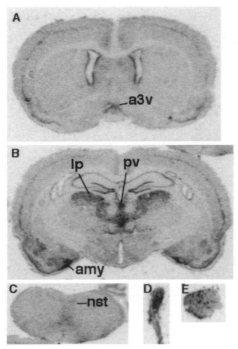

Fig. 9. Distribution of EP3 mRNA in the rat brain (A–C), nodose ganglion (D), and trigeminal ganglia (E). *In situ* hybridization was made with a ^{35}S-labeled cRNA probe directed to rat EP3 mRNA.

secretion of α-MSH (Matsumura et al., 1995). Since α-MSH acts as an anti-inflammatory substance, suppression of its secretion by PGE_2 may lead to an enhancement of inflammation. This response could take place in the initial stage of inflammation at which full actions of inflammatory cytokines may be required.

$PGF_{2\alpha}$ receptor

The presence of $PGF_{2\alpha}$ receptor in the brain was suggested by the binding of $[^3H]PGF_{2\alpha}$ to the membrane fraction of rat brain (Malet et al., 1982). Cloning and expression of cDNA for the $PGF_{2\alpha}$ receptor (FP receptor) revealed its structure and functions (Sugimoto et al., 1994). As in the case of other PG receptors, FP has seven transmembrane domains and shows coupling to G protein. Intracellular Ca^{2+} increases when the FP receptor is stimulated by an agonist. The location of $[^3H]PGF_{2\alpha}$ binding sites in the brain was demonstrated by Watanabe et al. (1989), who found a high level of binding in the paraventricular and supraoptic nuclei of the monkey hypothalamus. No corresponding *in situ* hybridization study has been reported.

PGI_2 receptor

PGI_2 (or prostacyclin) was first discovered by Vane's group as a vasodilator (Bunting et al., 1976). PGI_2 also possesses platelet anti-aggregatory action. Thus, its profound action on the blood vessels and platelets led researchers to consider PGI_2 as a prostanoid in the cardiovascular system. As far as we understand, no study has reported the binding of $[^3H]PGI_2$ or its analogue to the membrane fraction of the brain. The cloned PGI_2 receptor (IP) had seven transmembrane domains and was coupled to G protein. The mRNA was abundant in the thymus, spleen, and heart but was scant in the brain (Namba et al., 1994). Stimulation of IP receptor increased either cAMP or Ca^{2+} depending on the dose of the agonist (Namba et al., 1994).

There is, however, some evidence suggesting possible roles of PGI_2 in the nervous system. For example, PGI_2, when injected intravenously, not only reduced vascular tone but also modified cardiovascular reflex probably through its action on the central neuronal network involved in cardiovascular regulation (Chapple et al., 1980). Also, PGI_2 sensitized peripheral pain receptors to potentiate the response to pain stimulation (Birrell et al., 1991). In order to investigate the possible involvement of PGI_2 in brain function, we conducted *in vitro* receptor autoradiography using $[^3H]$iloprost, a stable agonist for PGI_2 receptor (Matsumura et al., 1995), as PGI_2 itself degrades with a half-life of a few minutes. Dense concentrations of iloprost binding sites were observed in the caudal and commisural parts of the NST and in the superficial layers of the trigeminal spinal nucleus and of the dorsal horn of the spinal cord. Low but significant specific binding was also observed in the thalamus, cerebral cortex, and dorsal cochlear nucleus. The three regions possessing a high density of iloprost binding sites were common in that they all receive primary sensory afferents: the NST receives viscerosensory inputs via the vagus, whereas the other two receive somatosensory inputs via the trigeminal nerve and spinal nerves, respectively. When these nerves were transected at a point between their sensory ganglia and brain or spinal cord, iloprost binding in the corresponding brain or spinal cord region was reduced ipsilaterally. The ligation of the vagus nerve between the nodose ganglion and brain also decreased iloprost binding in the NST. Instead, iloprost binding sites accumulated at the ligation site proximal to the nodose ganglion. From these results, we concluded that PGI_2 receptors were synthesized in the sensory ganglia and transported to both central and peripheral terminals of the primary sensory system. In line with this idea, Oida et al. (1995) showed that mRNA for IP was present in the neurons of dorsal root ganglia.

Central type of PGI_2 receptor

When another prostacyclin analogue, [^{3}H]isocarbacyclin, was used as a ligand for receptor autoradiography, the binding in the cerebral cortex, striatum, thalamus and hippocampus was apparently higher than that obtained with [^{3}H]iloprost; whereas the binding associated with the primary sensory afferents, i.e. those in the NST, spinal trigeminal nucleus, and dorsal horn, did not differ from those obtained with [^{3}H]iloprost. This finding suggested that brain has a novel subtype of PGI_2 receptor to which isocarbacyclin, but not iloprost, can bind with high affinity. To confirm this, Takechi et al. (1996) performed Scatchard plot analysis of the binding of either [^{3}H]isocarbacyclin or [^{3}H]iloprost to frozen sections of the thalamus and the NST. As expected, isocarbacyclin bound to the thalamus with high affinity ($K_d = 7.8$ nM) while iloprost bound to it with low affinity ($K_d = 159$ nM). In contrast, in the NST, both of these ligands had comparable affinity (3.9 nM for isocarbacyclin and 6.8 nM for iloprost). Binding of [^{3}H]iso-

carbacyclin in the thalamus was displaced by several prostaglandin analogues in the order of isocarbacyclin = 15R-16-(m-tolyl)-isocarbacyclin > carbacyclin > iloprost > PGE_2 > PGE_1 = cicaprost > PGD_2 = $PGF_{2\alpha}$. In contrast, in the NST, the order was isocarbacyclin = cicaprost = iloprost > carbacyclin > PGE_1 > 15R-16-(m-tolyl)-isocarbacyclin > PGE_2 > PGD_2 = $PGF_{2\alpha}$. The order in the NST is similar to that reported for the cloned prostacyclin receptor (Namba et al., 1994). IP is widely expressed in peripheral tissues (Oida et al., 1995), and the primary sensory afferents are also peripheral nerves. In this sense, IP is preferably expressed in the peripheral tissues. The isocarbacyclin-specific binding sites in the brain seem to represent another type of PGI_2 receptor expressed preferentially in the central nervous system. We designated it as IP2 with the former IP as IP1. Its signal transduction mechanism and cDNA sequence are now under investigation.

The isocarbacyclin binding sites are likely neurons. One intriguing feature of IP2 is its abundant expression in the brain. In the thalamus, the B_{max} value, which corresponds to receptor density, is 230 fmol/mg tissue. This implicates a significant role of PGI_2 and IP2 in the brain functions. This possibility is supported by an electrophysiological experiment on hippocampal brain slices (Takechi et al., 1996). Both application of 0.3 to 1 μM isocarbacyclin increased by two- to threefold the slope of the excitatory postsynaptic potential in the CA1 region evoked by electrical stimulation of the Schaffer collateral.

At present we have no firm evidence that IP2 is expressed only in the central nervous system partly because we have had no receptor ligand specific for IP2; isocarbacyclin binds to both IP1 and IP2 equipotently. However, in the search for a prostacyclin receptor ligand suitable for positron emission tomography (PET), we found that one of the isocarbacyclin analogues, (15R)-16-m-Tolyl-17,18,19,20- tetranorisocarbacyclin, selectively binds to IP2 (Suzuki et al., 1996; Takechi et al., 1996). This molecule will be a useful tool for the investigation of IP2 function in the future.

Concluding remarks

Recent biochemical studies, especially those that employed molecular biological techniques, have provided a great deal of information on the molecular nature of individual components of the PG system. The final goal should be, however, to understand the mode of regulation of this system and its functions *in vivo*, and to apply this knowledge for clinical purposes. Although in vitro experiments are perhaps less complicated, *in vivo* ones based on recent biochemical information are indispensable for the final goal. Knockout mice lacking one of the genes in the PG system are also becoming available and are expected to facilitate the study of the PG system *in vivo*. As for the brain, the heterogenous localization of PG system components is of importance for the understanding of their functions. We hope the present review has been informative and will stimulate further *in vivo* investigations.

Acknowledgments

We would like to thank Dr Larry D. Frye for critical reading of the manuscript, Dr Kanato Yamagata for providing the cDNA of rat COX-2, and Dr Kazuhisa Takeuchi for providing the cDNA of rat EP3 receptor.

References

Akaike, A., Kaneko, S., Tamura, Y., Nakata, N., Shiomi, H., Ushikubi, F. and Narumiya, S. (1994) Prostaglandin E_2 protects cultured cortical neurons against *N*-methyl-D-aspartate receptor-mediated glutamate cytotoxicity. *Brain Res.*, 663: 237–243.

Batshake, B., Nilsson, C. and Sundelin, J. (1995) Molecular characterization of the mouse prostanoid EP1 receptor gene. *Eur. J. Biochem.*, 231: 809–814.

Bazan, N.G., Rodriguez de Turco, E.B. and Allan, G. (1995) Mediators of injury in neurotrauma: intracellular signal transduction and gene expression. *J. Neurotrauma*, 12: 791–814.

Birrell, G.J., McQueen, D.S., Iggo, A., Coleman, R.A. and Grubb, B.D. (1991) PGI_2-induced activation and sensitization of articular mechanonociceptors. *Neurosci. Lett.*, 124: 5–8.

Bonventre, J.V. and Koroshetz, W.J. (1993) Phospholipase A_2 (PLA_2) activity in gerbil brain: characterization of cytosolic and membrane-associated forms and effects of ischemia and reperfusion on enzymatic activity. *J. Lipid Mediators*, 6: 457–471.

Breder, C.D., Dewitt, D. and Kraig, R.P. (1995) Characterization of inducible cyclooxygenase in rat brain. *J. Comp. Neurol.*, 355: 296–315.

Breder, C.D. and Saper, C.B. (1996) Expression of inducible cyclooxygenase mRNA in the mouse brain after systemic administration of bacterial lipopolysaccharide. *Brain Res.*, 713: 64–69.

Breder, C.D., Smith, W.L., Raz, A., Masferrer, J., Seibert, K., Needleman, P. and Saper, C.B. (1992) Distribution and characterization of cyclooxygenase immunoreactivity in the ovine brain. *J. Comp. Neurol.*, 322: 409–438.

Breitner, J.C.S., Gau, B.A., Welch, K.A., Plassman, B.L., McDonald, W.M., Helms, M.J. and Anthony, J.C. (1994) Inverse association of anti-inflammatory treatments and Alzheimer's disease: initial results of a co-twin control study. *Neurology*, 44: 227–232.

Bunting, S., Gryglewski, R., Moncada, S. and Vane, J.R. (1976) Arterial walls generate from prostaglandin endoperoxides a substance (prostaglandin X) which relaxes strips of mesenteric and coeliac arteries and inhibits platelet aggregation. *Prostaglandins*, 12: 897–913.

Cao, C., Matsumura, K., Yamagata, K. and Watanabe, Y. (1995) Induction by lipopolysaccharide of cyclooxygenase-2 mRNA in rat brain; its possible role in the febrile response. *Brain Res.*, 697: 187–196.

Cao, C., Matsumura, K., Yamagata, K. and Watanabe, Y. (1996) Endothelial cells of the rat brain vasculature express cyclooxygenase-2 mRNA in response to systemic interleukin-1β: a possible site of prostaglandin synthesis responsible for fever. *Brain Res.*, 733: 263–272.

Cao, C., Matsumura, K. and Watanabe, Y. (1997) Involvement of cyclooxygenase-2 in LPS-induced fever and its regulation in the brain. *Am. J. Physiol.*, 272: R1712–R1725.

Chapple, D.J., Dusting, G.J., Hughes, R. and Vane, J.R. (1980) Some direct and reflex cardiovascular actions of prostacyclin (PGI_2) and prostaglandin E_2 in anaesthetized dogs. *Br. J. Pharmacol.*, 68: 437–447.

Clark, J.D., Lin, L.L., Kriz, R.W., Ramesha, C.S., Sultzman, L.A., Lin, A.Y., Milona, N. and Knopf, J.L. (1991) A novel arachidonic acid-selective cytosolic PLA_2 contains a Ca^{2+}-dependent translocation domain with homology to PKC and GAP. *Cell*, 65: 1043–1051.

Clark, J.D., Milona, N. and Knopf, J.L. (1990) Purification of a 110-kilodalton cytosolic phospholipase A_2 from the human monocytic cell line U937. *Proc. Natl. Acad. Sci. USA*, 87: 7708–7712.

Coleman, R.A., Smith, W.L. and Narumiya, S. (1994) International union of pharmacology classification of prostanoid receptors: properties, distribution, and structure of the receptors and their subtypes. *Pharmacol. Rev.*, 46: 205–229.

Exton, J.H. (1994) Phosphatidylcholine breakdown and signal transduction. *Biochim. Biophys. Acta*, 1212: 26–42.

Fletcher, B.S., Kujubu, D.A., Perrin, D.M. and Herschman, H.R. (1992) Structure of the mitogen-inducible TIS10 gene and demonstration that the TIS10-encoded protein is a functional prostaglandin G/H synthase. *J. Biol. Chem.*, 267: 4338–4344.

Fujimoto, N., Kaneko, T., Eguchi, N., Urade, Y., Mizuno, N. and Hayaishi, O. (1992) Biochemical and immunohistochemical demonstration of a tightly bound form of prostaglandin E_2 in the rat brain. *Neuroscience*, 49: 591–606.

Futaki, N., Arai, I., Hamasaka, Y., Takahashi, S., Higuchi, S. and Otomo, S. (1993) Selective inhibition of NS-398 on prostanoid production in inflamed tissue in rat carrageenan-air-pouch inflammation. *J. Pharm. Pharmacol.*, 45: 753–755.

Futaki, N., Takahashi, S., Yokoyama, M., Arai, I., Higuchi, S. and Otomo, S. (1994) NS-398, a new anti-inflammatory agent, selectively inhibits prostaglandin G/H synthase/cyclooxygenase (COX-2) activity *in vitro*. *Prostaglandins*, 47: 55–59.

Futaki, N., Yoshikawa, K., Hamasaka, Y., Arai, I., Higuchi, S., Iizuka, H. and Otomo, S. (1993) NS-398, a novel nonsteroidal anti-inflammatory drug with potent analgesic and antipyretic effects, which causes minimal stomach lesions. *Gen. Pharmacol.*, 24: 105–110.

Glaser, K.B., Mobilio, D., Chang, J.Y. and Senko, N. (1993) Phospholipase A_2 enzymes: regulation and inhibition. *Trends Pharmacol. Sci.*, 14: 92–98.

Goppelt-Struebe, M. (1995) Regulation of prostaglandin endoperoxide synthase (cyclooxygenase) isozyme expression. *Prostaglandins Leukotrienes Essent. Fatty Acids*, 52: 213–222.

Hara, S., Miyata, A., Yokoyama, C., Inoue, H., Brugger, R., Lottspeich, F., Ullrich, V. and Tanabe, T. (1994) Isolation and molecular cloning of prostacyclin synthase from bovine endothelial cells. *J. Biol. Chem.*, 269: 19897–19903.

Hirata, M., Hayashi, Y., Ushikubi, F., Yokota, Y., Kageyama, R., Nakanishi, S. and Narumiya, S. (1991) Cloning and expression of cDNA for a human thromboxane A_2 receptor. *Nature*, 349: 617–620.

Hirata, M., Kakizuka, A., Aizawa, M., Ushikubi, F. and Narumiya, S. (1994) Molecular characterization of a mouse prostaglandin D receptor and functional expression of the cloned gene. *Proc. Natl. Acad. Sci. USA*, 91: 11192–11196.

Honda, A., Sugimoto, Y., Namba, T., Watabe, A., Irie, A., Negishi, M., Narumiya, S. and Ichikawa, A. (1993) Cloning and expression of a cDNA for mouse prostaglandin E receptor EP2 subtype. *J. Biol. Chem.*, 268: 7759–7762.

Kawasaki, M., Yoshihara, Y., Yamaji, M. and Watanabe, Y. (1993) Expression of prostaglandin endoperoxide synthase in rat brain. *Mol. Brain Res.*, 19: 39–46.

Kim, D.K., Rordorf, G., Nemenoff, R.A., Koroshetz, W.J. and Bonventre, J.V. (1995) Glutamate stably enhances the activity of two cytosolic forms of phospholipase A_2 in brain cortical cultures. *Biochem. J.*, 310: 83–90.

Kujubu, D.A., Fletcher, B.S., Varnum, B.C., Lim, R.W. and Herschman, H.R. (1991) TIS10, a phorbol ester tumor promoter-inducible mRNA from Swiss 3T3 cells, encodes a novel prostaglandin synthase/cyclooxygenase homologue. *J. Biol. Chem.*, 266: 12866–12872.

Kurzrok, R. and Lieb, C.C. (1930) Biochemical studies of human semen. II. The action of semen on the human uterus. *Proc. Soc. Exp. Biol. Med.*, 28: 268–272.

Lauritzen, I., Heurteaux, C. and Lazdunski, M. (1994) Expression of group II phospholipase A_2 in rat brain after severe forebrain ischemia and in endotoxic shock. *Brain Res.*, 651: 353–356.

Li, S.R., Wu, K.K., Anggard, E. and Ferns, G. (1993) Localization of prostaglandin G/H synthase gene expression in rat brain by *in situ* hybridization. *Biol. Signals*, 2: 77–83.

Malet, C., Scherrer, H., Saavedra, J.M. and Dray, F. (1982) Specific binding of [^{3}H]prostaglandin E_2 to rat brain membranes and synaptosomes. *Brain Res.*, 236: 227–233.

Masferrer, J.L., Zweifel, B.S., Manning, P.T., Hauser, S.D., Leahy, K.M., Smith, W.G., Isakson, P.C. and Seibert, K. (1994) Selective inhibition of inducible cyclooxygenase 2 *in vivo* is antiinflammatory and nonulcerogenic. *Proc. Natl. Acad. Sci. USA*, 91: 3228–3232.

Matsumura, H., Nakajima, T., Osaka, T., Satoh, S., Kawase, K., Kubo, E., Kantha, S.S., Kasahara, K. and Hayaishi, O. (1994) Prostaglandin D_2-sensitive, sleep-promoting zone defined in the ventral surface of the rostral basal forebrain. *Proc. Natl. Acad. Sci. USA*, 91: 11998–12002.

Matsumura, K., Mochizuki-Oda, N., Watanabe, Y., Onoe, H. and Watanabe, Y., (1995) Function of prostaglandin E_2 receptor in the intermediate lobe of the pituitary gland. In: T. Nagasaka and A.S. Milton (Eds.), *Body Temperature and Metabolism*, IPEC, Tokyo, pp. 41–44.

Matsumura, K., Watanabe, Y., Imai-Matsumura, K., Connolly, M., Koyama, Y., Onoe, H. and Watanabe, Y. (1992) Mapping of prostaglandin E_2 binding sites in rat brain using quantitative autoradiography. *Brain Res.*, 581: 292–298.

Matsumura, K., Watanabe, Y., Onoe, H., Koyama, Y. and Watanabe, Y. (1992) *In vitro* receptor autoradiography: a map for exploring the hypothalamus. *Physiol. Res.*, 41: 95–97.

Matsumura, K., Watanabe, Y., Onoe, H. and Watanabe, Y. (1995) Prostacyclin receptor in the brain and central terminals of the primary sensory neurons: an autoradiographic study using a stable prostacyclin analogue [^{3}H]iloprost. *Neuroscience*, 65: 493–503.

Matsumura, K., Watanabe, Y., Onoe, H., Watanabe, Y. and Hayaishi, O. (1990) High density of prostaglandin E_2 binding sites in the anterior wall of the 3rd ventricle: a possible site of its hyperthermic action. *Brain Res.*, 533: 147–151.

Milton, A.S., (1982) Prostaglandins in fever and the mode of action of antipyretic drugs. In: A.S. Milton (Ed.), *Pyretics and Antipyretics*, Springer, Berlin, pp. 259–267.

Morii, H., Ozaki, M. and Watanabe, Y. (1994) 5'-flanking region surrounding a human cytosolic phospholipase A_2 gene. *Biochem. Biophys. Res. Commun.*, 205: 6–11.

Namba, T., Oida, H., Sugimoto, Y., Kakizuka, A., Negishi, M., Ichikawa, A. and Narumiya, S. (1994) cDNA cloning of a mouse prostacyclin receptor. *J. Biol. Chem.*, 269: 9986–9992.

Namba, T., Sugimoto, Y., Negishi, M., Irie, A., Ushikubi, F., Kakizuka, A., Seiji, I., Ichikawa, A. and Narumiya, S. (1993) Alternative splicing of C-terminal tail of prostaglandin E receptor subtype EP3 determines G-protein specificity. *Nature*, 365: 166–170.

Ogawa, H., Kassell, N.F., Sasaki, T., Hongo, K., Tsukahara, T., Hudson, S.B., Asban, G.I., Tuan, H.L. and Torner, J.C. (1988) Immunohistochemically demonstrated increase of prostaglandin F$_2$-alpha in neurons after reoxygenation in anoxic rats. *Prostaglandins*, 36: 891–900.

Ogorochi, T., Narumiya, S., Mizuno, N., Yamashita, K., Miyazaki, H. and Hayaishi, O. (1984) Regional distribution of prostaglandins D$_2$, E$_2$, and F$_{2\alpha}$ and related enzymes in postmortem human brain. *J. Neurochem.*, 43: 71–82.

Oida, H., Namba, T., Sugimoto, Y., Ushikubi, F., Ohishi, H., Ichikawa, A. and Narumiya, S. (1995) *In situ* hybridization of prostacyclin receptor mRNA expression in various mouse organs. *Br. J. Pharmacol.*, 116: 2828–2837.

Oka, S. and Arita, H. (1991) Inflammatory factors stimulate expression of group II phospholipase A$_2$ in rat cultured astrocytes. *J. Biol. Chem.*, 266: 9956–9960.

Oka, T., Aou, S. and Hori, T. (1994) Intracerebroventricular injection of prostaglandin E$_2$ induces thermal hyperalgesia in rats: the possible involvement of EP3 receptors. *Brain Res.*, 663: 287–292.

Owada, Y., Tominaga, T., Yoshimoto, T. and Kondo, H. (1994) Molecular cloning of rat cDNA for cytosolic phospholipase A$_2$ and the increased gene expression in the dentate gyrus following transient forebrain ischemia. *Mol. Brain Res.*, 25: 364–368.

Ozaki, M., Morii, H., Qvist, R. and Watanabe, Y. (1994) Interleukin-β induces cytosolic phospholipase A$_2$ gene in rats C6 glioma cell line. *Biochem. Biophys. Res. Commun.*, 205: 12–17.

Planas, A.M., Soriano, M.A., Rodríguez-Farré, E. and Ferrer, I. (1995) Induction of cyclooxygenase-2 mRNA and protein following transient focal ischemia in the rat brain. *Neurosci. Lett.*, 200: 187–190.

Qvist, R., Morii, H. and Watanabe, Y. (1995) Interleukin-β stimulates phospholipase A$_2$ activity in rat C6 glioma cells. *Biochem. Mol. Biol. Int.*, 35: 363–370.

Rogers, J., Kirby, L.C. and Hempelman, S.R. (1993) Clinical trial of indomethacin in Alzheimer's disease. *Neurology*, 43: 1609–1611.

Sasaki, T., Nakagomi, T., Kirino, T., Tamura, A., Noguchi, M., Saito, I. and Takakura, K. (1988) Indomethacin ameliorates ischemic neuronal damage in the gerbil hippocampal CA1 sector. *Stroke*, 19: 1399–1403.

Sharma, H.S., Olsson, Y. and Cervós-Navarro, J. (1993a) Early perifocal cell changes and edema in traumatic injury of the spinal cord are reduced by indomethacin, an inhibitor of prostaglandin synthesis; Experimental study in the rat. *Acta Neuropathol.*, 85: 145–153.

Sharma, H.S., Olsson, Y., Nyberg, F. and Dey, P.K. (1993b) Prostaglandins modulate alterations of microvascular permeability, blood flow, edema and serotonin levels following spinal cord injury: an experimental study in the rat. *Neuroscience*, 57: 443–449.

Sharma, H.S., Olsson, Y., Persson, S. and Nyberg, F. (1995) Trauma-induced opening of the blood-spinal cord barrier is reduced by indomethacin, an inhibitor of prostaglandin biosynthesis. Experimental observations in the rat using [^{131}I]-sodium, evans blue and lanthanum as tracers. *Restor. Neurol. Neurosci.*, 7: 207–215.

Sharma, H.S., Westman, J., Nyberg, F., Cervos-Navarro, J. and Dey, P.K. (1994) Role of serotonin and prostaglandins in brain edema induced by heat stress. An experimental study in the young rat. *Acta Neurochir.*, Suppl. 60: 65–70.

Shimizu, T. and Wolfe, L.S. (1990) Arachidonic acid cascade and signal transduction. *J. Neurochem.*, 55: 1–15.

Shimizu, T., Yamashita, A. and Hayaishi, O. (1982) Specific binding of prostaglandin D$_2$ to rat brain synaptic membrane. Occurrence, properties, and distribution. *J. Biol. Chem.*, 257: 13570–13575.

Smith, W.L., Marnett, L.J. and DeWitt, D.L. (1991) Prostaglandin and thromboxane biosynthesis. *Pharmacol. Ther.*, 49: 153–179.

Stephenson, D.T., Manetta, J.V., White, D.L., Chiou, X.G., Cox, L., Gitter, B., May, P.C., Sharp, J.D., Kramer, R.M. and Clemens, J.A. (1994) Calcium-sensitive cytosolic phospholipase A$_2$ (cPLA$_2$) is expressed in human brain astrocytes. *Brain Res.*, 637: 97–105.

Sugimoto, Y., Hasumoto, K., Namba, T., Irie, A., Katsuyama, M., Negishi, M., Kakizuka, A., Narumiya, S. and Ichikawa, A. (1994) Cloning and expression of a cDNA for mouse prostaglandin F receptor. *J. Biol. Chem.*, 269: 1356–1360.

Sugimoto, Y., Shigemoto, R., Namba, T., Negishi, M., Mizuno, N., Narumiya, S. and Ichikawa, A. (1994) Distribution of the mRNA for the prostaglandin E receptor subtype EP3 in the mouse nervous system. *Neuroscience*, 62: 919–928.

Sugimoto, Y., Namba, T., Honda, A., Hayashi, Y., Negishi, M., Ichikawa, A. and Narumiya, S. (1992) Cloning and expression of a cDNA for mouse prostaglandin E receptor EP3 subtype. *J. Biol. Chem.*, 267: 6463–6466.

Suzuki, M., Kato, K., Noyori, R., Watanabe, Y., Takechi, H., Matsumura, K., Långström, B. and Watanabe, Y. (1996) (15R)-16-m-Tolyl-17,18,19,20-tetranorisocarbacyclin: a stable ligand with high binding affinity and selectivity for a prostacyclin receptor in the central nervous system. *Angew. Chem. Int. Ed. Engl.*, 35: 334–336.

Takechi, H., Matsumura, K., Watanabe, Y., Kato, K., Noyori, R., Suzuki, M. and Watanabe, Y. (1996) A novel subtype of the prostaglandin receptor expressed in the central nervous system. *J. Biol. Chem.*, 271: 5901–5906.

Takeuchi, K., Abe, T., Takahashi, N. and Keishi, A. (1993) Molecular cloning and intrarenal localization of rat prostaglandin E$_2$ receptor EP3 subtype. *Biochem. Biophys. Res. Commun.*, 194: 885–891.

Takeuchi, K., Takahashi, N., Abr, T. and Abe, K. (1994) Two isoforms of the rat kidney EP3 receptor derived by alternative RNA splicing: intrarenal expression and co-localization. *Biochem. Biophys. Res. Commun.*, 199: 834–84.

Tokumoto, H., Watanabe, Y., Yamashita, A., Arai, Y. and Hayaishi, O. (1986) Specificity of prostaglandin D$_2$ binding to synaptic membrane fraction of rat brain. *Brain Res.*, 362: 114–121.

Tsubokura, S., Watanabe, Y., Ehara, H., Imamura, K., Sugimoto, O., Kagamiyama, H., Yamamoto, S. and Hayaishi, O. (1991) Localization of prostaglandin endoperoxide synthase in neurons and glia of monkey brain. *Brain Res.*, 543: 15–24.

Ueno, R., Osama, H., Urade, Y. and Hayaishi, O. (1985) Changes of enzymes involved in prostaglandin metabolism and prostaglandin binding proteins in rat brain during development and aging. *J. Neurochem.*, 45: 483–489.

Urade, Y., Fujimoto, N., Kaneko, T., Mizuno, N. and Hayaishi, O. (1987) Postnatal changes in the localization of prostaglandin D synthase from neurons to oligodendrocytes in the rat brain. *J. Biol. Chem.*, 262: 15132–15136.

Urade, Y., Watanabe, K. and Hayaishi, O. (1995) Prostaglandin D, E, and F synthases. *J. Lipid Mediators Cell Signalling*, 12: 257–273.

Ushikubi, F., Hirata, M. and Narumiya, S. (1995) Molecular biology of prostanoid receptors; an overview. *J. Lipid Mediators*, 12: 343–359.

van Dam, A.-M., Brouns, M., Man-A-Hing, W. and Berkenbosch, F. (1993) Immunocytochemical detection of prostaglandin E$_2$ in microvasculature and in neurons of rat brain after administration of bacterial endotoxin. *Brain Res.*, 613: 331–336.

Watabe, A., Sugimoto, Y., Honda, A., Irie, A., Namba, T., Negishi, M., Ito, S., Narumiya, S. and Ichikawa, A. (1993) Cloning and expression of cDNA for a mouse EP1 subtype of prostaglandin E receptor. *J. Biol. Chem.*, 268: 20175–20178.

Watanabe, K., Fujii, Y., Nakayama, K., Ohkubo, H., Kuramitsu, S., Kagamiyama, H., Nakanishi, S. and Hayaishi, O. (1988) Structural similarity of bovine lung prostaglandin F synthase to lens ε-crystallin of the European common frog. *Proc. Natl. Acad. Sci. USA*, 85: 11–15.

Watanabe, K., Urade, Y., Mader, M., Murphy, C. and Hayaishi, O. (1994) Identification of b-trace as prostaglandin D synthase. *Biochem. Biophys. Res. Commun.*, 203: 1110–1116.

Watanabe, Y., Watanabe, Y., Hamada, K., Bommelaer-Bayt, M.-C., Dray, F., Kaneko, T., Yumoto, N. and Hayaishi, O. (1989) Distinct localization of prostaglandin D$_2$, E$_2$, and F$_{2\alpha}$ binding sites in monkey brain. *Brain Res.*, 478: 143–148.

Watanabe, Y., Watanabe, Y. and Hayaishi, O. (1988) Quantitative autoradiographic localization of prostaglandin E$_2$ binding sites in monkey diencephalon. *J. Neurosci.*, 8: 2003–2010.

Watanabe, Y., Yamashita, A., Tokumoto, H. and Hayaishi, O. (1983) Localization of prostaglandin D$_2$ binding protein and NADP-linked 15-hydroxyprostaglandin D$_2$ dehydrogenase in the Purkinje cells of miniature pig cerebellum. *Proc. Natl. Acad. Sci. USA*, 80: 4542–4545.

Xie, W., Chipman, J.G., Robertson, D.L., Erikson, R.L. and Simmons, D.L. (1991) Expression of a mitogen-responsive gene encoding prostaglandin synthase is regulated by mRNA splicing. *Proc. Natl. Acad. Sci. USA*, 88: 2692–2696.

Yamagata, K., Andreasson, K.I., Kaufmann, W.E., Barnes, C.A. and Worley, P.F. (1993) Expression of a mitogen-inducible cyclooxygenase in brain neurons: regulation by synaptic activity and glucocorticoids. *Neuron*, 11: 371–386.

Yamashita, A., Watanabe, Y. and Hayaishi, O. (1983) Autoradiographic localization of a binding protein(s) specific for prostaglandin D$_2$ in rat brain. *Proc. Natl. Acad. Sci. USA*, 80: 6114–6118.

Yokoyama, C., Miyata, A., Ihara, H., Ullrich, V. and Tanabe, T. (1991) Molecular cloning of human platelet thromboxane A synthase. *Biochem. Biophys. Res. Commun.*, 178: 1479–1484.

Yoshihara, Y. and Watanabe, Y. (1990) Translocation of phospholipase A$_2$ from cytosol to membranes in rat brain induced by calcium ions. *Biochem. Biophys. Res. Commun.*, 170: 484–490.

Yumoto, N., Watanabe, Y., Watanabe, K., Watanabe, Y. and Hayaishi, O. (1986) Solubilization and characterization of prostaglandin E$_2$ binding protein from porcine cerebral cortex. *J. Neurochem.*, 46: 125–132.

H.S. Sharma and J. Westman (Eds.)
Progress in Brain Research, Vol 115
© 1998 Elsevier Science BV. All rights reserved.

CHAPTER 16

Nitric oxide and carbon monoxide in the brain pathology of heat stress

Hari Shanker Sharma[1]*, Per Alm[2] and Jan Westman[1]

[1]*Laboratory of Neuroanatomy, Department of Anatomy, Box 571, Biomedical Centre, Uppsala University, S-751 23 Uppsala, Sweden*
[2]*Department of Pathology, University Hospital, Lund University, S-221 85 Lund, Sweden*

Introduction

During recent years nitric oxide (NO) and carbon monoxide (CO) have emerged as important new chemical messenger molecules which can influence physiological and pathological processes in both central nervous system (CNS) and in the peripheral nervous system (PNS) (Tables 1 and 2) (Maines, 1988, 1992, 1996; Bredt and Snyder, 1992; Snyder, 1992; Choi, 1993; Verma et al., 1993; Chiueh et al., 1994; Dawson and Dawson, 1994; Schuman and Madison, 1994; Garthwaite and Boulton, 1995; Whittle, 1995; Abraham et al., 1996). NO is a free radical gaseous molecule and is a highly unstable compound (Bredt et al., 1991; Dawson and Snyder, 1994). Its half-life is extremely short (about 5 s) (Dawson et al., 1992; Feldman et al., 1993). The biological action of NO does not require its binding to the membrane receptors (Bredt, 1995), whereas CO is a byproduct of heme degradation and serves as a messenger molecule like NO (Maines, 1992, 1996; Verma et al., 1993; Abraham et al., 1996). There is evidence that CO mimics many actions of NO in both *in vivo* and *in vitro* situations (Table 2)

(Verma et al., 1993; Dawson and Snyder, 1994; Maines, 1996). However the details of their biological function in health and diseases is not yet well understood.

These two gaseous molecules are now considered as putative neurotransmitters because they influence intracellular signal transduction mechanisms by freely diffusing from one cell to another. However, unlike conventional neurotransmitters, these molecules are not stored in synaptic vesicles and their release is not influenced by exocytosis following membrane depolarisation (Verma et al., 1993; Dawson and Snyder, 1994; Dawson and Dawson, 1996; Kimura and Steinbusch, 1996). It appears that NO and CO are synthesised on demand by their respective synthesising enzymes nitric oxide synthase (NOS) and heme oxygenase (HO) normally found in the CNS (Abraham et al., 1996; Maines, 1996; Dawson and Dawson, 1996).

Since NO and CO are very short-lived molecules their involvement in various physiological and pathological conditions involving the CNS is difficult to ascertain. Thus, most investigations are confined to studying the expression of their synthesising enzymes NOS and HO respectively in various experimental or clinical conditions (Dawson et al., 1991; Bredt et al., 1992; Ewing and Maines, 1992; Maines, 1992). Activation of

---

*Corresponding author. Tel: +46 18 4714433; Fax: +46 18 243899; e-mail: sharma@anatomi.uu.se

NOS and HO is associated with production of NO and CO in the biological system (Bredt et al.,

TABLE 1

Pathophysiological functions of nitric oxide in the CNS *in vivo* and *in vitro*

Basic functions of NO
 Messenger molecule in the CNS and in PNS
 Induces relaxation of vascular smooth muscle (known as EDRF)
 Increases cGMP on acting GC
 Regulation of CBF
  Maintenance of cellular memory process
  Long-term potentiation (LTP) in hippocampus
  Long-term depression (LTD) in cerebellum
 Synaptic plasticity
 Thermoregulation
 Control of drinking behaviour
 Learning
 Pain and analgesia
 Narcotic dependence and withdrawal
 Stress mechanisms
 Neuromodulation[a,b]
 Ageing
 Cortical arousal
 Long-term habituation
 Apoptosis

NO is neurotoxic
 Glutamate induced neurotoxicity in cell culture is prevented
  by inhibitors of NOS (no neuroprotection by NOS
  inhibitors in neurotoxicity induced by quisqulate or kainate)
 Intracellular accumulation of Ca^{2+} [i] mediates neurotoxic
  effects of NO and induces cell death
 Pretreatment with NOS inhibitors has some neuroprotective effects

NO production
 Synthesised from NOS
 Released from neurons, astrocytes, endothelial cells,
 macrophages, blood

NO and neurodegeneration
 NO production is influenced in following diseases of the
  CNS
  Alzheimer's
  Parkinson's
  Huntington's
  Amyotrophic lateral sclerosis
  Epilepsy
  Stroke
  Ischemia

(Continued)

TABLE 1   *(Continued)*

NO production is influenced in following experimental conditions
 Brain injury[a,b]
 Spinal cord injury[a,b]
 Axotomy
 Motor neuron diseases
 Spinal root avulsion
 Spinal nerve lesion
 Neuropathic pain[a,b]
 Heat stress[a,b]
 LPS induced fever[a,b]
 Ischemia
 Stroke
 Infarction
 Hypoxia
 Haemorrhagic hypotension

Compiled from various sources (see text).
[a]Authors own investigations.
[b]Unpublished observations by authors.

1990; Ewing and Maines, 1991; Dawson et al., 1993a, 1994a; McCoubrey and Maines, 1994; Fukuda et al., 1995). Thus by assessing the expression of NOS and HO in different pathological conditions, one can get information regarding the involvement of NO and CO in such disease processes (Bredt et al., 1990; Alm et al., 1993; Chiueh et al., 1994; Beesley, 1995; Dwyer et al., 1995; Abraham et al., 1996; Fukuda et al., 1996; Sharma et al., 1996a–d, 1997a–d). Based on this information, data accumulated in the last 6–8 years implicate the involvement of NO and CO in many brain diseases (Tables 1 and 2) (Chiueh et al., 1994; Kimura and Steinbusch, 1996; Dawson and Dawson, 1996). However, involvement of NO and CO in hyperthermic brain injury is still a new subject which has not been well studied in the past.

This review is focused on the involvement of NO and CO in the brain pathology of heat stress which is based on our immunohistochemical investigations of NOS and HO expression in a rat model. In addition, new knowledge regarding modulation of brain function by NO and CO which has emerged recently, is briefly reviewed. Finally, to understand the contribution of NO and CO in brain pathology, the influence of selec-

TABLE 2

Physiological and pathological functions of CO

Heme oxygenase (HO), the enzyme responsible for the synthesis of CO is altered in various states
  Ischemia
  Hypoxia
  Oxidative stress
  Heat stress[a,b]
  Heat shock
  Brain injury
  Spinal cord injury[a,b]
  Subarachnoid haemorrhage
Inducers of HO
  Interleukin-1
  Tumor necrosis factor α
  Reactive oxygen species
  Metals
  Degeneration and ageing processes
  Cellular defence mechanism
  Hypertension
  Developmental processes
  Hormonal regulation
  Hematopoiesis
  Infections (malaria and other parasites)
  Inflammation
  Phagocytosis
  Alcoholism
  Tobacco smoking
  Environmental pollutants
  AIDS
  Regeneration and repair mechanisms?[a,b]

Similarities between NO and CO in many physiological functions
  Modulation of endothelial cell function
  Powerful vasodilator
  Activation of guanylyl cyclase
  Inhibitor of platelet aggregation
  Increases K^+ current in smooth muscle
  Functions as neurotransmitter?
  Involved in signal transduction mechanisms
  Long-term potentiation
  Regulates cell function and communication

Few notable differences in NO and CO function
  NO mediates glutamate-induced NMDA receptors
  CO mediates glutamate-induced metabotropic receptors
  CO influence metabotropic receptor-induced conductance
    of ion channels via cGMP
  NO does not influence agonist-induced increase in channel
    conductance

Compiled from various sources (for details see text). ? = further research is needed.
[a]Authors own investigations.
[b]Unpublished observations by authors.

tive neuroprotective drugs on NOS and HO expression was also examined in this model. These pharmacological observations in hyperthermic brain injury opened a new strategy in the field of NO and CO research which is very important in our understanding of the brain function in health and disease.

Nitric oxide is a new class of neurotransmitter in the CNS

Discovery of NO as a messenger molecule has revolutionised the concept of neuronal communication in the CNS (Dawson and Snyder, 1994). NO is freely permeable to the plasma membrane and thus does not need a biological receptor to influence the intracellular communication or signal transduction mechanisms (Galea et al., 1992; Dawson et al., 1992; Dinerman et al., 1994; Wood and Garthwaite, 1994; Bredt, 1995). Once generated, the cell cannot regulate the local concentration of NO. Thus, the other way to influence NO activity is to control its synthesis (Dawson and Snyder, 1994; Garthwaite and Boulton, 1995; Dawson and Dawson, 1996). The action of NO is terminated when it reacts chemically with a substrate (Lonart et al., 1992; Marletta, 1993; Förstermann, 1994; Kimura and Steinbusch, 1996). NO is involved in many physiological and pathophysiological processes (Table 1) and can influence a wide range of biological functions (Table 3) (Verge et al., 1992; Wu and Li, 1993; Zhuo et al., 1993; Wu et al., 1994a,b; Yu, 1994; Zhang et al., 1994a,b; Wildemann et al., 1995; Ueta et al., 1995; Dawson and Dawson, 1996; Kimura and Steinbusch, 1996; Sharma et al., 1996a, 1997a,b; Yamada et al., 1996). Abnormal production of NO in large quantities is associated with neurotoxicity; however small quantities of NO production can regulate cerebral blood flow (CBF) and local brain metabolism (Chiueh et al., 1994; Lipton et al., 1994). However, the mechanisms of NO production and its biological consequences in the CNS are not known in great detail.

TABLE 3

Involvement of NO in some pathophysiological functions within the CNS is emerging

---

NO seems to be involved in the following functions

Cell swelling and edema[a]
  Vasogenic edema[a]
  Cytotoxic edema?
Microvascular permeability disturbances
  Blood–brain barrier[a]
  Blood–spinal cord barrier[a]
  CSF–brain barrier?
  Blood–CSF barrier?
Cell injury and cell death
  Neuronal injury[a,b]
  Glial injury[b]
  Myelin injury?
Stress response
  HSP response[b]
  Gene expression?
Neurochemical metabolism[a,b]
Interaction with neurochemicals[c]
  Carbon monoxide
  Serotonin[a]
  Prostaglandins?
  Histamine[b]
  Opioids (dynorphin)[a,b]
  Catecholamines?
  Amino acid neurotransmitters
    GABA
    Glycine?
    Glutamate
    Aspartate?
    Taurine?
  Growth factors
Regeneration and repair mechanisms[a]
Modulation of ion channels
  Calcium
  Potassium?
  Sodium?
  Chloride
Bioelectricity
  Action potential
  Synaptic potential
  Evoked potentials?
    Somatosensory evoked potentials
    Motor evoked potentials
    Spinal cord evoked potentials[a]
    Cerebellar evoked potentials

(Continued)

TABLE 3   *(Continued)*

  Electroencephalogram?
    Cortical electroencephalogram
    Spinal electroencephalogram?
    Intracerebral electroencephalogram?

Compiled from various sources (for details see text). ? = further research is needed.
[a]Authors own investigations.
[b]Unpublished observations by authors.

Nitric oxide synthase and its isoforms in the CNS

The enzyme responsible for NO synthesis is NOS which is present in the CNS and in the periphery (Dawson et al., 1991; Lambert et al., 1991; Cho et al., 1992; Springall et al., 1992; Stuehr and Griffith, 1992; Alm et al., 1993; Baek et al., 1993; Ceccatelli et al., 1993; Drapier et al., 1993; Fiallos-Estrada et al., 1993; Koprowski et al., 1993; Marletta, 1993; Dinerman et al., 1994; Förstermann, 1994; Kadowaki et al., 1994; Klatt et al., 1994; Bredt, 1995; Mayer, 1995; Loesch and Burnstock, 1996; Magnusson et al., 1996). Recently, a new molecular approach has expanded our knowledge of the biochemistry of NO and NOS in greater detail. According to the normal occurrence and ability of NO formation, NOS is present in two principal isoforms (a) the constitutive NOS (cNOS) which is further subdivided into the neuronal NOS (nNOS; type I) and the endothelial NOS (eNOS; type III) according to its localization; and (b) the inducible NOS (iNOS, type II) also referred as immunologic NOS (for review see Dawson and Snyder, 1994; Dawson and Dawson, 1994, 1996; Kimura and Steinbusch, 1996). This nomenclature is principally based on the tissue from which they were first cloned; however all three isoforms of NOS are expressed in the CNS (Chiueh et al., 1994; Bredt, 1995; Dawson and Dawson, 1996).

The expression of these isoforms of NOS and

their relation with particular biological functions is still unclear. eNOS which is expressed in the cerebral endothelial cells critically regulates the cerebral blood flow (CBF); however its expression is not limited to the cerebral vessels only (Dalkara et al., 1994; Dawson and Dawson, 1994; Dawson et al., 1994a; Dinerman et al., 1994). Most NOS neurons express the neuronal isoform of the enzyme (nNOS); however, a small population of neurons in the pyramidal cells of CA1, CA2 and CA3 subfields of the hippocampus and granule cells of the dentate gyrus express eNOS immunostaining (Dinerman et al., 1994). The functional significance of this finding is not clear at the moment. The neuronally produced NO is involved in synaptic plasticity, neuronal signalling and neurotoxicity (Table 2) (Dawson et al., 1994a,b; Dinerman et al., 1994; Dawson and Dawson, 1996).

Genetic homology between various NOS isoforms

The nNOS, sometimes denoted as brain NOS (bNOS), is purified from human, mouse, porcine and rat cerebellum (Bredt, 1995). The molecular mass of the human cerebellar NOS is 160 kDa, which is similar to that purified from rat cerebellum and exhibits a 94–95% homology with NOS obtained from human or mouse cerebellum (Bredt and Snyder, 1992; Förstermann, 1994). The C-terminal part contains the recognition sites for nicotineamide adenine dinucleotide phosphate diaphorase (NADPH), flavine adenine dinucleotide (FAD), flavin mononucleotide (FMN) and tetrahydrobiopterin (H_4B) and shows a 36% homology to cytochrome P-450 reductase (Förstermann, 1994; Garthwaite and Boulton, 1995). The N-terminal part contains sites for phosphorylation (White and Marletta, 1992; Schuman and Madison, 1994; Garthwaite and Boulton, 1995; Mayer, 1995). eNOS, purified from bovine aortic endothelial cells has a lower molecular mass (133–135 kDa), and shows about 60% homology with the rat cerebellar NOS (Snyder, 1992; Springall et al., 1992; Stuehr and Griffith, 1992).

Cloning of iNOS from murine macrophages revealed a 93% homology with iNOS from rat vascular smooth muscle and 82% homology with human hepatocytes (Alm et al., 1993; Baek et al., 1993). iNOS which has a molecular mass of 130–135 kDa, exhibits 65% homology with eNOS and nNOS (Bredt and Snyder, 1992; Bredt, 1995). In addition to macrophages, the presence of iNOS has been demonstrated in mast cells, granulocytes, mesangial cells, hepatocytes, Kupfer cells, chondrocytes, osteoclasts and vascular smooth muscle (Baek et al., 1993; Bredt, 1995).

Co-localisation of NOS with other neurotransmitters in the CNS

NOS is often co-localised with many other neurotransmitters (for details see Kimura and Steinbusch, 1996; Yamada et al., 1996) which is not comparable to any other classical neurotransmitters in the CNS (for details see Table 4). Thus NOS is apparently not co-localised with any one neurotransmitter. However, most of the nNOS neurons identified are mainly co-localised with the histochemical stain NADPH diaphorase (Hope et al., 1991; Vincent and Kimura, 1992; Wolf et al., 1992; Fiallos-Estrada et al., 1993; Matsumoto et al., 1993; Kharazia et al., 1994; Vizzard et al., 1994; Wallace and Bisland, 1994).

Both immunohistochemistry and *in situ* hybridisation studies show that nNOS is co-localised with glutaminergic granule cells and GABergic basket cells in the cerebellum, and in the cerebral cortex with somatostatin, neuropeptide Y and GABA (Dawson and Dawson, 1996). In the corpus striatum, NOS is co-localised with somatostatin and neuropeptide Y and in the brain stem pedunculopontine tegmental nucleus, the enzyme is found with choline acetyltransferase (Dawson et al., 1991). In the hypothalamus, NOS immunoreactive neurons are co-localised with substance P and enkephalins (Yamada et al., 1996; Kimura and Steinbusch, 1996). However, in some hypothalamic nuclei NOS immunoreactive neurons are located with cholecystokinin, oxytocin, corticotropin releasing factor, galanin and so-

TABLE 4

Co-localisation of NOS with other neurotransmitters in the CNS

Brain region	NOS type	Neurotransmitters/enzymes
Cerebellum	nNOS	Glutaminergic granule cells, GABAergic basket cells
Cerebral cortex	nNOS	Somatostatin, neuropeptide Y, GABA
Corpus striatum	nNOS	Somatostatin, neuropeptide Y
Pedunculopontine tegmental nucleus	nNOS	Choline acetyltransferase
Hypothalamus	nNOS	Substance P, enkephalins, cholecystokinin, somatostatin, oxytocin, galanin, corticotropin releasing factor
CNS	nNOS	NADPH diaphorase
CNS	nNOS	CO[a]

Compiled from various sources (for details see Dawson and Dawson, 1996; Kimura and Steinbusch, 1996; Yamada et al., 1996). Based on *in situ* hybridisation signals or immunohistochemical staining.
[a] Found in some neurons in the CNS (for details see Vincent et al., 1994).

matostatin (Table 4) (for details see Yamada et al., 1996).

The functional significance of this co-localisation of nNOS with many neurotransmitters in different brain regions is not clear. However, it seems quite likely that nNOS is involved in various neuromodulatory functions in the CNS, a feature which however requires additional investigation.

Upregulation of NOS and NO production

Upregulation of NOS is seen in many experimental or clinical conditions involving brain pathology (Table 1) (Chao et al., 1992; Hyman et al., 1992; Vallance et al., 1992b; Dawson et al., 1993a,b,c; Herdegen et al., 1993; Koprowski et al., 1993; Merrill et al., 1993; Mollace et al., 1993; Wu and Li, 1993; Bo et al., 1994; Carreau et al., 1994; Chiueh et al., 1994; Dalkara et al., 1994; Huang et al., 1994; Kadowaki et al., 1994; Santiago et al., 1994; Sharkey and Butcher, 1994; Visser et al., 1994; Wu et al., 1994a,b; Yu, 1994; Zhang et al., 1994a; Novikov et al., 1995; Resink et al., 1995; Ueta et al., 1995; Wildemann et al., 1995; Przed-

borski et al., 1996; Sharma et al., 1996a–d, 1997a–c). Thus, upregulation of nNOS can be seen in the CNS neurons not normally showing this activity in ischemia (Dalkara et al., 1994; Huang et al., 1994; Dawson and Dawson, 1996), acute spinal cord injury (Sharma et al., 1996a,d, 1997b,c) or in chronic spinal lesion caused by peripheral axotomy or root avulsions (Verge et al., 1992; Fiallos-Estrada et al., 1993; Herdegen et al., 1993; Wu et al., 1994a,b; Yu, 1994; Sharma et al., 1996b). Induction of iNOS occurs in various tissues following heat shock (Maines, 1996), and in cultured peripheral ganglia during conditions of regeneration (Magnusson et al., 1996).

Activation of NOS produces NO as a free radical (NO·). The free radical (NO·) will react with carrier molecules and releases NO in oxidised (NO^+) or reduced (NO^-) forms (Lipton et al., 1994; Stamler, 1994). All three valance states are found in the CNS which seems to be responsible for different biological effects (Dawson and Dawson, 1994, 1996). This may partially explain the controversial effects of NO in the CNS.

The NO produced by iNOS is sustained for long time periods and most probably is responsible for neurodegeneration in several clinical or experimental conditions (Murphy et al., 1993; Dawson and Dawson, 1996). On the other hand, the constitutive isomers are expressed constantly which is not dependent on transcriptional induction of protein synthesis like the inducible isomer (Chiueh et al., 1994; Dawson and Snyder, 1994; Bredt, 1995; Kimura and Steinbusch, 1996).

Molecular mechanisms of NOS activation

Activation of different isoforms of NOS in biological systems requires various factors and co-factors. Increase in intracellular calcium is a prerequisite for activation of eNOS and nNOS which forms calcium/calmodulin complexes in order to exhibit its action after binding to the dimers (Cho et al., 1992; Bolanos et al., 1995). However, the iNOS differs in both expression and function compared to eNOS or nNOS (Dawson et al., 1994a). nNOS has a predominant cytosolic location whereas the iNOS is totally located in the cytosol (Dawson et al., 1992; Drapier et al., 1993) and eNOS is bound to the plasma membrane by N-terminal myristylation (Pollock et al., 1992). For full activity, iNOS is dependent on various cofactors for electron transfer in the oxidation process, such as e.g. NADPH, FAD, FMN and H_4B, for which there are recognition sites on the reductase domain of the enzyme molecule (Förstermann, 1994; Garthwaite and Boulton, 1995).

eNOS and nNOS are also dependent on cofactors such as H_4B, FAD, FMN and NADPH, the recognition sites for which are present on the reductase domain of the enzyme molecule like iNOS (Klatt et al., 1994; Koch et al., 1994; Mayer, 1995). In addition, in the middle part of the molecule of eNOS and nNOS, there are binding sites for calmodulin (Galea et al., 1992; White and Marletta, 1992).

In addition to these cofactors, other regulatory mechanisms have been suggested to influence the activity of the constitutive isoform of NOS (see review by Mayer, 1995). Thus, cNOS can be phosphorylated by various protein kinases which leads to a diminished catalytic activity by the influence of cyclic AMP- and GMP-dependent protein kinases, protein kinase C and calcium/calmodulin dependent kinases (Förstermann, 1994). Increased catalytic activity of NOS is also influenced by protein phosphatase and calcineurin (Bredt, 1995; Mayer, 1995).

In contrast to nNOS and eNOS, iNOS can bind to calmodulin even at a very low concentration of intracellular calcium (Cho et al., 1992; Baek et al., 1993), although recognition sites with tightly bound calmodulin have been demonstrated in the middle of the enzyme molecule (Bredt et al., 1992; Mayer, 1995; Whittle, 1995). Thus, iNOS can be expressed as a functionally active dimer without any increase in intracellular calcium (Dawson and Dawson, 1996). However, antagonists of calcium binding proteins do not block the synthesis of iNOS.

In general, iNOS is not expressed in normal CNS; however an increased expression in astrocytes and microglia occurs following viral infections and trauma (Dawson and Dawson, 1996). Activation of iNOS requires gene transcription and induction can be influenced by endotoxin and cytokines (interleukin-1, interleukin-2, lipopolysaccharide, interferon-γ, tumor necrosis factor). This activation can be blocked by anti-inflammatory drugs (dexamethasone, hydrocortisone), inhibitory cytokines (interleukin-4, interleukin-10, macrophage deactivating factor, tissue growth factors) or inhibitors of protein synthesis, e.g. cyclohexamide (see reviews by Stuehr and Griffith, 1992; Feldman et al., 1993).

Inhibitors of NOS

Several specific and non-specific inhibitors of NOS are commercially available (see reviews by Stuehr and Griffith, 1992; Mayer, 1995; Whittle, 1995). In general, N-substituted derivatives of arginine such as NG-monomethyl-L-arginine (L-NMMA, L-Met-Arg), NG-nitro-L-arginine (NARG) and L-nitro arginine methyl ester (L-NAME) are commonly used as NOS inhibitors (McCal et al., 1990; Corbett et al., 1992; Babbedge et al., 1993; Carreau et al., 1994; Mayer et al., 1994). However, these substances differ in inhibitory effects and selectivity with regard to the various isoforms of NOS. L-NMMA exerts a long-lasting inhibitory effects on the iNOS- and nNOS isoforms, whereas, L-NNA and L-NAME (its corresponding methyl ester) exert their selective inhibitory effects on nNOS and eNOS isomers (Mayer et al., 1994; Mayer, 1995).

Depending on the dose, these compounds can inhibit various other isoforms of NOS as well. Thus, low concentrations of L-NNA inhibits nNOS and to some extent the eNOS activity, without having any influence on iNOS (Mayer, 1995). This effect of L-NNA on eNOS (cultured bovine aortic cells) and nNOS (rat cerebellar) is 30- to 200-fold more efficient (Gross et al., 1991) as compared to L-NMMA. On the other hand, the inhibitory effect of L-NNA on iNOS is 20-fold less potent as compared with L-NMMA (Gross et al., 1990, Lambert et al., 1991).

Compounds which are not analogues of arginine are also found to be potent inhibitors of NOS. 7-Nitro indazol (7-NI) is one compound which shows a specific selectivity for inhibition of nNOS by competition with arginine (McCal et al., 1990; Babbedge et al., 1993; Moore et al., 1993a,b) and its binding with the cofactor H_4B (Klatt et al., 1994). The other compounds, such as L-canavanine and aminoguanidine which are not true derivatives of arginine, can readily inhibit iNOS activity in neutrophils, vascular tissue and insuloma cells of pancreas (McCal et al., 1990; Corbett et al., 1992; Umans and Samsel, 1992).

Drugs influencing enzymes other than NOS can also influence the NO activity. These compounds include dichlorophenol which interferes with NADPH-requiring enzymes, diphenyl ioidonium which inhibits the enzymes utilising nucleotide flavoproteins as cofactors; and other antagonists of calmodulin or calmodulin-dependent enzymes (for review, see Mayer, 1995).

Methylated arginines which are capable of inhibiting nitric oxide synthesis are found in plasma of healthy volunteers. The levels of these com-pounds are increased in patients with chronic renal failure (Vallance et al., 1992a,b). However, the functional significance of these endogenous inhibitors of NOS activity is not well known at this moment.

Pathophysiological functions of NOS and NO in the CNS

Based on diffusion studies, there are some assumptions that NO once generated can diffuse up to 300 μm from its origin (Wood and Garthwaite, 1994). A rough estimate suggests that NO by this way can influence about 2×10^6 synapses in the CNS (Peters et al., 1991). Thus NO can influence a large sphere of the brain if activated either following glutamate excitotoxicity, stroke, ischemia, infarction or trauma. However, the detailed molecular mechanisms of NO-induced cell injury is not known.

Recent evidence suggests that the upregulation of NOS is harmful and is somehow related to cell injury. This is evident by two independent observations in experimental models of trauma and ischemia. Experiments done in our laboratory for the first time demonstrated that application of nNOS antiserum in high concentrations on the traumatised spinal cord is neuroprotective (Sharma et al., 1994a, 1995a). In these experiments trauma induced edema formation and cell injury are attenuated by application of nNOS antiserum (Sharma et al., 1994a, 1995a) which correlates well with nNOS upregulation in the traumatised spinal cord (Sharma et al., 1996a). This observation suggests that upregulation of NOS is related to edema and cell injury.

The other line of evidence came from studies on ischemia in nNOS null mice (Huang et al., 1994) which demonstrated that nNOS knockout mice exhibited significantly less infarction and cell damage following ischemia compared to the wild-type controls. These two independent observations strongly point out that upregulation of NOS is harmful and NO is involved in cell injury.

This idea is further supported in various animal

models using a pharmacological approach. Thus, in stroke, neuroprotection can be achieved by compounds which are potential inhibitors of nNOS rather than eNOS or both (Dawson and Dawson, 1994). Thus a selective inhibition of nNOS by 7-NI significantly reduced the infarct volume (Dalkara et al., 1994), whereas non-selective inhibition or partial inhibition of eNOS using other NOS inhibitors increases the infarct volume. This is because these non-selective NOS inhibitors inhibit the eNOS activity resulting in a reduction in CBF which will aggravate cell injury during ischemia and stroke (for details, see Dawson and Snyder, 1994).

The potential benefit of pharmacological agents in achieving neuroprotection thus depends on their ability to influence specific isoform of NOS in animal experiments. A failure of NOS inhibitors in inducing neuroprotection described by many workers may be due to the fact that most NOS inhibitors are non-selective and can inhibit all isoforms of NOS with different potency (Dawson and Dawson, 1996).

Cerebral infarction induces upregulation of nNOS and increases NO production via stimulation of NMDA receptors (Dawson et al., 1994b). Some gangliosides which inhibit or bind with calmodulin can offer neuroprotection by decreasing NOS catalytic activity (Dawson et al., 1995). This neuroprotection is due to inhibition of nNOS which parallels the binding of ganglioside with calmodulin (Dawson et al., 1995). Another line of evidence with regard to a neurodestructive role of NO came from studies using immunosuppressants FK 506 and cyclosporin-A which offer good neuroprotection in animal models or in cell culture studies (Dawson et al., 1993c). These immunosuppressants inhibit calcium-activated phosphatase, calcineurin. Inhibition of calcineurin with immunosuppressants prevents dephosphorylation and activation of nNOS resulting in neuroprotection (Dawson et al., 1993c; Sharkey and Butcher, 1994; Dawson and Dawson, 1996). These observations strongly suggest that generation of NO from the activated NOS is contributing to cell injury.

NO in brain diseases

Overproduction of NO seems to be instrumental in various brain diseases (Tables 1 and 3). Induction of human iNOS occurs in multiple sclerosis which is mainly found in the areas exhibiting demyelination (Bo et al., 1994). It seems quite likely that NO exerts a neurotoxic effect on oligodendrocytes which are responsible for myelination (Merrill et al., 1993). NO production is increased in bacterial meningitis (Visser et al., 1994) and sufferers of migraine are supersensitive to NO (Thomsen et al., 1993).

In cell culture studies, NO is involved in the pathogenesis of Alzheimer's disease and AIDS dementia. Thus, NOS inhibitors offer neuroprotection following cell damage induced by fragments of human amyloid protein in cortical cell cultures (Resink et al., 1995). Neurotoxicity induced by HIV protein gp 120 is related to activation of NOS in cell culture and studies of human cases of AIDS dementia exhibited a profound increase in iNOS activity (Wildemann et al., 1995) indicating the involvement of NO in AIDS (Dawson et al., 1993b). NO neurotoxicity is seen in animal models of Parkinson's disease. Thus nNOS null transgenic mice are resistant to MPP^+ induced depletion of dopamine in striatum (Przedborski et al., 1996). In animal model of Huntington's disease, NOS inhibitors are neuroprotective against 3-nitroprorionic acid or malonate-induced lesions (Schultz et al., 1995a,b).

These observations support the idea that NO is involved in many brain diseases. However, in the *in vivo* situation, no single chemical compound is responsible for all the observed changes. Thus it seems quite likely that the regulation of NO by other neurotransmitter substances and interaction of NO with many endogenous molecules are of vital importance in the pathogenesis of various brain diseases (Table 3). Thus efforts should be made to influence NOS upregulation using various pharmacological strategies.

Carbon monoxide influences CNS function in health and diseases

In the CNS, apart from NO, there are some other small diffusible signalling molecule such as CO (Maines, 1988, 1992, 1996; Ewing and Maines, 1991; Verma et al., 1993; Abraham et al., 1996) and OH (Zoccarato et al., 1989; Beckman, 1994; Chiueh et al., 1994). These freely diffusible molecules allow for a better co-ordinated communication between neurons not offered by the conventional neurotransmitters. The activity of these molecules is controlled by different short half lives and different diffusible constants (Schuman and Madison, 1994). Out of these gaseous molecules, CO has recently emerged as one of the important new neurotransmitter candidates regulating some important aspects of CNS function in health and diseases (Table 2) (Dawson and Snyder, 1994; Abraham et al., 1996).

CO is a by-product of heme degradation (Maines, 1988, 1992, 1996). Heme is a complex of the transition metal iron linked to the four nitrogen atoms of a tetrapyrrole macrocycle and is involved in neurite outgrowth, protein synthesis as well as cell differentiation and development (Maines et al., 1995; Maines, 1996). Degradation of heme to biliverdin releases iron and generates CO. This reaction is catalysed by the enzyme heme oxygenase (HO) which appears to be of major importance in the regulation of various cellular phenomena (for review, see Abraham et al., 1996).

The heme oxygenase enzyme

The rate limiting enzyme, HO responsible for heme degradation was first described in 1968 by Tenhunen and co-workers (Tenhunen et al., 1968). This enzyme was initially though to be a species of cytochrome P-450 but was found later to be a separate protein capable of degradation of heme to biliverdin and iron with a concomitant release of CO. This enzyme is highly conserved throughout evolution and is found in all prokaryotes, higher species and even in plants (Abraham et al., 1996).

HO was first purified from rat liver and pig spleen and has a molecular weight of about 32 kDa (Maines et al., 1977). Recent studies showed that this enzyme exists in two isoforms. The original enzyme studied is designated type 1 (HO-1) and the recently discovered isoenzyme is designated type 2 (HO-2) (Maines, 1992, 1996).

Isoforms of heme oxygenase

HO is present in various tissues with the highest activity in the brain, liver, spleen and testes (Vincent et al., 1994; Vollerthun et al., 1995, 1996; Yamanaka et al., 1996; Zakhary et al., 1996). HO occurs in two isoforms (HO-1, inducible and HO-2, constitutive) and requires the same cofactors (NADPH cytochrome P450-reductase and NADPH), like NO and is located in the smooth endoplasmic reticulum (Shibahara et al., 1993). However, the formation of the two isomers is transcribed from two separate genes. The HO-1 differs from HO-2 in molecular weight (HO-1 $\gg$ 30 kDa, HO-2 $\gg$ 36 kDa), biochemistry (e.g. loss of enzyme activity by heat, ability of precipitation by ammonium sulphate, electrophoretic mobility, sequence and composition of amino acids) and in immunological functions (Shibahara et al., 1993; Abraham et al., 1996). The antisera raised against these two isomers do not recognise opposite antigenic epitopes (Maines, 1996; Affiniti Research Products, 1996).

Genetic homology between isoforms of HO

The genes for human, mouse, pig and rat HO-1 have been well characterised and cloned recently (Shibahara et al., 1993). The HO-1 genes are organised into four introns and five exons. The 5'-untranslated region of the genes contains different regulatory sites. The complete nucleotide sequences for human rat and rabbit HO-2 has been published (McCoubrey et al., 1992) and like HO-1, HO-2 genes also consist of five exons and four entrons. HO-2 has a molecular weight of 34 kDa and exhibits 40% homology of amino acid sequence with HO-1 (Maines, 1988, 1992). The most discriminating character of the two HO isomers is their method of formation (Rotenberg and Maines, 1990).

Inducers of HO

The HO-1 is inducible by many diverse inducers, such as chemical compounds (heme substances, alkylating agents, halogenated hydrocarbons, organic solvents), therapeutic agents (H_2-receptor antagonists), hormones (adrenaline, insulin, glucagon), bacterial toxins or antigenic substances, various neoplastic states and conditions such as heat shock, oxidative stress and many other forms of cellular stress (Table 2) (see review by Maines, 1992, 1996).

On the other hand, the role of HO-2 in cells is not well understood. There is evidence that HO-2 is constitutively expressed with a more or less constant level and it may play important roles in signal transduction mechanisms in the nervous tissues (Verma et al., 1993; Dawson and Snyder, 1994).

HO and heat shock proteins response

There is evidence that HO-1 may act as a heat shock protein (HSP) known as HSP 32 and can be induced by cellular stress caused by oxidative damage (Marcuccilli and Miller, 1994; for details see review by Westman and Sharma, this volume) which seems to be protective in nature (for review, see Marcuccilli and Miller, 1994). Induction of HO-1 occurs together with HSP in the brain during various experimental conditions involving oxidative stress, hyperthermia, ischemia and trauma (Ewing and Maines, 1991; Fukuda et al., 1995, 1996) and a focal lesion of the spinal cord (Sharma H.S., unpublished observations).

The mechanisms of HO-1 or HSP induction is unclear. However, in hyperthermia, corticosteroids seem to induce upregulation of HO-1 in hippocampus (Maines et al., 1995). It appears that induction of HO-1 and HSP response is dependent on the newly discovered heat shock factors (HSFs) (for details, see review by Marcuccilli and Miller, 1994 and Westman and Sharma, this volume).

Regional variations in HO expression

There is great variability in the tissue distribution of the two isoforms of HO and the basal levels of HO-2 expression vary considerably from one tissue to another. Thus HO-1 is mainly concentrated in peripheral tissues such as spleen and the liver whereas, HO-2 occurs in high concentrations in the CNS (Verma et al., 1993; Sharma et al., 1996b, 1997d). High concentrations of HO-2 are present in hippocampal pyramidal and granule cells. In the cerebellum, large concentrations of HO-2 are present in granule and Purkinje cell layers. In addition HO-2 is also found in pyriform cortex, tenia tecta, olfactory tubercle and islands of Callejae (Verma et al., 1993). Highest concentrations of HO-2 in brain are found in neurons of olfactory epithelium and in neuronal and granule cell layers of the olfactory bulb. There is some evidence that a few neurons in the spinal cord are also positive for HO-2. However, the detailed mapping of HO-2 positive cells in the CNS is not completely known. Preliminary results suggest that induction of HO-1 can occur without any change in HO-2 expression at least in cultured rat autonomic ganglia (Alm et al., unpublished observations).

Pathophysiological functions of HO

The detailed pathophysiological role of HO is not completely known. However, with the identification of the HO gene, it is possible to follow the cascade of intracellular events following changes in HO expression (Abraham et al., 1996; Maines, 1996) in order to understand the involvement of HO/CO in health and disease (Table 2).

Alteration in HO occurs during a wide range of pathophysiological conditions (Table 2) (for review see Abraham et al., 1996; Maines, 1996). However, it is not yet certain whether an upregulation of HO expression is beneficial or injurious to the cell. There are some suggestions that generation of CO from the activated HO may counterbalance some of the injurious effects of NO (Zhuo et al., 1993; Vincent et al., 1994); however no concrete evidence is available to either accept or reject this hypothesis.

It seems quite likely that CO is involved in the mechanism of cell injury (Fukuda et al., 1996; Panizzon et al., 1996; Soltesz, 1996). This is evident from the fact that CO binds to heme in guanylyl cyclase (GC) to activate cGMP (Gräser et al., 1990). This affinity of CO for heme is mainly accounted for the lethality of the cells because after binding to heme, CO prevents haemoglobin from delivering oxygen to the tissues. Using olfactory neurons in cell culture studies, it has been found that CO is responsible for maintaining endogenous levels of cGMP. This effect is blocked by potent HO inhibitors but not by NOS inhibitors (Verma et al., 1993; Maines, 1996).

Based on endogenous distribution of HO enzyme in the CNS it has been suggested that CO can influence neurotransmission like NO (Verma et al., 1993; Dawson and Snyder, 1994). CO appears to be involved as a retrograde messenger in LTP because one potent HO inhibitor, ZnPP-9 blocks the induction of LTP in hippocampal slices (Stevens and Wang, 1993). Furthermore long-lasting increases in the amplitude of evoked potentials are observed when CO is applied at the same time as a weak tetanic stimulation (Zhuo et al., 1993).

Experimental evidence indicates that CO is involved in mediating glutamate action at metabotropic receptors (Gräser et al., 1990; Verma et al., 1993; Dawson and Snyder, 1994). This is evident from the fact that metabotropic receptor activation in the brain stem regulates the conductance of specific ion channels via a cGMP dependent mechanism. This effects is blocked by HO inhibitors (Glaum and Miller, 1993).

CO vs. NO

Experimental evidence suggests that CO plays a similar role like NO in the signal transduction mechanism for the regulation of cell function and cell to cell communication (Abraham et al., 1996; Maines, 1996) (Table 2). Thus CO serves as a modulator of endothelial cell function and is a powerful vasodilator substance (Gräser et al., 1990). CO also inhibits platelet aggregation, increases K^+ current in smooth muscles and activates GC (Dawson and Snyder, 1994). Thus, CO shares some of the chemical and biological properties of NO.

There are also some similarities between HO and NOS function. Thus HO resembles NOS in that the electrons for CO synthesis are donated by cytochrome P450 reductase which is 60% homologous at the amino acid level to the carboxylterminal half of NOS (White and Marletta, 1992). CO like NO binds to iron in heme in GC to activate cGMP (Dawson and Snyder, 1994). However, there are some differences in function of CO compared to NO (Table 2). Thus NO mainly mediates glutamate effects at NMDA receptors while CO is primarily responsible for glutamate action at metabotropic receptors (Table 2). Taken together, it appears that CO and NO play an important role in the regulation of CNS function at both cellular and molecular levels and derangements of NO and CO metabolism are somehow associated with abnormal brain function (see below).

HO expression in disease states

Involvement of HO in various diseases states is evident from the fact that expression of either HO protein or HO mRNA is altered in many diverse but clinically relevant conditions (Table 2) (Maines, 1988, 1992; Ewing and Maines, 1991; 1992; Verma et al., 1993; Dawson and Snyder, 1994; Meffert et al., 1994; Raju and Maines, 1994; Fukuda et al., 1995; Maines et al., 1995; Fukuda et al., 1996; Ny et al., 1996; Panizzon et al., 1996; Sharma et al., 1996b; Soltesz, 1996; Sharma et al., 1997d). HO-1 mRNA expression is increased in ischemia and hypoxia which seems to have a protective effect (Abraham et al., 1996; Fukuda et al., 1995, 1996). Further evidence of HO in cell protection is evident in some forms of oxidative stress such as exposure to light, free radicals, irradiation and other forms of degenerative diseases and ageing processes in which enhanced HO activity seems to have an anti-oxidant effect (Abraham et al., 1996; Maines, 1996).

The induction of HO is well known to exert a pronounced effect on hormonal regulation (Maines, 1992) and is regarded as a general response to cellular stress (Fukuda et al., 1996). The level of HO mRNA is elevated in peripheral blood in patients with AIDS compared to normal subjects (for details see review by Abraham et al., 1996) and the HO expression is also altered in other diseases such as jaundice and diabetes (Abraham et al., 1996; Maines, 1996). In hypertension, inducers of renal HO exert a profound antihypertensive effect (Abraham et al., 1996). The functional significance of such findings is not yet clear. However, it appears that HO inducers and inhibitors may have some new therapeutic potentials in future, a subject which requires additional investigation.

Inhibitors of heme oxygenase enzyme

In general, metalloporphyrins in which the central iron atom is replaced either by Co, Cr, Mn, Sn or Zn act as competitive inhibitors of the enzyme (Glaum and Miller, 1993; Meffert et al., 1994). On the other hand, metalloporphyrins such as Cu, Mg and Ni protoporphyrins, which also bind to the catalytic site of HO have a much lesser inhibitory effect on heme degradation.

Potent metalloproporphyrins currently used as specific inhibitors of HO are zinc-protoporphyrins IX (Zn-PP-9) or tin-protoporphyrins (Sn-PP) (Glaum and Miller, 1993; Verma et al., 1993; Dawson and Snyder, 1994; Panizzon et al., 1996; Soltesz, 1996). However, there are reports that both Sn-PP and Zn-PP have adverse side effects and they interfere with many other biological processes as well (Meffert et al., 1994; Maines, 1996; Ny et al., 1996).

Morphological detection of HO and NOS

Detection of the sites and molecular mechanisms of CO and NO formation in the CNS is crucial in order to understand their involvement in health and disease. Histochemical localization of NOS and HO is one of the great tools utilised currently by many workers to understand the function of NO and CO in the CNS (Dawson et al., 1991; Ewing and Maines, 1991, 1992; Aoki et al., 1993; Ceccatelli et al., 1993; Dinerman et al., 1994; Beesley, 1995; Dwyer et al., 1995; Maines et al., 1995; Fukuda et al., 1995, 1996). In addition, *in situ* hybridisation methods for localising these enzymes in the CNS have been developed recently (for review, see Vincent et al., 1994; Maines, 1996). In brief, the following techniques are widely used to detect NOS and HO in the CNS at present.

NADPH-diaphorase enzyme histochemistry for NOS detection

NADPH-diaphorase is one of the cofactors of NOS and catalyses a reaction which precipitates as an insoluble and dark-blue to black formazan-Nitro Blue reaction product. The similarity between nNOS and NADPH-diaphorase (Dawson et al., 1991; Hope et al., 1991) is examined in a large number of studies which led to the use of NADPH-diaphorase as a marker for nNOS.

However, there are some reports describing differences in the distribution of nNOS and NADPH-diaphorase activity, suggesting that this staining is not a specific marker for NOS (Kharazia et al., 1994; Vizzard et al., 1994). Some similarities between NOS and NADPH-diaphorase reaction products can be seen by NOS-immunolabelled sections that are sequentially stained using the NADPH-diaphorase method (for details see Alm et al., 1993; Wallace and Bisland, 1994; Dawson and Dawson, 1996).

However with this method, it is not possible to identify the different isoforms of NOS or cytochrome P450 reductase because both use NADPH-diaphorase as a cofactor. This reaction is non-specific as it stains other forms of diaphorases as well. Most workers still use this method because NADPH-diaphorase which is not associated with NOS is more sensitive to formalin. The other disadvantage of this method is that the intensity and number of the dark-blue reaction products diminish with advancement of post-fixation period. This is particularly true in the case of nNOS (Matsumoto et al., 1993). However, the NADPH-diaphorase technique is still in use due to the simplicity and rapidity in the performance of this method.

Immunohistochemistry for NOS and HO expression

Immunohistochemical techniques are most frequently used to localise HO and NOS in either perfusion- and/or immersion-fixed materials. The advantage of this method is that these fixed tissues can be stored in the same fixative at 4°C for quite a long period of time. Many workers prefer cryostat or vibratome sectioning (for details see Alm et al., 1993; Sharma et al., 1995b, 1996a, 1997a); however, in some laboratories, paraffin embedding works equally well (Pollock et al., 1995). The immunostaining of NOS on vibratome sections (40–60 μm) or cryostat sections (10–50 μm) is done either attached to glass slides (in the case of frozen sections) or in a free-floating condition (vibratome sections). The sites for antibodies are then revealed by immunoenzyme- or immunofluorescence-detection techniques. These immunoreaction products obtained by immunoenzyme techniques are quite stable and can be quantified using semiquantitative techniques (Fukuda et al., 1995; Sharma et al. 1996a, 1997d). Thus the immunohistochemical methods of NOS and HO detection offer a specific, reliable and reproducible technique.

The technique of immunofluorescence-detection in combination with double- or triple-immunolabelling allows evaluation of the relationship between several compounds of interest in the same section. Thus a simultaneous evaluation of

the relationship between HO or NOS with other neurochemical substances is possible. It is easy to determine if these compounds are co-localised within the same structure by using confocal microscopy (for review, see Ny et al., 1996).

The main issue in these techniques is to use a good antiserum in order to detect specific immunolabelling. A few years ago, antiserum to NOS was raised by a few research laboratories and were inaccessible to many other workers. But nowadays antiserum to almost all isoforms of NOS are commercially available. However, there are overt differences in sensitivity, specificity and cross-reactivity in different tissues and species between various antibodies available commercially. One reason for this could be related to the method of production of these antibodies. It has been found that nNOS antiserum raised against a specific sequence of the enzyme molecule gives a specific labelling to only neuronal structures (Springall et al., 1992; Alm et al., 1993). Whereas, nNOS antiserum raised against the whole enzyme molecule can also bind to epitopes of the cofactors, which are in common in different isoforms of NOS. Thus, using this type of antisera, it is not possible to detect immunolabelling of structures containing only nNOS because other isoforms of NOS will be stained as well (cf. Bredt et al., 1990). For this reason, we have used nNOS antiserum raised by ourselves in the present investigation (for details see Alm et al., 1993; Sharma et al., 1996a).

Compared to NOS immunostaining, immunohistochemical studies localising HO enzyme in the CNS are not common. This is because of the fact that antiserum to HO were not commercially available until a few years ago. The first antisera was raised against HO-1 and HO-2 by Maines and her co-workers about 5 years ago. Using these rabbit polyclonal antisera, a differential distribution of HO-1- and HO-2-immunoreactivity in the rat brain was described (Ewing and Maines, 1992). The results show that though the HO-2-immunoreactivity can be seen in some brain regions, the presence of HO-1-immunoreactivity is normally not found in control rats (Ewing and Maines, 1992). However, an increase in the HO-1 immunoreactivity was observed in neurons and more markedly in glial cells following hyperthermia.

Recently, antisera against HO have become commercially available (StressGen, Victoria, BC, Canada; Affiniti Research Products, Exter, UK), and have been used in various laboratories with reliable and reproducible results in both CNS as well as in PNS. Yamanaka et al. (1996) using a rabbit antiserum raised against a peptide sequence corresponding to the amino-terminal region of HO-2 cloned from rat testis (Rotenberg and Maines, 1990) detected HO-2-immunoreactivity in dendrites and somata of Purkinje cells and basket cells of the rat cerebellum. In the PNS, HO-2-immunoreactivity is found in most neuronal cell bodies (but not in nerve fibres), in autonomic ganglia (Vollerthun et al., 1995, 1996; Zakhary et al., 1996) as well as in intramural ganglia of the gastrointestinal (Zakhary et al., 1996) and genito-urinary tracts (Alm et al., unpublished observations). In autonomic ganglia, the HO-1-immunoreactivity was not detected in normal rats; however HO-1-immunoreactivity was expressed in some neurons and in satellite cells during cell culture (Alm et al., in preparation). These results indicate that the immunohistochemical staining of HO-1 and HO-2 is a quite reliable tool to assess the functional significance of CO in health and disease.

Though the exact relationship between NOS and HO is still unclear, there is some evidence that co-expression of NOS and HO occurs in a very limited number of neurons as examined using the immunofluorescence technique in combination with NADPH-diaphorase histochemistry (Vincent et al., 1994). A few NOS and HO-2 immunoreactive neurons are also co-localised in the rat spinal cord (Dwyer et al., 1995). The functional significance of such co-localisation is not yet clear.

Ultrastructural localization of HO and NOS

Ultrastructural localisation of NOS immuno-labelling has been examined in some studies previously; however, to our knowledge no report on the ultrastructural localisation of HO is available so far. Thus, in a few investigations NOS immunolabelling is compared by both light and electron microscopy using a pre-embedding technique (Llewellyn-Smith et al., 1992; Aoki et al., 1993; Ceccatelli et al., 1993; Kummer and Mayer, 1993; Loesch and Burnstock, 1996; Sharma et al., 1996a) described in detail elsewhere (for review see Beesley, 1995; Sharma et al., 1995b, 1996a).

In brief, tissue specimens were fixed either by perfusion- and/or immersion techniques, using fixatives quite similar to those used for light microscopy. In most cases the same immunostained vibratome sections (thickness about 60 μm) were used for ultrastructural investigations. For this purpose, the free floating vibratome sections were incubated in the presence of NOS antiserum, which is followed by standard procedures of immunoperoxidase labelling, plastic embedding and ultrathin sectioning. Only the most outer parts of the tissue specimens were taken for evaluation, as the ability of penetration of antibodies is limited (Pickel, 1981; Sharma et al., 1996a).

Another pre-embedding technique with some modification was used by Kummer and Mayer (1993). After perfusion fixation in buffered 4% formaldehyde without the addition of glutaraldehyde like in some other studies, the tissue specimens were cryoprotected in 18% sucrose in phosphate buffer and then shock frozen. The fresh-frozen, free-floating cryostat sections (40 μm) were immunolabelled and plastic embedded. Using this technique, NOS immunolabelling was found intracellularly diffused and widespread without exhibiting any ultrastructural details. This indicates the limitation of the frozen method for routine use.

In some studies, NOS was visualised using NADPH-diaphorase as a marker at an ultrastructural level. In these investigations, NADPH-diaphorase activity was found to be localised on membrane structures (Wolf et al., 1992; Wang et al., 1996).

In situ hybridisation for detection of NOS and HO expression

This technique has now emerged as a valuable tool, revealing the synthesising machinery and the activity of NO and CO which can be demonstrated concomitantly by immunohistochemistry or radiolabelled ligands. The relevant methodology for the detection of NOS gene expression and a comprehensive discussion of various methodological problems have been recently described (Ewing and Maines, 1992; for review see Beesley, 1995; Norris et al., 1995).

A detailed protocol for *in situ* hybridisation methodology for the detection of HO-2 mRNA using digoxigenin-labelled oligonucleotide probes was originally described by Ewing and Maines (1992). In a preliminary study, using a radioactively labelled oligonucleotide probe we did not find either HO-1 mRNA expression or HO-1 immunoreactivity detectable in normal cervical or nodose ganglia. However, 24 or 48 h following culture there were pronounced expressions of HO-1 mRNA and HO-1 immunoreactivity in ganglion cells of various types (Alm et al., in preparation).

Thus technically, it is feasible to demonstrate NOS and HO expression in the CNS using several techniques. The published results are in good agreement regarding similar localisation and distribution of NOS and HO in the CNS either using *in situ* hybridisation or immunohistochemical techniques (Verma et al., 1993; Dawson and Dawson, 1996). Thus it appears that histochemical techniques are equally sensitive in detecting NOS and HO expression in CNS like *in situ* hybridisation studies.

NOS and HO expression in hyperthermia

Until now, very little, if anything is known regarding the function of these gaseous molecules in brain pathology caused by heat stress or heat-related disorders (Milton, 1994; Blatteis, 1997). Previously, there were only a few sporadic reports on NOS and HO expression following hyperthermia in animals exposed to very high ambient temperature (for review see Maines, 1992, 1996; Abraham et al., 1996). Thus, exposure of rats to 45°C for 1 h resulted in upregulation of NOS and HO in many organs of the body including some parts in the brain. It is important to note that the exposure temperatures used in these investigations are far beyond the physiological range of thermoregulatory mechanisms (Milton, 1994; Blatteis, 1997). Thus, these changes may represent the exhaustive state of thermal stress mechanisms (Blatteis, 1997). Furthermore, in these studies, the CNS is not considered in great detail and cell changes in the brain, if any, are not described. Thus, the expression of NOS and HO in the CNS following hyperthermic brain injury is still a new subject and the involvement of NO and CO in the brain pathology of heat stress is not completely understood.

A few reports indicate that hyperthermia produced by systemic injection of bacterial endotoxin induces upregulation of NOS in some brain regions (Gross et al., 1991; Dawson and Dawson, 1996). This observation suggests that the physiological range of hyperthermia influences NOS upregulation (for details see Blatteis, 1997). However studies on HO expression in the physiological range of hyperthermia and/or fever simulating clinical conditions are still lacking. Thus, it would be interesting to examine NOS and HO expression in the CNS following systemic hyperthermia comparable to clinical situations frequently encountered during high fever following bacterial or viral infections (Milton, 1994; Blatteis, 1997); radiotherapy for cancer treatment (Sminia et al., 1994); and/or short term exercise in hot environment (Glowes and O'Donnell, 1974; Sterner, 1990).

Problems of heat stress

Heat stress and associated hyperthermia due to fever, radiotherapy for tumours, or exercise in hot environment is a serious clinical problem in many parts of the world (Malamud et al., 1946; Austin and Berry, 1956; Glowes and O'Donnell, 1974;

Sharma and Dey, 1986, 1987; Sterner, 1990; Sminia et al., 1994). The symptoms of heat stress include hyperpyrexia, delirium, coma, unconsciousness and eventually death in more than 50% of the victims. Post-mortem findings show micro-haemorrhages, edema and tissue softening in many parts of the brain (Malamud et al., 1946). The probable mechanisms of brain pathology in heat stress are not well understood.

Experiments carried out in our laboratory in the past suggest that hyperthermia-induced brain damage is mainly due to occurrence of ischemia, anoxia, haemorrhages, alteration in microvascular permeability and vasogenic edema (Sharma and Dey, 1986, 1987; Sharma and Cervós-Navarro, 1990; Sharma et al., 1992a,b, 1994b, 1996e). These changes are mediated by hyperthermia-induced release of several neurochemicals (Milton, 1994; Blatteis, 1997; Sharma et al., 1996e, 1997a,e,f). This is apparent with the finding that pretreatment with various drugs modifying serotonin, prostaglandins, opioids and histamine metabolism is neuroprotective in nature (Sharma and Dey, 1987; Sharma and Cervós-Navarro, 1990; Sharma et al., 1992a,b, 1994b, 1996e, 1997a,e,f). Likewise drugs which are capable of reducing oxidative stress and/or cellular stress also offer good neuroprotection (Mustafa et al., 1995; Sharma et al., 1997a). These observations suggest that hyperthermia-induced brain damage is mediated by neurochemicals as well as cellular and oxidative stress. However, in heat stress, like many other experimental or clinical situations, no single chemical compound is responsible for all the observed changes. Thus, a possibility exists that a wide spectrum of neurochemicals or compounds influencing various signal transduction mechanisms are also involved.

NO and CO are involved in neuronal communication and participate in various forms of cell injury occurring in different experimental or clinical conditions such as neurodegenerative diseases, excitotoxicity, ischemia, epilepsy, and many other forms of acute and chronic injuries to the CNS caused by either mechanical trauma or peripheral nerve lesion, spinal nerve lesion or spinal

root avulsion (Abraham et al., 1996; Maines, 1996; Kimura and Steinbusch, 1996; Dawson and Dawson, 1996; Yamada et al., 1996; Sharma et al., 1996a).

Since molecular mechanisms of brain injury in various experimental or clinical conditions are very similar in nature, it seems quite likely that NO and CO may play a significant role in hyperthermic brain injury caused by heat stress.

Our investigations in hyperthermia

In order to test the above hypothesis, in the present investigation we examined the role of NO and CO in the CNS in heat stress using immunohistochemistry of constitutive isoforms of NOS (nNOS) and HO (HO-2) expression in various regions of the CNS. Furthermore, in order to understand the contribution of NOS and HO expression in the brain pathology of heat stress, the influence of selected neuroprotective drugs on NOS and HO immunohistochemistry was also examined.

Exposure to heat stress

Experiments were carried out on conscious male Wistar rats (9–10 weeks old, body weight 100–140 g) kept at room temperature ($21 \pm 1°C$) with a 12 h light, 12 h dark schedule and free access to food and tap water before experiments.

Animals were exposed to heat stress for 4 h in a biological oxygen demand (BOD) incubator (relative humidity, 50–55%; wind velocity, 20–25 cm/s) maintained at 38°C (Sharma and Dey, 1986, 1987). Animals kept at room temperature served as controls (Sharma and Cervós-Navarro, 1990). This experimental condition was approved by the Ethical Committee of Banaras Hindu University, Varanasi, India; Uppsala University, Uppsala; and Lund University, Lund, Sweden.

Influence of drug treatments

In separate groups of rats, the effects of pretreatment of a serotonin synthesis inhibitor drug, *p-*

chlorophenylalanine p-CPA; an antistress drug, diazepam; or an anti-oxidant compound, H-290/51 on heat stress induced alterations in NOS and HO expression were examined (Table 5) (Sharma and Dey, 1987; Sharma and Cervós-Navarro, 1990; Sharma et al., 1992a,b, 1997a,e).

Immunohistochemistry of NOS and HO

The NOS and HO immunoreactivity was examined on perfusion fixed vibratome (60 μm thick) sections obtained from several regions of the brain and spinal cord in controls, heat-stressed and drug-treated heat-stressed rats as described earlier (Alm et al., 1993; Sharma et al., 1995b, 1996a, 1997d).

NOS and HO antibodies

The NOS antiserum was raised in rabbits against an amino acid sequence (FIEESKKADA-DEVFSS) of the C-terminal end of cloned cere-bellar NOS (Alm et al., 1993; Sharma et al., 1996a). The HO-2 antiserum was obtained from StressGene Laboratory (Canada) (Sharma et al., 1996b, 1997d).

Light microscopy

NOS and HO-2 immunohistochemistry was done in normal rats, and in 4 h heat-stressed rats with or without treatment with drugs as described earlier (Sharma et al., 1995b,c, 1996a,b, 1997a,e). In brief, the sections were incubated for 36 h at room temperature in a solution of rabbit NOS antiserum or HO-2 antiserum (1:5000 in PBS) and normal swine serum (1:30 in PBS). Following repeated rinsing in PBS, the sections were incubated for 60 min at room temperature in swine anti-rabbit immunoglobulins (1:30 in PBS) and incubated in rabbit PAP complex (1:20 in PBS). To reveal peroxidase activity, the sections were incubated for 6–7 min in a solution containing 75 mg of DAB and 30 μl of 30% H_2O_2/100 ml of

TABLE 5

Heat stress-induced upregulation of nNOS and HO-2 upregulation in the CNS and their modification with drugs

Type of experiment	n	Cortex[a]		Hippocampus[b]		Cerebellum[c]	
		nNOS	HO-2	nNOS	HO-2	nNOS	HO-2
Control	5	+ +	−	+	+	+ +	+ +
p-CPA	3	+ +	+	+	− /?	+	+
H-290/51	4	+ /?	+ /?	+	+	+ +	+ +
Diazepam	3	+ +	−	+ /?	+	+ +	+
4 h HS	6	+ + + +	+ + +	+ + + +	+ + +	+ + + +	+ + + +
p-CPA + HS	5	+ /?	+	+ +	+	+ /?	+ + /?
H-290/51 + HS	5	+ /− ?	+ /?	+ /?	+	+ /?	+
Diazepam + HS	5	+ +	+ /?	+ +	+ /?	+ +	+ +

The nNOS and HO-2 immunostaining were made on free floating 40–60-μm thick sections using peroxidase-antiperoxidase technique (for details see Sharma et al., 1996a). The immunoreaction products in various groups of animals were examined by at least two independent workers and assessed in a blind fashion. In this semiquantitative estimation of immunolabelling, a 25% error is possible due to overlap in the assessment. + = positive; − = negative; ? = not seen in all animals; + + = mild; + + + = moderate; + + + + = intense.
[a] Examined mainly in parietal and cingulate cortex.
[b] Examined in dentate gyrus and CA1–CA4 subfields.
[c] Examined in vermis region only.

Tris–HCl buffer. The reaction was terminated by transferring the sections to Tris–HCl buffer, whereupon the sections were then washed in 0.15 M sodium cacodylate buffer. To serve as controls, consecutive sections were incubated in parallel in the absence of NOS or HO antiserum. Sections from all types of experiments were processed simultaneously.

Electron microscopy

For ultrastructural investigation of labelled neurons, osmicated Vibratome sections were used. One half of the section was attached to an Epon block and part of the tissue containing labelled neurons was trimmed out. Semithin sections were stained with toluidine blue and examined under light microscopy and photographed. Ultrathin sections were cut, collected on a one hole grid and stained with uranyl acetate and lead citrate (Sharma et al., 1996a, 1997a). Some of the sections were examined unstained under a Philips 300 or Hitachi transmission electron microscope. Since, the penetration of the antibodies was limited, serial sections (beginning from the surface of the Vibratome sections) were examined from a level of poor preservation and strong immunolabelling to a level at which the preservation was good and immunolabelling was still visible.

nNOS and HO-2 immunoreactivity in normal animals

Only a few neurons showed NOS immunostaining in the cerebral cortex, hippocampus, thalamus, hypothalamus and brain stem in normal rats (Fig. 1). The spinal cord in general did not show NOS positive neurons. This pattern of NOS immunoreactivity is in agreement with previously published reports (Novikov et al., 1995; Dawson and Dawson, 1996).

As described by many workers in the past, only a few HO-2 immunolabelled nerve cells are present in some brain regions in normal rats (for details, see Maines, 1996; Abraham et al., 1996;

Fukuda et al., 1996; Panizzon et al., 1996). Thus, few HO-2 positive cells can be identified in the spinal cord (Fig. 2), cerebellum, cerebral cortex, thalamus and hypothalamus. The number of HO-2 positive cells are considerably less compared to NOS positive cells in control group.

nNOS and HO-2 immunoreactivity in heat-stressed animals

Subjection of animals to a 4 h heat stress resulted in profound upregulation of nNOS and HO-2 positive neurons in many brain regions compared to normal rats (Figs. 1 and 2). Upregulation of NOS immunoreactivity was found in many parts of the cortex, hippocampus, cerebellum, thalamus, hypothalamus and spinal cord which do not normally exhibit nNOS activity. However, in some brain regions, the NOS activity appears to be less intense compared to the normal rats. The immunostaining of NOS is clearly visible in neuronal cytoplasm. In some neurons, immunostaining of the cell nucleus is quite common (Fig. 1). A representative example of NOS upregulation is shown in Fig. 1. As evident in this figure, many NOS positive neurons can be seen after 4 h heat stress in the cerebral cortex, hippocampus, and brain stem (b,d,f) compared to the control group (a,c).

Similar to NOS upregulation, many nerve cells exhibited profoundly increased expression of HO-2 immunoreactivity following 4 h heat stress in different brain regions (Fig. 2). A marked increase in HO-2 immunostaining is seen in the brain stem, hypothalamus, thalamus and in cerebellum (Fig. 2a–d). The HO-2 immunoreactivity is often seen in the cell cytoplasm and in many cases the cell nucleus and the karyoplasm remain unstained. The control group exhibited only a few HO-2 positive cells (Fig. 2e,f).

It appears that both NOS and HO-2 positive cells are located in the edematous regions of the brain. This is evident from the fact that in similar brain regions showing upregulation of NOS and HO expression, Nissl staining exhibited many damaged nerve cells compared to the control group

316

cNOS immunostaining

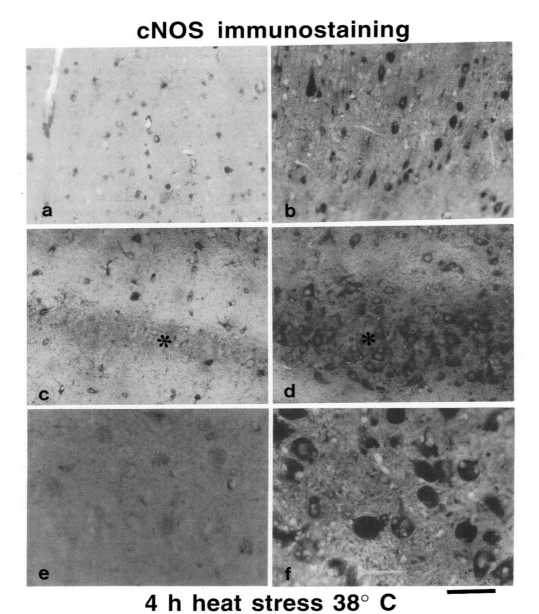

4 h heat stress 38° C

Fig. 1. Representative example of upregulation of constitutive isoform of neuronal NOS in one 4 h heat-stressed rat (b,d,f) compared to controls (a,c). Only a few nNOS immunolabelling can be seen in the cerebral cortex (a) and hippocampus (c) in normal rat. However profound upregulation of nNOS is evident in corresponding regions of brain in heat-stressed rat. The NOS immunoreactivity is mainly localised in the cell cytoplasm; however, in some cases, the cell nucleus is also stained. Many NOS positive neurons can be seen in the cerebral cortex (b), hippocampus (d) and brain stem (f) in stressed rats. It is apparent from the figure that in heat stress, NOS positive neurons can be seen in the cortex and hippocampus (*) in regions which normally do not exhibit NOS activity. Likewise NOS activity is mainly evident in distorted neurons located in edematous areas. e = negative control section obtained from brain stem of a 4 h heat-stressed rat (bar a,c = 50 μm; b,d = 30 μm; e,f = 20 μm; Vibratome sections 50–60 μm thick).

HO II immunostaining

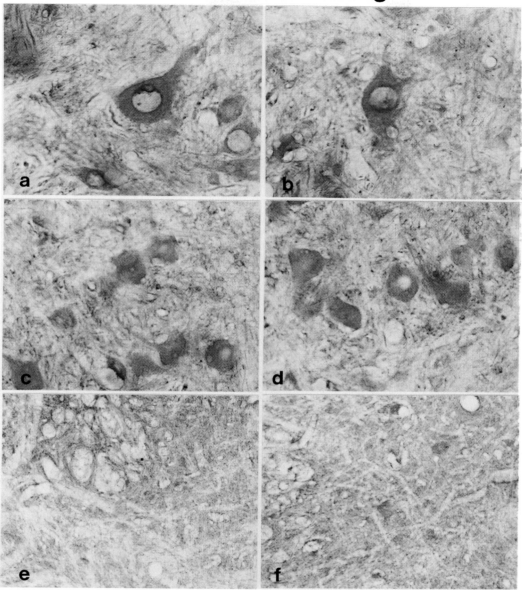

4 h heat stress 38° C

Fig. 2. Representative example of upregulation of constitute isoform of heme oxygenase-2 (HO II) immunostaining in one 4 h heat-stressed rat (a–d) compared to controls (e,f). Only a few HO-2 immunolabelling can be seen in the brain stem (e) and thalamus (f) in normal rat. However profound upregulation of HO-2 is evident in several brain regions in heat-stressed rat. The HO immunoreactivity is mainly localised in the cell cytoplasm; however, in a few cases, the cell nucleus is also stained. Many HO positive neurons can be seen in the thalamus (a), hypothalamus (b), brain stem (c) and cerebellum (d) in stressed rat. HO positive neurons can be seen mainly in the brain regions which normally do not exhibit HO activity. HO immunolabelling is mainly evident in distorted neurons located in edematous areas (bar a,b = 10 μm; c,d = 20 μm; e,f = 50 μm; Vibratome sections 50–60 μm thick).

(Fig. 3). This indicates that induction of NOS or HO is somehow associated with cell injury. Without the use of double immunostaining and confocal microscopy in heat stress, it is difficult to

Neuronal damage

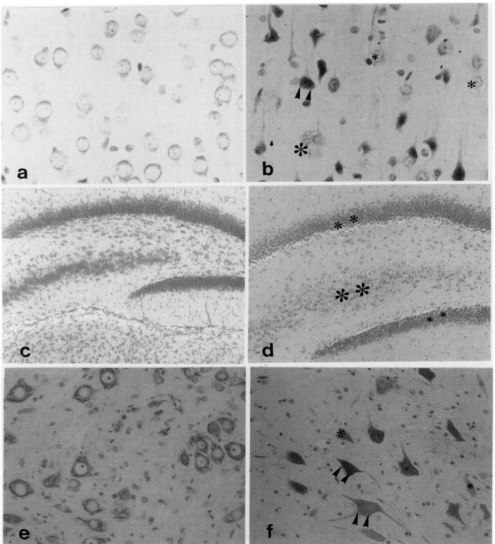

4 h heat stress 38° C

Fig. 3. Representative example of Haemotoxylin Eosin (a–d) and Nissl (e,f) stained sections from control (a,c,e) and heat stressed rat (b,d,f) showing marked cell changes in the cerebral cortex (b), hippocampus (d) and brain stem (f) after 4 h heat stress. General sponginess, edema (*), distortion of nerve cells (arrow heads) are clearly evident in heat-stressed rats compared to corresponding regions in control group (bar a,b = 30 μm; c,d = 50 μm; e,f = 25 μm; paraffin sections 3 μm thick).

discern at this moment whether NOS and HO-2 immunostaining are co-expressed in a few nerve cells in some brain regions, a feature which will require additional investigation.

Pharmacological manipulation of nNOS and HO-2 immunoreactivity

To further confirm the involvement of NOS and HO upregulation in cell injury caused by heat stress, we used pretreatment of a few selected neuroprotective drugs known to attenuate brain pathology in this model earlier (Sharma and Cervós-Navarro, 1990; Sharma et al., 1992a,b, 1997e). Pretreatment with these drugs significantly attenuated the upregulation of NOS and HO-2 immunostaining in the CNS of heat-stressed

animals (Table 5). However, these drug treatments in normal rats did not influence NOS or HO-2 expression (Table 5).

Our results suggest that prior treatment with drugs which are capable of reducing edema and cell changes in heat stress are also able to attenuate hyperthermia-induced upregulation of neuronal NOS and HO activity. These observations for the first time demonstrate a positive involvement of NOS and HO upregulation in brain pathology caused by heat stress.

Ultrastructural localisation of nNOS and HO-2 immunoreactivity

The intracellular localisation of NOS and HO immunolabelling at ultrastructural levels was ex-

cNOS immunostaining

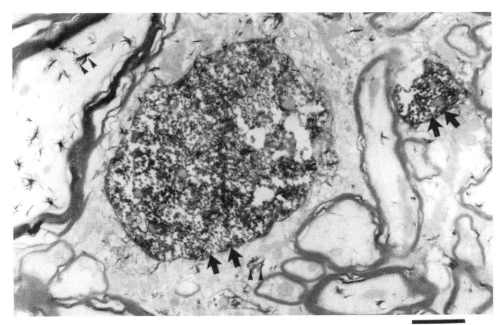

4 h heat stress 38° C

Fig. 4. Ultrastructural localisation of constitutive isoform of neuronal NOS in the brain stem of a 4 h heat-stressed rat. The dark black immunolabelled profiles (arrows) representing NOS activity is confined in two dendrites. Few scattered crystal like non-specific black particles (arrow heads) represent artefacts. This unstained ultrathin section is not contrasted with lead citrate or uranyl acetate (bar = 600 nm).

Spinal cord

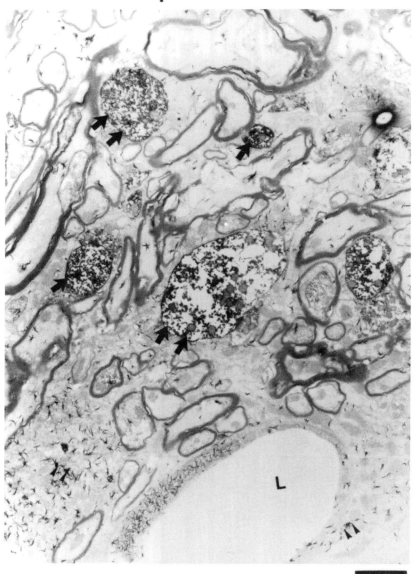

4 h heat stress 38° C

Fig. 5. Ultrastructural localisation of constitutive isoform of heme oxygenase-2 immunoreactivity in the spinal cord of a 4 h heat stressed rat. The dark black immunolabelled profiles (arrows) representing HO activity are confined to several dendrites of various diameters. Few scattered crystal like non-specific black particles (arrow heads) represent artefacts. This unstained ultrathin section is not contrasted with lead citrate or uranyl acetate. L = lumen of one capillary (bar = 1 μm).

amined using electron microscopy as described earlier (Sharma et al., 1996a, 1997a). Electron

microscopy of NOS and HO immunostained material obtained from brain stem and spinal cord in heat-stressed rats show that the immunoreactivity is mainly confined within the cytoplasm of the neurons and in dendrites. A representative example of NOS immunoreactivity can be seen in the cytoplasm of dendrites in the brain stem (Fig. 4).

Like NOS, the HO immunolabelling is also present in the cytoplasm of nerve cells and dendrites. Figure 5 shows immunolabelling of HO-2 at an ultrastructural level in the spinal cord of a heat-stressed rat. The dark black profiles representing HO-2 immunostained material can be seen in several dendrites. In a few cases, the HO immunostaining was also found in the nucleus and karyoplasm (results not shown).

This immunolabelling of NOS and HO seen at the ultrastructural level is in line with the biochemical studies showing localisation of NOS and HO enzymes at the membrane level in neuronal cytoplasm attached to the endoplasmic reticulum (Ewing and Maines, 1992; Llewellyn-Smith et al., 1992; McCoubrey et al., 1992; White and Marletta, 1992; Aoki et al., 1993; Kummer and Mayer, 1993; Verma et al., 1993; Klatt et al., 1994; Koch et al., 1994; Bolanos et al., 1995; Dwyer et al., 1995; Yamanaka et al., 1996).

We also used routine transmission electron microscopy in similar brain regions to find a relationship between ultrastructural localisation of NOS and HO with morphological alterations in heat stress (Sharma and Cervós-Navarro, 1990). The results show that many nerve cells in the area associated with upregulation of NOS and HO exhibit profound cell damage, vacuolation and edema. A representative example of ultrastructural changes in one heat-stressed rat from the cerebellum and brain stem is shown in Figs. 6 and 7. As evident in the figures, the nerve cells showed marked changes in structure in both cerebellum (Fig. 6) and in brain stem (Fig. 7). Vacuolation, edema and membrane damage are quite frequent in the neuropil (Fig. 7). Swelling of glia, granule cell and purkinje cell is clearly visible in the cerebellum (Fig. 6) and morphological alteration in cell nucleus is apparent in the brain stem (Figs. 7 and 8). A high power electron micrograph of one nerve cell nucleus from the brain stem showed marked structural changes (Fig. 8). Thus

the nuclear membrane is abnormally folded and the nucleolus showed signs of degeneration and vacuolation (Fig. 8). These cell changes in the nucleus and nucleolus represent the symptoms of cellular stress associated with the abnormal production of heat shock proteins (for details see Westman and Sharma, this volume). These observations strongly indicate that NOS or HO upregulation occurs in cells showing profound stress and are located in the regions exhibiting injury, edema and membrane damage.

This idea is further supported by ultrastructural studies in drug-treated rats. Thus, in drug-treated and heat-stressed rats, the structural changes in NOS and HO immunolabelling are mainly absent (results not shown) indicating that the neuroprotective compounds have the capacity to inhibit the upregulation of NOS and HO upregulation at the ultrastructural level as well. The detail mechanisms of drug-induced inhibition of NOS and HO expression in heat stress are not known. However, it appears that reduction in cellular or oxidative stress, injury or edema by these drugs play an important role.

Mechanisms of NOS and HO upregulation in hyperthermic brain injury

The probable mechanisms by which hyperthermia induces NOS and HO upregulation is not clear from this investigation. However, it appears that heat stress-induced alteration in microvascular permeability, vasogenic edema and cell injury are important factors involved in NOS and HO induction.

There is evidence that heat stress can induce release of several neurochemicals and is associated with lipid peroxidation and generation of free radicals (Milton, 1994; Blatteis, 1997; Sharma et al., 1997a,e). These neurochemicals are known mediators of microvascular permeability and vasogenic edema (Wahl et al., 1988; Bradbury, 1992). It seems quite likely that generation of free radicals will trigger opening of cation permeable channels resulting in an increased accumulation of intracellular Ca^{2+} in the brain microenvironment (Cho et al., 1992; Darley-Usmar et al., 1992;

cell reaction and edema
cerebellar cortex

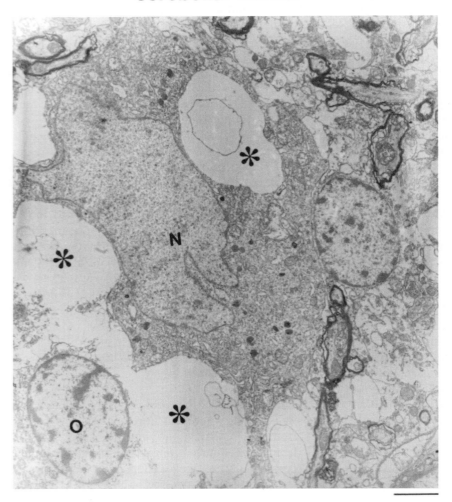

4 h heat stress 38° C

Fig. 6. Ultrastructural changes in nerve cell and edema in the cerebellar cortex of a 4 h heat-stressed rat. The purkinje cells (N) showed marked distortion with pericellular edema (*). One swollen oligodendrocyte (o) is seen in the lower left corner of the figure. Distortion of granule cell and myelin vesiculation is apparent (bar = 600 nm).

Hirsch et al., 1993; Dawson et al., 1994a; Kurenny et al., 1994). The intracellular Ca^{2+} will then bind to calmodulin, a cofactor of NOS and stimulates NOS activity (Dawson and Snyder, 1994; Koch et al., 1994; Dawson and Dawson, 1994, 1996).

NO generated from activated NOS will react with the superoxide anion to produce the potent oxidant, peroxynitrite ($ONOO^-$) (Radi et al., 1991; Koppenol et al., 1992) which inhibits DNA synthesis, liberates iron from the iron storage

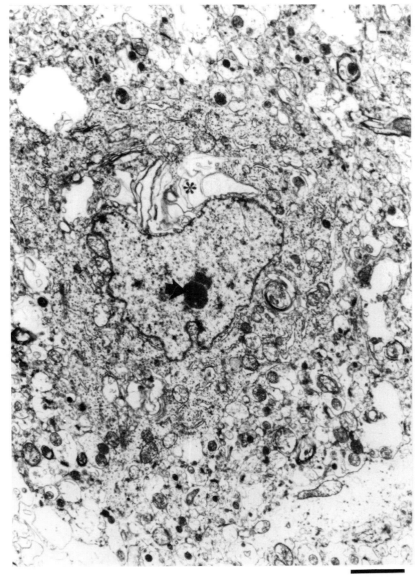

Fig. 7. Ultrastructural changes in the nerve cell and edema in the brain stem reticular formation of a 4 h heat-stressed rat. Membrane vacuolation, edema (*) and cell damage is quite prominent. The nerve cell cytoplasm is vacuolated and the cell nucleus appears shrunken with an eccentric nucleolus (arrow) (bar = 2 μm).

protein ferritin and influences iron metabolism at the post-transcription level (Oury et al., 1992, for details see Dawson and Dawson, 1996). Overproduction of NO thus contributes to the neuronal injury by cytotoxic cascade via oxidant compounds peroxynitrite and superoxide anion (Oury et al., 1992; Lipton et al., 1994; Stamler, 1994). This is evident from the fact that superoxide dismutase offers neuroprotection in cell cultures from both glutamate and other NO donors (Dawson and

324

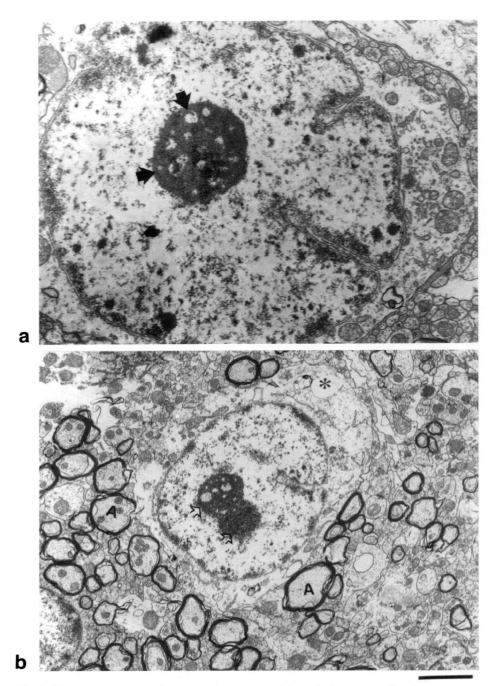

Fig. 8. High power electron micrograph of one nerve cell from the brain stem of a 4 h heat-stressed rat. a = the nerve cell nucleus and nucleolus (filled arrows) in brain stem of stressed rat showing marked degenerative changes. b = vacuolation, edema (*) and axonal (A) damage is quite prominent in the neuropil surrounding another nerve cell in the same region following heat stress. Damage of nerve cell and cell nucleus is quite prominent and disintegration of karyoplasm containing nucleolus (blank arrows) is clearly visible (bar a = 200 nm; b = 800 nm).

Dawson, 1996). The other possibility that NO and ONOO$^-$ will damage DNA with the subsequent activation of the nuclear enzyme poly ADP ribose synthetase (PARS), is also quite likely (Lautier et al., 1993; Beckman, 1994; Dawson et al., 1994a; Bolanos et al., 1995). Activation of PARS can cause cell death by rapid depletion of cell energy and PARS inhibitors protect cortical cell cultures from glutamate and NO neurotoxicity (Zhang et al., 1994a,b).

One of the important targets of NO in the biological system is the iron in heme moieties. NO binds to the heme-iron protein in guanylyl cyclase to elicit cGMP formation which is known to influence microvascular permeability disturbances (Kubes and Granger, 1992; Ochoa et al., 1993; Stamler, 1994; Garthwaite and Boulton, 1995). It seems quite likely that NO-induced disturbances in microvascular permeability are instrumental in edema formation and cell injury (Sharma et al., 1995c, 1996a, 1997a,b,d,e).

It appears that similar mechanisms responsible for NOS induction may also contribute to upregulation of HO in the CNS (Verma et al., 1993; Dawson and Snyder, 1994; Vincent et al., 1994; Abraham et al., 1996). There is some evidence that oxidative stress, haemorrhage and/or ischemia are important factors in induction of HO response following fluid percussion brain injury in rats (Fukuda et al., 1996; Panizzon et al., 1996; Soltesz, 1996). Since heat stress is frequently associated with ischemia, microhaemorrhages and oxidative stress (for review see Sharma, Westman and Nyberg, this volume) it appears that these factors are also responsible for HO induction in the CNS following hyperthermia.

HO-2 is a constitutive isoenzyme present in neurons in the normal brain (Ewing and Maines, 1992; Verma et al., 1993). However, the functional significance of activation of HO-2 following trauma or stress is not well known. Induction of HO-1, the inducible form of the enzyme, occurs in astrocytes 6 h to several days after the initial brain trauma (Fukuda et al., 1996). This upregulation of HO-1 following brain injury is considered to be protective in nature. This idea is based on

the hypothesis that activation of glial cells is neuroprotective because they are involved in regulation of the fluid microenvironment of the brain (Peters et al., 1991). Thus activation of astrocytes and induction of HO-1 (mainly in glial cells) seems to be associated with cell protection. However, activation of astrocytes does not necessarily mean neuroprotection (Sharma et al., 1992a). Activation of astrocytes is a common feature in various forms of trauma and stress and mainly represents a sign of glial cell injury (for details see Cervós-Navarro et al., this volume; Sharma et al., 1995c). Thus upregulation of HO-1 in glial cells following injury is not sufficient to assume that this induction is related to neuroprotection.

On the other hand, it seems quite likely that activation of HO is associated with neuronal injury (Panizzon et al., 1996). Activation of HO is responsible for production of CO which is associated with induction of LTP, a feature commonly known to mediate neuronal injury in many pathophysiological conditions (Meffert et al., 1994). Another possibility of HO/CO induced neuronal damage may be due to the release of free iron which acts as a catalyst for the production of free radicals and therefore amplifies the neuronal damage (Maines, 1988, 1992). Thus generation of CO like NO is also related to cell injury.

One of the strongest arguments which favours the idea that upregulation of HO is harmful to the neurons came from the studies in brain trauma using HO inhibitors by Panizzon et al. (1996). These authors used an *in vitro* model of anoxia and fluid percussion injury to examine the effects HO inhibitors, metalloporphyrins (Sn-PP or Zn-PP). Their results suggest that HO-2 isoforms which are found in CA1 pyramidal neurons appear to be most active during brain trauma in inducing neuronal injury. This is evident from the fact that trauma-induced neuronal injury is significantly attenuated by HO inhibitors (Sn-PP or Zn-PP). The mechanisms by which HO inhibitors offer neuroprotection are not yet clear. One possibility would be that these inhibitors exert some anti-inflammatory effects which is apparent from the finding that Zn-PP reduces infarct size and edema following cerebral ischemia (Kadoya et al., 1995). On the basis of these observations it appears that upregulation of HO-2 is also associated with cell injury and neurodestruction via generation of CO.

Abnormal production of NO and CO in pathological conditions thus can lead to neuronal death. However, there are some reports speculating that NOS upregulation is accompanied by HO expression in order to counterbalance the harmful effects of NO (Vincent et al., 1994). Though the idea is interesting in itself, further clear experimental evidence is needed either to support or reject this hypothesis.

Neuroprotection vs. neurodestruction by NOS and HO expression in hyperthermia

Our new experimental evidence using pharmacology in heat stress clearly shows that upregulation of both NOS and HO expression is responsible for cell injury probably via production of NO and CO from the activated forms of these enzymes. Thus, pretreatment with neuroprotective drugs in heat stress which attenuated the stress response, microvascular permeability disturbances, edema and cell reaction in the CNS also prevented the upregulation of NOS and HO expression.

This indicates that signals responsible for stress reaction, disruption of the BBB, edema and cell changes are important in inducing an upregulation of NOS and HO. It appears that cellular stress caused by hyperthermia can play an important role in expression of NOS and HO. Obviously, a reduction in cellular stress by pharmacological means is responsible for less disturbances in intracellular signal transduction mechanisms responsible for NOS and HO expression in heat stress (Kubes and Granger, 1992; Marcuccilli and Miller, 1994; Mustafa et al., 1995; Sharma et al., 1996e; for details see Sharma, Westman and Nyberg, this volume). A direct effect of these drugs on NOS or HO metabolism is unlikely because these drugs did not influence the upregulation of NOS and HO expression in normal rats.

Microvascular permeability disturbances and NOS and HO induction

Pharmacological manipulation of NOS and HO expression in heat stress are in line with the idea that the microvascular permeability disturbances play an important role in cell injury. Breakdown of the BBB permeability by neurochemical mediators following secondary injury cascade will allow access of many serum factors or other vasoactive compounds into the cerebral compartment (Wahl et al., 1988; Bradbury, 1992). This will lead to profound alterations in extracellular fluid microenvironment of the cellular compartments in the brain. As a result marked disturbances in the ionic, chemical, immunological and metabolic environment of the nerve cells and glial cells will occur which are mainly responsible for alterations in the bioelectrical activity and axonal conduction (Wahl et al., 1988; Bradbury, 1992; Sharma et al., 1995b, 1996a, 1997a,e). All these macro and micromolecular events will lead to profound cellular stress in the brain resulting in abnormal expression of many proteins including NOS and HO expression. This idea is in line with the observation that these compounds also inhibited the HSP induction (for details see Westman and Sharma, this volume) and attenuated the GFAP immunoreactivity (see Cervós-Navarro et al., this volume). Obviously a mild stress response is responsible for less disturbances in the brain fluid microenvironment. This hypothesis gets further support from the observation that pretreatment with drugs in heat stress which significantly attenuated the NOS and HO induction are also capable of preventing the breakdown of the BBB permeability.

Conclusion

Our results demonstrate that hyperthermia associated with heat exposure has the capacity of inducing upregulation of nNOS and HO-2 immunoreactivity in the CNS. This induction of NOS and HO in neurons can be prevented by prior treatment with several neuroprotective drugs influencing microvascular permeability, edema and cell reaction. This indicates an important contribution of microvascular permeability disturbances, edema formation and cell injury as important regulatory signals for NOS and HO induction in the CNS, not reported earlier.

Future direction

Studies are in progress in our laboratory to further understand the role of NO and CO in brain injury caused by heat stress. Currently we are engaged in evaluating the influence of selective and specific inhibitors of NOS and HO on heat stress-induced microvascular permeability disturbances, edema formation, cell injury, HSP expression and GFAP immunoreactivity. Based on these findings, it would be interesting to see whether these drug treatments can also influence the expression of mRNA levels of NOS and HO in various brain regions following heat stress.

Acknowledgements

This investigation is supported by grants from the Swedish Medical Research Council nos. 2710, 11205; Astra Hässle, Mölndal, Sweden; Magnus Bergvall, Crafoord and Åke Wiberg Stiftelse, Sweden; Alexander von Humboldt Foundation, Bonn, Germany; and The University Grants Commission, New Delhi, India. The skilful technical assistance of Ingamarie Olsson, Kärstin Flink, Elisabeth Scherer, Franziska Drum, Katja Deparade and Hanna Pluckhän is highly appreciated. The secretarial assistance of Aruna Misra is acknowledged with thanks.

References

Abraham, N.G., Drummond, G.S., Lutton, J.D. and Kappas, A. (1996) The biological significance and physiological role of heme oxygenase. Cell. Physiol. Biochem., 6: 129–168.

Affiniti Research Products Ltd. (1996) Heme Oxygenase Research, December, 1996, Issue 2, pp. 1–3, Affiniti, Exeter, UK.

Alm, P., Larsson, B., Ekblad, E., Sundler, F. and Andersson, K.-E. (1993) Immunohistochemical localization of periph-eral nitric oxide synthase-containing nerves using antibodies raised against synthesized C- and N-terminal fragments of a cloned enzyme from rat brain. Acta Physiol. Scand., 148: 421–429.

Aoki, C., Fenstenmaker, S., Lubin, M. and Go, C.G. (1993) Nitric oxide in the visual cortex of monocular monkeys as revealed by light and electron microscopic immunocytochemistry. Brain Res., 620: 97–113.

Austin, M.G. and Berry, J.W. (1956) Observation on one hundred cases of heatstroke. J. Am. Med. Assoc., 161: 1525–1529.

Baek, K.J., Thiel, B.A., Lucas, S. and Stuehr, D.J (1993) Macrophage nitric oxide subunits. Purification, characterization, and the role of prosthetic groups and substrate in regulating their association into a dimeric enzyme. J. Biol. Chem., 268: 21120–21129.

Babbedge, R.C., Bland-Ward, P.A., Hart, S.L. and Moore, P.K. (1993) Inhibition of rat nitric oxide synthase by 7-nitro indazole and related substituted indazoles. Br. J. Pharmacol., 110: 225–228.

Beckman, J.S. (1994) Peroxynitrite vs. hydroxyl radical: the role of nitric oxide in superoxide-dependent cerebral injury. In: C.C. Chiueh, D.L. Gilbert and C. Colton (Eds.), The Neurobiology of NO and OH, Ann. New York Acad. Sci., pp. 69–75.

Beesley, J.E. (1995) Histochemical methods for detecting nitric oxide synthase. Histochem. J., 27: 757–769.

Blatteis, C. (1997) Thermoregulation: Recent progress and new frontiers, Ann. New York Acad. Sci., 813: 1–865.

Bo, L., Dawson, T.M., Wesslingh, S., Mork, S., Choi, S., Kong, P.A., Pardo, C., Hanley, D. and Trapp, B.D. (1994) Induction of nitric oxide synthase in demyelinating regions of multiple sclerosis brains. Am. Neurol., 36: 778–786.

Bolanos, J.P., Heales, S.J.R., Land, J.M. and Clark, J.B. (1995) Effect of peroxynitrite on the mitochondrial respiratory chain: differential susceptibility of neurones and astrocytes in primary culture. J. Neurochem., 64: 1965–1972.

Bradbury, M.W.B. (1992) Physiology and pharmacology of the blood-brain barrier. Handbook Exp. Pharmacol., 103: 1–450, Springer, Heidelberg.

Bredt, D.S. (1995) Molecular characterization of nitric oxide synthase. In: S. Vincent (Ed)., Nitric Oxide Synthase in the Nervous System, Academic Press, New York, pp. 1–19.

Bredt, D.S. and Snyder, S.H. (1992) Nitric oxide, a novel neuronal messenger. Neuron, 8: 3–11.

Bredt, D.S., Hwang, P.M. and Snyder, S.H. (1990) Localization of nitric oxide synthase indicating a neuronal role for nitric oxide. Nature, 347: 768–770.

Bredt, D.S., Glatt, C.E., Hwang, P.M., Fotuhi, M., Dawson, T.M. and Snyder, S.H. (1991) Nitric oxide synthase protein and mRNA are discretely localized in neuronal populations of the mammalian CNS together with NADPH diaphorase. Neuron, 7: 615–624.

328

Bredt, D.S., Ferris, C.D. and Snyder, S.H. (1992) Nitric oxide synthase regulatory sites. *J. Biol. Chem.*, 267: 10976–10981.

Carreau, A., Duval, D., Poignet, H., Scatton, B., Vige, X. and Nowicki, J.-P. (1994) Neuroprotective efficacy of Nw-nitro-L-arginine after focal cerebral ischemia in the mouse and inhibition of cortical nitric oxide synthase. *Eur. J. Pharmacol.*, 256: 241–249.

Ceccatelli, S., Hulting A.L., Zhang, X., Gustafsson, L., Villar, M. and Hökfelt, T. (1993) Nitric oxide synthase in the rat anterior pituitary gland and the role of nitric oxide in regulation of luteinizing hormone secretion. *Proc. Natl. Acad. Sci. USA*, 90: 11292–11296.

Cervós-Navarro, J., Sharma, H.S., Westman, J. and Bongcam-Rudloff, E. (1998) Glial cell reactions in the central nervous system following heat stress, In: H.S. Sharma and J. Westman (Eds.), *Brain Functions in Hot Environment*, Vol. 115, *Progress in Brain Research*, Elsevier, Amsterdam, pp. 297–333.

Chao, C.C., Hu, S., Molitor, T.W., Shaskan, E.G. and Peterson, P.K. (1992) Activated microglia mediate neuronal cell injury via a nitric oxide mechanism. *J. Immunol.*, 149: 2736–2741.

Chiueh, C.C., Gilbert, D.L. and Colton, C.A. (1994) The Neurobiology of NO· and ·OH. *Ann. New York Acad. Sci.*, 738: 1–471.

Cho, H.J., Xie, Q.W., Calaycay, J., Mumford, R.A., Swiderek, K.M., Lee, T.D. and Nathan, C. (1992) Calmodulin is a subunit of a nitric oxide synthase from macrophages. *J. Exp. Med.*, 176: 599–604.

Choi, D.W. (1993) Nitric oxide: Foe or friend to the injured brain. *Proc. Natl. Acad. Sci. USA*, 90: 9741–9743.

Corbett, J.A., Tilton, R.G., Chang, K., Hasan, K.S., Ido, Y., Wang, J.L., Sweetland, M.A., Lancaster, J.R. Jr, Williamson, J.R. and McDaniel, M.L. (1992) Aminoguanidine, a novel inhibitor of nitric oxide formation prevents diabetic vascular dysfunction. *Diabetes*, 41: 552–556.

Dalkara, T., Yoshida, T., Irikura, K. and Moskowitz, M. (1994) Dual role of nitric oxide in focal cerebral ischemia. *Neuropharmacology* 33: 1447–1452.

Darley-Usmar, V.M., Hogg, N., O'Leary, V.J., Wilson, M.T. and Moncada, S. (1992) The simultaneous generation of superoxide and nitric oxide can initiate lipid peroxidation in human low density lipoprotein. *Free Radic. Commun.*, 17: 9–20.

Dawson, T.M. and Dawson, V.L. (1994) Nitric oxide: actions and pathological roles. *Neuroscientist*, 1: 9–20.

Dawson, T.M. and Snyder, S.H. (1994) Gases as biological messenger: nitric oxide and carbon monoxide in the brain. *J. Neurosci.*, 14: 5147–5159.

Dawson, V.L. and Dawson, T.M. (1996) Nitric oxide neurotoxicity. *J. Chem. Neuroanat.*, 10: 179–190.

Dawson, T.M., Bredt, D.S., Fotuhi, M., Hwang, P.M. and Snyder, S.H. (1991) Nitric oxide synthase and neuronal NADPH diaphorase are identical in brain and peripheral tissues. *Proc. Natl. Acad. Sci. USA*, 88: 7797–7801.

Dawson, T.M., Dawson, V.L. and Snyder, S.H. (1992) A novel neuronal messenger molecule in brain: the free radical, nitric oxide. *Ann. Neurol.*, 32: 297–311.

Dawson, V.L., Dawson, T.M., Bartley, D.A., Uhl, G.R. and Snyder, S.H. (1993a) Mechanisms of nitric oxide mediated neurotoxicity in primary brain cultures. *J. Neurosci.*, 13: 2651–2661.

Dawson, V.L., Dawson, T.M., Uhl, G.R. and Snyder, S.H. (1993b) Human immunodeficiency virus type 1 coat protein neurotoxicity mediated by nitric oxide in primary cortical cultures. *Proc. Natl. Acad. Sci. USA*, 90: 3256–3259.

Dawson, T.M., Steiner, J.P., Dawson, V.L., Dinerman, J.L., Uhl, G.R. and Snyder, S.H. (1993c) Immunos enhances phosphorylation of nitric oxide synthase and protects against glutamate neurotoxicity. *Proc. Natl. Acad. Sci. USA*, 90: 9808–9812.

Dawson, T.M., Dawson, V.L. and Snyder, S.H. (1994a). Molecular mechanisms of nitric oxide actions in the brain. *Ann. New York Acad. Sci.*, 738: 76–85.

Dawson, V.L., Brambhatt, H.P., Mong, J.A. and Dawson, T.M. (1994b) Expression of inducible nitric oxide synthase causes delayed neurotoxicity in primary mixed neuronal-glial cortical cultures. *Neuropharmacology*, 33: 1425–1430.

Dawson, T.M., Hung, K., Dawson, V.L., Steiner, J.P. and Snyder, S.H. (1995) Neuroprotective effects of gangliosides may involve inhibition of nitric oxide synthase. *Ann. Neurol.*, 37: 115–118.

Dinerman, J.L., Dawson, T.M., Schell, M.J., Snowman, A. and Snyder, S.H. (1994) Endothelial nitric oxide synthase localized to hippocampal pyramidal cells: implications for synaptic plasticity. *Proc. Natl. Acad. Sci. USA*, 91: 4214–4218.

Drapier, J.-C., Hirling, H., Wietzerbin, J., Kaldy, P. and Kuhn, L.C. (1993) Biosynthesis of nitric oxide activates iron regulatory factor in macrophages. *EMBO J.*, 12: 3643–3649.

Dwyer, B.E., Nishimura, R.N. and Lu, S.-Y. (1995) Differential localization of heme oxygenase and NADPH-diaphorase in spinal neurons. *NeuroReport*, 6: 973–976.

Ewing, J.F. and Maines, M.D. (1991) Rapid induction of heme oxygenase 1 mRNA and protein by hyperthermia in rat brain: heme oxygenase 2 is not a heat shock protein. *Proc. Natl. Acad. Sci. USA*, 88: 5364–5368.

Ewing, J.F. and Maines, M.D. (1992) *In situ* hybridisation and immunohistochemical localization of heme oxygenase-2 mRNA and protein in normal rat brain: Differential distribution of isozyme 1 and 2. *Mol. Cell. Neurosci.*, 3: 559–570.

Feldman, P.L., Griffith, O.W. and Stuehr, D.J. (1993) The surprising life of nitric oxide. *Chem. Eng. News*, 71: 28–38.

Fiallos-Estrada, C.E., Kummer, W., Mayer, B., Bravo, R., Zimmermann, M. and Herdegen, T. (1993) Long lasting increase of nitric oxide synthase immunoreactivity, NADPH-diaphorase reaction and c-JUN co-expression in rat dorsal root ganglion following sciatic nerve transaction. *Neurosci. Lett.*, 150: 169–173.

Förstermann, U. (1994) Biochemistry and molecular biology of nitric oxide synthase. *Arzenmittelforschung*, 44: 402–407.

Fukuda, K., Panter, S.S., Sharp, F.R. and Noble, L.J. (1995) Induction of heme oxygenase-1 (HO-1) after traumatic injury in the rat. *Neurosci. Lett.*, 199: 127–130.

Fukuda, K., Richman, J.D., Sato, M., Sharp, F.R., Panter, S.S., and Noble, L.J. (1996) Induction of heme oxygenase-1 (HO-1) in glia after traumatic brain injury. *Brain Res.*, 736: 68–75.

Galea, E., Feinstein, D.L. and Reis, D.J. (1992) Induction of calcium dependent nitric oxide synthase activity in primary rat glial cultures. *Proc. Natl. Acad. Sci. USA*, 89: 10945–10949.

Garthwaite, J. and Boulton, C.L. (1995) Nitric oxide signalling in the central nervous system. *Annu. Rev. Physiol.*, 57: 683–706.

Glaum, S.R. and Miller, R.J. (1993) Zinc protoporphyrin-IX blocks the effects of metabotropic glutamate receptor activation in the rat nucleus tractus solitarii. *Mol. Pharmacol.*, 43: 965–969.

Glowes, G.H.A. Jr. and O'Donnell, T.F. Jr. (1974) Heat stroke-current concepts. *New Engl. J. Med.*, 291: 564–566.

Gräser, T., Vedernikov, Y.P. and Li, D.S. (1990) Study on the mechanism of carbon monoxide induced endothelium-independent relaxation in porcine coronary artery and vein. *Biomed. Biochim. Acta*, 49: 293–296.

Gross, S.S., Stuehr, D.J., Aisaka, K., Jaffe, E.A., Levi, R. and Griffith, O.W. (1990) Macrophage and endothelial cell nitric oxide synthesis: cell-type selective inhibition of N^G-aminoarginine, N^G-nitroarginine and N^G-methylarginine. *Biochem. Biophys. Res. Commun.*, 170: 96–103.

Gross, S.S., Jafe, E.A., Levi, R. and Kilbourn, R.G. (1991) Cytokine-activated endothelial cells express an isotype of nitric oxide synthase which is tetrahydrobiopterin-dependent, calmodulin-independent and inhibited by arginine analogs with a rank-order of potency characteristic of activated macrophages. *Biochem. Biophys. Res. Commun.*, 178: 823–829.

Herdegen, T., Brecht, S., Kummer, W., Mayer, B., Leah, J., Bravo, R. and Zimmermann, M. (1993) Long lasting expression of JUN and KROX transcription factors and nitric oxide synthase in intrinsic neurons of the rat brain following axotomy. *J. Neurosci.*, 13: 4130–4146.

Hirsch, D.B., Steiner, J.P., Dawson, T.M., Mammen, A., Hayek, E., and Snyder, S.H. (1993) Neurotransmitter Release Regulated by Nitric Oxide in PC-12 Cells and Brain Synaptosomes. *Curr. Biol.*, 3: 749–754.

Hope, B.T., Michael, G.J., Knigge, K.M. and Vincent, S.R. (1991) Neuronal NADPH diaphorase is a nitric oxide synthase. *Proc. Natl. Acad. Sci. USA*, 88: 2811–2814.

Huang, Z., Huang, P.L., Panahian, N., Dalkara, T., Fishman, M.C. and Moskowitz, M.A. (1994) Effects of cerebral ischemia in mice deficient in neuronal nitric oxide synthase. *Science*, 265: 1883–1885.

Hyman, B.T., Marzloff, K., Wenninger, J.J., Dawson, T.M., Bredt, D.S. and Snyder, S.H. (1992) Relative sparing of nitric oxide synthase-containing neurons in the hippocampal formation in Alzheimer's disease. *Ann. Neurol.*, 32: 818–820.

Kadowaki, K., Kishimoto, J., Leng, G. and Emson, P.C. (1994) Up-regulation of nitric oxide synthase (NOS) gene expression together with NOS activity in the rat hypothalamo-hypophysial system after chronic salt loading: evidence of a neuromodulatory role of nitric oxide in arginine vasopressin and oxytocin secretion. *Endocrinology*, 134: 1011–1017.

Kadoya, C., Domino, E.F., Yang, G.Y., Stern, J.D. and Betz, A.L. (1995) Preischemic but not postischemic zinc protoporphyrin treatment reduces infarct size and edema accumulation after temporary focal cerebral ischemia in rats. *Stroke*, 26: 1035–1038.

Kharazia, V.N., Schmidt, H.H.H.W. and Weinberg, R.J. (1994) Type I nitric oxide synthase fully accounts for NADPH-diaphorase in rat striatum, but not cortex. *Neuroscience*, 62: 983–987.

Kimura, H. and Steinbusch, H.W.M. (1996) The role of nitric oxide in the central nervous system. From basic to therapeutic aspect. *J. Chem. Neuroanat.*, 10: 179–322.

Klatt, P., Schmid, M., Leopold, E., Schmidt, K., Werner, E.R. and Mayer, B. (1994) The pteridine binding site of brain nitric oxide synthase. Tetrahydrobiopterin binding kinetics, specificity, and allosteric interaction with the substrate domain. *J. Biol. Chem.*, 269: 13861–13866.

Koch, K.W., Lambrecht, H.G., Haberecht, M., Redburn, D. and Schmidt, H.H. (1994) Functional coupling of a Ca^{2+}/calmodulin-dependent nitric oxide synthase and a soluble guanylyl cyclase in vertebrate photoreceptor cells. *EMBO J.*, 13: 3312–3320.

Koppenol, W.H., Moreno, J.J., Pryor, W.A., Ischiropoulos, H. and Beckman, J.S. (1992) Peroxynitrite, a cloaked oxidant formed by nitric oxide and superoxide. *Chem. Res. Toxicol.*, 5: 834–842.

Koprowski, H., Zheng, Y.M., Heber-Katz, E., Fraser, N., Rorke, L., Fu, Z.F., Hanlon, C. and Dietzschold, B. (1993) *In vivo* expression of inducible nitric oxide synthase in experimentally induced neurologic diseases. *Proc. Natl. Acad. Sci. USA*, 90: 3024–3027.

Kubes, P. and Granger, D.N. (1992) Nitric oxide modulates microvascular permeability. *Am. J. Physiol.*, 262: H611–H615.

Kummer, W. and Mayer, B. (1993) Nitric oxide synthase-immunoreactive axons inervating the guinea-pig lingual artery: an ultrastructural immunohistochemical study using elastic bright field imaging. *Histochemistry*, 99: 175–179.

Kurenny, D.E., Moroz, L.L., Turner, R.W., Sharkey, K. and Barnes, S. (1994) Modulation of ion channels in rod photoreceptors by nitric oxide. *Neuron*, 13: 315–324.

Lambert, L.E., Whitten, J.P., Baron, B.M., Cheng, H.C., Doherty, N.S. and McDonald, I.A. (1991) Nitric oxide synthesis in the CNS, endothelium and macrophages differs in its sensitivity to inhibition by arginine analogues. *Life Sci.*, 48: 69–75.

Lautier, D., Lagueux, J., Thibodeau, J., Menard, L. and Poirier, G.G. (1993) Molecular and biochemical features of poly (ADP-ribose) metabolism. *Mol. Cell. Biochem.*, 122: 171–193.

Llewellyn-Smith, I.J., Song, Z.M., Costa, M., Bredt, D.S. and Snyder, S.H. (1992) Ultrastructural location of nitric oxide synthase immunoreactivity in guinea-pig enteric neurons. *Brain Res.*, 577: 337–342.

Lipton, S.A., Singel, D.J. and Stamler, J.S. (1994) Neuroprotective and neurodestructive effects of nitric oxide and redox congeners. *Ann. New York Acad. Sci.*, 738: 382–387.

Loesch, A. and Burnstock, G. (1996) Ultrastructural localization of nitric oxide synthase and endothelin in rat pulmonary artery and vein during postnatal development and ageing. *Cell. Tissue Res.*, 283: 355–366.

Lonart, G., Wang, J. and Johnson, K.M. (1992) Nitric oxide induces neurotransmitter release from hippocampal slices. *Eur. J. Pharmacol.*, 220: 271–272.

Magnusson, S., Alm, P. and Kanje, M. (1996) Inducible nitric oxide synthase in regenerating rat ganglia. *NeuroReport*, 7: 2046–2050.

Maines, M.D. (1988) Heme oxygenase: function, multiplicity, regulatory mechanisms and clinical applications. *FASEB J.*, 2: 2557–2568.

Maines, M.D. (1992) *Heme Oxygenase. Clinical Applications and Functions*, CRC Press, Boca Raton, FL.

Maines, M.D. (1996) The heme oxygenase system; a regulator of second messenger gases. *Annu. Rev. Pharmacol. Toxicol.*, in press.

Maines, M.D., Abraham, N.G. and Kappas, A. (1977) Solubilization and partial purification of heme oxygenase from rat liver. *J. Biol. Chem.*, 252: 5900–5903.

Maines, M.D., Eke, B.C., Weber, C.M. and Ewing, J.F. (1995) Corticosterone has a permissive effect on expression of heme oxygenase-1 in CA1-CA3 neurons of hippocampus in thermal stressed rats. *J. Neurochem.*, 64: 1769–1779.

Malamud, N., Haymaker, W. and Custer, R.P. (1946) Heat stroke: a clinicopathologic study of 125 fatal stroke. *Milit. Surg.*, 99: 397–449.

Marcuccilli, C.J. and Miller, R.J. (1994) CNS stress response: too hot to handle. *Trends Neurosci.*, 17: 135–138.

Marletta, M.A. (1993) Nitric oxide synthase structure and mechanism. *J. Biol. Chem.*, 268: 12231–12234.

Matsumoto, T., Nakane, M., Pollock, J.S., Kuk, J.E. and Förstermann, U. (1993) A correlation between soluble brain nitric oxide synthase and NADPH-diaphorase activity is only seen after exposure of the tissue to fixative. *Neurosci. Lett.*, 155: 61–64.

Mayer, B. (1995) Biochemistry and molecular pharmacology of nitric oxide synthases. In: S. Vincent (Ed.), *Nitric Oxide in the Nervous System*, Academic Press, New York, pp. 21–42.

Mayer, B., Klatt, P., Werner, E.R. and Schmidt, K. (1994) Molecular mechanisms of inhibition of porcine brain nitric oxide synthase by the antinociceptive drug 7-nitro indazole.

Neuropharmacology, 33: 1253–1259, and *Neuropharmacology*, 34: 243.

McCal, T., Palmer, R.M., Boughton-Smith, N., Whittle, B.J.R. and Moncada, S. (1990) The L-arginine nitric oxide pathway in neutrophils. In: S. Moncada and E.A. Higgs (Eds.), *Nitric Oxide from L-Arginine: A Bioregulatory System*, Elsevier, Amsterdam, pp. 257–65.

McCoubrey, K. and Maines, M.D. (1994) The structure, organisation and differential expression of gene encoding rat heme oxygenase-2. *Gene*, 139: 155–161.

McCoubrey, W.K. Jr, Ewing, J.F. and Maines, M.D. (1992) Human heme oxygenase-2: characterisation and expression of a full-length cDNA and evidence suggesting that the two HO-2 transcripts may differ by choice of a polyadenylation signal. *Arch. Biochem. Biophys.*, 295: 13–20.

Meffert, M.K., Haley, J.E., Schuman, E.M., Schulman, H. and Madison, D.V. (1994) Inhibition of hippocampal heme oxygenase, nitric oxide synthase, and long-term potentiation by metalloporphyrins. *Neuron*, 13: 1225–1233.

Merrill, J.E., Ignarro, L.J., Sherman, M.P., Melinek, J. and Lane, T.E. (1993) Microglial cell cytotoxicity of oligodendrocytes is mediated through nitric oxide. *J. Immunol.*, 151: 2132–2141.

Milton, A.S. (1994) *Physiology of Thermoregulation*, Birkhauser, Basel, pp. 1–405.

Mollace, V., Colasanti, M., Persichini, T., Bagetta, G., Lauro, G.M. and Nistico, G. (1993) HIV gp 120 glycoprotein stimulates the inducible isoform of NO synthase in human cultured astrocytoma cells. *Biochem. Biophys. Res. Commun.*, 194: 439–445.

Moore, P.K., Babbedge, R.C., Wallace, P., Gaffen, Z.A. and Hart, S.L. (1993a) 7-Nitro indazole, an inhibitor of nitric oxide synthase, exhibits anti-nociceptive activity in the mouse without increasing blood pressure. *Br. J. Pharmacol.*, 108: 296–297.

Moore, P.K., Wallace, P., Gaffen, Z., Hart, S.L. and Babbedge, P.C. (1993b) Characterization of the novel nitric oxide synthase inhibitor 7-nitro indazole and related indazoles: antinociceptive and cardiovascular effects. *Br. J. Pharmacol.*, 110: 219–224.

Murphy, S., Simmons, M.L., Agullo, L., Garcia, A., Feinstein, D.L., Galea, E., Reis, D.J., Minc-Golomb, D. and Schwartz, J.P. (1993) Synthesis of nitric oxide in CNS glial cells. *Trends Neurosci.*, 16: 323–328.

Mustafa, A., Sharma, H.S., Olsson, Y., Gordh, T., Thóren, P., Sjöquist, P.-O., Roos, P., Adem, A. and Nyberg, F. (1995) Vascular permeability to growth hormone in the rat central nervous system after focal spinal cord injury. Influence of a new antioxidant, H. 290/51 and age. *Neurosci. Res.*, 23: 185–194.

Norris, P.J., Charles, I.G., Scorer, C.A. and Emson, P.C. (1995) Studies on the localization and expression of nitric oxide synthase using histochemical techniques. *Histochem. J.*, 27: 745–756.

Novikov, L., Novikova, L. and Kellerth, J.-O. (1995) Brain-derived neurotrophic factor promotes survival and blocks nitric oxide synthase expression in adult rat spinal motoneurons after ventral nerve root avulsion. *Neurosci. Lett.*, 200: 45–48.

Ny, L., Alm, P., Ekström, J., Larsson, B., Grundemar, L. and Andersson, K.-E. (1996) Localization and activity of heme oxygenase and functional effects of carbon monoxide in the feline lower oesophageal sphincter. *Br. J. Pharmacol.*, 118: 392–399.

Ochoa, L.F., Pinheiro, J.M.B., Siflinger-Birnboim, A. and Malik, A.B. (1993) Effects of nitric oxide (NO) on endothelial barrier function. *FASEB J.*, 7: A770.

Oury, T.D., Ho, Y.-S., Piantadosi, C.A. and Crapo, J.D. (1992) Extracellular superoxide dismutase, nitric oxide and central nervous system O_2 toxicity. *Proc. Natl. Acad. Sci. USA*, 89: 9715–9719.

Panizzon, K.L., Dwyer, B.E., Nishimura, R.N. and Wallis, R.A. (1996) Neuroprotection against CA1 injury with metalloporphyrins. *NeuroReport*, 7: 662–666.

Peters, A., Palay, S.L. and de Webster, H.F. (1991) *The Fine Structure of the Nervous System*, Oxford University Press, London.

Pickel, V.M. (1981) Immunocytochemical methods. In: L. Heimer and M.J. Robards (Eds.), *Neuroanatomical Tract-tracing Methods*, Plenum Press, New York, pp. 483–509.

Pollock, J.S., Klinghofer, V., Förstermann, U. and Murad, F. (1992) Endothelial nitric oxide is myristylated. *FEBS*, 309: 402–404.

Pollock, J.S., Förstermann, U., Tracey, W.R. and Nakane, M. (1995) Nitric oxide synthase isozymes antibodies. *Histochem. J.*, 27: 738–744.

Przedborski, S., Jackson-Lewis, V., Yokoyama, R., Shibata, T., Dawson, V.L. and Dawson, T.M. (1996) Role of neuronal nitric oxide synthase in 1-methyl-4-phenyl-1,2,3,6-tetrahydrophyridine (MPTP)-induced dopaminergic neurotoxicity. *Proc. Natl. Acad. Sci. USA*, 93: 4565–4571.

Radi, R., Beckman, J.S., Bush, K.M. and Freeman, B.A. (1991) Peroxynitrite oxidation of sulfhydryls. The cytotoxic potential of superoxide and nitric oxide. *J. Biol. Chem.*, 266: 4244–4250.

Raju, V.S. and Maines, M.D. (1994) Coordinated expression and mechanism of induction of HSP-32 (heme oxygenase-1) mRNA by hyperthermia in rat organs. *Biochim. Biophys. Acta*, 1217: 273–280.

Resink, A.M., Brambhatt, H.P., Cordell, B., Dawson, V.L. and Dawson, T.M. (1995) Nitric oxide mediates a component of amyloid neurotoxicity in cortical neuronal cultures. *Soc. Neurosci.*, Abstr. 21, 1010.

Rotenberg, M.O. and Maines, M.D. (1990) Isolation, characterization and expression in *Escherichia coli* of a cDNA encoding rat heme oxygenase-2. *J. Biol. Chem.*, 205: 7501–7506.

Santiago, M., Nachado, A. and Cano, J. (1994) Effect of l-arginine/nitric oxide pathway on MPP(+)-induced cell injury in the stratum of rats. *Br. J. Pharmacol.*, 111: 837–842.

Schultz, J.B., Matthews, R.T., Jenkins, T., Ferrante, R.J., Siwek, D., Henshaw, D.R., Cipolloni, P.B., Mecocci, P., Kowall, N.W., Rosen, B.R. and Beal, M.F. (1995a) Blockade of neuronal nitric oxide synthase protects against excitotoxicity *in vivo*. *J. Neurosci.*, 15: 8419–8429.

Schultz, J.B., Matthews, R.T., Muqit, M.M.K., Browne, S.E. and Beal, M.F. (1995b) Inhibition of neuronal nitric oxide synthase by 7-nitroindazole protects against MPTP induced neurotoxicity in mice. *J. Neurochem.*, 64: 936–939.

Schuman, E.M. and Madison, D.V. (1994) Nitric oxide and synaptic function. *Annu. Rev. Neurosci.*, 17: 153–183.

Sharkey, J. and Butcher, S.P. (1994) Immunophillins mediate the neuroprotective effects of FK506 in focal cerebral ischemia. *Nature*, 371: 336–339.

Sharma, H.S. and Dey, P.K. (1986) Probable involvement of 5-hydroxytryptamine in increased permeability of blood–brain barrier under heat stress. *Neuropharmacology*, 25: 161–167.

Sharma, H.S. and Dey, P.K. (1987) Influence of long-term acute heat exposure on regional blood–brain barrier permeability, cerebral blood flow and 5-HT level in conscious normotensive young rats. *Brain Res.*, 424: 153–162.

Sharma, H.S. and Cervós-Navarro, J. (1990) Brain oedema and cellular changes induced by acute heat stress in young rats. *Acta Neurochir. (Wien)*, Suppl. 51: 383–386.

Sharma, H.S., Zimmer, C., Westman, J. and Cervós-Navarro, J. (1992a) Acute systemic heat stress increases glial fibrillary acidic protein immunoreactivity in brain. An experimental study in the conscious normotensive young rats. *Neuroscience*, 48: 889–901.

Sharma, H.S., Nyberg, F., Cervós-Navarro, J. and Dey, P.K. (1992b) Histamine modulates heat stress induced changes in blood-brain barrier permeability, cerebral blood flow, brain oedema and serotonin levels: An experimental study in conscious young rats. *Neuroscience*, 50: 445–454.

Sharma, H.S., Alm, P., Olsson, Y., Gordh, T., Nyberg, F. and Westman, J. (1994a) Topical application of antibodies to nitric oxide synthase reduces a focal trauma induced alterations in microvascular permeability, edema and cell changes in the rat spinal cord. An experimental study in the rat. In: *Nitric Oxide in the Nervous System*, satellite symposium IUPHAAR, Montreal, Toronto, p. 32.

Sharma, H.S., Westman, J., Nyberg, F., Cervós-Navarro, J. and Dey, P.K. (1994b) Role of serotonin and prostaglandins in brain edema induced by heat stress. An experimental study in the rat. *Acta Neurochir. (Suppl.)* 60: 65–70.

Sharma, H.S., Alm, P., Olsson, Y., Gordh, T., Nyberg, F. and Westman, J. (1995a) Topical application of antibodies to nitric oxide synthase reduces edema and cell changes of the traumatised spinal cord. An experimental study in the rat. *J. Neurotrauma*, 12: 370.

Sharma, H.S., Olsson, Y. and Westman, J. (1995b) A serotonin synthesis inhibitor, p-chlorophenylalanine reduces the heat shock protein response following trauma to the spinal cord. An immunohistochemical and ultrastructural study in the rat. *Neurosci. Res.*, 21: 241–249.

Sharma, H.S., Olsson, Y. and Nyberg, F. (1995c) Influence of dynorphin-A antibodies on the formation of edema and cell changes in spinal cord trauma. In: F. Nyberg, H.S. Sharma and Z. Wissenfeld-Halin (Eds.), *Prog. Brain Res.*, Vol. 104, Elsevier, Amsterdam, pp. 401–416.

Sharma, H.S., Westman, J., Olsson, Y. and Alm, P. (1996a) Involvement of nitric oxide in acute spinal cord injury: an immunohistochemical study using light and electron microscopy in the rat. *Neurosci. Res.*, 24: 373–384.

Sharma, H.S., Gordh, T., Alm, P., Lindholm, D. and Westman, J. (1996b) Involvement of nitric oxide and carbon monoxide in a rat model of neurodegenerative disease. Annual Meeting of American Association of Advancement of Science, AMSIE'96, February 8–13, 1996, Baltimore, Maryland, USA, 161 pp.

Sharma, H.S., Westman, J., Cervós-Navarro, J. and Alm, P. (1996c) Involvement of nitric oxide in hyperthermic brain injury. Clinical Neuropathology, 5th European Congress of Neuropathology, April 23–27, 1996, Paris. *Neuropathol. Appl. Neurobiol.*, 22, Suppl. 1: 14–15.

Sharma, H.S., Lindholm, D., Alm, P., Gordh, T., Olsson, Y. and Westman, J. (1996d) Topical application of brain-derived neurotrophic factor reduces upregulation of neuronal nitric oxide synthase following focal trauma to the rat spinal cord. Swiss International Winter Meeting, St. Mauritz, March 20–23, 1996, pp. 16–17.

Sharma, H.S., Westman, J., Cervós-Navarro, J. and Nyberg, F. (1996e) A 5-HT$_2$ receptor mediated breakdown of the blood-brain barrier permeability and brain pathology in heat stress. An experimental study using cyproheptadine and ketanserin in young rats. In: P. Couraud and A. Scherman (Eds.), *Biology and Physiology of the Blood-Brain Barrier*, Plenum Press, New York, pp. 117–124.

Sharma, H.S., Westman, J., Alm, P., Sjöquist, P.-Ö., Cervós-Navarro, J. and Nyberg, F. (1997a) Involvement of nitric oxide in the pathophysiology of acute heat stress in the rat. influence of a new antioxidant compound H 290/51. *Ann. New York Acad. Sci.*, 813: 581–590.

Sharma, H.S., Westman, J. Nyberg, F., Alm, P. and Lindholm, D. (1997b) Nitric oxide in spinal cord injury and repair mechanisms. In: E. Stålberg, H.S. Sharma and Y. Olsson (Eds.), *Spinal Cord Monitoring, Basic and Clinical Aspects*, Springer, New York (in press).

Sharma, H.S., Nyberg, F., Gordh, T., Alm, P. and Westman, J. (1997c) Topical application of insulin like growth factor-1 reduces edema and upregulation of neuronal nitric oxide synthase following trauma to the rat spinal cord. *Acta Neurochir. (Wien)*, Suppl. 71: 130–133.

Sharma, H.S., Alm, P. and Westman, J. (1997d) Upregulation of heme oxygenase-II in the rat spinal cord following heat stress, *Proc. Int. Thermal Physiol. Symp.*, 1997 Copenhagen, The August Krogh Institute, pp. 135–138.

Sharma, H.S., Westman, J., Cervós-Navarro, J., Dey, P.K. and Nyberg, F. (1997e) Opioid receptor antagonists attenuate heat stress induced reduction in cerebral blood flow, increased blood-brain barrier permeability, vasogenic edema and cell changes in the rat. *Ann. New York Acad. Sci.*, 813: 559–571.

Sharma, H.S., Westman, J. and Nyberg, F. (1998) Pathophysiology of Brain Edema and Cell Changes following Hyperthermic Brain Injury. In: H.S. Sharma and J. Westman (Eds.), *Brain Functions in Hot Environment, Vol. 115, Progress in Brain Research*, Elsevier, Amsterdam, pp. 351–412.

Shibahara, S., Yoshizawa, M., Suzuki, H., Takeda, K., Meguro, K., and Endo, K. (1993) Functional analysis of cDNA for two types of human heme oxygenase and evidence for their separate regulation. *J. Biochem.*, 113: 214–218.

Sminia, P., van der Zee, J., Wondergem, J. and Haveman, J. (1994) Effect of hyperthermia on the central nervous system: a review. *Int. J. Hypertherm.*, 10: 1–30.

Snyder, S.H. (1992) Nitric oxide: first in a new class of neurotransmitters. *Science*, 257 (5069): 494–496.

Soltesz, I. (1996) Heme oxygenase inhibitors in neurotrauma. A commentary. *NeuroReport*, 7: 385–386.

Springall, D.R., Riveros-Moreno, V., Suburo, A., Bishop, A.E., Merrett, M., Moncada, S. and Polak, J.M. (1992) Immunological detection of nitric oxide synthase(s) in human tissues using heterologous antibodies suggesting different isoforms. *Histochemistry*, 98: 259–266.

Stamler, J.S. (1994) Redox signalling: nitrosylation and related target interactions of nitric oxide. *Cell*, 78: 931–936.

Sterner, S. (1990) Summer heat illnesses. Conditions that range from mild to fatal. *Postgrad. Med.*, 87: 215–217.

Stevens, C.F. and Wang, Y. (1993) Reversal of long-term potentiation by inhibitors of heme oxygenase. *Nature*, 364: 147–148.

Stuehr, D.J. and Griffith, O.W. (1992) Mammalian nitric oxide synthases. *Adv. Enzymol.*, 65: 287–346.

Tenhunen, R., Marver, H.S. and Schmid, R. (1968) The enzymatic conversion of heme to bilirubin by microsomal heme oxygenase. *Proc. Natl. Acad. Sci. USA*, 61: 748–755.

Thomsen, L.L., Iversen, H.K., Brinck, T.A. and Olesen, J. (1993) Arterial super sensitivity to nitric oxide (nitroglycerin) in migraine sufferers. *Cephalalgia*, 13: 395–399.

Ueta, Y., Levy, A., Chowdrey, H.S. and Lightman, S.L. (1995) Water deprivation in the rat induces nitric oxide synthase (NOS) gene expression in the hypothalamic paraventricular and supraoptic nuclei. *Neurosci. Res.*, 23: 317–319.

Umans, J.G. and Samsel, R.W. (1992) L-Canavanine selectively augments contraction in aortas from endotoxemic rats. *Eur. J. Pharmacol.*, 210: 343–346.

Vallance, P., Leone, A., Calver, A., Collier, J. and Moncada, S. (1992a) Endogenous dimethylarginine as an inhibitor of nitric oxide synthesis. *J. Cardiovasc. Pharmacol.*, 20 (Suppl. 12): S60–62.

Vallance, P., Leone, A., Calver, A., Collier, J. and Moncada, S. (1992b) Accumulation of an endogenous inhibitor of nitric oxide synthesis in chronic renal failure. *Lancet*, 339: 572–575.

Verge, V.M., Xu, Z., Xu, X.J., Wiesenfeld-Hallin, Z. and Hökfelt, T. (1992) Marked increase in nitric oxide synthase mRNA in rat dorsal ganglia after peripheral axotomy: *in situ* hybridization and functional studies. *Proc. Natl. Acad. Sci. USA*, 89: 11617–11621.

Verma, A., Hirsch, D.J., Glatt, C.E., Ronnett, G.V. and Snyder, S.H. (1993) Carbon monoxide: a putative neural messenger. *Science*, 295: 381–384.

Vincent, S.R. and Kimura, H. (1992) Histochemical mapping of nitric oxide synthase in the rat brain. *Neuroscience*, 46: 755–784.

Vincent, S.R., Das, S. and Maines, M.D. (1994) Brain heme oxygenase isoenzymes and nitric oxide synthase are co-localized in select neurons. *Neuroscience*, 63: 223–231.

Visser, J.J., Scholten, R.J.P.M. and Hoeckman, K. (1994) Nitric oxide synthesis in meningoccal meningitis. *Ann. Int. Med.*, 120: 345–346.

Vizzard, M.A., Erdman, S.L., Roppolo, J.R., Förstermann, U. and deGroat, W.C. (1994) Differential localization of neuronal nitric oxide synthase immunoreactivity and NADPH-diaphorase activity in cat spinal cord. *Cell Tissue Res.*, 278: 299–309.

Vollerthun, R., Höhler, B. and Kummer, W. (1995) Guinea pig sympathetic postganglionic neurones contain heme oxygenase-2. *NeuroReport*, 7: 173–176.

Vollerthun, R., Höhler, B. and Kummer, W. (1996) Heme oxygenase-2 in primary afferent neurons of the guinea-pig. *Histochem. Cell Biol.*, 105: 453–458.

Wahl, M., Unterberg, A., Baethmann, A. and Schilling, L. (1988) Mediators of blood-brain barrier dysfunction and formation of vasogenic brain edema. *J. Cereb. Blood Flow Metab.*, 8: 621–634.

Wallace, M.N. and Bisland, S.K. (1994) NADPH-diaphorase activity in activated astrocytes represents inducible nitric oxide synthase. *Neuroscience*, 59: 905–919.

Wang, X.-Y., Wong, W.-C. and Ling, E.-A. (1996) Localization of choline acetyltransferase and NADPH diaphorase activities in the submucous ganglia of the guinea pig colon. *Brain Res.*, 712: 107–116.

Westman, J. and Sharma, H.S. (1997) Heat shock protein response in the CNS following heat stress. In: H.S. Sharma and J. Westman (Eds.), *Brain Functions in Hot Environment. Progress in Brain Research*, Elsevier, Amsterdam, this volume.

White, L.A. and Marletta, M.A. (1992) Nitric oxide is a cytochrome *P*-450 hemoprotein. *Biochemistry*, 31: 6627–6631.

Whittle, B.J.R. (1995) Nitric oxide in physiology and pathology. *Histochem. J.*, 27: 727–737.

Wildemann, B., Dawson, V.L., Adamson, D.C., McArthur, J., Glass, J. and Dawson, T.M. (1995) Immunologic nitric oxide synthase is elevated in HIV infected individuals with dementia. *Soc. Neurosci.*, Abstr. 21: 1520.

Wolf, G., Würdig, S. and Schünzel, G. (1992) Nitric oxide synthase is predominantly located at neuronal endoplasmic reticulum: an electron microscopic demonstration of NADPH-diaphorase activity. *Neurosci. Lett.*, 147: 63–66.

Wood, J. and Garthwaite, J. (1994) Models of the diffusional spread of nitric oxide: implication for neural nitric oxide signalling and its pharmacological properties. *Neuropharmacology*, 33: 1235–1244.

Wu, W. and Li, L. (1993) Inhibition of nitric oxide synthase reduces motoneuron death due to spinal root avulsion. *Neurosci. Lett.*, 153: 121–124.

Wu, W., Liuzzi, F.J., Schinco, F.P., Depto, A.S., Li, Y., Mong, J.A., Dawson, T.M. and Snyder, S.H. (1994a) Neuronal nitric oxide synthase is induced in spinal neurons by traumatic injury. *Neuroscience*, 61: 719–726.

Wu, W., Han, K., Li, L. and Schinco, F.P. (1994b) Implantation of PNS graft inhibits the induction of neuronal nitric oxide synthase and enhances the survival of spinal motoneurons following root avulsion. *Exp. Neurol.*, 129: 335–339.

Yamada, K., Emson, P. and Hökfelt, T. (1996) Immunohistochemical mapping of nitric oxide synthase in the rat hypothalamus and colocalization with neuropeptides. *J. Chem. Neuroanat.*, 10: 295–316.

Yamanaka, M., Yamabe, K., Saito, Y., Katoh-Semba, R. and Semba, R. (1996) Immunocytochemical localization of heme oxygenase-2 in the rat cerebellum. *Neurosci. Res.*, 24, 403–407.

Yu, W.-H.A. (1994) Nitric oxide synthase in motor neurons after axotomy. *J. Histochem. Cytochem.*, 42: 451–457.

Zakhary, R., Gaine, S.P., Dinerman, J.L., Ruat, M., Flavahan, N.A. and Snyder S.H. (1996) Heme oxygenase 2: Endothelial and neuronal localization and role in endothelium-dependent relaxation. *Proc. Natl. Acad. Sci. USA*, 93: 795–798.

Zhang, Z.G., Chopp, M., Gautam, S., Zaloga, C., Zhang, R.L., Schmidt, H.H., Pollock, J.S. and Förstermann, U. (1994a) Upregulation of neuronal nitric oxide synthase-containing neurons after focal cerebral ischemia in rat. *Brain Res.*, 654: 85–95.

Zhang, J., Dawson, V.L., Dawson, T.M. and Snyder, S.H. (1994b) Nitric oxide activation of poly (ADP-ribose) synthase in neurotoxicity. *Science*, 263: 687–689.

Zhuo, M., Small, S.A., Kandel, E.R. and Hawkins, R.D. (1993) Nitric oxide and carbon monoxide produce activity-dependent long-term synaptic enhancement in hippocampus. *Science*, 260: 1946–1950.

Zoccarato, F., Deana, R., Cavallini, L. and Alexandre, A. (1989) Generation of hydrogen peroxide by cerebral cortex synaptosomes. *Eur. J. Biochem.*, 180: 473–478.

SECTION IV

Pathophysiological aspects

H.S. Sharma and J. Westman (Eds.)
Progress in Brain Research, Vol 115
© 1998 Elsevier Science BV. All rights reserved.

CHAPTER 17

Hyperthermia and the central nervous system

Peter Sminia* and Maarten C.C.M. Hulshof

Academic Medical Center, University of Amsterdam, Department of Radiotherapy, P.O. Box 22700, 1100 DE Amsterdam, The Netherlands

Introduction

Hyperthermia in oncotherapy indicates heat treatment at 40–46°C for 30–60 min, aiming to destroy tumour cells. The clinical strategy is directed to safely applying heat to the tumour target volume while avoiding normal tissue heating. Hyperthermia is generally applied as adjuvant to radiotherapy or chemotherapy for either potentiation of the effects of radiation or drugs or for its complementary effects (Hahn, 1982; Dahl, 1995; Konings, 1995). Since 1985, improved tumour control rates were reported in a number of clinical studies (see Seegenschmiedt and Feldmann, 1995, for an overview). Furthermore, hyperthermia additive to irradiation can increase resectability and prolong palliation for inoperable or recurrent tumours (González González et al., 1995). A European multicentre randomized trial on patients with malignant melanoma revealed an increase in the 5-year actuarial local tumour control from 28% after radiation alone to 46% after radiation combined with hyperthermia (Overgaard et al., 1995, 1996). Radiotherapy with or without hyperthermia in a randomized trial on recurrent or inoperable breast cancer proved to be advantageous for the combined treatment arm.

The overall complete tumour response rate for radiotherapy alone was 41% vs. 59% with hyperthermia (International Collaborative Hyperthermia Group, 1996).

Long-term prognosis for patients with primary brain- or intraspinal neoplasms is very poor with local progression as the main cause of failure (González González et al., 1987; Halperin et al., 1988). For that reason, there is increasing interest in the use of hyperthermia additional to radiotherapy in the treatment of such tumours. Information on the heat sensitivity of the normal human brain is therefore required. Data on the thermal effects on neural tissue from animals might serve as an indication for the heat response of the human CNS. In laboratory studies, several heating methods have been used and experiments have been performed on various animal species. Anatomically different parts of the brain and spinal cord have been locally exposed to heat at different temperatures and durations and effects were evaluated using electro-physiological, neurological or histological endpoints (Sminia et al., 1994). In this chapter the biological effects of hyperthermia on the CNS are reviewed with regard to the maximum tolerable heat dose, i.e. the temperature and duration of heat exposure above which injury can result in persistent functional impairment. The kinetics of functional and histopathological changes are described. An overview on the effects of the combination of heat and

---

*Corresponding author. Tel: +31 20 5664231; fax: +31 20 6091278; e-mail: P.SMINIA@AMC.UVA.NL

irradiation on the rodent spinal cord is included, since such detailed data are scarce for the brain. On the basis of morphological similarities between both parts of the CNS it may be justified to extrapolate the spinal cord data to the brain. Clinical observations regarding toxicity after hyperthermic exposure of human brain tissue are summarized. First clinical experiences of brain tumor treatment with brachytherapy alone or combined with interstitial hyperthermia are shown. In the last paragraph of this chapter, conclusions are drawn on the current state of knowledge with regard to the effects of hyperthermia on the CNS.

Hyperthermia studies on experimental animals

Animal brain studies

Resistance to localized heating of (part of) the normal brain was studied in dog, cat, rabbit and minipig, as summarized in Table 1. Harris et al. (1962) showed that the limit of heat tolerance after warm blood perfusion of one of the brain hemispheres was 42–43°C for 30 min. However, it was not tested whether animals could tolerate this temperature for a longer duration. Hyperthermia of one brain hemisphere at 44–46°C for 30 min was found to be lethal. Silberman et al. (1982) studied whole brain hyperthermia in the rabbit. Heating for 60 min at 42–43°C (average 42.4°C) was well tolerated, but animals died within minutes at a brain temperature of 45°C. Neither physiological effects nor histopathological changes were however reported by Samaras et al. (1982) after interstitial heating of a small part of cat forebrain to 45°C for 30 min. Because of the rapid temperature fall-off from the microwave antenna towards the surrounding brain tissue, a precise heat dose could not be given. Acute histopathological changes after heat exposure of cat and dog brain were investigated by, respectively Britt et al. (1983) and Lyons et al. (1984). Cerebral oedema and pyknotic cortical neurons were observed after 50–70 min heating at 42.2°C, while temperatures exceeding 43°C led to neuronal cell

death. Disruption of myelin tracts in the white matter became apparent at 43.0–43.5°C (Britt et al., 1983). Lyons et al. (1986) studied histopathological changes for a period of 56 days following brain hyperthermia. The organization and resolution of thermal damage were characterized by three stages of histopathological changes. The acute stage (days 1 to 3) was defined by extensive coagulation necrosis, pyknosis of neuronal elements in the grey matter, oedema and vacuolation in the white matter, and polymorphonuclear leucocyte infiltration. The subacute stage (days 4 to 21) was characterized by the appearance of lipid-laden macrophages, liquefaction of the necrotic regions, fibroblastic proliferation, and vascular proliferation with some perivascular lymphocyte infiltration. The chronic stage (days 22 to 56) was defined by fibrosis (reticulin and collagen formation) and gliosis (reactive astrocytic proliferation) occurring around the fluid-filled necrotic centre. A threshold heat dose of 41.0°C for 50 min was derived from these observations, above which damage was irreversible. This threshold value was even 1.0–1.5°C lower than reported for the acute histological effects (Britt et al., 1983; Lyons et al., 1984). The authors commented that caution is required when interpreting the data on chronic effects because of the lack of statistical significance. Neurological symptoms however were only observed in a few out of 75 animals up to 56 days after treatment, even after 50 min at 48°C, indicating that the small heated volume was not responsible for vital functions.

Interstitial microwave heating of dog brain tissue at 43°C or 44°C for 30 min resulted in hemiparesis in all five treated animals (Sneed et al., 1986). Four animals recovered within 24 h following heat treatment, but in the other animal (30 min at 44°C) a stable slight left hemiparesis persisted. Röntgenological examination after one week showed a focus of low density at the position of the antenna, surrounded by a thin ring of contrast enhancement in all five dogs. Histology at one week showed frank coagulation necrosis at the implantation site, surrounded by a variety of prominent vascular changes including marked en-

TABLE 1

Data on the effects of localized hyperthermia on normal animal brain

Part of heated brain/animal	Heating method	Heat dose	Observation time	Neurological observations	Pathological findings	Maximum tolerated dose	Reference
One of the brain hemispheres dog	Warm blood perfusion	42–46°C 30 min	68 days	No changes at 42–43°C; at 44–46°C hemiparesis, death within 36 h	No gross changes at 42–43°C; at 44–46° oedema, haemorrhages	30 min 42–43°C	Harris et al. (1962)
Whole brain rabbit	Radiofrequency 13.56 MHz	42–43°C, 60 min; 45°C few min	5 months	No changes after 42–43°C, death after few min at 45°C	No changes after 42–43°C	60 min 42.4°C	Silberman et al. (1982)
Small part of fore-brain cat	Interstitial microwave antenna 2450 MHz	45°C 30 min	Immediate	—	No significant difference between shamtreated brain and heated brain	30 min 45°C	Samaras et al. (1982)
Part of the occipital cortex cat	Ultrasound 2.06 MHz	42–48°C 50 min	Immediate	—	Damage to grey and white matter after 50 min 43°C	50 min 42°C	Britt et al. (1983)
Part of the occipital cortex dog	Interstitial microwave heating 915 MHz	42–43.5°C 50–70 min	Immediate	—	Damage to grey and white matter after 50 min 43°C	50–70 min 42–42.5°C	Lyons et al. (1984)
Part of the occipital cortex cat	Ultrasound 2.06 MHz	41–48°C 50 min	56 days	Minor symptoms in few animals	Necrosis, inflammation	50 min 41°C	Lyons et al. (1986)
Part of one of the hemispheres dog	Interstitial microwave heating 915, 2450 MHz	43–44°C 30 min	16 weeks	Transient hemiparesis in 4/5 dogs; persistent hemiparesis in 1/5 dogs	Necrosis, inflammation	< 30 min 43°C	Sneed et al. (1986)
Part of the frontal white matter of one hemisphere dog	Interstitial microwave heating 2450 MHz	40–44°C 30 min	6 weeks	Transient left-sided weakness during first 2 days after treatment	Focal coagulation necrosis (1–2 wks) neovascularization, gliosis, fibrosis (3–6 weeks)	30 min 43.9 ± 1.5°C	Fike et al. (1991)
Small part of left hemisphere minipig	Interstitial microwave heating 2450 MHz	43–> 44.5°C 45 min	1 week	No symptoms	Necrosis after 45 min > 44.5°C, minor changes after 45 min 44°C	45 min 43°C	Eddy et al. (1992)
Part of brain dog	Interstitial radio-frequency heating 8 MHz	42–44°C 15–60 min	Immediate	—	Coagulation necrosis. Neuronal death in grey matter oedema in white matter	45 min 42°C 15 min 43°C	Ikeda et al. (1994)

dothelial and medial wall hypertrophy and hyperplasia (the zone of contrast enhancement). Peripheral to this region, there was a zone of vacuolation, axonal damage, demyelination and increased cellularity, and oedema that varied from dog to dog. By 16 weeks, histology showed fibrosis and vascular proliferation around and within the previously necrotic area (hyperdense on precontrast CT scans). Fike et al. (1991) inserted a microwave antenna in the frontal white matter of dog brain to investigate the focal heat effects of 40–44°C for 30 min. Heat injury, evaluated with CT, was well tolerated and the neurological sequelae were minimal and transient in nature in all animals. Heat doses exceeding 43.9 ± 1.5°C for 30 min led to necrosis within one week following treatment. Eddy et al. (1992) also studied acute histopathological changes one week following interstitial hyperthermia in the minipig. Heat treatment at temperatures greater than about 44.5°C for 45 min of a small volume of the left cerebral brain hemisphere resulted in necrosis. No significant damage was observed at temperatures lower than about 43.5°C for 45 min. Ikeda et al. (1994) characterized acute thermal damage induced by interstitial heating of dog brain. After 43°C for 45 min, coagulation necrosis was present in most grey matter lesions, with less severe reaction in the white matter. At 44°C, necrosis was observed in both grey and white matter of the brain. Threshold tolerable heat doses were 42°C for 45 min and 43°C for 15 min.

Rodent spinal cord studies

Table 2 lists rodent data on the maximum tolerated heat dose after a single localized heat treatment of different anatomical parts of the spinal cord. Neurology after heat exposure of rat cervical spinal cord was evaluated by Sminia et al. (1987). The cervical vertebral column including the spinal cord was heated by means of a microwave ring applicator. One day after 41.5°C for 120 min or 42.3°C for 60 min neither neurological symptoms nor deaths were observed. Treatment at 42.3°C for 75 min resulted in minor motor

dysfunction. The incidence and severity of the neurological symptoms, ranging from uncoordinated use of the forelegs to complete paralysis and lethality, increased with increasing heat dose applied. Fig. 1 shows the incidence of foreleg paralysis after heat exposure of the spinal cord. The figure illustrates a steep increase in thermal damage with increasing duration of exposure as well as with increasing temperature between 42°C and 43°C. In all surviving rats suffering from neurological symptoms after treatment, recovery from motor dysfunction took place within one month. Histological sectioning of the spinal cord was performed up to 28 days following 42.9°C for 38 min (Sminia et al., 1989).

Immediately and 4 h after treatment, neurons in the grey matter of the cord were affected and vacuolization was observed in the white matter. In paralysed animals, neuronal degeneration was noticed with myelin pallor and sometimes haemorrhagic foci in white and grey matter. As a reaction to the thermal injury, between day 3 and 14, gliosis was observed and invasion of macrophages and lymphocytes (Fig. 2). Animals with severe neurological symptoms immediately after hyperthermia but that had recovered at day 28 after treatment showed focal scarring and demyelination in the spinal cord.

Kumano et al. (1989) evaluated heat injury to the rat thoracic spinal cord. The thermal dose threshold for neurological hind leg complications was either 30 min at 43.3°C or 15 min at 44.2°C. Effects of hyperthermia of the thoracolumbar mouse spinal cord were described by Goffinet et al. (1977), Lo (1989), Sasaki and Ide (1989) and Froese et al. (1990, 1991). Goffinet et al. (1977) heated murine spinal cord at 42°C for 60 min by immersing the whole thoracolumbar area of the animal in a 44°C waterbath. This heat dose was well tolerated. Heat doses resulting in partial paralysis within days after exposure were 84 min at 42°C, 61 min at 42.5°C and 41 min at 43°C (Lo, 1989). Most animals that were severely paralysed by heat died within a few days, the lethal dose for 50% of the animals was 89 min at 42°C, 62 min at 42.5°C and 42 min at 43°C. Survivors recovered

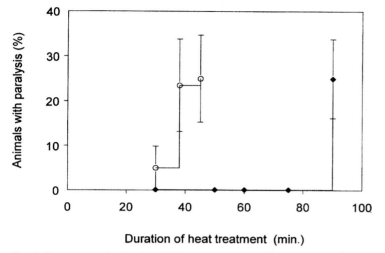

Fig. 1. Percentage of animals with foreleg paralysis one day after hyperthermia of the cervical rat spinal cord. Heat was applied with a microwave applicator to obtain a spinal cord temperature of 42.3°C (♦) and 42.9°C (○). Data points with error bars indicate mean ± S.E. of 8–24 animals.

within one month. Various degrees of neuronal injury, demyelination as well as vascular damage were noticed in spinal cord sections from animals with severe paralysis. Histopathological changes after 48–50°C contact heating for 1 h of a very small part (< 1 mm³) of the dorsal white matter of rat thoracolumbar spinal cord were studied in detail by Sasaki and Ide (1989). Microscopical examination of the spinal cord sections showed widespread damage to myelin sheaths but not to axons. Between 2 and 4 weeks, the denuded axons were remyelinated by either oligodendrocytes or Schwann cells. Froese et al. (1990, 1991) studied the neurological response of mice after heating of the thoracolumbar spinal cord and part of the dorsal musculature. Heat doses resulting in reflex leg extension > 40% in half of the treated animals were 60 min at 43.1°C or 11 min at 45°C.

Localized microwave heating of the rat lumbar region including the lumbosacral cord and cauda equina at 42.6°C for 60 min however, did not induce any neurological effect (Franken et al., 1992). Motor dysfunction of the hind legs was found after 60 min at 43.0°C or 43.8°C. In addition, 24 h after treatment at 43.8°C for 60 min, loss of tail tonus was observed as well as loss of

sensory functions. Recovery from motor disorders except for loss of tail tonus occurred within 2 weeks after treatment. Histopathological changes included haemorrhagic necrosis of both white and grey matter.

Thermal enhancement of radiation response of the central nervous system

Hyperthermia combined with irradiation can enhance the radiosensitivity of malignant tissue as well as that of surrounding normal tissue. The Thermal Enhancement Ratio (TER), i.e. the ratio of the radiation dose to achieve a certain effect without and with heat, is dependent on the sequence and time interval between both modalities, and on the type of tissue (e.g. Konings, 1995). There are no data on thermal enhancement of radiation effects in the brain. A number of detailed studies is however available on the effects of hyperthermia in combination with irradiation on anatomically different parts of rodent spinal cord (Table 3). In all studies, hyperthermia was applied in the well tolerated heat dose range, and animals were observed for neurological late effects. Goffinet et al. (1977) were the first investi-

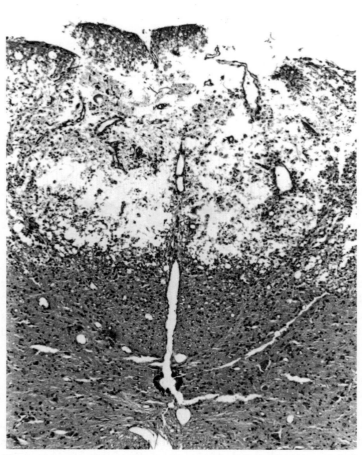

Fig. 2. Extensive thermal damage in the dorsal funiculi of the cervical spinal cord of a paralysed animal 7 days following hyperthermia, showing necrosis and a reactive cellular infiltrate (haematoxilin and eosin staining; magnification approx. ×60).

gators who performed a complete dose-response study on the murine spinal cord. Single radiation doses to the thoracolumbar spinal cord immediately before or after locoregional hyperthermia at 42°C for 60 min shortened the post irradiation latent period for expression of myelitis. In combination with hyperthermia, significantly lower radiation doses produced myelitis. From their data, a TER of 1.19 for the 'early delayed' paralysis up to 6 months after irradiation and 1.15 for the 'late delayed' paralysis 9–12 months post irradiation was calculated. Heat applied two weeks prior to irradiation affected neither the latent period nor the incidence of myelitis. Lo (1989) confirmed the observations of Goffinet et al. (1977). Mice were irradiated on the thoracolumbar spinal cord with 12–35 Gy and heated shortly thereafter at 42.5°C for 40 min, resulting in a TER of 1.27 for paralysis. Sminia et al. (1991) showed that hyperthermia applied 5–10 min after X-rays enhanced the radi-

TABLE 2

Localized hyperthermia of normal rodent spinal cord

Spinal cord segment and animal	Heating method	Heat dose	Neurological observations	Pathological findings	Maximum tolerated dose
Cervical rat spinal cord Sminia et al., 1987	Microwave	41.2–43.2°C 30–120 min	Uncoordinated use of forelegs, paralysis and death above 60 min 42.3°C	Neuronal damage, white matter necrosis, gliosis, vascular damage	60 min 42.3°C
Lower thoracic rat spinal cord Kumano et al., 1989	Radio-frequency 8 MHz	43.3–46°C 15–30 min	—	—	< 30 min 43.3°C
Thoracolumbar mouse spinal cord Goffinet et al., 1977	Waterbath	42°C 60 min	—	—	> = 60 min 42°C
Lo, 1989	Waterbath	42–43.5°C 20–100 min	Neurological complications and death above 40 min 42–42.5°C	Neuronal damage, demyelination, vascular damage	40 min 42–42.5°C
Froese et al., 1990/91	Radio-frequency	41.2–45.2°C 60 min	Paralysis increases from 11% after 1 h 41.2°C to 50% after 1 h 43.1°C	—	< 60 min 42°C
Lumbosacral rat spinal cord Franken et al., 1992	Microwave	42.6–43.8°C 60 min	Motor dysfunction above 60 min 43.0°C	Haemorrhagic necrosis of both white- and grey matter	60 min 42.6°C

ation response of the rat cervical spinal cord. The TER for both the 'early delayed' (5–10 months) and 'late delayed' (10 months to the end of life) radiation response were in the range of 1.1–1.3 (Table 3). Latency for paralysis was shortened for animals in certain radiation dose groups in which radiation alone resulted in 'late paralysis' but radiation in combination with hyperthermia in 'early paralysis'. Biological effects of hyperthermia in combination with radiation on rat lumbosacral spinal cord were essentially the same as those observed after exposure of the cervical- and thoracolumbar spinal cord. Fig. 3 shows that local heat treatment of rat lumbosacral spinal cord

immediately after X-irradiation leads to enhancement of the radiation response and shortening of the latent period for expression of radiation myelopathy. No difference was found with regard to pathological changes between irradiation treatment alone and irradiation combined with heat (Sminia et al., 1995).

Clinical hyperthermia studies

A large number of phase I–II studies on heat delivery to brain tumours in humans have been published in the last decade. Tumour response and side effects are evaluated in patients with a

TABLE 3

Experimental data on the effects of the combined treatment of radiation (X) and hyperthermia (H) on rodent spinal cord

Spinal cord segment and animal	Heat dose	X-ray dose (Gy)	Time interval between X and H	Latent period	TER early	TER late
Cervical rat spinal cord	30 min 41.2°C 42.1°C	15–32	X 5–10 min after H	Shift from 'late' to 'early'	1.07 1.17	1.25 1.31
Sminia et al., 1991	42.9°C			response	1.12	
Thoracolumbar mouse spinal cord	60–70 min 42°C	30–80	X immediately before and after H	Shortened by 10–15%	1.19	1.15
Goffinet et al., 1977; Lo, 1989	40 min. 42.5°C	12–35	X 5 min after H	No difference between X and X + H		1.27
Lumbosacral rat spinal cord Sminia et al., 1995	30 min 41.1°C 42.3°C 42.6°C	15–32	X 5–10 min after H	Shortened by 10–40%		1.32 1.24 1.29

TER is the ratio of the radiation dose to achieve myelitis in 50% of the animals with radiation alone and with radiation combined with hyperthermia.

large variety of tumours and medical histories. The feasibility and clinical outcome of these stud-ies have been discussed (Seegenschmiedt et al., 1995; Sneed and Stea, 1995). This paragraph

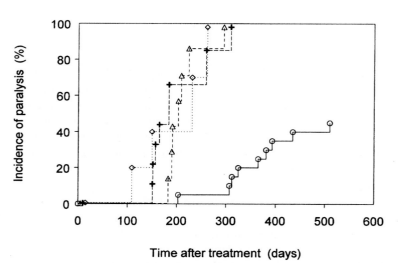

Fig. 3. Cumulative incidence of hind leg paralysis after local X-irradiation and hyperthermia of the lumbosacral rat spinal cord. 20 Gy alone (○) or combined with 30 min at 41.1°C (△), 30 min at 42.3°C (+) and 30 min at 42.6°C (◇). Treatment groups consisted of 5–20 animals. $P < 0.001$ for all three X-rays + hyperthermia groups vs. the X-rays alone group.

overviews the clinical studies, with emphasis on eventual adverse effects of the treatment and threshold tolerable heat dose of the normal brain tissue. First clinical results with brachytherapy combined with interstitial hyperthermia are summarized. Normal brain temperatures are however measured in a few studies for the reason that mainly interstitial heating techniques were used in which thermometry was limited to the tumour volume. Because hyperthermia has been used with either radiotherapy, chemotherapy or a combination of these treatment modalities, it is very difficult to clearly evaluate the response of the normal human brain to heat only.

Salcman and Samaras (1983) report on their limited experience with interstitial hyperthermia applied as sole treatment to six patients. Thermometry was restricted to the tumour volume. Two heat treatments at 45°C for 30–60 min tumour temperature appeared to be safe and were well tolerated in five patients, but transient worsening of pre-existing neurological deficit was observed in the other patient. In the study of Winter et al. (1985), tumour temperatures were maintained at 42.5°C for one hour. Normal brain temperatures were however not measured. They observed no adverse effects of repeated treatments in 12 patients. Silberman et al. (1986) administered hyperthermia non-invasively using a magnetrode to 13 patients that were treated in combination with chemotherapy. During the hyperthermia sessions, intracranial pressure (ICP) was measured. Maximum tumour temperatures achieved varied from 38.8°C to 46.3°C, whereas maximum normal brain temperature varied from 38.6°C to 43.4°C. Transient neurological complications were seen in two patients in whom the ICP exceeded 30 mm H_2O prior to hyperthermia.

Eighteen patients were treated with interstitial hyperthermia combined with brachytherapy and/or external beam radiotherapy by Roberts et al. (1986, 1989). The temperature was measured in the tumour only and reached 43°C at the periphery. The most frequent complication of treatment was that of worsening of pre-existent neurologic deficit, which was transient in five patients and persistent in four patients. Tanaka et al. (1989) combined interstitial hyperthermia with external beam radiotherapy, 40–50 Gy in 4–5 weeks and ACNU chemotherapy for 25 primary malignant glioma and heat alone for 15 recurrent tumours. Patients received hyperthermia twice weekly, 3 or 4 times at 42.5–43°C for 60 min at the tumour rim. Minor complications were observed in three patients, while a transient worsening of neurological symptoms was observed in five patients. Clinical response rates were promising, even among the patients that were treated with heat only (Tanaka et al., 1989).

Scanned focused ultrasound hyperthermia was combined with external beam radiation in the treatment of 15 patients with recurrent malignant tumours of the brain (Guthkelch et al., 1991). Therapeutic temperatures ($\geq$ 42.5°C) were achieved in approximately 50% of the measured points but significant intratumoural thermal gradients occurred. The number of heat sessions was 2–4 for 15 to 60 min duration. There was a smaller percentage of adequately heated points in the larger tumours. Although intracranial bleeding occurred in some patients due to the inserted temperature probes, no major complications attributed to the hyperthermia treatment were reported. Autopsy findings in five patients showed coagulation necrosis and vascular changes in the heated areas. In two patients necrosis extended into the peritumoural region, suggesting that treatment had been pursued to the limit of tolerance.

From 1987 to 1990, 41 patients with recurrent malignant gliomas after prior surgery and radiotherapy, were entered in BTRC protocol 8721 for treatment with combined brachytherapy and interstitial hyperthermia (Sneed et al., 1994). Brachytherapy was delivered by means of implant catheters housing Iodine 125 radiation sources. A typical example of the catheter geometry is shown in Fig. 4. The brachytherapy dose ranged from 32.4 to 63.3 Gy. A total of 78 hyperthermia treatments were performed with microwave antennas with a median T90, i.e. the temperature achieved in 90% of the thermocouple probes, of 41.1°C. Figure 5 shows that steady state temperatures ranged from 37.0 to 45.7°C, with an increase from

346

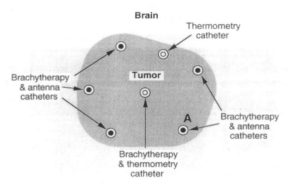

Fig. 4. A typical catheter arrangement for microwave hyperthermia antennas, brachytherapy and thermometry in a brain tumour. Antenna catheters were fairly evenly spaced, 1.2–1.5 cm apart from each other, about 3–5 mm inside the perimeter of the target volume [from Sneed et al. (1994), reprinted with kind permission of W.B. Saunders Company, Orlando, FL, USA].

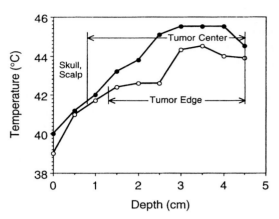

Fig. 5. Steady-temperatures vs. depth are shown for a recurrent glioblastoma heated with six microwave antennas. Temperatures were measured within two thermometry probes, including one through the centre of the tumour and one near an edge of the tumour. Vertical lines indicate the tumour margins for each temperature profile [from Sneed et al. (1994), reprinted with kind permission of W.B. Saunders Company, Orlando, FL, USA].

the tumour periphery towards the tumour centre. No correlation was found between T90 and tumour volume. Acute toxicity included 13 grade 1 complications (brief seizures and transient neurological changes), 5 grade 2 complications (seizures an neurological changes) and 5 grade 3 complications (2 infections, 1 deep venous thrombosis and 2 reversible neurological changes). The risk of grade 3 complications for combined brachytherapy and hyperthermia was greater than for brachytherapy alone (12% vs 6%). The reoperation rate for removal of necrosis was similar to that for brachytherapy alone (46%). A multivariate analysis identified histology, age and T90 as significant factors influencing survival (Sneed et al., 1992). This influence of T90 was also found by Seegenschmiedt et al. (1994) in their experience with 90 patients treated with interstitial thermoradiotherapy for advanced, recurrent or metastatic brain tumours. Both the T90 and average minimal temperature were of significant influence on survival ($P = 0.0006$).

Stea et al. (1994) compared survival and toxicity of patients with supratentorial high grade gliomas treated in Phase I/II protocols of interstitial thermoradiotherapy ($n = 25$) with that of a similar group of patients treated with interstitial

brachytherapy alone ($n = 33$). Hyperthermia was performed with a ferromagnetic seed implant and delivered for 60 min with the goal of heating as much of the implant volume to temperatures between 42°C and 45°C. Implant volumes were restricted to 110 cc. The analysis showed a significantly improved survival with the combination of hyperthermia and brachytherapy compared to brachytherapy alone ($P = 0.017$). Reversible grade 1 and 2 toxicities (seizures and transient neurological worsening) directly contributing to hyperthermia occurred in 11 patients. Three major complications after hyperthermia, i.e. a haemorrhage, hydrocephalus and pneumo-encephalous were attributed to the catheter implantations. One fatal complication occurred, resulting from oedema and mass effect secondary to both implantation and hyperthermia.

The NCOG protocol 6G-90-2 is the only trial which randomized interstitial thermoradiotherapy vs. brachytherapy alone additional to external radiotherapy with oral hydroxyurea in patients with newly diagnosed glioblastoma (Sneed et al., 1994). Interstitial hyperthermia was aimed at 42.5°C for 30 min using 915 MHz helical coil microwave

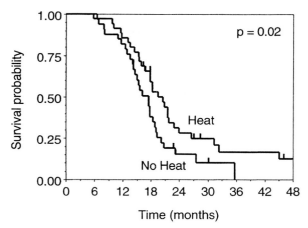

Fig. 6. Kaplan–Meier survival curves for evaluable patients who actually received brachytherapy, comparing 33 radiation alone patients with 35 radiation + hyperthermia patients (log rank, $P = 0.02$).

antennas before and after an interstitial dose of 60 Gy. Recently updated results for patients who actually underwent brachytherapy are presented in Fig. 6 (Sneed, 1997, personal communication). Median survival was significantly increased from 17.5 months after brachytherapy alone to 19.5 months for the thermoradiotherapy group, with 2-year survival probabilities of 14% vs. 31%, respectively. The median T90 achieved was 42.1°C, but no thermal parameter appeared to influence survival or complication rate. There were two grade 4 infections in the implant and hyperthermia group vs. none in the implant alone group. Both seizures (6 vs.. 4) and neurological changes (14 vs.. 1) were more frequent after hyperthermia.

Conclusions

In spite of the diversity of animal species studied, as well as endpoints for assessment of effects, brain structures treated, differences in anaesthesia procedures, thermometry and heating techniques applied, most animal data on the effects of localized hyperthermia on the brain indicate a maximum tolerable heat dose of 42–42.5°C for 40–60 min or 43°C for 10–30 min. Effects of hyperthermia are expressed immediately or within a few days after treatment. No late effects following heat treatment were reported. The dose response relationship for thermal doses exceeding the threshold is steep. Heat injury to neural tissue may result in neurological abnormalities which, unless lethal, are transient in most cases. Histological studies show irreversible lesions after high heat dose, characterized by coagulation necrosis. There is an indication that white matter is more heat resistant than grey matter. Thermal injury to normal neural tissue is repaired by fibrotic or gliotic scarring. Surviving neuronal elements may be responsible for functional recovery from heat injury, which is, however, dependent on the injured volume and anatomical site of the lesion. Hence, the data indicate a correlation between the exposed volume and toxicity of the heat treatment. The relatively high heat dose tolerated in interstitial heating can be ascribed to this volume effect, since the heated volume of normal neural tissue generally was small and not responsible for vital functions.

The spinal cord data concerning the response upon hyperthermia and maximum tolerable heat dose, point in the same direction as the above summarized data on the brain. The observations on neurology and heat sensitivity of the spinal cord in mice are very similar to those of the rat. Experimental data on the rat lumbosacral cord and cauda equina show that this part of the spinal cord is less sensitive to heat than the cervical and thoracolumbar spinal cord. This difference can be explained by the smaller volume of grey matter in the lumbosacral region. Experimental data demonstrate that heat injury to a small volume of the white matter of the cord does not inevitably result in functional impairment and can be repaired in about one month.

Data on the combined effects of X-ray irradiation and hyperthermia on rodent spinal cord, clearly show that the radiation response can be enhanced by a factor of 1.1–1.3. In all studies on thermal enhancement, a heat dose was administered in the tolerable range. The latent period for expression of late irradiation effects was slightly shortened in most of the studies. Histopathological changes after irradiation in combination with hyperthermia were not different from those after irradiation only.

Clinical experience obtained in over 400 patients shows that relatively safe hyperthermic treatment of brain tumours is feasible under appropriate technical conditions with adequate thermometry for careful control of the heating. Hyperthermia is often applied using interstitial heating techniques and in combination with brachytherapy. Promising results were obtained in Phase II studies with temperature controlled ferromagnetic implants. The first randomized clinical trial comparing brachytherapy alone vs. brachytherapy plus interstitial hyperthermia for primary or recurrent brain tumours has recently been closed resulting in a small but significant increase in survival for patients in the combined treatment arm. Early toxicity consisting of seizures and transient aggravation of neurological symptoms are more frequently observed after hyperthermia in combination with radiotherapy than after radiotherapy alone. Data on late effects are too scarce to draw conclusions. Toxicity seems to be acceptable in small implant volumes (< 100 cm^3). Thermometry generally is limited to the tumour, as it is expected that the increase in temperature outside the implant volume is not significant. Therefore, it is impossible to define a tolerable heat dose for nervous tissue from human data. It seems to be justified to assume that it is the same range as for animal brain, i.e. 40–60 min at 42–42.5°C or 10–30 min at 43°C. This relatively low threshold thermal dose however, does not hamper brain tumour hyperthermia, since the available interstitial heating techniques allow selective heating of the tumour with only limited heat dissipation in the surrounding normal brain.

Acknowledgements

The authors greatly appreciate and acknowledge Dr P.K. Sneed, Associate Professor in Residence at the Department of Radiation Oncology at the University of California, San Francisco, USA, for kindly providing us with Figs. 4, 5 and 6. Thanks are also due to Mrs A. Barten and Mrs A. Van der Graaff for preparation of the manuscript.

References

Britt, R.H., Lyons, B.E., Pounds, D.W. and Prionas, S.D. (1983) Feasibility of ultrasound hyperthermia in the treatment of malignant brain tumours. Med. Instrum., 17: 172–177.

Dahl, O. (1995) Interaction of heat and drugs in vitro and in vivo. In: M.H. Seegenschmidt, P. Fessenden and C.C. Vernon (Eds.), Thermoradiotherapy and Thermochemotherapy. Vol. 1: Biology, Physiology, and Physics, Springer, Berlin, pp. 103–121.

Eddy, H.A., Salazar, O.M., Amin, P.P., Better, W.E. and Ro, J. (1992) Acute histopathological changes in brain following interstitial hyperthermia and irradiation. Endocurietherapy / Hyperthermia Oncol., 8: 27–40.

Fike, J.R., Gobbel, G.T., Satoh, T. and Stauffer, P.R. (1991) Normal brain response after interstitial microwave hyperthermia. Int. J. Hyperthermia, 7: 795–808.

Franken, N.A.P., De Vrind, H.H., Sminia, P., Haveman, J., Troost, D. and González González, D. (1992) Neurological complications after 434 MHz microwave hyperthermia of the rat lumbar region including the spinal cord. Int. J. Radiat. Biol., 69: 229–238.

Froese, G., Dunscombe, P.B., Das, R.M. and Mclellan, J. (1990) Thermal dosimetry of spinal cord heating in the mouse. Int. J. Hyperthermia, 6: 319–332.

Froese, G., Das, R.M. and Dunscombe, P.B. (1991) The sensitivity of the thoracolumbar spinal cord in the mouse to hyperthermia. Radiat. Res., 125: 173–180.

Guthkelch, A.N., Carter, L.P., Cassidy, J.R., Hynynen, K.H., Iacono, R.P., Johnson, P.C., Obbens, E.A.M.T., Roemer, R.B., Seeger, J.F., Shimm, D.S. and Stea, B. (1991) Treatment of malignant brain tumors with focused ultrasound hyperthermia and radiation: results of a phase I trial. J. Neuro-Oncol., 10: 271–284.

Goffinet, D.R., Choi, K.Y. and Brown, J.M. (1977) The combined effects of hyperthermia and ionising radiation on the adult mouse spinal cord. Radiat. Res., 72: 238–245.

González González, D., Van der Werf, A.J.M., Van der Schueren, E. and Van Dijk, J.D.P. (1987) Results after radiotherapy in Gliomas. In: Proceedings of the fifth Varian European Clinac Users Meeting, Flims, Switzerland, pp. 99–104.

González González, D., Van Dijk, J.D.P. and Blank, L.E.C.M. (1995) Radiotherapy and Hyperthermia. Eur. J. Cancer, 31A: 1351–1355.

Hahn, G.M. (1982) Hyperthermia and Cancer, Plenum Press, New York.

Halperin, E.C., Burger, P.C. and Bullard, D.E. (1988) The

fallacy of the localized supratentorial malignant glioma. *Int. J. Radiat. Oncol. Biol. Phys.*, 15: 505–509.

Harris, A.B., Erickson, L., Kendig, J.H., Mingrino, S. and Goldring, S. (1962) Observations on selective brain heating in dogs. *J. Neurosurg.*, 19: 514–521.

Ikeda, N., Hayashida, O., Kameda, H., Ito, H. and Matsuda, T. (1994) Experimental study on thermal damage to dog normal brain. *Int. J. Hyperthermia*, 10: 553–561.

International Collaborative Hyperthermia Group (1996) Radiotherapy with or without hyperthermia in the treatment of superficial localized breast cancer: Results from five randomized controlled trials. *Int. J. Radiat. Oncol. Biol. Phys.*, 35: 731–744.

Konings, A.T.W. (1995) Interaction of heat and radiation in vitro and *in vivo*. In: M.H. Seegenschmidt, P. Fessenden and C.C. Vernon (Eds.), *Thermoradiotherapy and Thermochemotherapy*, Vol. 1: Biology, Physiology, and Physics, Springer, Berlin, pp. 89–102.

Kumano, K., Nakamura, T., Kadoya, S., Lizuka, H., Miyamora, T., Miyamura, J. and Kita, Y. (1989) Heat tolerance of the spinal cord in the rat by 8 MHz RF capacitive heating. In: T. Sugahara and M. Saito (Eds.), *Hyperthermic Oncology 1988*, Vol. 1, Taylor and Francis, London, pp. 306–307.

Lo, Y.-C. (1989) The effects of ionizing radiation and hyperthermia on mouse spinal cord. Thesis, University of California, Los Angeles. UMI, Michigan, USA.

Lyons, B.E., Britt, R.H. and Strohbehn, J.W. (1984) Localized hyperthermia in the treatment of malignant brain tumours using an interstitial microwave antenna array. *IEEE Trans. Biomed. Eng.*, 31: 53–62.

Lyons, B.E., Obana, W.G., Borchich, J.K., Kleinman R., Singh, D. and Britt, R.H. (1986) Chronic histological effects of ultrasonic hyperthermia on normal feline brain tissue. *Radiat. Res.*, 106: 234–251.

Overgaard, J., González González, D., Hulshof, M.C.C.M., Arcangeli, G., Dahl, O., Mella, O. and Bentzen, S.M. (1995) Randomised trial of hyperthermia as adjuvant to radiotherapy for recurrent or metastatic malignant melanoma. *Lancet*, 345: 540–543.

Overgaard, J., González González, D., Hulshof, M.C.C.M., Arcangeli, G., Dahl, O., Mella, O. and Bentzen, S.M. (1996) Hyperthermia as adjuvant to radiation therapy of recurrent or metastatic malignant melanoma. A multicentre randomized trial by the European Society for Hyperthermic Oncology. *Int. J. Hyperthermia*, 12: 3–20.

Roberts, D.W., Coughlin, C.T., Wong, T.Z., Ryan, T.P., Lyons, B.E., Douple, E.B. and Fratkin, J.D. (1986) Interstitial hyperthermia and iridium brachytherapy in the treatment of malignant glioma: a phase I clinical trial. *J. Neurosurg.*, 64: 581–587.

Roberts, D.W., Strohbehn, J.W., Coughlin, C.T., Ryan, T.P., Lyons, B.E., Douple, E.B. and Fratkin, J.D. (1989) Hyperthermia of brain tumor: The Dartmouth Experience. In: T.

Sugahara and M. Saito (Eds.), *Hyperthermic Oncology 1988*, Vol. 2. Taylor and Francis, London, pp. 476–479.

Salcman, M. and Samaras, G.M. (1983) Interstitial microwave hyperthermia for brain tumors: results of a phase I clinical trial. *J. Neuro-Oncol.*, 1: 225–236.

Samaras, G.M., Salcman, M., Cheung, A.Y., Abdo, H.S. and Schepp, R.S. (1982) Microwave-induced hyperthermia: An experimental adjunct for brain tumour therapy. *Natl. Cancer Inst. Monogr.*, 61: 477–482.

Sasaki, M. and Ide, C. (1989) Demyelination and remyelination in the dorsal funiculus of the rat spinal cord after heat injury. *J. Neurocytol.*, 18: 225–239.

Seegenschmiedt, M.H. and Feldmann, H.J. (1995) Clinical rationale for thermoradiotherapy. In: M.H. Seegenschmidt, P. Fessenden and C.C. Vernon (Eds.), *Thermoradiotherapy and Thermochemotherapy*, Vol. 2: Clinical Applications, Springer, Berlin, pp. 3–23.

Seegenschmiedt, M.H., Martus, P., Fietkau, R., Iro, H., Brady, L.W. and Sauer, R. (1994) Multivariate analysis of prognostic parameters using interstitial thermoradiotherapy (IHT-IRT): tumor and treatment variables predict outcome. *Int. J. Radiat. Oncol., Biol. Phys.*, 29: 1049–1063.

Seegenschmiedt, M.H., Klautke, G., Grabenbauer, G.G. and Sauer, R. (1995) Thermochemotherapy for malignant brain tumors: Review of biological and clinical studies. *Endocuritetherapy / Hyperthermia Oncol.*, 11: 201–221.

Silberman, A.W., Morgan, D.F., Storm, F.K., Rand, R.W., Bubbers, J.E., Brown, W.J. and Morton, D.L. (1982) Localized magnetic-loop induction hyperthermia of the rabbit brain. *J. Surg. Oncol.*, 20: 174–178.

Silberman, A.W., Rand, R.W., Krag, D.N., Storm, K., Benz, M., Drury, B. and Morton, D.L. (1986) Effect of localized magnetic-induction hyperthermia on the brain. *Cancer*, 57: 1401–1404.

Sminia, P., Haveman, J., Wondergem, J., Van Dijk, J.D.P. and Lebesque, J.V. (1987) Effects of 434 MHz microwave hyperthermia applied to the rat in the region of the cervical spinal cord. *Int. J. Hyperthermia*, 3: 441–452.

Sminia, P., Troost, D. and Haveman, J. (1989) Histopathological changes after 434 MHz microwave hyperthermia in the region of the rat cervical spinal cord. *Int. J. Hyperthermia*, 5: 85–98.

Sminia, P., Haveman, J., Van Dijk, J.D.P. and Hendriks, J.J.G.W. (1991) Enhancement by hyperthermia of the 'early delayed' and 'late delayed' radiation response of the rat cervical spinal cord. *Int. J. Radiat. Biol.*, 59: 259–271.

Sminia, P., Van der Zee, J., Wondergem, J. and Haveman, J. (1994) Effect of hyperthermia on the central nervous system: a review. *Int. J. Hyperthermia*, 10: 1–30.

Sminia, P., Hendriks, J.J.G.W., Van der Kracht, A.H.W., Rodermond, H.M., Haveman, J., Jansen, W., Koedooder, C. and Franken, N.A.P. (1995) Neurological observations after local irradiation and hyperthermia of rat lumbosacral spinal cord. *Int. J. Radiat. Oncol., Biol. Phys.*, 32: 165–174.

Sneed, P.K. and Stea, B. (1995) Thermoradiotherapy for brain tumors. In: M.H. Seegenschmidt, P. Fessenden and C.C. Vernon (Eds.), *Thermoradiotherapy and Thermochemotherapy*, Vol. 2: Clinical Applications, Springer, Berlin, pp. 159–173.

Sneed, P.K., Matsumoto, K., Stauffer, P.R., Fike, J.R., Smith, V. and Gutin, P.H. (1986) Interstitial microwave hyperthermia in a canine brain model. *Int. J. Radiat. Oncol. Biol., Phys.*, 12: 1887–1897.

Sneed, P.K., Gutin, P.H., Stauffer, P.R., Phillips, T.L., Prados, M.D., Weaver, K.A., Suen, S., Lamb, S.A., Ham, B., Ahn, D.K., Larson, D.A. and Wara, W.M. (1992) Thermoradiotherapy of recurrent malignant brain tumors. *Int. J. Radiat. Oncol. Biol. Phys.*, 23: 853–862.

Sneed, P.K., Larson, D.A. and Gutin, P.H. (1994) Brachytherapy and hyperthermia for malignant astrocytomas. *Semin. Oncol.*, 21: 186–197.

Stea, B., Rossman, K., Kittelson, J., Lulu, B., Shetter, A., Cassady, J.R. and Hamilton, A. (1994) A comparison of survival between radiosurgery and stereotactic implants for malignant astrocytomas. *Acta Neurochir.* (Suppl.) 62: 47–54.

Tanaka, R., Takahashi, H., Nakajima, T., Watanabe, M., Suda, T., Kaminuma, K. and Saito, A. (1989) Clinical trials of RF interstitial hyperthermia for malignant gliomas. In: T. Sugahara and M. Saito (Eds.), *Hyperthermic Oncology 1988*, Vol. 2, Taylor and Francis, London, pp. 158–160.

Winter, A., Laing, J., Paglione, R. and Sterzer, F. (1985) Microwave hyperthermia for brain tumors. *Neurosurgery*, 17: 387–399.

H.S. Sharma and J. Westman (Eds.)
Progress in Brain Research, Vol 115

CHAPTER 18

Pathophysiology of brain edema and cell changes following hyperthermic brain injury

Hari Shanker Sharma[1]*, Jan Westman[1] and Fred Nyberg[2]

[1]*Laboratory of Neuroanatomy, Department of Anatomy, Post Box 571, Biomedical Centre, Uppsala University, S-751 23 Uppsala, Sweden*
[2]*Department of Pharmaceutical Biosciences, Post Box 591, Division of Biological Research on Drug Dependence, Biomedical Centre, Uppsala University, S-751 24 Uppsala, Sweden*

Introduction

Brain edema is a serious complication of various neurological diseases following traumatic, ischemic or hypoxic injuries to the central nervous system (CNS) (Bakay and Lee, 1965; Klatzo and Seitelberger, 1967; Reulen and Kreysch, 1973; Cervós-Navarro and Ferszt, 1980; Reulen et al., 1990; Ito et al., 1994; James et al., 1997). If untreated, a progressive brain edema will lead to compression of cerebral compartment resulting in an increased intracranial pressure and brain tissue softening (Davson, 1967; Aukland, 1973; Cervós-Navarro and Ferszt, 1980; Go and Baethmann, 1984). Excessive swelling of the brain in a closed cranial compartment will result in depression of vital centres leading to death (Klatzo et al., 1958, 1965; Rapoport, 1976). So increased understanding of progression, persistence and resolution of brain edema is very important in order to develop suitable therapeutic measures for such a common and serious complication of brain disease occurring under a wide variety of noxious insults to the CNS.

Although much attention has been paid to the development of brain edema following traumatic or ischemic injuries (Mohanty et al., 1985, 1989; Dey and Sharma, 1983, 1984; Reulen et al., 1990; Sharma and Olsson, 1990; Sharma et al., 1992a; Ito et al., 1994; Sharma et al., 1995a,b, 1996a; James et al., 1997), edema formation following hyperthermic insults to the brain is a new subject and has not been well studied either in clinical or experimental conditions. Experimental research done in our labouratory during the past one and half decades strongly suggests that hyperthermic brain injury is associated with profound edema development and is a key factor in brain pathology (Sharma and Dey, 1978, 1984, 1986a, 1987; Sharma, 1982; Sharma et al., 1986, 1991a,b; Sharma and Cervós-Navarro, 1990a,b, 1991). This review is focused on brain edema formation in heat stress and its contribution to cell injury. In addition, the basic concepts of brain edema formation including various biomechanical, biophysical factors and chemical mediators involved in this mechanism are reviewed. Finally, based on our experimental observations a new pharmacological approach to reduce edema formation and cell injury by modifying the breakdown of the blood−brain barrier (BBB) in heat stress is discussed.

---

*Corresponding author. Tel: +46 18 4714433; fax: +46 18 243899; e-mail: Sharma@anatomi.uu.se

Basic concepts of edema formation

Edema is defined as an increase in the water content of the nervous system which can occur in specific brain regions following a focal or global cerebral insult (Klatzo, 1967, 1972, 1987; Cervós-Navarro and Ferszt, 1980; Go and Baethmann, 1984; Joó, 1987; Sharma et al., 1993a). In due course of time, the edema fluid will spread and depending on the magnitude and severity of the primary insult, whole brain can be swollen within 24–72 h (Bakay and Lee, 1965; Klatzo et al., 1965; Hirano, 1971; Cervós-Navarro and Ferszt, 1980). A swollen brain in the closed cranial compartment will result in compression of vital centres resulting in death (Cervós-Navarro and Ferszt, 1980; Reulen et al., 1990; Cervós-Navarro and Urich, 1995).

The early clinical symptoms of brain edema comprise signs of headache, nausea, vomiting, disturbances of consciousness, and occasionally coma (Reulen et al., 1990; Ito et al., 1994; Cervós-Navarro and Urich, 1995). The situation is often complicated by raised intracranial pressure and papilledema (Davson, 1967; Cervós-Navarro and Ferszt, 1980; Go and Baethmann, 1984). Progression of edema leads to brain herniation and vascular infarction that are common causes of death (Rapoport, 1976; Bradbury, 1979).

Types of brain edema

Brain edema is classified into two categories by Klatzo (1967) as 'vasogenic' and 'cytotoxic' in origin (Klatzo, 1967, 1972). Vasogenic brain edema formation appears mainly due to leakage of plasma proteins and water into the cerebral extracellular space due to traumatic or osmotic insults to the blood vessels, whereas cytotoxic edema is developed mainly due to intracellular accumulation of water caused by alterations in cell metabolism (Klatzo et al., 1965; Klatzo, 1987). Originally cytotoxic edema was thought to represent swelling of glial cells or astrocytes; however, recent findings demonstrate that water accumula-

tion can also occur within the neurons, glial cells and vascular endothelial cells.

With the development of new techniques and tracers to study the mechanisms of brain edema formation recent observations show that a considerable overlap exists between these two types of brain edema (Joó, 1987; Klatzo, 1987; Bradbury, 1992). Depending on the magnitude and primary nature of the insult, brain edema of both vasogenic and cytotoxic origin develops following noxious stimulus to brain by ischemia, hypoxia and trauma (Cervós-Navarro and Ferszt, 1980; Ito et al., 1994). Thus in vasogenic brain edema intracellular accumulation of water can also be seen before the BBB opening takes place (Rapoport, 1976; Reulen et al., 1990).

Disturbances in the osmotic balance between plasma and brain will lead to osmotic edema and interference with brain metabolism may result in metabolic edema (Rapoport, 1976). Traumatic edema develops following trauma to the brain or cerebral vessels (Pappius, 1970). In general, the BBB remains intact in osmotic and metabolic edema, whereas leakage of plasma proteins correlates well with the development of traumatic brain edema (Bakay and Lee, 1965).

Osmotic edema develops when plasma osmolality falls and water enters into the cerebral compartment resulting in swelling of the brain at the expense of CSF or blood volumes and the intracranial pressure rises (Rosomoff and Zugibe, 1963). In this condition, usually the cell membranes at both cerebrovascular endothelium and brain cells are intact (Rymer and Fishman, 1973). The inflow of water into brain dilutes Na^+ and K^+ concentrations per gram wet weight but changes on a dry weight basis are not significantly affected (Van Harreveld and Dubrovsky, 1967).

Inhibition of brain metabolism by pharmacological agents, freezing lesion of the brain or ischemia cause cell swelling and induce metabolic edema (Stern et al., 1949; Stern, 1959). In metabolic edema the cells and subcellular organelles including mitochondria swell mainly due to inhibition of the active transport mechanisms at their membrane sites (Leaf, 1973). Inhibition of Na$^+$ pump results in intracellular accumulation of Na$^+$ and loss of K$^+$. To accompany excess of intracellular Na$^+$, Cl$^-$ and water enter into the cells (Rapoport, 1976). Administration of cyanide causes gray and white matter edema by inhibiting oxidative enzymes and a reduction in the cerebral blood flow (Hirano et al., 1967; Hirano, 1971; Rapoport, 1976). Glial cells swell at the expense of extracellular space and the cortical conductivity is reduced (Baethmann and Van Harreveld, 1973). The water content is increased by more than 3% of the wet weight (Reulen and Kreysch, 1973). White matter edema is accompanied by axonal swelling and vesiculation of myelin (Hirano, 1971). The water filled vacuoles appear between myelin lamellae seen at the ultrastructural level (Hirano et al., 1967). However, the cerebrovascular permeability to trypan blue or ^{131}I-albumin is not compromised (Pappius, 1970).

Traumatic brain edema develops following trauma involving various complex processes both at cerebral capillaries and brain cells resulting in a progressive and irreversible pathological and metabolic change (Cervós-Navarro et al., 1988; Cervós-Navarro and Urich, 1995). In traumatic edema, vasogenic factors predominate in which cytotoxic factors contribute because of damage to cell membranes and cell metabolism (Klatzo, 1972). There are several models of traumatic brain edema in the literature (Cervós-Navarro and Ferszt, 1980; Go and Baethmann, 1984). However the best studied model of traumatic edema is a freezing lesion of the cerebral cortex in which a cold probe (about −50°C) is applied over the dura underlying the cerebral cortex for 30−50 s (Clasen et al., 1957, 1963; Klatzo et al., 1958, 1965).

In this freeze lesion model, cortical vessels are severely damaged and leakage of plasma proteins (mainly albumin and globulin) occurs progressively in the underlying white matter in the affected hemisphere and reaches its maximum level 24−48 h after the lesion and then decreases (Bakay, 1968; Rapoport, 1976). After 10 days the protein leakage is mainly absent (Klatzo et al., 1958). The magnitude and severity of leakage of

edema fluid following freeze lesion is however dependent on the initial level of blood pressure (Pappius, 1970). Thus, if the blood pressure is elevated by about 100 torr before the lesion, the extent of plasma protein leakage reaches its maximal level 4 h after the insult. It is interesting to note that similar edema is caused by brain tumours, infarction and physical trauma to the brain (Plum et al., 1963; Rapoport, 1976). Experimental observations on various types of brain insults suggest that edema formation appears mainly either due to damage of cells and their metabolism (cytotoxic type) or by opening of the BBB associated with leakage of proteins (vasogenic type) (Rapoport, 1976; Bradbury, 1979; Joó, 1987). These observations indicate that the basic mechanisms underlying edema formation following various insults to the brain may be quite similar in nature.

Biomechanics of brain edema formation

Brain edema formation can be understood in terms of basic principles of capillary filtration. Thus, Starling (1896) originally suggested that edema can occur in any tissue when the rate of capillary filtration exceeds the rate of fluid removal from the perivascular interstitium. Brain does not contain the lymphatic system like peripheral tissues where lymphatics remove the excess fluid (Davson, 1967). Thus the accumulated fluid from cerebral capillaries percolates through the cerebral compartment in order to reach CSF spaces (Davson, 1967).

The rate of capillary filtration and the driving force of water across the membrane or capillary wall is dependent on the hydrostatic and osmotic pressure differences between the vascular and cerebral compartments (Wiederhielm, 1968). Since cerebral capillaries are continuous due to the presence of tight junctions, their physical properties are very similar to that of an extended plasma membrane (Rapoport, 1976). The cerebral capillaries are almost completely impermeable to proteins, electrolytes and water soluble nonelectrolytes (Aukland, 1973). This property of cerebral endothelium creates an effective osmotic pressure between plasma and brain compartments which is equal to the total sum of contributions from salts, impermeable nonelectrolytes and proteins (Lieb and Stein, 1971). There is some evidence of slight differences in the capillary permeability at the arterial and venous ends (Aukland, 1973). The venous beds are comparatively more permeable than the arterial beds; however the details are not known about local differences in the osmotic and/or hydrostatic pressure gradients across the intracerebrovascular beds (Staub, 1974).

The protein osmotic pressure in brain is almost zero because CSF protein is negligible and the CSF osmolality due to non-protein solutes is very similar to plasma osmolality (Davson, 1967; Klatzo and Seitelberger, 1967; Rapoport, 1976). Thus the driving force for water permeability in brain is mainly dependent on capillary hydrostatic pressure and protein osmotic pressure (Staub, 1974; Rapoport, 1976). Edema develops when fluid accumulates in the brain resulting in an increase of brain volume. The rate of fluid accumulation depends on brain compliance which is usually very low (Miller, 1976). However, compliance in the brain is not constant and depends on local tissue pressure which may vary in different regions of the brain (Guyton, 1963).

Biophysical factors influencing brain edema formation

Various insults to the brain or cerebral vessels can influence the different factors controlling the biomechanics of brain edema formation and thereby can together or separately influence the final outcome following brain injury (Table 1) (Rapoport, 1976). Brain edema develops as a result of increased capillary infiltration and metabolic water production if that exceeds the rate of fluid loss from the brain (Starling, 1896; Rapoport, 1976). The spread of edema fluid and accumulation depends on tissue compliance and time period following the primary insult (Clasen et al., 1963). A defective autoregulation of cere-

bral blood flow (CBF) can allow an increase of hydrostatic pressure and breakdown of BBB permeability and thus induce brain edema formation (Rapoport, 1976; Bradbury, 1979; Cervós-Navarro and Ferszt, 1980). However, the exact relationship between capillary filtration, driving force of water due to osmotic or hydrostatic gradients, hydraulic conductivity and tissue compliance under various pathological conditions and their influence on brain edema formation is still unknown (Rapoport, 1976; Reulen et al., 1990).

Biochemical mediators of brain edema formation

Apart from these biophysical factors influencing brain edema, recently several endogenous biochemical mediators have been suggested to play an important role in brain edema formation (for review, see Wahl et al., 1988; Olesen, 1989). A summary of various chemical agents known as mediators of brain edema are listed in Table 2. This list is by no means complete and many new factors will be added in coming years due to rapid advancement of research in this field.

In general, the factors responsible for brain edema formation are also known mediators of the breakdown of BBB permeability (Wahl et al., 1988; Olesen, 1989; Bradbury, 1992; Couraud and Scherman, 1996). Thus it seems quite likely that these mediators influence brain edema formation probably via increasing the blood-brain transport of many solutes, ions and proteins resulting in alterations of osmotic gradient across the cerebrovascular compartment (Sharma et al., 1990, 1995c). This will result in water transport from the vascular to the cerebral compartment.

This effect of chemicals on the cerebral microvessels leading to the breakdown of BBB permeability and edema could be a direct effect of endothelial cells inducing signal transduction mechanisms coupled to neurochemical receptors, or through some indirect mechanisms (Sharma et al., 1990; Bradbury, 1992; Couraud and Scherman, 1996). Thus neurochemicals may have some effect on vasomotor tone of the microvessels causing severe dilatation or constriction (Rapo-

TABLE 1

Physical factors influencing biomechanics of brain edema formation

Factor	Effect	Brain edema	Mechanisms
Plasma osmotic pressure	Reduction in osmolality	Swelling	Altered osmotic gradient
	Chronic hypotonicity	Normal brain volume	Loss of K^+, other salts
Tissue osmotic pressure	Accumulation of tissue proteins, lactate, products of cell cytolysis	Swelling	Increased capillary infiltration
Capillary permeability	Disturbances in autoregulation of CBF, leakage of plasma proteins	Swelling	Increased hydraulic conductivity, altered osmotic gradient, increased capillary infiltration
Capillary hydrostatic pressure	Defective autoregulation of CBF, breakdown of BBB permeability		Hypertension
Tissue hydrostatic pressure	Increased	Counter-balance edema	Interstitial pressure altered
Tissue compliance	Higher in white matter Low in gray matter	Swelling Swelling	Less glycoprotein High glycoprotein for cell adhesion

CBF = cerebral blood flow, BBB = blood–brain barrier, compiled after Rapoport (1976).

port, 1976; Edvinsson and McKenzie, 1977; Bradbury, 1979). Depending on the magnitude and severity of these responses, the autoregulation of CBF will be perturbed (Rapoport, 1976; Bradbury, 1979; Johansson et al., 1990). Vasoconstriction of cerebral vessels will lead to ischemia and may influence cerebral energy metabolism resulting in failure of cellular or membrane oxidative metabolism causing cell swelling (Johansson et al., 1990; Bradbury, 1992). In the case of dilatation, increase in transmural pressure of the capillaries or tension across the cerebrovascular wall will initiate a series of events leading to the increased vesicular transport or widening of tight junctions resulting in a breakdown of BBB permeability (Rapoport, 1976; Johansson et al., 1990).

Alternatively, a direct effect of chemicals on cerebrovessels will induce a variety of cascades influencing the second messenger system within the endothelial cells leading to several intracellular mechanisms resulting in the increased transport of various molecules across the BBB (Jóo et al., 1975, 1985; Westergaard, 1980). One possible intracellular mechanism of tracer transport is related to the activation of cAMP by various hormonal messengers in the cerebromicrovessels and in choroid plexus. These chemical mediators (Table 2) are known to increase cAMP synthesis in the endothelial cells. An increased

TABLE 2

Neurochemical mediators of brain edema formation

Neurochemical	Thermoregulation	BBB permeability	Brain edema
Serotonin[a]	+ +	+ +	+ +
Prostaglandins[a]	+ + +	+ + +	+ + +
Arachidonic acid	+ +	+ + +	+ + +
Bradykinin[a]	+	+ +	+ +
Histamine[a]	+ / −	+ + +	+ +
Leukotrienes	−	+	+
Opioids[a]	+	+ / −	+ / −
Catecholamines	+ + +	+ +	+ +
Free radicals	−	+ +	+ +
Nitric oxide[a]	+ / −	+	+ / −

Compiled from various sources (Sharma, 1982; Sharma and Dey, 1986a, 1987; Wahl et al., 1988; Olesen, 1989; Sharma et al., 1992d, 1997b,c); + / − = further research is needed, + = involved, + + = well known, + + + = established, − = not known.
[a]Authors own investigation.

synthesis of cAMP will enhance transendothelial transport across the cerebral vessels (Baca and Palmer, 1978; Black, 1995). This hypothesis is supported by the fact that intra-arterial infusion of cAMP enhances vesicular transport in cerebrovessels seen ultrastructurally (Jóo et al., 1975).

Further evidence of a chemically-mediated permeability of the BBB via intracellular mechanisms came from the studies of Sharma and his co-workers who showed that in various stress conditions the increased permeability of the BBB is associated with abnormal accumulation of plasma serotonin (Sharma and Dey, 1981, 1984, 1986a,b, 1987, 1988; Sharma et al., 1990). This serotonin-induced breakdown of BBB permeability can be reduced not only by antiserotonergic drugs but also by drugs interfering with prostaglandin metabolism or vesicular transport (Sharma and Dey, 1986a,b, 1987, 1988; Sharma and Cervós-Navarro, 1990c; Sharma et al., 1990). Based on these studies Sharma and his group proposed the hypothesis that when serotonin binds to cerebrovascular receptors it will enhance prostaglandin synthesis within the endothelial cells (Sharma, 1982; Sharma and Dey, 1986a,b, 1987; Sharma et al., 1990, 1996b). An increased

prostaglandin biosynthesis is well known to enhance intracellular cAMP synthesis (Baca and Palmer, 1978). This increased cAMP synthesis somehow enhances vesicular transport across the cerebrovessels (Jóo, 1985). This hypothesis gets further support from studies using a vesicular transport inhibitor vinblastine (Sharma and Dey, 1984, 1986a,b, 1987, 1988). Thus vinblastine pretreatment also attenuated the breakdown of BBB permeability without affecting the serotonin level in stressed animals (Sharma and Dey, 1986a,b; Sharma et al., 1991a, 1996b, 1997a).

Recent reports show that nitric oxide (NO), a gaseous molecule which is involved in intracellular mechanisms of signal transduction, can influence BBB permeability and edema formation under pathological conditions (Chiueh et al., 1994; Sharma et al., 1996a, 1997b). This is evident from the fact that a breakdown of BBB permeability and edema caused by a focal spinal cord trauma is inhibited by application of antiserum to nitric oxide synthase (NOS), an enzyme responsible for conversion of NO from its precursor L-arginine (Chiueh et al., 1994; Sharma et al., 1996a). There are few NOS positive neurons present in the CNS (Chiueh et al., 1994; for a detail review see Chapter 16 in this volume). This observation indicates that NO is somehow involved in the breakdown of BBB permeability and edema formation (Sharma et al., 1996a, 1997b). The detailed mechanisms of NO-induced breakdown of BBB permeability and edema formation however require additional investigation.

Thus, it appears that the mechanisms underlying brain edema are rather complex and involve many biophysical and biochemical factors. A detailed understanding of these mechanisms is of vital importance in order to develop suitable therapeutic approaches. Further research in these lines is highly warranted in order to save the lives of victims following various kinds of brain insults.

Brain edema in pathological conditions

Brain edema either produced by brain tumours, infarction, ischemia, disturbances of cerebral autoregulation, metabolic disturbances of brain, infections of the CNS due to viruses and bacteria, autoimmune diseases, hypertensive encephalopathy, traumatic injuries to the CNS, hypoxia, hyperoxia, hypercapnia, concussion, raised intracranial pressure, or hydrocephalus, etc., exhibits pathophysiology of cell injury and edematous swelling in the perifocal regions which is quite similar in nature (Rapoport, 1976; Cervós-Navarro and Ferszt, 1980; Dey and Sharma, 1983, 1984; Go and Baethmann, 1984; Mohanty et al., 1985, 1989; Reulen et al., 1990; Sharma and Olsson, 1990; Sharma et al., 1992a, 1993a,b, 1995a,b,d, 1996a; Ito et al., 1994; James et al., 1997). The spread of edema fluid and leakage of plasma proteins will progress with time as mentioned above. The magnitude and severity of edematous swelling and concurrently brain damage depends on the intensity and duration of the primary insult (Rapoport, 1976; Bradbury, 1979).

Brain edema in hyperthermic brain injury

Though the incidence of hyperthermic brain da-

mage and death due to heat stroke has been known since Biblical times (McKendrick, 1868; Messiter, 1897; Aron, 1911; Weisenburg, 1912; Gauss and Meyer, 1917; McKenzie and LeCount, 1918; Wilcox, 1920; Adolph and Fulton, 1924; Hall and Wakefield, 1927; Marsh, 1930; Hartman and Major, 1935; Weiner, 1938; Freeman and Dumoff, 1944; Malamud et al., 1946; Schickele, 1946; for review, see Knochel, 1974; Sterner, 1990), the pathophysiology of cell injury and edema in hyperthermic brain insult has not yet been investigated in details. Thus the mechanism of edema formation following heat injury are largely unknown.

There are only a few clinical studies and experimental findings reported in the past which suggest that cell reaction in the brain and edema formation will occur in hyperthermic brain injuries (Malamud et al., 1946; Sminia et al., 1994). However, no definite conclusions can be drawn from these studies because they are not comparable.

Clinical hyperthermia

The scientific literature on pathological findings in the CNS following heat illness is very limited (Table 3) (Malamud et al., 1946; Austin and Berry, 1956; Brahams, 1989; Hart et al., 1982). There are only a few sporadic case reports in the past showing brain pathology at the light microscopic level in the victims of heat stroke who died at various time intervals ranging from 6 h to several weeks after heat illness (Malamud et al., 1946; Austin and Berry, 1956). Most of the cases describe changes in the cerebral cortex and cerebellum but other brain regions were not examined systematically. Thus the understanding of pathological anatomy of the nervous system and a selective vulnerability of the CNS, if any, following heat illness is not clear from these studies.

These reports are based on either Cresyl violet staining or occasionally Haemotoxylin and Eosin staining of the paraffin embedded brain specimens and no special immunostaining was applied to identify glial cells or myelin damage. More-

TABLE 3

Effect of heat on central nervous system damage in clinical cases

Duration of heat illness	Brain region	Cell damage		
		Nerve cells	Glial cells	Myelin
11 h	Cerebral cortex	Edema congestion disintegration	Not known	Not known
18 h		Shrunken hyperchromatic		
276 h		Degeneration	Proliferation of microglia and astrocytes	
4 d		Haemorrhages in white matter		
5 h	Cerebellum	Purkinje cells swollen, disintegrated	Proliferation of oligodendrocytes	
5.5 h		Edema, swollen and loss of Purkinje cells		
72 h		Purkinje cells completely disappeared	Glial proliferation	
276 h		Loss of Purkinje cells granular cell layer	Glial proliferation	
		Degeneration of Purkinje cells	Phagocytosis by glial cells	
11 h	Dentate nucleus	Hyperchromatic, capillary engorgement		
276 h		Few shrunken neurons	Extensive gliosis	
276 h	Thalamus	Neuronal loss	Proliferation of glia	
4 h	Hypothalamus	Microhaemorrhages only in PVN		
8 h		No significant change		
130 h		No significant change		
14 h		No significant change		
5 h	Midbrain	Microhaemorrhages in the floor of IV ventricle, PAG, OM		

These pathological observations are based on light microscopy using Crersyl violet stain or Haemotoxylin and Eosin staining. No immunohistochemistry was applied and ultrastructural investigations were not done; compiled after Malamud et al. (1946); PAG = periaqueductal grey matter, PVN = paraventricular nucleus, OM = occulomotor nucleus, h = hours, d = days.

over, on these materials no electron microscopy was performed. Thus the detailed ultrastructural changes and damage of the fine structures of the nervous system following heat injury are still unknown.

Knowledge accumulated by these investigations suggests that the cerebral cortex and cerebellum are the most susceptible organs of the brain following heat damage. No published report examined e.g. hippocampus in heat illness (Malamud et al., 1946). In some cases thalamus was also found to be affected but a possible involvement of hypothalamus and brain stem in heat illness was not very clear from these studies.

Thus, the information on pathological anatomy of the CNS following heat damage is rudimentary and further studies using modern techniques to examine brain pathology are urgently needed.

Brain edema in clinical heat illness

Although edema is the most prominent feature of hyperthermic brain injury, little emphasis is given in these case reports to the significance of edema in underlying cell changes of the nervous system. A flattening of convolutions and a cerebellar pressure cone along with softening of the brain tissue are the prominent features of brain edema that can be well recognised in the brains of these victims (cf. Malamud et al., 1946; Austin and Berry, 1956). But these findings have largely been ignored.

In a few cases, brain weight was recorded and found to have increased by several hundred grams (Malamud et al., 1946). These observations strongly indicate that edema was a common manifestation of brain disease in patients who died from heat illness. Edema of the leptomeninges was also prominent in many cases.

Edema and congestion in the cerebral cortex with signs of degenerative changes in the neurons are very common in these histopathological studies (Morgan and Vonderahe, 1939; Malamud et al., 1946). Most of the nerve cells and their dendrites were swollen. The nerve cells often contain pyknotic nucleoli and the chromatolysis of cytoplasm and vacuolation is quite common (Malamud et al., 1946).

Pathological changes in the human brain

The following description is based on various case reports dealing with brain pathology in heat illness (Malamud et al., 1946; Austin and Berry, 1956; for review see Knochel, 1974; Sterner, 1990). It appears that post-mortem autolysis does not play any significant role in these findings because similar changes were observed in different cases 6–15 h after the death of the victims.

Cerebral cortex. In the cerebral cortex, edema, congestion and degenerative changes in the neu-

rons were quite prominent in some sections of the frontal cortex seen 11 h after heat injury. At this time, the nerve cells and their dendrites were swollen. The nucleus showed disintegration and chromatolysis. However, glial reaction was not evident at this time. After 18 h of heat injury in another case, the neurons had shrunk and the cytoplasm and nuclei were hyperchromatic. Pericellular edema was prominent but gliosis was still not apparent. Glial cells appeared to proliferate in the cases of 24 h heat injury and onwards. At this time, severe neuronal loss was seen.

These nerve and glial cell changes were more pronounced with further increase in the duration of heat illness. Thus, in cases of 6 and 12 days of heat illness, the neuronal loss was most severe and the glial proliferation was quite distinct. Microglial activation and an increase in their number were quite clear. These changes were most prominent in the upper layers of the cerebral cortex compared to the lower layers. Damage of the white matter and signs of demyelination or vesiculation of myelin were mainly absent. Increased lipid content in nerve cells and occasionally in the perivascular space is quite common.

Basal ganglia. Changes in basal ganglia are less severe than the cortex. Thus the corpus striatum and thalamus were not so much affected by heat injury. In short periods of heat illness, only a few nerve cells in the caudate nucleus and putamen were diffusely damaged. In longer durations of heat illness many degenerating neurons were present. In thalamus, focal collection of glia was seen and proliferation of microglia around the nerve cell was quite common. It is interesting to note that the globus pallidus was the least affected region of the brain in these cases and the periventricular system was devoid of glial proliferation.

Cerebellum. Pathological changes in the cerebellum of heat-injured victims were most prominent irrespective of the duration of heat injury. Thus within 24 h of heat injury, edema of the Purkinje cell layer was most marked and the number of

Purkinje cells were considerably reduced. Interestingly, the molecular and granular layers of the cerebellum were not affected except for some minor proliferation of the satellite oligodendroglia.

Twenty-four hours after heat illness, the Purkinje cell layer had almost completely disappeared and glial reactions were more prominent at this time particularly in the Bergmann layer followed by the molecular layer. These glial changes were progressive in nature and the Purkinje cell necrosis was quite common after 3 days of heat illness. In cases of heat illness for 12 days, hyperplastic changes were apparent in molecular and Bergmann layers and the few remaining Purkinje cells were almost consumed by macrophages. These changes in the cerebellum were found in both the cerebellar hemispheres as well as in the vermis. The dentate nucleus was the other structure sensitive to heat damage in the cerebellum which showed signs of degeneration of nerve cells and hyperchromatic reactions 12 h after heat illness. In the case of 12 days of heat injury, this nucleus was hard to identify because almost all nerve cells were replaced by proliferating microglia.

Hypothalamus. Hypothalamus is the main seat of thermoregulation (Alpers, 1936; Davison, 1940; Zimmerman, 1940), thus great attention has been paid to study this structure in heat-injured brains. Pathological findings in short durations of heat illness revealed a mild to moderate degree of edema of the hypothalamic nuclei but no further changes were seen in the hypothalamus except a mild loss of neurons and a slight increase in the number of glial cells. However, cases with longer duration of heat illness also showed similar changes.

Midbrain, pons, medulla oblongata and spinal cord. Only a few, mild changes in the nerve cells and a slight increase in the number of glial cells were observed in the quadrigeminal region, the inferior olivery nuclei and the reticular formation. No distinct cell changes or edema were seen in other parts of these structures.

Brain haemorrhages. Interestingly, microhaemorrhages in leptomeninges and in many brain regions were common in heat injury. The microhaemorrhages in brain were mainly confined to the perivascular space. The leptomeningeal haemorrhages were most diffuse and most severe particularly in short durations of heat illness. The regional distribution of haemorrhage varied in location but the most pronounced haemorrhage can be seen in the periventricular system particularly in the paraventricular nucleus, the supraoptic nucleus, medial parts of the ventromedial and dorsomedial hypothalamic nuclei and less frequently in the perifornical and septal regions and the medial portion of the thalamus. The caudal part of the hypothalamus was least affected. No haemorrhages were observed in the mamillary body. Haemorrhages of the pons and medulla oblongata were seen which were mainly confined to the floor of the fourth ventricle and sometimes near the dorsal efferent nucleus of the vagus.

Mechanisms of brain damage in hyperthermia

No comprehensive explanation for damaged nerve cells following hyperthermia has been offered to date and the basic mechanisms of cell injury in the brain following heat stress is still speculative. The disturbed brain function and hemiplegia in heat-injured victims was mainly supposed to be due to brain haemorrhages. Thus most emphasis in the literature was placed on brain haemorrhage which can result from hyperthermia. Hyperthermia can induce clot formation due to thrombocytopaenia seen in many cases and the presence of haemorrhages in vital organs could be the cause of death (Adolph and Fulton, 1924; Wilson and Doan, 1939; Wilson, 1940).

Emphasis was also given to nerve cell changes, however, some authors believed that this could be due to post-mortem artefacts. Since changes in nerve cells can be followed by mild to moderate or extensive cell loss and proliferation of glia were observed with prolonged illness, many authors ruled out the possibility of post-mortem artefacts. Malamud et al. (1946) who reported the most extensive brain damage in 125 cases following heat stress believed that these nerve cell changes were real and could be due to hyperthermia, whereas haemorrhages, congestion and edema could be a secondary phenomenon of heat shock. However, there was no direct correlation between hyperthermia and damage of nerve cells in many clinical cases. Edema, congestion and haemorrhages were not consistent with the degree of hyperthermia. In these cases a direct relation between the severity of haemorrhage and the degree of shock was absent. The magnitude of shock correlated well with the lowering of blood pressure; however, the hypothesis that hyperthermia is one of the causes of shock in thermal brain injury requires additional investigation.

Some authors believe that anoxia as evident from a reduction in partial oxygen pressure in the blood can contribute to the shock phase that occurs following heat stress (Blum, 1945). But this is still controversial because the findings are not consistent.

Thus there are two major opinions to explain brain damage following heat injury. According to one concept, the external environmental temperature and resulting hyperthermia can induce shock causing damage to the brain (Kopp and Solomon, 1937; Cournand et al., 1943; Wallace, 1943), whereas some authors believed that circulatory collapse followed by insufficient blood supply to the brain is the main cause of ischemia and brain damage (Marsh, 1930; Heilman and Montgomery, 1936; Chakravarti and Tyagi, 1938). It is interesting to note that the problem of breakdown of the BBB and brain edema as a major cause of cell injury is not discussed. The probable cause of microhaemorrhage is also not described. A direct effect of heat on the CNS damage was not mentioned because of the negative findings in the hypothalamus of the victims of heat injury (Morgan and Vonderahe, 1939; Zimmerman, 1940). Thus, the mechanisms behind brain damage in heat stress are still speculative.

Experimental hyperthermia

From the previous discussion on brain damage in clinical condition it appears that hyperthermia can induce cell changes in the brain (Adolph, 1947; Britt et al., 1983; Sminia et al., 1994). However, apart from heat stroke, hyperthermia is a common problem in many other clinical conditions like fever, infection and cancer therapy (Harris et al., 1962; Hahn, 1982; Sminia et al., 1994). Thus, hyperthermia is quite common following radiotherapy of tumours and a local increase in tissue temperature is one of the primary causes of abnormal cell reaction in the brain during this treatment. In order to understand the detailed mechanisms of this phenomena, various animal models using direct heat exposure of various brain regions were developed (for review see Sminia and Huschlof, this volume).

In brief, most of the experiments were performed to study the effects of localised brain heating produced either by microwave energy, radiofrequency or water bath application (cf. Hahn, 1982). These experiments were designed to understand the effects of local brain heating in order to simulate the clinical conditions of patients given radiotherapy for brain tumours. However, in these experiments, histopathology of the CNS was not well studied. In most cases, the pathological examination was conducted 4 h to 30 days after initial thermal insults (Table 4). Thus it is not clear from these studies whether hyperthermia can induce cell changes in the brain after short- or long-term heat exposure (Table 4).

The main drawback of this kind of investigation is that either the whole brain or a part of it was heated at a very high temperature for long periods which are usually beyond the physiological range (Milton, 1994; Zeisburger et al., 1994). In addition, the magnitude and severity of heating in one experiment is not comparable to the other study and in various animal experiments different brain regions were heated (for review see Sminia et al., 1994). Thus carefully controlled experi-

TABLE 4

Effect of heat on CNS damage in laboratory animals

Species	Exposure T°C	Tissue exposed	Duration (min)	Pathological findings
Dog	42–46[e]	Cerebral hemisphere	30	Edema, haemorrhages
	42–43.5[a]	Occipital cortex	50–70	Gray and white matter damage
	43–44[a]	Cerebral hemisphere	30	Necrosis, inflammation
	40–44[a]	Frontal cortex, cerebral hemisphere	30	Necrosis, gliosis, fibrosis
Cat	45[a]	Forebrain	30	No change
	42–48[c]	Occipital cortex	50	Gray and white matter damage
	41–48[c]	Occipital cortex	50	Necrosis, inflammation
Mouse	42[d]	Spinal cord	60	Not known
	41.2–45.2[b]	Spinal cord	60	Not known
	42–43.5[d]	Spinal cord	20–100	Neuronal and vascular damage, demyelination
Rat	41.2–43.2[a]	Spinal cord	30–120	Neuronal damage, white matter necrosis, gliosis
	43.4–46[b]	Spinal cord	15–30	Not known
	42.6–43.8[a]	Spinal cord	60	Not known
Rabbit	42–43[b]	Whole brain	60	No change
	45[b]		Few	Not known

These observations are based on a very crude pathological examination done from 4–24 h, 3, 7, 14 and 28 days after thermal insults. In some cases, details of pathological examination are not available; compiled after Sminia et al. (1994).

[a] Microwave.
[b] Radiofrequency.
[c] Ultrasound.
[d] Water bath.
[e] Warm blood infusion.

ments of local or regional brain heating within the physiological range and histopathological examination of the CNS using modern techniques are urgently needed to improve our understanding of this subject.

Effect of local hyperthermia on the CNS

There are only a few reports indicating that either local or regional heating of brain can induce edema and cell changes. However pathological findings in these investigations are not well characterised. In some cases haemorrhages, necrosis, inflammation and gliosis are described. In these experiments, lethality after hyperthermic insults to the brain was very common; however, the real cause of such phenomena is not known. There are reasons to believe that hyperthermia *per se* can induce such lethality although this issue is still controversial.

Experimental studies in dogs have demonstrated that thermal damage of the brain occurs after exposure of occipital cortex to 42–43.5°C for 50–70 min (Table 4). Cerebral edema and pyknotic cortical neurons were found after heating of the cortex at 42.5°C and at 43°C, neuronal cell lysis and disruption of myelin sheath in the white matter was noted. Exposure of microwave hyperthermia to dog brain tissue at 43–44°C for 30 min resulted in edematous swelling after 1 week of heat treatment. Sixteen weeks after thermal challenge, focal lesions containing central coagulation, necrosis and neovascularisation were apparent within the lesion. These changes were mainly confined within the exposure zone and were sometimes found in the perifocal regions (Harris et al., 1962; Sneed et al., 1986, 1991; Fike et al., 1991).

Heating at 41–41.5°C for 50 min is the threshold temperature required to induce the pathological changes in the cat brain. After this temperature, heat-induced cell damage was irreversible. Thus, microwave heating of cat brain at 45°C for 30 min did not show any signs of histopathology immediately. However, thermally damaged nerve cells can be seen 56 days after heat injury. On the other hand, heating of cat brain at 42°C for 50 min resulted in profound histopathological changes. Thus, 1–3 days after the insult, extensive coagulation necrosis and pyknosis of nerve cells in the gray matter, edema and vacuolation in the white matter along with polymorphonuclear leukocyte infiltration were quite common. Four to 21 days after the lesion, appearance of lipid-laden macrophages, liquefaction of the necrotic regions, fibroblastic proliferation, vascular proliferation with infiltration of perivascular lymphocytes can be seen. In the chronic stage (22–56 days after the lesion) fibrosis was seen with reticulin and collagen formation, and gliosis with proliferation of astrocytes and fluid filled necrotic centres were quite common. Since no lethality or other complications in these cat experiments were found after 56 days of heat treatment, it was concluded that heating of small volume of the brain is not responsible for alterations in vital functions (Samaras et al., 1982; Ryan, 1982; Britt et al., 1983; Lyons et al., 1986).

Studies on local heating of rodent brain showed profound neurological changes; however, histopathological data are not available in all these studies (cf. Sminia et al., 1994). Non-invasive electromagnetic heating of rabbit whole brain at 42–43°C for 60 min did not result in apparent histopathological damage or clinical symptoms, whereas, all animals died within minutes after heating the brain at a temperature of 45°C. Sminia and his group heated rat spinal cord by a double ring applicator placed on the cervical part of the vertebral column using microwave energy at 42.9°C for 38 min (Sminia et al., 1989). This resulted in histopathological changes after 4 h. Thus neurons in the gray matter showed mild damage and vacuolisation appeared in the white matter. Some animals were paralysed and in these animals neuronal degeneration, myelin damage and sometimes haemorrhagic foci in the white and gray matter were present. Gliosis, invasion of macrophages and lymphocyte were present after 3–14 days of thermal challenge. Some animals that recovered from neurological deficit after 28 days of heat treatment also showed demyelination in the spinal cord (cf. Sminia et al., 1994).

These observations of Sminia et al., were further extended by Sasaki and Ide (1989) who heated 1 mm^3 of the spinal cord dorsal white matter using water circulating tubes. Circulation of water at temperatures of 48–50°C for 1 h resulted in no neurological deficits. However ultrastructural studies showed profound myelin damage but no damage of the axons. Remyelination was observed 1 month after the heat treatment. This study suggests that heat treatment of small amounts of dorsal white matter is not associated with functional impairment and can be repaired within 1 month. However, other reports suggest that heating of thoracic vertebra at 44.2°C for 30 min will result in crawling with mild difficulties in all the animals.

Heating of mouse thoracolumbar spinal cord using water bath (42–43°C) for 80–160 min resulted in paralysis of animals. Most animals died within a few days. The survivors recovered within 1 month. Histopathological studies done only in a very few animals with paralysis showed neuronal injury, demyelination and vascular damage. These observations showed no difference in the heat sensitivity of the rat or mouse spinal cord in relation to cell changes or neurological damage (Goffinet et al., 1977; Lo, 1989; Froese et al., 1991).

Local heat treatment of CNS tumours in humans

Regarding the effect of local hyperthermia in human CNS, very little is known. Several studies were done to heat the CNS tumours using a 2450 MHz microwave antenna. In patients an antenna temperature of up to 45°C placed on the tumour appeared safe but heating of peritumoral brain regions was found to be unsafe. A tumour temperature of 42.5°C for 1 h was not found to be associated with any adverse effect; however, during this procedure normal tissue temperature was not measured (Winter et al., 1985). In a separate study by Tanaka et al. (1987) in which the tumour tissue was heated to 44–49°C, the normal tissue temperature did not exceed 38–40°C. In this study, the heat treatment resulted in aggravation of peritumoral edema and a focal brain swelling. In contrast to this study, deep heating was applied in many patients without apparent heat neurotoxicity (Petrovich et al., 1989).

One possibility why heat toxicity did not develop in these studies is that most of the experiments were conducted under anaesthesia. Thus, the passive heating of brain may be an entirely different phenomena rather than the stress associated with heating. It is important to note that most of the anaesthetics used in these investigations like pentobarbital and ketamine are known neuroprotective agents following various forms of ischemic or metabolic insults to the nervous system (Salzman, 1990). However, to get further clarification of the effects of anaesthetics on brain dysfunction following hyperthermia additional work is required.

Effect of whole body hyperthermia on the CNS

The potential benefit of whole body hyperthermia for tumour patients is that a uniform temperature of tumour tissue can be achieved. However, a disadvantage in this procedure is that heating of all the tissues including CNS will result in adverse effects. Therefore, only a few experimental studies have been directed to examining the histopathology of brain in whole body hyperthermia (for review, see Sminia et al., 1994).

Many workers did not observe heat toxicity in the brain after whole body hyperthermia although the treatment caused lethality (Thrall et al., 1992; for review see Sminia et al., 1994). Based on these observations it has been suggested that CNS is not an organ at risk after whole body hyperthermia. However electrophysiological studies showed profound alteration in brain electrical activity after whole body heating (Britt et al., 1984). This observation indicates that CNS is somehow influenced by whole body hyperthermia. Several reports suggest that the rise in brain temperature is not uniform after whole body heating, however, rectal temperature closely reflects the brain temperature in many cases (Dickson et al., 1979; Macy et al., 1985). Thus when a probe is deeply inserted into the rectum, no difference in brain or rectal temperature was noted following whole body hyperthermia in dogs and pigs (Dickson et al., 1979; Macy et al., 1985). In another study, dogs with brain tumours were exposed to 42°C for 60 min and it was found that the liver and brain temperatures were only 0.1° and 0.2° higher than the rectal temperature. Since histopathological studies in the CNS were not done after whole body heating, the subject of heat-induced brain damage still remains controversial.

Animal experiments

Dogs exposed to 60°C hot air in a cabin for 2 h showed no signs of edema as seen by changes in epidural pressure recordings. The rectal temperature in these dogs reached 42.5°C which is very close to the brain temperature. In this study histopathological studies show a generalised dilatation of the subarachnoid space in three out of four dogs but further details about brain damage was not examined. Based on these observations it is concluded that exposure of animals to whole body hyperthermia does not induce brain edema and cell changes (Eshel et al., 1990).

On the other hand, several studies on spontaneous electrical activity or the auditory brain stem evoked potentials in rats and cats suggest that the electrical activity is greatly affected after whole body hyperthermia. A significant reduction to complete flattening of the amplitude was seen in these experiments which correspond well with the observed rise in brain temperature. In rats a rise of rectal temperature from 36.75 to 42.65°C after whole body hyperthermia corresponded to a rise in brain stem temperature from 35.25 to 41.5°C. This heat treatment resulted in a marked reduction of the amplitude and increase in the latency of auditory brain stem evoked potentials. These observations clearly demonstrate that whole body hyperthermia significantly affects brain function (Bulochnik and Zyablov, 1978; Marsh et al., 1984).

In cats, elevation of cortical temperature by whole body hyperthermia up to 44–45°C caused different responses of electrical activity in different regions after cortical stimulation (Britt et al., 1984). On the basis of these observations it is concluded that the thermal sensitivity of the cortical cells is different in hyperthermia. In dogs microwave heating with 106.5 MHz for 60 min resulted in a left cardiac ventricle temperature of 42°C and the lumbar spinal canal temperature reached between 42.5° and 43°C. In these dogs, pelvic limb dysfunction was noted 12–24 h after hyperthermia and histopathological examination revealed severe haemorrhage and edema in the lumbar spinal cord (Eshel et al., 1990). It is interesting to note that in all these investigations the state of the BBB, CBF or edema was not examined. Thus the impact of hyperthermia on these important aspects of brain dysfunction is still lacking.

Clinical observations

Observations on whole body hyperthermia on human CNS are very rare. Mellergård and Nordström (1990) studied the brain temperature in neurosurgical patients having brain tumour during systemic hyperthermia. Their observation for 1–5 days showed that rectal temperature adequately reflects the epidural space temperature which is very similar to that of tympanic membrane temperature. However, in these reports biopsy findings or study of other brain functions like CBF or intracranial pressure following systemic hyperthermia are not available. Thus the effects of human whole body hyperthermia on brain function is not well known (Van der Zee, 1987). Several clinical investigations on traumatised brain patients showed that if systemic hyperthermia or brain temperature exceeds 39°C, the neurological outcome is worsened. However, the mechanisms behind such phenomenon are still unknown.

Our investigations of whole body hyperthermia in rats on brain dysfunction

Studies carried out in our labouratory during the last two decades show that the CNS is highly vulnerable to systemic hyperthermia induced by whole body heating of conscious animals (Sharma, 1982; Sharma and Dey, 1978, 1981, 1984, 1986a,b, 1987; Sharma et al., 1986, 1991a,b,c, 1992a,b,c,d,e, 1994a,b,c,d, 1996b, 1997a,b,c; Sharma and Cervós-Navarro, 1990a,b,c, 1991). Our observations further suggest that damage of CNS depends on the magnitude and severity of heat exposure, the amount of thermal load and the physiological states of animals prior to heat exposure (Sharma et al., 1991c, 1992e, 1994c).

We feel that stress caused by hyperthermia influences brain function by modifying the permeability of the BBB which is mediated by several neurochemicals (Sharma, 1982; Sharma and Dey, 1986a, 1987; Sharma et al., 1992c,d,g, 1994a,b, 1995e, 1996c, 1997a,b,c). An increased permeability of the BBB is responsible for vasogenic edema formation and cell injury (Sharma and Cervós-Navarro, 1990a,c; Sharma et al., 1992a,b,c,d).

Studies carried out by Sharma and his group for the first time showed that exposure of rats to summer heat or acute heat exposure in a biological oxygen demand (BOD) incubator is associated with increased permeability of the BBB in specific brain regions (Sharma and Dey, 1978; Sharma, 1982). Further studies carried out by Sharma and his co-workers demonstrated that BBB permeability is mediated by several neurochemical mediators and plays an instrumental role in brain edema formation and cell injury (Sharma and Dey, 1984, 1986a, 1987; Sharma and Cervós-Navarro, 1990a,b,c; Sharma et al., 1991a,b).

The rat model

Animal models of heat exposure to study pathophysiology of brain dysfunction were not well characterised in the past (Hall and Wakefield, 1927; Morgan, 1938; Weiner, 1938; Wilson and Doan, 1939; Adolph, 1947; for review see Selye, 1976; Haubbard et al., 1977; Bulochnik and Zyablov, 1978; Britt et al., 1984). Various workers used exposure temperatures varied from 32 to 46°C for a period of 30 min to 8 h in acute experiments and several days at 30–34°C for chronic studies. In some models, animals were exposed to extremely high temperature (usually 41–44°C) until they develop neurological symptoms of acute heat stroke. In these models the death rate is very high (more than 80%), thus study of brain dysfunction *in situ* is not possible (for review see Lee, 1964).

Keeping this in mind, we worked out a model situation in which animals develop symptoms of heat illness without heat stroke (Sharma and Dey, 1978, 1984, 1986a, 1987; Sharma, 1982). In this model, rats are exposed to heat at 38°C in a biological oxygen demand (BOD) incubator for 4 h. The relative humidity (45–50%) and wind velocity (20–25 cm/s) is kept constant (Sharma, 1982) (Table 5). This experimental set up resulted in stress symptoms and physiological variables (Table 6) very close to those in a clinical situation. However, exposure of rats to either 30° or 34°C in the BOD incubator resulted in only mild hyperthermia (Fig. 1) and minor stress symptoms. Our model is based on physiological aspects of noxious heat stimulus and is not associated with skin injury and has significantly less mortality (less than 20%, if any). The amount of thermal load imposed on animals in this model is shown in Table 5.

Validity of the model

Exposure of rats to 38°C for 4 h simulates a clinical situation of heat illness. This is evident from the development of stress symptoms and behavioural parameters in these rats (Table 6). The rise in body temperature in these rats following 1 h, 2 h or 4 h heat stress is linear (Fig. 1). Likewise exposure of rats to a mild thermal heat load, i.e. 30° or 34°C for 4 h also exhibited mild hyperthermia (Fig. 1). These observations indicate that the model can be used to induce a graded heat load in conscious rats as well (Sharma et al., 1986).

At the end of the 4 h heat exposure at 38°C, some rats lay prostrate in cages and did not move even after gentle pushing (Sharma and Dey, 1978; Sharma, 1982). However, these rats did not lose their righting reflex (Sharma, 1982). Some rats whose body temperature exceeded 42°C died either during or a few min after termination of heat exposure (Sharma, 1982; Sharma et al., 1986).

TABLE 5

Heat stress model in rat

Skin (T°C, T_s)	Exposure (T°C, T_e)	Heat load (°C $T_s - T_e$)	Rel. humidity (%)	Wind vel. (cm/s)	Exposure duration (h)
24–26	36–38	12–14	47–50	24–26	1–4 (acute)[a]
24–26	34–36	10–12	45–47	20–24	8–9 (1 week)[b]

After Sharma and Dey (1978) and Sharma (1982).
[a] Exposed in a biological oxygen demand (BOD) incubator.
[b] Kept at laboratory room temperature.

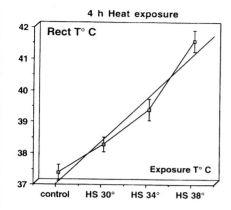

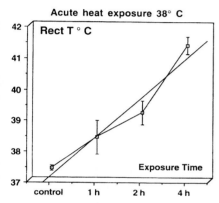

Fig. 1. Rectal temperature of control, 1 h, 2 h and 4 h heat-stressed rats exposed at 38°C (lower panel) or rats exposed for 4 h heat stress at 30°C, 34°C or 38°C (upper panel). Each point represents mean ± standard deviation of 6–12 rats. The straight line represents the mathematical curve fit superimposed on the actual data (StatView II™, Abacus Concepts Inc, USA). Rats were subjected to heat stress in a BOD incubator (for details see text). Animals kept at normal room temperature served as controls (data modified after Sharma, 1982).

The detailed mechanisms of heat-induced death is not clear (Sharma and Dey, 1984; Sharma et al., 1986). In few animals which survived 5–10 min after heat exposure, we measured physiological variables, BBB permeability and brain edema (Sharma et al., 1986). The results of such an investigation show that most of the dying rats have a low mean arterial blood pressure (MABP, 60–65 torr) very close to or below the critical lower limit of the cerebral autoregulation. This indicates that these rats developed brain ischemia due to poor brain perfusion as a result of defective autoregulation of the CBF (Rapoport, 1976). In these rats postmortem studies showed fluidity of all the cerebral components (Sharma et al., 1986; Dey et al., 1988). Measurement of BBB showed a greater degree of Evans blue extravasation and edema development was much more pronounced compared to those rats who survived after heat exposure (Sharma, 1982; Sharma et al., 1986; Dey et al., 1988, 1993). Damage of vital centres due to volume swelling of the brain in a closed cranial compartment is the main cause of death (Sharma et al., 1986).

Obviously, this model can be used to study brain pathology in heat stress and to explore new strategies of various therapeutic measures to achieve neuroprotection.

Effect of heat stress on brain dysfunction

Using our model, we studied the influence of both summer heat (Sharma and Dey, 1984, 1986a) and experimental heat exposure (Sharma and Dey, 1984, 1986a, 1987) on various parameters of brain dysfunction. The salient findings are described below.

Chronic summer heat exposure

During late May and throughout June, in many tropical countries and in northern parts of India the uncontrolled room air temperature gradually reaches to 34–36°C. In order to simulate chronic summer heat conditions, animals were exposed to this ambient air temperature of Varanasi (relative humidity 50–55%, wind velocity 24.5 cm/s) from 08:00 h to 18:00 h for 1 week (Sharma, 1982; Sharma and Dey, 1978, 1984, 1986a) and BBB permeability was examined using Evans blue albumin as exogenous protein tracer.

Exposure of five young rats to chronic summer heat at 31–33°C caused a mild thermal load as shown by the small rise in mean rectal temperature by 0.84 ± 0.23°C. In these animals no increase in the permeability of the BBB was observed. On the other hand when 18 young rats

TABLE 6

Stress symptoms and physiological variables in control and heat-stressed rats

Parameters examined	Control[a] n = 8	Heat stress at 38°C in BOD chamber		
		1 h n = 6	2 h n = 8	4 h n = 12
A. Stress symptoms				
Rectal T°C	37.42 ± 0.23	38.41 ± 0.32*	39.24 ± 0.21**	41.48 ± 0.23***
Salivation	Nil	+ +	+ + +	+ + + +
Prostration	Nil	Nil	Nil	+ + + +
Gastric haemorrhage	Nil	4 ± 3	8 ± 3	34 ± 8 (microhaemorrhages)
B. Physiological variables				
MABP torr	101 ± 6	94 ± 8	124 ± 8**	76 ± 4**
Arterial pH	7.38 ± 0.04	7.36 ± 0.03	7.33 ± 0.10	7.34 ± 0.08
$PaCO_2$ torr	33.46 ± 1.04	33.56 ± 0.76	34.13 ± 0.24	32.12 ± 0.11*
PaO_2 torr	78.24 ± 1.22	79.12 ± 0.54	79.34 ± 0.26	82.14 ± 0.23**

Control rats kept at room temperature (21 ± 1°C); rats exposed in a biological oxygen demand (BOD) incubator at 38°C for heat stress (for details see text); nil = absent, + + = mild, + + + = moderate, + + + + = severe; data modified after Sharma (1982), Sharma and Dey (1986a, 1987). *$P < 0.05$; **$P < 0.01$; ***$P < 0.001$, Student's unpaired t-test.

(age 8–9 weeks old) were exposed chronically to summer heat at 34–36°C, the permeability of the BBB increased in 11 animals. These rats experienced a greater degree of thermal stress and the mean rectal temperature was increased by 2.5 ± 0.46°C. This increased permeability was limited to young rats only because eight old rats (age 24–32 weeks) when subjected to similar exposure at 34–36°C did not show any increase in BBB permeability. These rats showed a rise in mean rectal temperature of 1.8 ± 0.23°C (Sharma and Dey, 1984, 1986a).

These results showed for the first time that chronic summer heat can induce a breakdown of BBB permeability, a feature which is most prominent in young age groups (Sharma and Dey, 1978; Sharma, 1982). We further observed that in animals following heat exposure, only 50% dose of urethane is required to achieve stage IV anaesthesia (Sharma, 1982; Sharma and Dey, 1986a). This indicates that stress can enhance the susceptibility of drugs acting on the CNS, probably due to a defective BBB. Our results opened a new

vista of brain research indicating that the metabolism and pharmacokinetics of drug transport to the brain is altered in summer heat conditions, a finding which was confirmed by several independent workers (for review see Lomax and Schönbaum, this volume).

Sharabi et al. (1991) discovered a threefold increase in the frequency of CNS stress symptoms like headaches, insomnia, drowsiness, nervousness, distraction, and impaired capacity to conduct simple calculations following pyridostigmine (a carbamate inhibitor of acetylcholinesterase which is used in military personal as antidote of nerve gas poisoning) ingestion by 213 Israeli soldiers treated during the Persian Gulf War. These soldiers serving in the Gulf War may have developed leaky barrier due to hot weather conditions in that region (Hanin, 1996). This was confirmed recently by the findings of Friedmann et al. (1996) who observed that in stressed mice due to forced swimming exercise, only 1/100th dose of the peripherally administered pyridostigmine is necessary to inhibit brain acetylcholinesterase by

50% compared to the control group (Friedmann et al., 1996). These results confirmed the original observations of Sharma and strongly support the idea that the pharmacokinetics of drug transport in the CNS are altered under stressful situations.

Acute heat exposure

Since summer heat resulted in a leaky BBB, we further examined the effect of thermal stress in a controlled manner by exposing rats in a biological oxygen demand (BOD) incubator (Sharma, 1982; Sharma and Dey, 1984, 1986a, 1987; Sharma et al., 1986; Dey et al., 1988, 1993). The influence of controlled heat exposure on various brain function is described below.

Stress symptoms and physiological variables. Exposure of young rats in a BOD incubator at 34°C or 36°C for 4 h resulted in a small rise in their rectal temperature ($+1.8 \pm 0.12$°C and $+2.4 \pm 0.18$°C, respectively) and exhibited only minor salivation. Few animals exhibited microhaemorrhages in their stomach wall (Sharma, 1982).

Exposure of rats for 4 h at 38°C in the BOD chamber resulted in profound stress symptoms. The rise of rectal temperature in these rats was about 3.64 ± 0.57°C. These animals showed profuse salivation and behavioural prostration. Postmortem examination showed many haemorrhagic petachae in the stomach wall. In these animals, MABP fell by 20 torr from the basal value. The PaO_2 showed mild increase, whereas the $PaCO_2$ and arterial pH were slightly decreased (Table 6).

On the other hand, rats exposed to 38°C for 1 or 2 h showed a mild degree of stress symptoms. The MABP in these rat was significantly increased by 28 torr at the end of a 2 h period following heat exposure, whereas the arterial pH, PaO_2 or $PaCO_2$ were not altered significantly (Sharma and Dey, 1986a, 1987). These observations suggest that the magnitude and severity of stress symptoms is dependent on the amount of thermal load and duration of heat exposure.

Blood–brain barrier permeability. Exposure of rats at 34° or 36°C in a BOD incubator did not result in breakdown of BBB permeability (Sharma, 1982; Sharma and Dey, 1978). We examined BBB permeability in heat stress using two exogenous protein tracers, i.e. Evans blue (0.3 ml of a 2% solution, pH 7.4) and radioactive iodine ^{131}I-sodium (100 μCi/kg) (Sharma, 1982; Sharma and Dey, 1984). These tracers will bind to serum albumin when injected into the circulation. A leakage of these tracers across the BBB will thus represent extravasation of tracer-protein complex (Rapoport, 1976; Bradbury, 1979; Sharma, 1982). We administered both tracers into the right femoral vein 5 min before termination of heat stress through an indwelling catheter placed aseptically 2 days before the experiments (Sharma and Dey, 1986a; Sharma, 1987). Five minutes after tracer injection, the animals were anaesthetised with urethane (0.8 g/kg, i.p.) and the brains were perfused via the heart with 0.9% saline for 45 s in order to remove intravascular tracers. After visual inspection of Evans blue dye extravasation, the brains were removed and bisected in the midline. One half of the brain was dissected into the 14 anatomical regions (Sharma and Dey, 1986a,b), weighed immediately and the radioactivity was determined in a gamma counter. The other half of brain was dissolved in a mixture of acetone and sodium sulphate (0.5%, pH 7.4) in order to extract the Evans blue dye entered into the brain. The extracted dye was measured using colourimetry (Sharma and Dey, 1981). The radioactivity in the brain was expressed as percentage of the activity in the whole blood using the formula: counts/min/mg brain tissue over counts/min/mg blood $\times$ 100 (Sharma and Dey, 1986a,b). The blood sample was taken from the heart immediately before perfusion. There was no significant difference in whole blood tracer concentration between controls and heat-stressed rats either following 1, 2 or 4 h periods of heat stress (Sharma and Dey, 1987).

Rats exposed to 4-h heat stress at 38°C showed a marked increase in BBB permeability to Evans blue and radioactive iodine (Fig. 2). This increase in BBB permeability was absent in animals subjected to 1 h or 2 h periods of heat exposure (Fig.

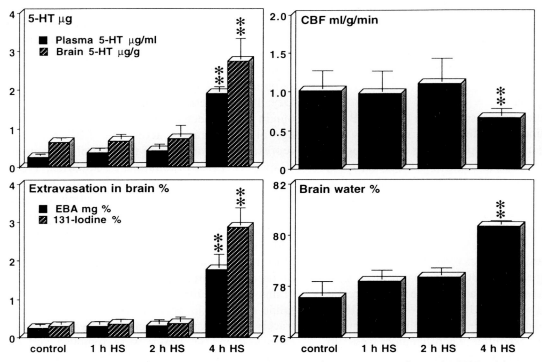

Fig. 2. Blood–brain barrier permeability, brain edema (lower panel), cerebral blood flow and 5-HT level (upper panel) in control and heat-stressed rats. Values represent mean ± standard deviation of 8–12 rats. ** $P < 0.001$ Student's unpaired t-test, compared to the control group (data modified after Sharma and Dey, 1987; Sharma et al., 1986).

2). Our observations demonstrate that heat stress has the capacity to induce a widespread increase in the permeability of the BBB to protein tracers depending on its magnitude and duration.

Regional BBB permeability. In order to detect selective vulnerability of brain regions sensitive to heat, the regional increase in the permeability of the BBB was examined following heat stress (Fig. 3).

We determined the regional BBB permeability in 14 areas of rat brain subjected to 4 h heat exposure. The pattern of extravasation of dye showed minor differences in individual animals. However in general, the Evans blue staining was noted in eight brain regions only. In order of decreased frequency these brain regions ($n = 24$) are cingulate cortex (99%), occipital cortex (96%),

parietal cortex (94%), cerebellum (90%), temporal cortex (88%), frontal cortex (85%), hypothalamus (78%) and thalamus (64%). The other brain regions were mainly devoid of blue staining.

On the other hand, a significant increase in radioactivity was noted in all 14 brain regions examined (Fig. 3). Thus, besides the eight blue-stained regions, another six brain regions viz., hippocampus, caudate nucleus, superior colliculus, inferior colliculus, pons and medulla also showed an increase in ^{131}I-sodium extravasation (Fig. 3).

This extensive increase in the permeability of the radiotracer compared to Evans blue dye appears to be due to differences in the protein binding capacity of the former tracer or due to differences in proteins to which these tracers adhere in the circulation (Sharma and Dey, 1987).

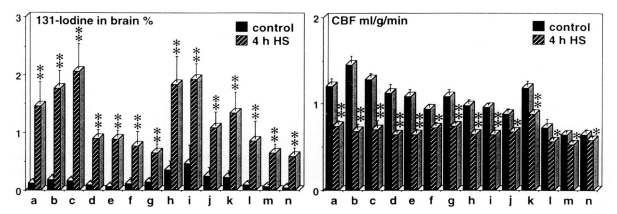

Fig. 3. Regional blood–brain barrier permeability and regional cerebral blood flow in control and 4 h heat-stressed rats. Values are mean ± S.D. of 12–14 rats. = frontal cortex, b = parietal cortex, c = ocipital cortex, d = cingulate cortex, e = hippocampus, f = caudate nucleus, = halamus, h = hypothalamus, i = superior colliculus, j = inferior colliculus, k = cerebellum, l = pons, m = medulla. *P < 0.05, **P < 0.01, compared to controls (ANOVA followed by Dunnett test) (data modified after Sharma and Dey, 1987).

These observations clearly show that heat stress has the capacity to induce a selective increase in BBB permeability not described earlier (Sharma and Dey, 1978, 1986a,b, 1987).

Cerebral blood flow changes. The changes in BBB permeability are often accompanied by changes in the CBF; however a direct relationship between these two factors has not yet been fully established (Rapoport, 1976; Bradbury, 1979, 1992). Studies concerning CBF changes in heat stress are not well attended in the past and regional changes in the CBF are not described. Thus, in order to gain new insight regarding the contribution of cerebral circulation in BBB dysfunction, we examined changes in global and regional CBF in heat stress using tracer microspheres (Sharma, 1987; Sharma and Dey, 1987).

The CBF was measured only once in each animal at the end of a 1, 2 and 4 h period following heat exposure using tracer microspheres (15 ± 0.6 μm in diameter) labelled with ^{125}I-iodine suspended in 0.05% Tween 80 in 0.7% NaCl solution (Sharma, 1987; Sharma and Dey, 1987). About 100 μl of this suspension (containing approximately 78 000–87 000 microspheres)

was injected over 20–30 s into the left cardiac ventricle. The reference sample from right femoral artery was withdrawn at the rate of 0.8–1.211 ml/min starting from 30 s before infusion and continuing up to 90 s after infusion (Sharma and Dey, 1986b).

For determination of regional CBF, animals were decapitated after 90 s of microsphere infusion and the brains were removed. The large superficial veins were removed and the brain was bisected at the mid line (Sharma, 1987). Each half was divided into the 14 anatomically identical brain regions (Fig. 3) and the radioactivity determined in a gamma counter (Sharma and Dey, 1987). The blood samples were divided into aliquots to provide counting geometry similar to that for tissue samples (Sharma and Dey, 1986b). The CBF (ml/g) was calculated from the equation: $CBF = C_B \times RBF \div C_R$, where C_B = counts/min/g brain, RBF = reference blood flow (rate of withdrawal of blood samples from reference artery) and C_R = total counts in the reference blood samples (for details, see Sharma, 1987).

The measurement of CBF showed that subjection of rats to 4 h heat stress significantly reduced the global CBF by 30%, whereas heat exposure of

1 h or 2 h did not influence the CBF changes significantly compared to the control value (Fig. 3). These observations suggest that CBF is influenced by heat stress, which in turn depends on the duration of heat exposure.

Regional CBF. In order to determine a relationship between regional BBB permeability changes and regional CBF we examined changes in the blood flow in identical 14 brain regions in rats subjected to 4 h heat stress (Sharma and Dey, 1987). Our results showed that the regional CBF declined significantly in all the 14 brain regions examined at the end of the 4 h period of heat exposure (Fig. 3). This decrease in regional CBF in cortical regions was 38–53%, in subcortical regions, 23–31% and in cerebellum and brain stem was 15–22% (Fig. 3) (Sharma and Dey, 1987). These results show that the regional CBF changes showed marked variation in heat stress. The probable mechanisms of such variation in the regional CBF are not known.

Relationship between changes in regional CBF and BBB permeability. Our observation on regional CBF changes showed marked ischemia in many brain regions as evident from a general reduction in the CBF following heat stress. However, this ischemia associated with 4 h heat exposure is not sufficient to induce a breakdown of the regional BBB permeability (Sharma et al., 1990). This is further evident from the fact that although the decline in the CBF was seen in almost all the regions exhibiting increased BBB permeability, the regional changes in the CBF and the BBB were unrelated. In five cortical and six subcortical brain regions the regional CBF was significantly reduced by 38–53% and 23–31%, whereas BBB permeability in these regions increased by 87–1366% and 318–590% (Fig. 3). On the other hand, in cerebellum and brain stem, though the regional CBF declined only by 15–22%, the regional BBB permeability increased by 844–1350% (Fig. 3). Thus the intensity of flow reduction was not correlated with the magnitude of increased BBB permeability. A reduction in CBF however

may influence brain metabolism and can contribute to the local cerebral energy changes (Siesjö, 1978) in heat stress which require further investigation.

Brain edema formation. An increased permeability of the BBB resulting in extravasation of protein tracers in many brain regions is associated with vasogenic brain edema formation (Rapoport, 1976; Cervós-Navarro and Ferszt, 1980; Go and Baethmann, 1984). Thus it seems quite likely that breakdown of BBB permeability following heat exposure will result in brain edema formation (Sharma et al., 1986). To test this hypothesis, we examined brain edema in rats subjected to heat stress (Sharma and Cervós-Navarro, 1990a,b).

Brain edema was evaluated from changes in the brain water content and volume swelling (Rapoport, 1976; Bradbury, 1979). The brain water content was measured in each animal using the differences in wet and dry weight of the brain (Dey and Sharma, 1983, 1984). The brain samples were rapidly removed after decapitation following heat stress and weighed immediately (Dey and Sharma, 1983, 1984). The samples were dried in an oven maintained at 90°C for 72 h or till the dry weight became constant in at least two subsequent determinations (Sharma and Cervós-Navarro, 1990a; Sharma et al., 1991a,c). The percentage volume swelling (% f) was determined from the changes in brain water content between control and heat-stressed animals using the formula of Elliott and Jasper (1949) as follows: % water in control + $f/100$ + f = % water in experiment/100. Thus small increments in water represent much larger volume increases. In general, an increase of 1% water content will reflect about a 3% increase in volume swelling (Rapoport, 1976; Cervós-Navarro and Ferszt, 1980; Sharma and Cervós-Navarro, 1990a, 1991).

Our results from heat stress studies support the idea that brain edema formation is closely associated with breakdown of BBB permeability. Thus, rats did not show either edema development or leakage of BBB permeability at the end of 1 or 2 h periods of heat exposure (Fig. 2). However, 4 h heat exposure significantly resulted in the breakdown of BBB permeability and lead to profound brain edema formation (Fig. 2). In these rats, the brain water content increased by 4% corresponding to about 16% increase in volume swelling (Sharma et al., 1986). Our results are the first to show that acute heat exposure can induce brain edema formation (Sharma et al., 1986) and the magnitude and severity of brain swelling in the closed cranial compartment is responsible for heat-induced deaths (Sharma et al., 1986).

Regional brain edema. In order to find out a regional difference in brain edema formation, we examined regional changes in the brain water content following heat stress (Fig. 4). The results show that there was a significant increase in the brain water content in the cerebral cortex (3%, volume swelling 12%), whereas the hippocampus showed approximately 5% increase in water content representing about 20% increase in volume swelling. The cerebellum exhibited a 4% increase in the water content and the brain stem showed about 5% increase in brain water content compared to the control group. These observations are the first to suggest that heat stress has the capacity to induce a selective increase in the regional brain water content. This may reflect a selective vulnerability of these brain regions by heat, a subject which requires further investigation.

Neurochemical mediators of brain dysfunction

Our results show that heat stress-induced brain edema formation seems to be closely associated with breakdown of the BBB to proteins. The detailed mechanisms underlying BBB permeability and brain edema formation in heat stress are still unknown. However, it appears that heat stress-induced alteration in neurochemicals may play an important role (Wahl et al., 1988; Olesen, 1989; Sharma et al., 1990, 1995a,b,c,e; Sharma and Cervós-Navarro, 1991; Black, 1995).

There are various known neurochemical mediators involved in thermoregulation (Milton, 1994;

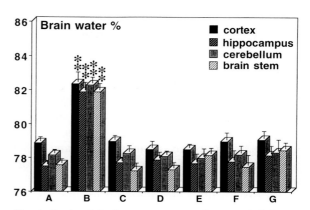

Fig. 4. Regional brain water content in control (A), 4 h heat-stressed (B) rats and its modification with various pharmacological agents (C–G). All drugs were given before heat stress (for details see Table 7). Values are mean ± standard deviation of 6–8 rats *$P < 0.01$, Student's unpaired t-test, compared to the control group. A = control, B = 4-h heat stress, C = p-CPA + heat stress, D = indomethacin + heat stress, E = diazepam + heat stress, F = cyproheptadine + heat stress, G = vinblastine + heat stress.

Zeisburger et al., 1994; Blatteis, 1997), brain edema formation (Wahl et al., 1988; Olesen, 1989) and breakdown of BBB permeability (Bradbury, 1992; Black, 1995; Couraud and Scherman, 1996) (Table 2). Most of these neurochemicals are also known mediators of stress reaction (Selye, 1976; Chrousos et al., 1995). Thus a possibility exists that the same neurochemicals participating in stress reaction or thermoregulatory mechanisms can also influence BBB permeability and brain edema formation probably via a receptor-mediated mechanism (Bradbury, 1992; Black, 1995). The receptors to various neurochemicals are present on the cerebral microvessels and on neuronal, glial and synaptic membranes. Thus alteration in metabolism of these neurochemicals by heat exposure can influence molecular machinery of both neural and non-neural cells causing disturbances in brain function.

In the *in vivo* situation, no single chemical compound appears to be responsible for all the changes seen in any particular stress condition (Sharma et al., 1993a,b, 1995a, 1997a,b,c; Chrousos et al., 1995; Cervós-Navarro and Urich,

1995). Thus it seems that also in heat stress a wide spectrum of neurochemicals are involved (Wahl et al., 1988; Olesen, 1989; Blatteis, 1997). Neurochemicals are suggested to work in synergy to achieve homeostasis which is profoundly disturbed under situations of stress (Selye, 1976). The potential neurochemicals involved in the biology of stress are biogenic amines, prostaglandins, endogenous opioids and many other neuropeptides as well as excitatory and inhibitory amino acid neurotransmitters.

We first focused our attention on the involvement of serotonin in the pathophysiology of heat stress. This is because this amine is the phylogenetically oldest neurochemical present in the mammalian CNS which is often co-localised with various neuropeptides and amino acid neurotransmitters (Hökfelt et al., 1978; Essman, 1978). Serotonin interacts with almost all neurotransmitters or neuromodulators *in vivo* and influences the molecular mechanisms of neuronal transmission via more than seven receptors types and several subtypes (Chaouloff, 1993; Hoyer and Martin, 1996). Under situations of stress, this amine plays an important role in adaptation mechanisms (Lee, 1964; Sharma et al., 1991c, 1992e). Recent observations show that the amine is also involved in the pathophysiology of ischemia, hypoxic and traumatic injuries of the CNS (Sharma and Olsson, 1990; Faden and Salzman, 1992; Sharma et al., 1992a, 1993a,b, 1995d). The basic mechanisms of cell injury following trauma, hypoxia or ischemia are quite similar in nature (Cervós-Navarro and Urich, 1995). Thus, it seems quite likely that this amine is playing an important role in the pathophysiology of heat stress as well.

Serotonin in heat stress

To understand the role of serotonin in the pathophysiology of heat stress we measured the amine content in plasma and brain using a very sensitive and specific spectrophotofluorometric method (Snyder et al., 1965; Sharma and Dey, 1981). Our results show that the serotonin level was increased in the plasma from 0.25 ± 0.04 to 1.89 ± 0.12 $\mu g/ml$ and in brain 0.64 ± 0.06 to 2.74 ± 0.54 $\mu g/g$ after 4 h heat stress (from the control values, respectively, Fig. 2). On the other hand, subjection of rats to either 1- or 2-h periods of heat exposure did not result in any significant increase in the level of this amine in plasma or brain (Fig. 2). These observations suggest that heat stress has the capacity to influence serotonin metabolism in rats which depends on the duration of heat exposure.

Regional brain serotonin. Since serotonergic neurons from raphé, nucleus projects to almost every part of the brain, we wanted to know if there is any selective influence of heat on regional serotonin levels in the brain. For this purpose we measured serotonin concentrations in four major brain regions, i.e. cerebral cortex, hippocampus, cerebellum and brain stem 1, 2 and 4 h after heat stress. In order to find out whether changes in plasma levels of the amine can influence brain serotonin activity in heat stress, the plasma serotonin in these animals were also measured (Essman, 1978; Sharma et al., 1986; Dey et al., 1993).

Serotonin levels of various brain regions in normal animals showed a wide variation which is in agreement with the other workers who used a similar technique or the radioimmunoassay method (Essman, 1978; Chauoloff, 1993). The effect of heat exposure on brain serotonin levels in various regions, however, exhibited different effects dependent on the duration of heat stress. Thus 1 h after heat exposure, the serotonin level was diminished in the cortex, mid brain and hippocampus but not in the cerebellum where a significant increase was found (Fig. 5). Two hours after heat exposure the serotonin level was very similar to that of the control value in all the brain regions. However, at the end of 4 h after heat exposure, the serotonin level showed a significant increase in all the regions except the mid brain (Fig. 5). Taken together, these results indicate that serotonergic transmission in the brain is greatly affected by heat stress.

The plasma concentration of serotonin closely follows the changes in brain serotonin level (Toh, 1960; Fernstrom and Wurtman, 1971). Thus, an

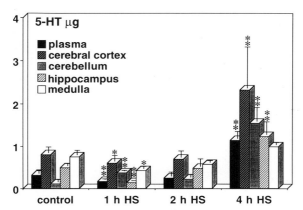

Fig. 5. Plasma and regional brain serotonin content in control and 1 h, 2 h or 4 h heat-stressed rats. Values are mean ± S.D. of 6–8 rats. *$P < 0.05$, **$P < 0.01$, ANOVA followed by Dunnett test, compared to control group (data modified after Sharma, 1982; Dey et al., 1988, 1993).

increased level in brain serotonin at the end of 4 h heat exposure was closely associated with a high rise in plasma serotonin levels. This indicates that a breakdown of the BBB at this time period also contributes to the rise in brain serotonin levels apart from a direct effect of heat on central serotonergic transmission. In order to further clarify the contribution of neuronal serotonin in different brain regions after heat exposure, additional studies using destruction of central serotonergic neurons by 5,7-dihydroxytryptamine (5,7-DHT) are needed.

Heat-induced brain dysfunction: Stress component vs. passive heating

Our observations clearly demonstrate that acute heat exposure has the capacity to induce hyperthermia, breakdown of BBB permeability and brain edema formation. However, it is not clear from these investigations whether the neurological symptoms following heat exposure are due to stress associated with heat or due to the effect of passive heating alone.

To answer this question, we exposed rats to 4 h heat stress at 38°C under urethane or equithesin anaesthesia (Sharma et al., 1994c; Sharma, H.S., unpublished observations). The results are shown in Fig. 6. These anaesthetised rats did not develop stress symptoms (Fig. 6). In these rats, disturbances of BBB permeability, brain edema, CBF or 5-HT levels were not observed (Fig. 6). There was no difference in the results obtained following heat stress in rats anaesthetised either with urethane or equithesin. These observations clearly demonstrate that the stress associated with heat is the key factor in causing brain dysfunction.

Obviously, the feeling of discomfort and stress due to heat exposure is significantly attenuated or prevented by anaesthetics (Selye, 1976; Salzman, 1990). The effect of anaesthetics is very similar to the anxiolytic or pschycopharmacologic drugs in reducing the perception of stress at the level of CNS (Selye, 1976). Due to a reduction in the perception of stress, anaesthetic compounds apparently offer a certain degree of neuroprotection (Salzman, 1990), a subject which encourages additional investigation.

Brain pathology in heat stress

Our results show that heat stress can induce widespread alterations in the permeability of the BBB and leakage of plasma proteins in various brain regions. An increase of protein transport into the cerebral compartment will induce alterations in the osmotic gradient across the cerebrovascular wall (Rapoport, 1976). As a result water from the vascular compartment will enter into the cerebral compartment resulting in vasogenic edema formation (Rapoport, 1976; Cervós-Navarro and Ferszt, 1980; Reulen et al., 1990). Opening of the BBB will also enhance transport of many other vasoactive substances which can influence the neuronal function directly or indirectly via their receptors (Bradbury, 1992). Altered fluid microenvironment of the brain and impaired cellular energy states can contribute to cytotoxic edema, abnormal cell reaction or cell death (Siesjö, 1978; Cervós-Navarro and Urich, 1995). Perturbed ionic, chemical and immunologic microenvironments of the brain will result in neuronal, glial and myelin reactions leading to brain pathology in heat stress. Thus, we examined neuronal, glial, axonal and vascular reaction in various brain regions after heat stress using modern histopathological techniques. The results are described below.

General methodology

For morphology, the animals were perfused under anaesthesia with about 100 ml of a glutaraldehyde-based fixative (2.5% paraformaldehyde, 0.5% glutaraldehyde in 0.1 M phosphate buffer (pH 7.4), containing 2.5% picric acid) preceded with a brief saline (about 50 ml of 0.9%

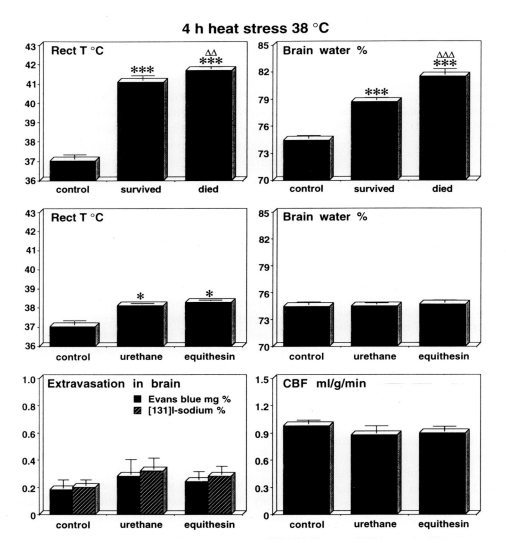

Fig. 6. Effect of 4 h heat stress on brain hyperthermia and brain function in conscious (upper panel), urethane or equithesin anaesthetised rats (middle and lower panels). Values represent mean ± S.D. of 5–6 rats. *$P < 0.05$, ***$P < 0.001$ compared to control group, $\Delta\Delta\Delta = P < 0.001$ compared to survived group (upper panel) (data modified after Sharma, 1982; Sharma et al., 1986).

NaCl solution) rinses thorough the heart (Sharma and Cervós-Navarro, 1990a,b,c). To examine the permeability of the BBB across cerebral vessels at the ultrastructural level, ionic lanthanum (lanthanum chloride), an electron dense tracer was used (Sharma and Cervós-Navarro, 1990a,b; Sharma et al., 1991b,c). This compound was added to the fixative (2.5% lanthanum chloride) immediately before perfusion. The perfusion pressue was effectively maintained at 100 torr throughout the period of perfusion. Immediately after perfusion, the brains were removed and kept in the same fixative for 3–4 days at 4°C in a refrigerator (Sharma et al., 1991a,b,c).

For light microscopy, the desired pieces of brain were embedded in paraffin. About 3 μm-thick multiple sections were cut and stained with routine Haemotoxylin Eosin and Nissl staining as well as glial fibrillary acidic protein (GFAP) and myelin basic protein (MBP) immunostaining (Sharma et al., 1992b,d). For ultrastructural level, the small tissue pieces were postfixed in osmium tetraoxide (OsO_4) and embedded in Epon 812 (Sharma and Cervós-Navarro, 1990a,b,c). About one micron thick multiple sections were cut, stained with toluidine blue and examined under the light microscope. The desired area was then trimmed from the blocks and ultrathin sections were cut using a diamond knife on an LKB ultramicrotome (Sweden). The ultrathin sections were counterstained with uranyl acetate and lead citrate and examined under a Phillips transmission electron microscope (Sharma and Cervós-Navarro, 1990a).

Light microscopy

Since 4 h heat stress induced marked changes in BBB permeability and development of brain edema formation, the morphological examination was done in animals subjected to 4 h heat stress only. Light microscopy revealed marked changes in the heat-stressed brain compared to the control group.

Neuronal changes. Four-hour heat stress resulted in profound neuronal changes as evident from Nissl staining in many parts of the brain compared to the control group (Fig. 7). Dark and distorted neurons were present in the cerebral cortex (Fig. 8), brain stem, cerebellum, thalamus and hypothalamus. Edematous expansion of the neuropil and sponginess in these brain regions was clearly observed. In some regions loss of neurons is very common (Sharma et al., 1991a). These results suggest that neurons are particularly vulnerable to heat stress in many brain regions (Sharma et al., 1992f).

In hippocampus, the most severe changes in the nerve cells were noted in the CA-4 subfield compared to other regions (Fig. 9). Although edematous cells and general sponginess were present in the whole hippocampus, loss of neurons and degenerated nerve cells were most frequent in the phylogenetically oldest part of the hippocampus (i.e. CA-4). The functional significance of this finding is unclear. However our results demonstrate that CA-4 subfield of hippocampus is particularly vulnerable to heat stress (Figs. 9 and 13) which has not been reported earlier (Sharma et al., 1994c,d, 1997a,b).

Glial changes. Glial cells outnumber the neurons and are responsible for CNS homeostasis (Davson, 1967; Cervós-Navarro and Urich, 1995). Thus it is quite likely that glial cells are sensitive to heat stress (Sharma et al., 1992b). We examined glial reaction following heat stress using immunostaining of a specific marker for astrocytes, the glial fibrillary acidic protein (GFAP). Our results show that profound upregulation of GFAP can be seen in many parts of the brain after 4-h heat stress (Fig. 10). This indicates that glial cells are vulnerable to heat-induced damage of the CNS (for details see review by Cervós-Navarro et al., this volume). In general, the glial reactivity was more pronounced in brain stem, cerebellum, thalamus and hypothalamus. A representative example of increased GFAP immunostaining is shown in Fig. 10. However, the cerebral cortex and hippocampus showed only a mild increase in the GFAP activity after heat stress. This observation suggests a regional difference in neuronal

Nissl staining

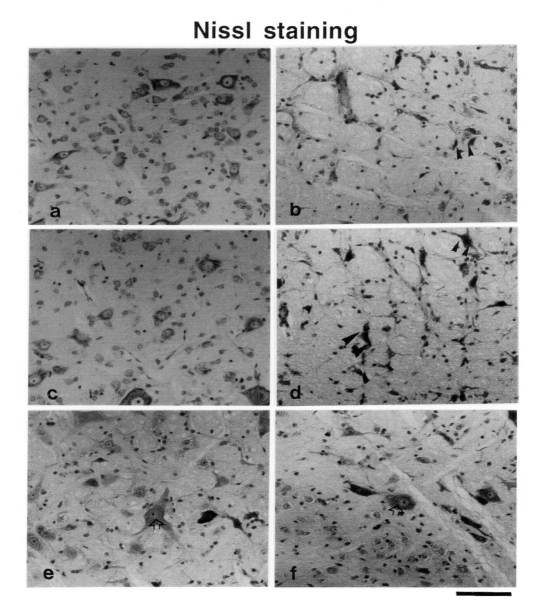

4 h heat stress 38° C

Fig. 7. Nissl-stained nerve cells in one control (a,c) and one 4 h heat-stressed (b,d,e,f) rat. In control rat many healthy nerve cells with distinct nucleus containing centrally located nucleolus can be seen in thalamus (a) and brain stem (c). In heat-stressed rat many dark stained nerve cells without showing a nucleus or nucleolus are very common in many parts of brain including brain stem reticular formation (b,d). In thalamus (e,f) many dark and distorted nerve cells (arrow heads) containing vacuolated cytoplasm (blank arrows) are common. A general sponginess, edema and loss of neurons are quite common (scale bar a,c,e,f = 50 μm; b,d = 80 μm).

Cortical damage

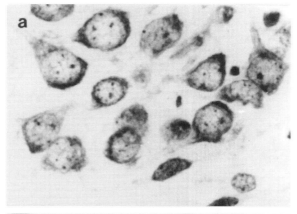

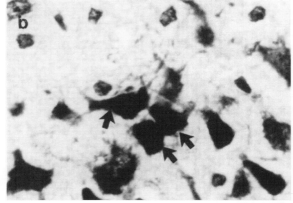

4 h heat stress 38° C

Fig. 8. Nissl-stained nerve cells in the cerebral cortex of one control (a) and one 4 h heat-stressed (b) rat. In normal rat many nerve cells are densely packed and show a distinct nucleus. In heat-stressed rat many damaged and dark stained nerve cells (arrows) are present. Nerve cell loss, a general sponginess and edema are apparent (bar = 30 μm).

and glial responses to heat stress, a subject which requires further careful investigation.

Myelin changes. The myelin changes were examined using myelin basic protein (MBP) immunostaining in rats subjected to 4 h heat stress. MBP is an important protein of myelin (Driscoll et al., 1974). Vesiculation or degradation of myelin

is usually associated with a loss of MBP immunostaining. The MBP appears red in colour and a loss of MBP will result in less intense red staining compared to the controls (Sharma et al., 1991a,c, 1992d). Our results with MBP in heat stress showed a significant reduction in red staining representing a degradation of MBP following heat stress in many brain regions. This decrease in MBP immunostaining was most pronounced in the brain stem reticular formation, pons and medulla. A representative example of a decrease in MBP staining following heat stress compared to controls in pons and medulla is shown in Fig. 11. A marked decrease in MBP immunostained fibre groups in the spinal cord can also be seen after heat stress. These changes were most marked in the spinal cord dorsal and ventral horn.

These observations suggest that heat stress has the capacity to influence myelin damage. Damage of myelin in many experimental or clinical conditions is associated with profound neurological symptoms and alterations in various motor or sensory functions. Further studies aimed at establishing the specific pathways of myelin damage in the CNS and its impact on loss of other motor or sensory functions in heat stress will be of great importance in this field.

Electron microscopy

To examine cellular changes in the brain following heat stress at the ultrastructural level, we used electron microscopy. These observations revealed widespread changes in the nerve cells, axons, synapses, glial cells, myelin and microvessels throughout the brain and spinal cord. Our studies are the first to demonstrate structural changes in neuronal and non-neuronal components in various brain regions at the ultrastructural level following heat stress in rats (Sharma and Cervós-Navarro, 1990a; Sharma et al., 1991a,b,c, 1992a,d,e). This section describes cell changes at the ultrastructural level in heat stress.

Neuronal damage. Nerve cell changes are seen in many parts of the brain in heat stress. Thus damaged nerve cells, and degenerated nucleus

380

Hippocampal damage

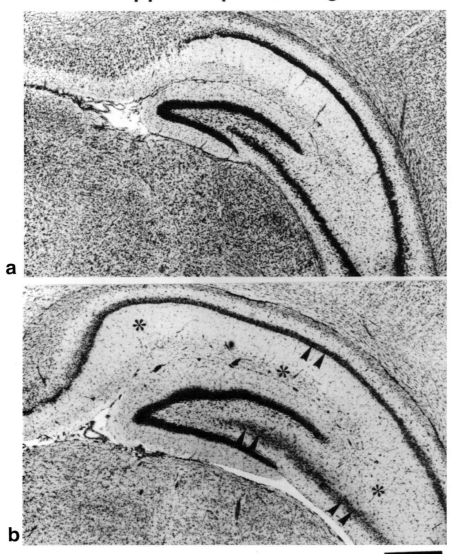

4 h heat stress 38° C

Fig. 9. Low power Haemotoxylin and Eosin stained celloidin section (5 μm thick) of hippocampus in one control (a) and one 4 h heat-stressed (b) rat. In control, densely packed nerve cells are evident in the hippocampal regions CA1, CA2, CA3, CA4, dentate gyrus and in the surrounding brain regions. In heat-stressed rats, general sponginess and loss of nerve cells in the hippocampus and the surrounding brain regions are quite distinct. Edematous expansion of the hippocampus (*) and loss of nerve cells (arrow heads) in the CA1, CA2, CA3 and CA4 are clearly visible. The most prominent nerve cell loss in the hippocampus of heat-stressed rat is seen in the CA4 region (bar = 200 μm).

GFAP immunostaining

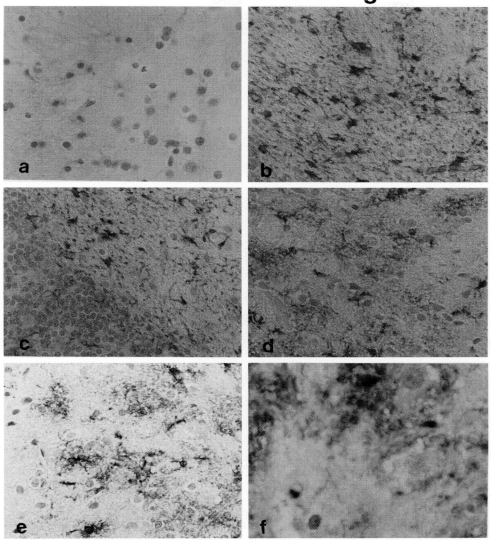

4 h heat stress 38° C

Fig. 10. Glial fibrillary acidic protein (GFAP) immunostaining seen as brown reaction product in one control (a) and one 4 h heat-stressed (b–f) rat. In control rat GFAP immunostaining is almost negative in many brain regions including thalamus (a), whereas marked upregulation of GFAP immunostaining is evident in thalamus (b), cerebellum (c), brain stem (d) spinal cord (e) and striatum (f) (bar a,b,c,d = 80 μm; e = 50 μm; f = 40 μm).

382

MBP immunostaining

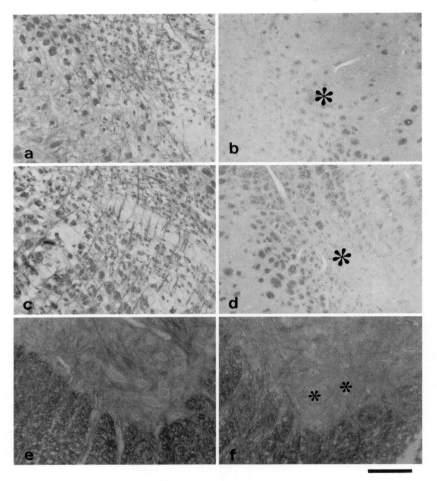

4 h heat stress 38° C

Fig. 11. Myelin basic protein (MBP) immunostaining seen as red reaction product in one control (a,c,e) and one 4 h heat-stressed (b,d,f) rat. In control rat many nerve fibres and bundles are stained dark red in the brain stem reticular formation (a,c) or spinal cord (e), whereas in heat-stressed rat loss of MBP staining in corresponding brain and spinal cord regions (*) is quite distinct (bar = 100 μm).

often accompanied with eccentric nucleolus can be seen in the cerebral cortex (Fig. 12), hippocampus (Fig. 13), cerebellum (Fig. 14), thalamus (Fig. 15), hypothalamus, and brain stem (Fig. 12). Many nerve cells are dark in appearance and contain vacuolated cytoplasm. The nuclear membrane exhibits much irregular folding and the nucleolus often showed signs of degeneration. In

some nerve cells the nucleolus is attached to one end of the nuclear membrane. Many dark and dense structures are present in the nuclear or nerve cell cytoplasm. Some nerve cells are shrunk and some are swollen.

A representative example of one dark neuron in the III layer of the parietal cerebral cortex is shown in Fig. 12b. This nerve cell has an eccentric

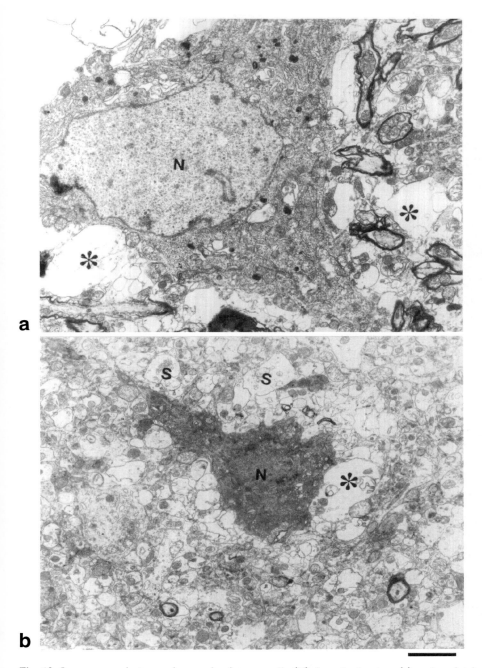

Fig. 12. Low power electron micrograph of nerve cells (N) from brain stem (a) and parietal cerebral cortex (b) of one 4 h heat-stressed rat. Degeneration of nerve cells, cytoplasmic vacuolation (a) and increased density of cytoplasm and karyoplasm (b) are clearly visible. In these nerve cell nucleus, nucleolus is completely degenerated. Signs of vacuolation, edema (*) and synaptic damage (S) are quite frequent (bar a = 500 nm; b = 1 μm).

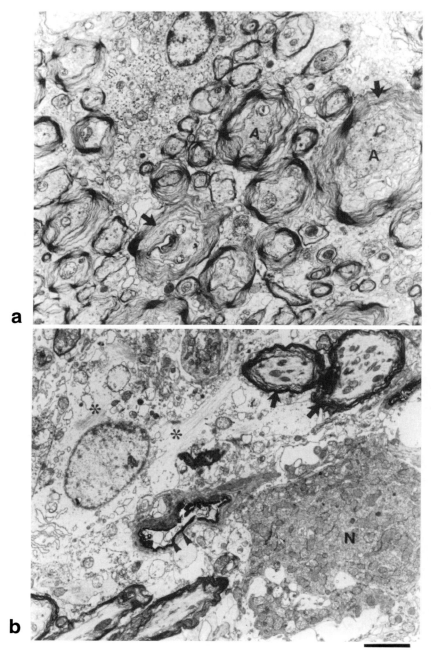

Fig. 13. Low power electron micrograph of medulla (a) and hippocampus CA4 subfield (b) of a 4 h heat-stressed rat. Many myelinated axons (A) exhibit vesiculation of myelin (arrows), membrane disruption and edema (a). In the hippocampus (b) one nerve cell (N) is almost completely disintegrated as evident with loss of distinct nucleus and appearance of many vacuoles and dense cytoplasmic bodies within the nerve cell. A partially collapsed vessel (arrow heads) showing signs of perivascular edema and diffuse exudation of lanthanum across the endothelium is apparent near the nerve cell. Damage to myelinated (arrows) axons, astrocytic edema (*), vacuolation and membrane degeneration are quite frequent in the CA4 subfield of hippocampus (bar = 1 μm).

Cerebellum

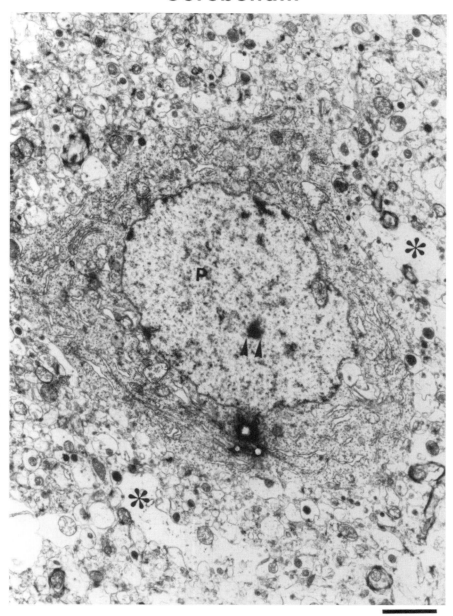

4 h heat stress 38° C

Fig. 14. Low power electron micrograph of one Purkinje cell (P) in the cerebellum of a 4 h heat-stressed rat. This nerve cell cytoplasm is dense and contains many vacuoles. The nuclear membrane shows some abnormal folding in this cell and the nucleolus (arrow heads) is almost completely disintegrated. In the periphery of the nerve cell, vacuolation (*) and edema are clearly evident (bar = 600 nm).

Thalamus

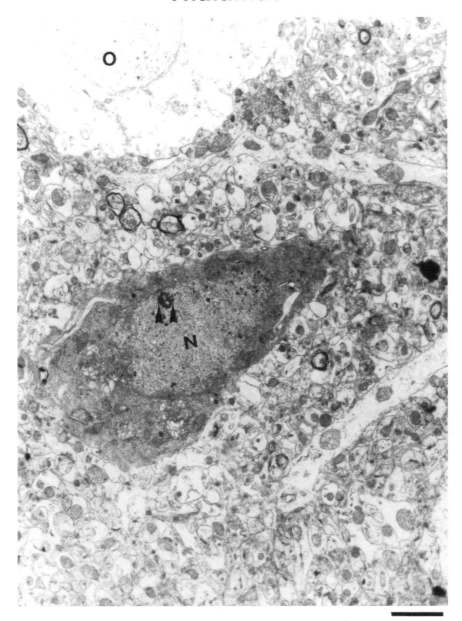

4 h heat stress 38° C

Fig. 15. Electron micrograph of one nerve cell (N) located in the massa intermedia of one rat subjected to 4 h heat stress. This nerve cell is dark in appearance and contains many electron dense granules distributed throughout the cytoplasm as well as in the nucleus. The eccentric nucleolus (arrow heads) is clearly evident. In the periphery of this nerve cell one oligodendrocyte (O) shows complete degeneration, and signs of membrane damage, vacuolation and edema are quite frequent throughout the neuropil (bar = 1 μm).

nucleolus and electron dense cytoplasm. The surroundings of the nerve cells showed vacuolation, membrane disruption and edema.

An example of nerve cell damage in hippocampus (Fig. 13), cerebellum (Fig. 14), thalamus (Fig. 15) and brain stem (Fig. 12a) following 4-h heat stress suggests that the magnitude and severity of cell damage at the ultrastructural level vary in different brain regions. Thus the signs of vacuolation, damage of membrane, edema, swollen synapse, collapsed microvessels and vesiculation of myelin are most widespread and prominent in the brain stem reticular formation followed by thalamus and cerebellum. The hippocampus showed selective cell damage. The CA-4 subfield showed most extensive damage (Fig. 13b) within the hippocampus compared to other subfields. In the cerebral cortex, superficial cell layers (II to III) show the most pronounced damage compared to deeper layers (IV to VI).

Interestingly in many parts of the brain such as hippocampus, cerebellum and brain stem and in some regions of the cerebral cortex, often one nerve cell can be seen as dark with condensed cytoplasm whereas the adjacent nerve cell is quite normal in appearance. This indicates a selective vulnerability of nerve cells following heat exposure. The detailed mechanisms of such selectivity are unknown and require further investigation.

Synaptic damage. Most of the synapses examined in many parts of the brain including cerebral cortex, hippocampus, thalamus, brain stem and cerebellum showed profound structural damage. Swollen synapses with damage to both pre- and post-synaptic membranes are quite common (Fig. 16). This synaptic damage is most pronounced in thalamus, brain stem, hypothalamus, cerebellum, hippocampus and in cerebral cortex. The salient features of synaptic damage include edema, membrane damage, vacuolation, degenerated and damaged synaptic vesicles (Fig. 16). In some regions damage of post-synaptic dendrites and disruption of synaptic membrane are most pronounced.

Axonal damage. Heat stress induces widespread axonal damage, demyelination and vesiculation in many parts of the brain. However, the most extensive damage can be seen in the regions rich in white matter. Thus brain stem reticular formation (Fig. 13a), pons, medulla and spinal cord exhibit most pronounced damage to myelin. The vesiculation of myelin and swollen axons are common findings. Many unmyelinated axons are also swollen. These observations support the idea that heat can induce axonal damage (for details see Lynch and Pollock, this volume).

Vascular reaction

Vascular reaction following heat stress is most pronounced in many parts of the brain. The vascular changes include partial or complete collapse of microvessels indicating ischemia, perivascular edema and disruption of the BBB as seen by infiltration of lanthanum tracer across the cerebral endothelium (Figs. 17 and 18). It is interesting to note that in some vessels the above changes were most pronounced in one brain region while the adjacent vessel may appear quite normal in appearance or show only minor changes. The possible mechanism of such selectivity is unknown. The salient features of vascular changes are described below.

Permeability of the cerebral endothelium: new aspect. Disruption of the BBB at the ultrastructural level is the most common finding in heat stress. Thus many microvessels in several brain regions exhibit leakage of lanthanum across the cerebral endothelium (Fig. 18). However this leakage of lanthanum is not evident in all the vessels in any particular brain region. In one brain region it is possible that one particular vessel or often one endothelial cell shows leakage of lanthanum whereas the rest of the vessel or the adjacent endothelial cell do not show any evidence of increased microvascular permeability. These observations are the first direct evidence of the highly selective nature of the endothelial cell membrane permeability, not described earlier.

The probable mechanism responsible for such a selective increase in microvascular permeability

Synaptic damage

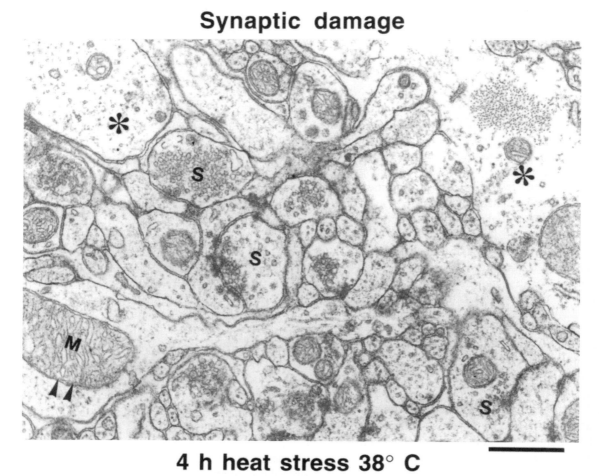

4 h heat stress 38° C

Fig. 16. High power electron micrograph of synaptic (S) damage in the cerebral cortex of one 4 h heat-stressed rat. Many synapses (S) showed swelling and degeneration. Membrane disruption and edema (*) are clearly visible. However the mitochondria (M) appears quite well preserved (arrow heads) (bar = 300 nm).

confined to a small part of the vessel is not clear from our studies. It appears that selective activation of various endothelial cell transporters, permeability factors, neurochemical receptors or ions channels located on the the specific area of the cell membrane could contribute to such a selective increase in lanthanum permeability. However, this is an entirely new concept in the light of recently discovered permeability factors and further studies on this aspect are highly warranted.

Permeability of the tight junctions: New facet. We

examined about 400 vascular profiles at the ultrastructural level from various brain regions of heat-stressed rats using lanthanum tracer. In general, we did not observe widening of tight junctions containing lanthanum in any vascular profile (Fig. 17). However, we observed a completely new phenomenon of permeability increase involving tight junctions in heat stress, which is not known from earlier studies (Fig. 18).

Our observation of this new and interesting aspect of vascular permeability across the tight junctions is summarised in Figs. 17 and 18. Thus, many microvessels showed infiltration of lan-

Tight junction permeability

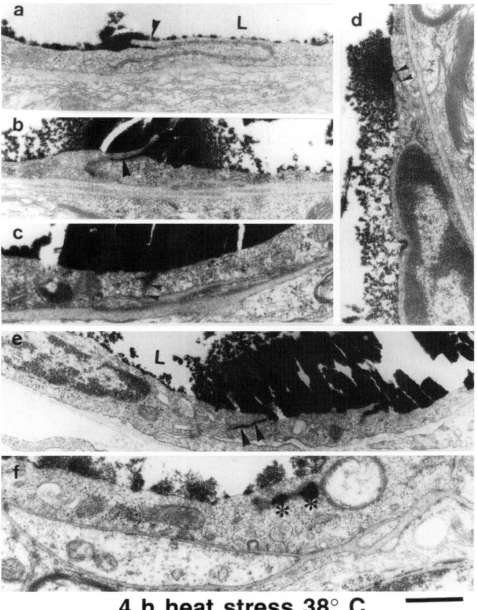

4 h heat stress 38° C

Fig. 17. Electron micrograph showing microvascular permeability to lanthanum, an electron dense tracer (seen as dark black particles) across the tight junctions between the cerebral endothelium located in various parts of the rat brain in control (a) and 4 h heat-stressed rats (b–f). In both control and heat-stressed rats, lanthanum is stopped at the first tight junction (arrow heads) between the apposed plasma membranes of the adjacent endothelium. On the other hand lanthanum is seen within the endothelial cell cytoplasm (*) in many vessels without apparently widening the tight junctions (bar a,b,c,e = 300 nm; d,f = 200 nm).

390

Tight junction permeability

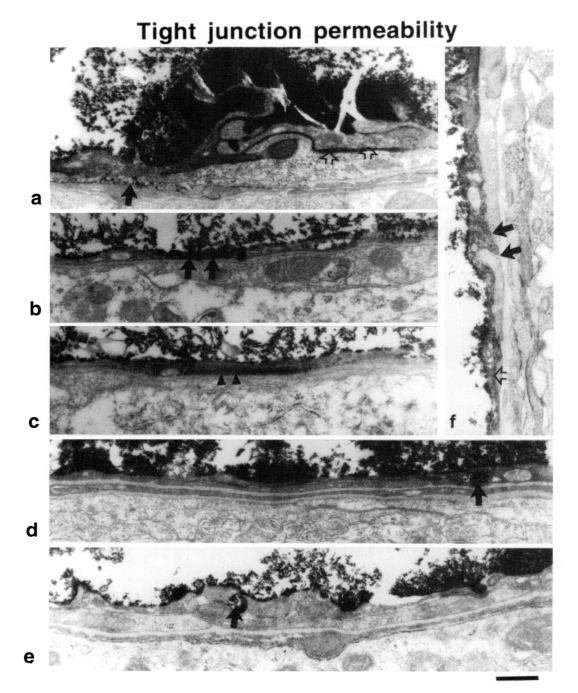

4 h heat stress 38° C

Fig. 18. Electron micrograph showing microvascular permeability of lanthanum across the cerebral endothelial cell membrane and containing tight junctions in 4 h heat-stressed rats. In some cases lanthanum is seen diffusely infiltrated within the cell membranes

thanum across the endothelial cells that are connected with tight junctions. In some cases the membrane permeability across the tight junctions was increased without apparent deformation of these junctions (Fig. 18). This evidence of increased permeability of the tight junctions to lanthanum in heat stress without widening them is a new phenomenon of vascular permeability which has not been described in the literature before.

Tight junctions are formed between two opposing endothelial cell membrane layers (Davson, 1967; Bakay, 1968; Brightman and Reese, 1969; Rapoport, 1976; Bradbury, 1979, 1992). An increase in the endothelial cell membrane permeability (as above) in those regions containing tight junctions can occur without apparently widening them. Our ultrastructural evidence in heat stress points towards this idea which however requires additional research.

In many vascular profiles, lanthanum is stopped between tight junctions (Fig. 17) whereas in other vessels the endothelial membrane is infiltrated with lanthanum in a very selective and specific manner as described above (Fig. 18). Thus, one endothelial cell is completely infiltrated with lanthanum while the adjacent one is entirely normal. These observations support the idea of a specific receptor-mediated increase in microvascular permeability. Since receptors can also be present on the membranes apposing tight junctions, increased microvascular permeability around the junctions is possible via activation of such receptors.

Significance of ultrastructural observations in hyperthermic brain injury

The ultrastructural changes confirm our observation with light microscopy and further support the pathophysiological findings obtained in *in vivo* studies following heat stress. Thus, vascular changes in heat stress seen at the ultrastructural level using lanthanum confirm the breakdown of BBB permeability to protein tracers (Figs. 17 and 18). The collapse of microvessels in many brain regions seen by electron microscopy is in line with the CBF results obtained using microsphere techniques (Fig. 19). These ultrastructural changes support the hypothesis that reduction in the CBF is unrelated to the breakdown of BBB permeability. This is evident from the findings that in several brain regions following heat stress many vessels are completely collapsed but they do not show signs of leakage of lanthanum across the cerebral endothelium. Edematous swelling of astrocytes, nerve cells, vacuolation and membrane degeneration seen at the ultrastructural level is well correlated with the measurement of water content to demonstrate edema formation. Perivascular swelling of astrocytes supports the findings obtained with glial fibrillary acidic protein (GFAP) immunostaining and further confirms the idea of glial activation in heat stress (Fig. 19). Myelin vesiculation seen at the ultrastructural level fits very well with loss of MBP immunostaining (Fig. 13).

We found evidence of both vasogenic and cytotoxic types of edema formation using electron microscopy in heat stress (Figs 16 and 19). Thus apart from membrane damage and vacuolation due to water filled spaces, cell swelling due to intracellular accumulation of water is also observed. This indicates that hyperthermic brain edema is very similar to that of traumatic edema in which vasogenic factors are primarily responsi-

---

of tight junction complex and endothelial cell cytoplasm covering the apposed plasma membranes connected with the tight junctions (a). However in these cases the tight junctions are not found opened because lanthanum within the intercellular cleft is stopped at the tight junction (blank arrows, a); whereas lanthanum can be seen in the basal lamina under the portion of the cerebral endothelium where the cell membrane is completely infiltrated with lanthanum (filled arrow, a). In most cases a portion of the endothelial cell membrane is found completely infiltrated with lanthanum (b: filled arrows, c: arrow heads) or occasionally found within the vesicles of endothelial cell cytoplasm (d,e: filled arrow). In some cases only one endothelial cell membrane covering tight junction is found diffusely infiltrated with lanthanum (filled and blank arrows) leaving its counterpart completely intact (f: filled arrows) (bar a,e,f = 200 nm; b,c,d = 300 nm).

vascular reaction and edema

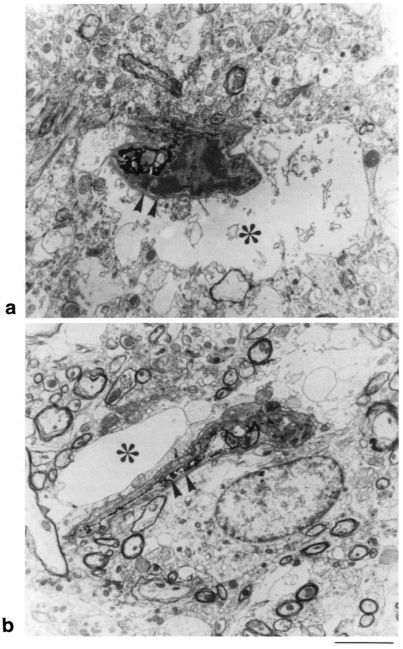

4 h heat stress 38° C

Fig. 19. Low power electron micrograph showing completely collapsed microvessel in the thalamus (a) and in the brain stem (b) of a 4 h heat-stressed rat. Lanthanum as black dark particles is confined within the lumen (arrows). Perivascular edema (*) and membrane damage is quite frequent (bar = 2 μm).

ble but get further complicated by various cyto-toxic factors.

Pharmacological manipulation of hyperthermic brain dysfunction

As indicated above, our results strongly suggest that breakdown of BBB permeability is one of the important factors in brain dysfunction following heat stress. This breakdown of the BBB appears to be associated with increased plasma and brain serotonin levels. Obviously a breakdown of BBB permeability will induce vasogenic brain edema formation and allow many restricted substances to enter into the cerebral compartment. Thus alterations in ionic, chemical, or immunological microenvironments of the cerebral compartment due to breakdown of the BBB will precipitate nerve cell, glial cells or myelin reaction in the brain (see above).

In order to test this hypothesis, we used various pharmacological tools to modify BBB permeability, serotonin metabolism, stress response or cellular transport in rats before heat stress and examined the state of brain edema formation and the cell changes according to the standard protocol (as above). A summary of drugs used in heat stress is shown in Table 7. In the following section, the influence of these drugs on various parameters in heat stress is described.

Pharmacological manipulation of BBB permeability, CBF and serotonin levels

Our results show that pretreatment with p-chlorophenylalanine (p-CPA, a serotonin synthesis inhibitor), indomethacin (a prostaglandin synthesis inhibitor) and diazepam (anxiolytic drug) significantly attenuated the increase of BBB permeability (Fig. 20) and plasma and brain serotonin levels following heat stress (Fig. 21). No significant difference in either total or regional CBF was noted in these drug treated-stressed animals compared to heat-stressed controls (Figs. 21 and 22). On the other hand, pretreatment with cyproheptadine (a serotonin$_2$ receptor antagonist) and vinblastine (a vesicular transport inhibitor), though markedly attenuating the increased BBB permeability following heat stress (Fig. 20) the plasma and brain serotonin levels continued to remain high (Fig. 21). However, the CBF values were restored near normal values in cyproheptadine pretreated heat-stressed animals (Fig. 22) whereas in vinblastine pretreated rats no significant difference in the CBF values was found from the untreated stressed group (Fig. 22).

Thus it appears that all the above drugs significantly reduced BBB permeability following heat stress and this ability of the drugs mainly depends on their capacity to either reduce the serotonin levels (p-CPA, indomethacin, di-

TABLE 7

Pharmacotherapy of rats subjected to 4 h heat stress

Drug	Dosage	Route	No. of injections	Schedule	Source
p-CPA	100 mg/kg/day	i.p.	3	24 h before HS	Sigma
Indomethacin	10 mg/kg	i.p.	1	30 min before	Sigma
Diazepam[a]	4 mg/kg	s.c.	1	30 min before	Glaxo, UK
Cyproheptadine	10 mg/kg	i.p.	1	30 min before	MSD, UK
Vinblastine[a]	0.8 mg/kg	i.v.	1	24 h before	Eli, Lily

Doasage of drugs selected after Sharma (1982); Sharma and Dey (1986a, 1987); i.p. = intraperitoneal, s.c. = subcutaneous, i.v. = intravenous.
[a]Ampoule; other drugs in powder form were dissolved in physiological saline and adjusted to pH 7.4 before administration.

394

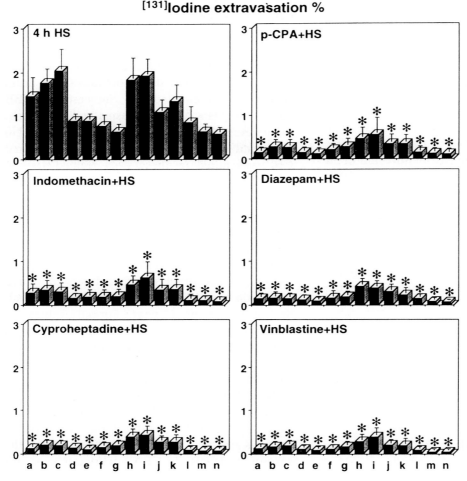

[131]Iodine extravasation %

Fig. 20. Shows regional blood–brain barrier permeability in 4-h heat-stressed rats and its modification with various drugs. All drugs were given before the onset of heat stress (for details see Table 7). Values are mean ± S.D. of 6–8 rats. a = frontal cortex, b = parietal cortex, c = occipital cortex, d = cingulate cortex, e = hippocampus, f = caudate nucleus, g = thalamus, h = hypothalamus, i = superior colliculus, j = inferior colliculus, k = cerebellum, l = pons, m = medulla. *P < 0.01, ANOVA followed by Dunnett test, compared to 4-h heat-stressed rats (data modified after Sharma and Dey, 1986a, 1987).

azepam) or its action on the cerebrovasculature (cyproheptadine) except vinblastine which inhibits the vesicular transport of tracer substances at the cerebral microvessels.

Mechanisms of BBB breakdown in heat stress. Our pharmacological studies clearly indicate that an increased level of serotonin in heat stress is a contributing factor to the breakdown of BBB permeability either directly or through some indirect mechanisms (Sharma and Dey, 1987; Sharma et al., 1996a,b,c). Thus in p-CPA treated rats, heat stress is not able to induce an increase in serotonin because the amine was not available for release from its stores due to decreased synthesis. Pretreatment with p-CPA has been reported to reduce the level of serotonin in almost all tissues of the body including brain (Essman, 1978).

395

On the other hand, indomethacin and diazepam which are not inhibitors of serotonin synthesis also reduced the increase of serotonin following heat stress. Diazepam is a well known anxiolytic drug and pretreatment with this drug prevents altered EEG changes and behaviour following immobilization stress in primates (Bouyer et al., 1978). In addition, diazepam reduces the synthesis and utilisation of serotonin in brain by reducing the activity of serotonergic neurons (Stein et al., 1973) which is believed to be relevant to its anxiolytic action (Haefely et al., 1981).

Our results further suggest that this drug probably inhibited the stress response and therefore no increase in the serotonin level following heat stress was noted.

The prevention of BBB dysfunction with indomethacin suggest that prostaglandins are also involved. Prostaglandins are implicated as first mediators of stress (Hanukoglu, 1977) and inhibition of their release with indomethacin prevents the stress-induced release of corticosterone. In addition, prostaglandins are known stimulators of serotonin synthesis (Haubrich et al., 1973). Thus

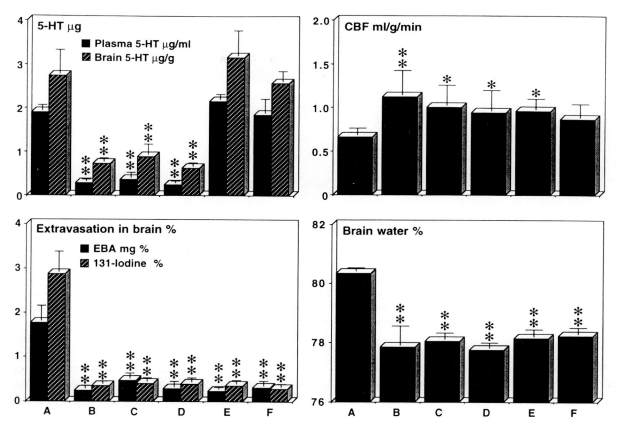

Fig. 21. Blood–brain barrier permeability, brain edema (lower panel), cerebral blood flow and 5-HT levels (upper panel) in 4 h heat-stressed rats and their modification with various drugs. All drugs were given before the onset of heat stress (for details see Table 7). Values are mean ± standard deviation of 6–8 rats. *$P < 0.05$, **$P < 0.01$, ANOVA followed by Dunnett test, compared to 4-h heat-stressed rats. A = 4 h heat stress; B = p-CPA + heat stress; C = indomethacin + heat stress; D = diazepam + heat stress; E = cyproheptadine + heat stress; F = vinblastine + heat stress (data modified after Sharma, 1982; Sharma and Dey, 1986a, 1987; Sharma and Cervós-Navarro, 1990a).

rCBF (ml/g/min)

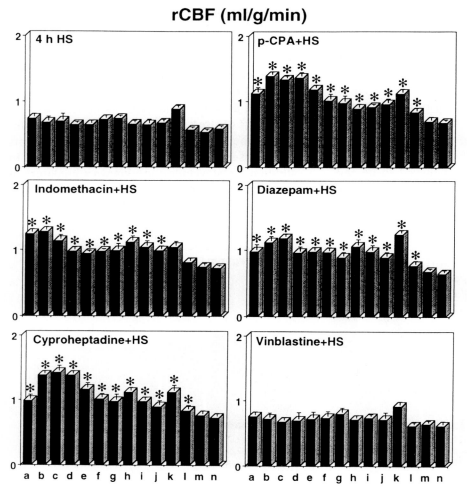

Fig. 22. Regional cerebral blood flow in 4-h heat-stressed rats and their modification with various drugs. All drugs were given before the onset of heat stress (for details see Table 7). Values are mean ± S.D. of 6–8 rats. a = frontal cortex, b = parietal cortex, c = occipital cortex, d = cingulate cortex, e = hippocampus, f = caudate nucleus, g = thalamus, h = hypothalamus, i = superior colliculus, j = inferior colliculus, k = cerebellum, l = pons, m = medulla. $^*P < 0.05$, ANOVA followed by Dunnett test, compared to 4 h heat-stressed rats (data modified after Sharma and Dey, 1987).

it seems quite likely that indomethacin prevents the release of prostaglandins following heat stress resulting in a lower increase in serotonin level in this group.

The cerebral capillary walls contain prostaglandin and cAMP synthesis and catabolizing enzymes (Hagen et al., 1979; Goehlert et al., 1981; Joó, 1985), and a local accumulation of prostaglandins and cAMP in cerebral microves-

sels leads to an increase in vesicular transport of tracer substances (Eakins, 1977). It seems quite likely that increased plasma and brain serotonin levels stimulate prostaglandin biosynthesis in cerebral microvessels which in turn stimulates cAMP biosynthesis (Baca and Palmer, 1978). The increased cAMP level then stimulates vesicular transport resulting in a breakdown of BBB permeability (Joó, 1985).

The above hypothesis is well supported by the results obtained with vinblastine, a compound which inhibits the vesicular transport (Larsson et al., 1980). Thus vinblastine pretreatment attenuated the breakdown of BBB permeability in spite of the very large rise in plasma and brain serotonin levels indicating that vesicular transport is playing a major role in tracer transport, a feature which is well supported by our ultrastructural observations (see above). The idea that increased serotonin level in plasma is important for the breakdown of BBB permeability is supported by the results obtained with cyproheptadine treatment. This compound is a specific serotonin$_2$ receptor antagonist and blockade of this receptor resulted in attenuation of BBB breakdown. This observation suggests a receptor-mediated breakdown of BBB permeability in heat stress (Sharma and Dey, 1986a,b, 1987; Sharma et al., 1990a,b, 1992b,d, 1994a,b, 1996c, 1997a,b,c).

Pharmacological manipulations of brain edema formation

The hypothesis that breakdown of the BBB is associated with vasogenic edema formation was further confirmed in this model by measuring brain water content in rats subjected to heat stress with pretreatment of the above drugs (Fig. 4). It is interesting to note that all the drugs which prevented BBB permeability following heat stress were able to significantly thwart the brain edema formation. In addition we used drugs modifying either opioid receptors (naloxone) or inhibitors of free radical formation (H 290/51, Astra Hässle, Mölndal, Mustafa et al., 1995) which also reduced BBB permeability and prevented brain edema formation in heat stress (Sharma et al., 1997b). These observations strongly support the idea that breakdown of the BBB is a key factor in brain edema formation.

Additional support for this hypothesis came from drugs modifying catecholaminergic or histaminergic transmission in the nervous system (Sharma, 1982; Sharma et al., 1992g; Sharma, H.S., unpublished observations). Thus pretreatment with phenoxybenzamine (an α-receptor blocker), propranolol (a β-receptor blocker), 6-hydroxydopamine (6-OHDA, a catecholaminergic neurotoxin) and mepyramine (histamine H$_1$ receptor blocker) did not prevent BBB permeability. These rats also did not show a reduction in brain edema formation. In fact 6-OHDA and mepyramine pretreatment resulted in a greater degree of protein extravasation across the BBB and resulted in an aggravation of brain edema formation in heat-stressed rats (Sharma, 1982; Sharma et al., 1992g; Sharma, H.S., unpublished observations). Thus there was a good correlation ($r^2 = 0.968, < 0.001$) between breakdown of the BBB permeability and development of edema in heat stress (Fig. 23). These results for the first time provide new direct evidence that the breakdown of BBB permeability is related to brain edema formation.

Pharmacological manipulations of brain pathology

In order to understand the role of BBB permeability and brain edema formation in cell injury, we used a morphological approach to examine cell changes in heat stress under selective drug treatments as described above. Our results showed that the drugs which reduced BBB permeability and brain edema formation (p-CPA, ketanserin, cyproheptadine, indomethacin, naloxone) were able to reduce cell injury either seen at light or electron microscopic level. An example of p-CPA (Fig. 24), indomethacin and cyproheptadine pretreated (Fig. 25) and heat-stressed animal showing markedly less cell changes at the ultrastructural level is shown in Figs. 24 and 25. Thus the neuropil appears to be quite compact and membrane vacuolation, edema, collapse of vessels, synaptic damage are less frequent in the drug-treated rats following heat stress. On the other hand, drugs (memyramine, 6-OHDA) which aggravated brain edema formation and BBB permeability disturbances resulted in significantly more adverse cell changes compared to untreated stressed rats (Sharma, H.S., unpublished observations). One example of ultrastructural cell changes in heat-stressed rats treated with 6-OHDA is shown in Fig. 26. Edema, membrane damage, vacuolation

398

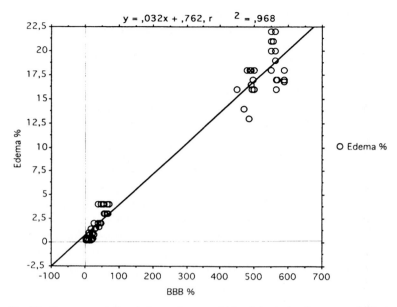

Fig. 23. Shows correlation between increased blood–brain barrier permeability to Evans blue albumin (%, X-axis) and increased brain water content (%, Y-axis) in control, 4 h heat stress and drug-treated heat-stressed rats. The regression line showed strong correlation between breakdown of the BBB permeability in heat stress with brain edema development irrespective of treatment or no treatment ($r^2 = 0.968$, P < 0.001).

and collapsed vessels are quite frequent in this group.

This pharmacological evidence at the ultrastructural level provides new direct evidence that breakdown of the BBB is the key factor in inducing brain edema formation and subsequently adverse cell reaction in heat stress.

Effect of age on heat stress-induced brain pathology

Age is one of the important factors influencing stress response (Selye, 1976) and induces desensitisation of various neurochemical receptors in the CNS (Sharma and Dey, 1988; Dey et al., 1988). To find out if heat-induced brain dysfunction is influenced by age, in separate investigations we examined the effect of age on heat stress-induced alterations in BBB permeability, serotonin metabolism, CBF, brain edema and cell changes (Sharma et al., 1992d).

For this purpose we exposed adult rats (age

24–32 weeks) to 4 h heat stress at 38°C and compared the results obtained with heat exposure in young rats (age 8–9 weeks). Our results showed that young rats are most susceptible to heat stress-induced changes in BBB permeability, brain edema and cell changes compared to adult rats (Sharma et al., 1992d).

Other important observations from this study are that the plasma and brain serotonin levels correlated very well with the breakdown of BBB permeability, brain edema and cell changes. Thus young rats showing profound changes in brain function in terms of breakdown of BBB permeability, development of edema formation and occurrence of cell changes throughout the brain exhibited a marked increase in plasma (687%) and brain (267%) serotonin levels. However, adult animals showed only minor changes in the amine content in plasma (141%) or brain (20%) compared to the normal control group (Sharma et al., 1992d). This observation suggests that serotonin

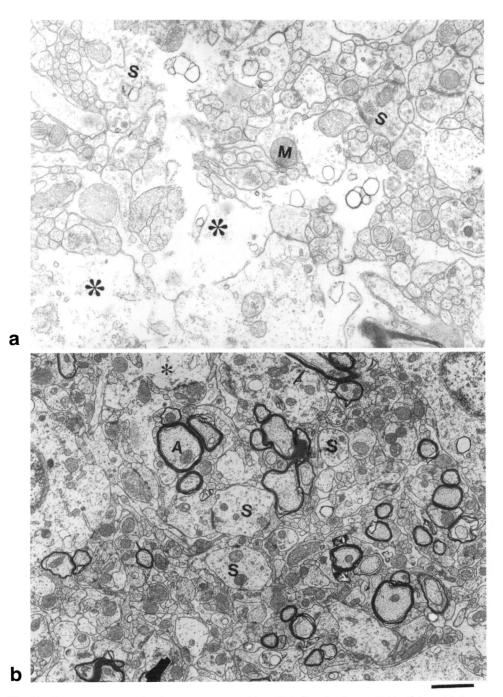

Fig. 24. Shows neuroprotection by pretreatment with p-CPA (for details see Table 7) in a 4 h heat-stressed rat (b) compared to untreated heat-stressed rat (a). The signs of edema (*) and synaptic damage (S) are less evident in the p-CPA pretreated heat-stressed rat. Vesiculation of myelin in myelinated axons (A) is less severe (bar a = 800 nm; b = 1 μm).

400

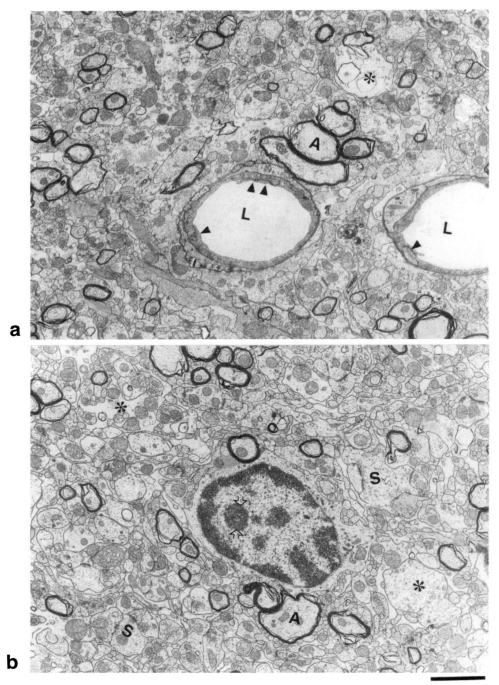

Fig. 25. Neuroprotection offered by indomethacin (a) and cyproheptadine (b) in a 4 h heat-stressed rat. The cerebral vessels are round in shape and perivascular edema is not evident. The tight junctions (arrow heads) are intact. Other signs of edema (*), synaptic damage (S), vesiculation of myelin in the myelinated axons (A) are minimal. One microglia with distinct nucleus and nucleolus (blank arrows) looks quite normal in appearance in cyproheptadine-treated heat-stressed rat (bar = 1 μm).

4 h Heat Stress

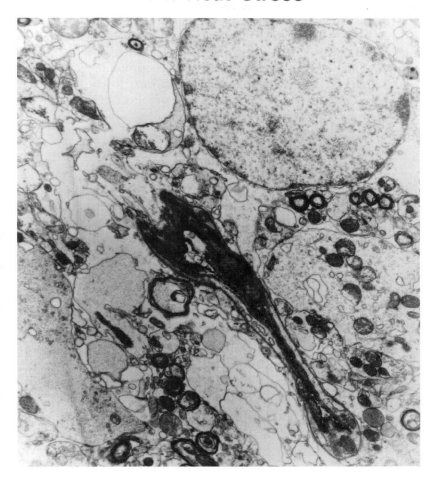

6-OHDA icv treated

Fig. 26. Electron micrograph from cerebellar cortex of a 4 h heat-stressed rat pretreated with 6-OHDA (for details see text). As apparent from the figure, signs of vascular reaction, edema, vacuolation and cell damage are prominent in this heat-stressed rat pretreated with 6-OHDA. The neuropil shows marked cell damage, perivascular edema and a completely collapsed microvessel (bar = 1 μm).

could be one of the important neurotransmitters involved in the pathophysiology of brain function in heat stress.

The probable mechanisms of such alterations in serotonin levels following heat stress in young and adult rats subjected to heat stress are not well known. However, it appears that the intensity of stress, its perception at the cellular level and elicitation of stress response will decrease with advancing age (Selye, 1976). Another possibility would be that the processing of thermoregulatory information in the CNS at thermoregulatory effectors are more efficient in adult animals compared to young rats (see review by Kanosue et al., Ch. 4).

Lung monoamine oxidase activity and circulating serotonin level. The mechanisms underlying the increased level of serotonin in plasma following heat stress are unknown. However, it appears that lung monoamine oxidase (MAO) activity may play an important role in serotonin accumulation in the circulation following heat stress (Sharma et al., 1986; Youdim et al., 1980). This is evident from the fact that apart from central serotonergic regulation, the blood serotonin level is controlled by lung monoamine oxidase (MAO) activity (Youdim and Holzbauer, 1980). More than 90% of the circulating serotonin is cleared by MAO located in the pulmonary endothelium (Alabaster, 1977). This enzyme activity is saturable and dependent on substrate concentration as well as temperature (optimum activity $38 \pm 0.05°C$) and pH (optimum 7.4) of the incubation medium (Youdim et al., 1980; Sharma et al., 1986; Dey et al., 1988).

Heat stress induces profound hyperthermia thus one possibility of accumulation of serotonin in plasma would be due to a decrease in lung MAO activity. In order to test this hypothesis we measured MAO activity in lung homogenates in heat-stressed rats (Sharma et al., 1986). Our results indicated that the circulating serotonin level and lung MAO activity showed a good correlation in both young and adult rats following heat stress. Thus in young rats there was a significant retardation in lung MAO activity by 56–64% compared to the control group. However, in adult animals the enzyme activity did not diminish. In fact, there was an increase in lung MAO activity by 50–132% compared with the control group (Sharma et al., 1986, 1992d). These observations provide the first experimental evidence that a reduction in lung MAO activity may be one of the major mechanisms leading to the accumulation of serotonin in circulation following heat stress in young rats.

Serotonin has the capacity to influence microcirculation in brain and can induce breakdown of BBB permeability (Sharma et al., 1990). An increased permeability of the BBB will induce vasogenic edema and may result in subsequent cell damage (Sharma and Olsson, 1990; Sharma et al., 1990; Sharma and Cervós-Navarro, 1990a). Thus, a lower accumulation of serotonin in adult rats following heat stress appears to be instrumental in causing minimal disturbances of brain function (Sharma et al., 1992d).

Brain pathology in chronic experimental heat exposure

Our results obtained in adult rats suggest that a significant attenuation of BBB breakdown following heat stress is one important factor in inducing less cell changes and edema. A minor breakdown of the BBB appears to be associated with a small rise of plasma and brain serotonin levels in these rats (Sharma et al., 1992e). To further examine this hypothesis we used an experimental model for chronic heat exposure (Sharma et al., 1991c, 1992e; Dey et al., 1993). This is because the effect of acute stress gradually diminishes following repeated short-term exposure of a mild degree of particular stress (Selye, 1976; Sharma et al., 1992g; Chrousos et al., 1995). Thus subjection of similar stress to these adapted individuals will then elicit very mild or no symptoms (Selye, 1976). This condition is known as state of adaption. Adaptation to heat is a common phenomenon which depends on prior physiological or environmental conditions (Lee, 1964; Prosser, 1964; Selye, 1976; Chrousos et al., 1995).

To find out whether a prior adaptation to heat influences the magnitude or severity of hyperthermic brain injury, we examined the effect of heat stress in rats either exposed to repeated short-term heat exposures or which were adapted to heat by rearing at mild or moderately hot environments (Sharma et al., 1991c, 1992e; Dey et al., 1993).

Influence of repeated short-term heat exposure
To examine the effect of short-term repeated heat exposure on the consequences of hyper-

thermic brain injury we exposed separate group of rats to 1 or 2 h heat stress daily at 38°C for 7 days. On the eighth day these rats were subjected to 4 h heat stress (as above). Control group of rats were also exposed daily to heat stress but were not subjected to 4 h heat stress on the 8th

brain stem

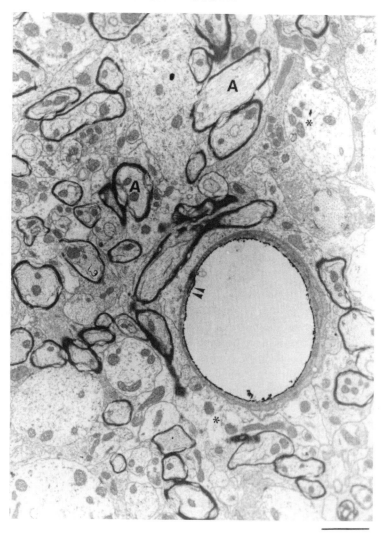

chronic heat exposure

Fig. 27. Shows electron micrograph of one microvessel from the brain stem of a chronically heat-stressed rat showing signs of heat adaptation (for details see text). Rats were exposed to repeated short-term heat exposure for 1 h daily for 7 days. On the 8th day, these rats were subjected to a 4 h heat stress session. Subjection of rats to heat stress in heat-adapted rats did not induce any prominent cell damage. The lanthanum is mainly confined within the lumen and the signs of perivascular edema, membrane damage, vesiculation of myelin are mainly absent (bar = 1200 nm).

day. The results showed that subjection of rats to 1 or 2 h HS daily for 7 days did not result in symptoms (Sharma et al., 1992e). Their rectal temperature and plasma and brain serotonin levels were slightly but significantly elevated on the 7th day compared to the intact rats kept at normal room temperature. Exposure of these rats to an additional 4 h heat stress on the 8th day did not elicit any further rise in either the rectal temperature or the serotonin level. In these rats no breakdown of BBB permeability was observed as seen with Evans blue and ^{131}I-sodium tracers (Sharma et al., 1992). The brain water content was within the normal range. Morphological examination showed almost normal appearance of the neuropil (Fig. 27).

These findings suggest that a slight but significant increase in the basal serotonin level and rectal temperature following animals subjected to repeated heat stress induces heat tolerance and plays an important role in heat adaptation (Sharma et al., 1992e). The other important finding of this investigation is that in heat-adapted animals, BBB breakdown does not occur. As a result brain edema formation is also absent. Obviously with the absence of BBB breakdown and brain edema formation, the cell changes in the brain following heat stress cannot be seen. These observations strongly support the hypothesis that BBB breakdown in heat stress is instrumental in precipitating brain edema formation and cell injury.

Influence of rearing at high ambient temperature

To further confirm the above hypothesis we examined the influence of rearing at ambient temperature on the consequences of heat stress-induced changes in BBB permeability, brain edema formation and cell injury in a separate group of rats (Sharma et al., 1991c). For this purpose, we placed separate groups of rats immediately after weaning (on the day 21) at warm (28 ± 1°C) or hot (34 ± 1°C) ambient air temperatures, respectively for 6 weeks. The control group of rats were kept at normal room temperature (21 ± 1°C). At the age of 9 weeks these rats were exposed to 4 h heat stress at 38°C and development of stress symptoms, BBB permeability, brain edema and cell changes were examined (Sharma et al., 1991c).

Subjection of these rats to heat stress showed that in rats exposed to warm ambient temperatures, the development of stress symptoms were only mild whereas rats reared at hot ambient temperature did not show any symptoms. In these rats the extravasation of tracers across the BBB or increase in the brain water content were mainly absent. The decline in the CBF was limited to only 12%. Interestingly, though the basal levels of plasma and brain serotonin levels showed a mild increase in rats reared at warm or hot ambient temperatures respectively, subjection of heat stress to these rats did not further increase the amine content in plasma or brain significantly.

Morphological examination in these rats showed no apparent distortion of nerve cells, glial cells or myelin damage seen at both light and electron microscopy (Sharma et al., 1991c). These observations further confirm the idea that BBB breakdown is instrumental in inducing cell injury in the CNS. Brain edema formation and alteration of the microenvironment of the brain are primarily responsible for cell injury in the brain of heat-stressed rats.

Since thermal adaptation plays an important role in heat stress induced symptoms, our results indicate the important role of basal physiological mechanisms prior to heat exposure in CNS injury caused by heat stress. The probable mechanisms of such heat adaptation at the cellular or molecular level in the CNS is not well understood. However, a possibility exists that exposure to prior heat stimulus may induce upregulation of heat shock proteins in the CNS which could play an important neuroprotective role, a feature which requires additional study.

General conclusion

Our study shows that hyperthermia if accompanied by breakdown of BBB permeability is associated with profound edema and cell changes.

This increase in BBB permeability is mediated by various neurochemicals. The effects of hyperthermia on brain dysfunction is reduced by advancing age, anaesthesia or prior heat experience indicating that the age and physiological states of the animals before heat exposure are important determining factors for the outcome of thermal brain damage.

Significance of our findings

Our experimental observations on hyperthermia-induced brain edema and cell changes have added a new dimension in the field of heat stress and CNS injury. Our results clearly show that brain edema formation can occur in heat stress, the mechanisms of which are quite comparable to that of traumatic edema. Thus breakdown of BBB permeability is mainly responsible for the hyperthermic brain edema and cell changes. This breakdown of the BBB in hyperthermia can be prevented by many pharmacological agents either interfering with the stress mechanisms or influencing the metabolism of various neurochemical mediators. Thus the functional significance of our findings using a new approach of hyperthermic brain injury suggests that the mechanisms underlying cellular injury in the CNS following various types of insults such as ischemia, hypoxia, trauma, etc. are quite similar in nature. The magnitude and severity of the primary insult to the CNS mainly determines the final outcome of cell injury in a particular situation. The second most important point that has come from this study is that in any pathological condition, no single chemical compound or factor is responsibl for all the neuropathological changes seen in the CNS. In fact the final outcome is due to a combination of many factors and neurochemicals exerting a synergistic influence on the CNS. Thus to achieve a goal of neuroprotection these multiple factors must be considered in order to develop a suitable therapeutic strategy to treat the problems of CNS injury.

Future perspectivs

In order to understand the molecular mechanisms of heat stress-induced brain injury in detail, further investigations on additional factors involved in CNS injury and repair mechanism in our model are needed. Studies in our labouratory are thus in progress to examine brain damage and repair mechanisms in hyperthermia in relation to neurochemical metabolism, expression of immediate early genes, cytokines, growth factors and their receptors. Currently we are engaged in mapping of various neuropeptides, amino acids and their receptors at the protein as well as their mRNA levels in the CNS using immunohistochemistry and *in situ* hybridisation techniques in our model of hyperthermic brain injury.

Acknowledgements

This work is supported by grants from the Swedish Medical Research council no. 2710, 9459; Göran Gustafsson Foundation, Sweden, Astra Hässle, Mölndal, Sweden; Alexander Humboldt Foundation, Bonn, Germany; The University Grants Commission, New Delhi; Indian Council of Medical Research, New Delhi, India. The authors are grateful to Jorge Cervós-Navarro, Institute of Neuropathology, Free University Berlin, Germany and Prasanta Kumar Dey, Neurophysiology Research Unit, Department of Physiology, Banaras Hindu University, Varanasi, India where parts of the work reported in this review were carried out by HSS. The technical assistance of Aftab Ahmed, R.K. Gupta, Deep Chand Lal, Mohammad Siddiqqui (Varanasi), Katja Deparade, Elisabeth Scherer, Franziska Drum (Berlin), Ingmarie Olsson, Kärstin Flink, Madeleine Thörnwall, Madelien Jarild, Gunilla Tibling (Uppsala) and secretarial assistance of Kishori Ram, R.K. Ganguli (Varanasi), Angela Jan, Katherin Kern (Berlin), Aruna Misra, Gunilla Åberg, Gun Britt Lind, Agneta Bergström, Sigrid Pettersson, Eva Lundberg (Uppsala) are highly appreciated. We are grateful to Tord Loving for providing outstanding help in library facilities. The skilful assistance in photographic work by Frank Bittkowski (Uppsala), R.K. Srivastav (Varanasi), L. Schindler (Berlin) and computer assistance of Mathia Korves (Berlin), William Schannong (Uppsala) are acknowledged with thanks.

References

Adolph, E.F. (1947) Tolerance to heat and dehydration in several species of mammals. *Am. J. Physiol.*, 151: 564–757.

Adolph, E.F. and Fulton, W.B. (1924) The effects of exposure to high temperatures upon the circulation in man. *Am. J. Physiol.*, 67: 573–588.

Alabaster, V.A. (1977) Inactivation of endogenous amines in the lung. In: Y.S. Bakhle and J.R. Vanes (Eds.), *Metabolic Functions of the Lung*, Vol. 4, Marcel Dekker, New York, pp. 3–31.

Alpers, B.J. (1936) Hyperthermia due to lesions in the hypothalamus. *Arch. Neurol. Psychiatry*, 35: 30–42.

Aron, H. (1911) Investigation on the action of the tropical sun on men and animals. *Philippine J. Sci. B. Med. Sci.*, 6: 101–132.

Aukland, K. (1973) Autoregulation of interstitial fluid volume: Edema-preventing mechanisms. *Scand. J. Clin. Lab. Invest.*, 31: 247–254.

Austin, M.G. and Berry, J.W. (1956) Observation on one hundred case of heatstroke. *J. Am. Med. Assoc.*, 161: 1525–1529.

Baethmann, A. and Van Harreveld, A. (1973) Water and electrolyte distribution in grey matter rendered edematous with a metabolic inhibitor. *J. Neuropathol. Exp. Neurol.*, 32: 408–423.

Baca, G.M. and Palmer, G.C. (1978) Presence of hormonally-sensitive adenylate cyclase receptors in capillary enriched fraction from rat cerebral cortex. *Blood Vessels*, 15: 286–296.

Bakay, L. (1968) Changes in barrier effect in pathological states. *Prog. Brain Res.*, 29: 315–339.

Bakay, L. and Lee, J.C. (1965) *Cerebral Edema*, Thomas, Springfield, IL.

Black, K.L. (1995) Biochemical opening of the blood–brain barrier. *Adv. Drug Deliv. Rev*, 15: 37–52.

Blatteis, C. (1997) Thermoregulation: Recent Progress and New Frontiers. *Ann. New York Acad. Sci*, 813: 1–865.

Blum, H.F. (1945) The physiological effects of sunlight on man. *Physiol. Rev.*, 25: 483–530.

Bouyer, J.-J., Dedet, L., Debray, O. and Rougeul, A. (1978) Restraint in primate chair may cause unusual behaviour in baboons; electroencephalographic correlates and corrective effects of diazepam. *Electroencephalogr. Clin. Neurophysiol.*, 44: 562–567.

Bradbury, M.W.B. (1979) *The Concept of a Blood–Brain Barrier*, Chicester, London.

Bradbury, M.W.B. (1992) Physiology and Pharmacology of the Blood-Brain Barrier. In: *Handbook Exp. Pharmacol.*, 103: 1–450, Springer, Heidelberg.

Brahams, D. (1989) Heat stroke in training: a fatal case in Massachusetts. *Lancet*, ii, 1167.

Brightman, M.W. and Reese, T.S. (1969) Junctions between intimately apposed cell membranes in the vertebrate brain. *J. Cell Biol.*, 40(26): 99–123.

Britt, R.H., Lyons, B.E., Pounds, D.W. and Prionas, S.D. (1983) Feasibility of ultrasound hyperthermia in the treatment of malignant brain tumours. *Med. Instrum.*, 17: 172–177.

Britt, R.H., Lyons, B.E., Ryan, T., Saxer, E., Obana, W. and Rossi, G. (1984) Effect of whole body hyperthermia on auditory brainstem and somatosensory and visual evoked potentials. In: J.R.S. Hales (Ed.), *Thermal Physiology*, Raven, New York, pp. 519–523.

Bulochnik, E.D. and Zyablov, M.P. (1978) Effect of hyperthermia induced by a high ambient temperature on the direct cortical response. *Byulleten 'Eksperimental'noi Biologii i Meditsiny*, 84: 657–660.

Chakravarti, D.N. and Tyagi, N. (1938) Studies on effects of heat. *Indian J. Med. Res.*, 25: 791–827.

Cervós-Navarro, J. and Ferszt, R. (1980) Brain edema: Pathology, diagnosis and therapy. *Adv. Neurol.*, 20: 1–450.

Cervós-Navarro, J., Kannuki, S. and Nakagawa, Y. (1988) Blood–brain barrier (BBB): review from morphological aspect. *Histol. Histopathol.*, 3: 203–213.

Cervós-Navarro, J. and Urich, H. (1995) *Metabolic and Degenerative Diseases of the Central Nervous System: Pathology, Biochemistry and Genetics*, Academic Press, New York, pp. 1–775.

Chaouloff, F. (1993) Physiopharmacological interactions between stress hormones and central serotonergic systems. *Brain Res. Rev.*, 18: 1–32.

Chiueh, C.C., Gilbert, D.L. and Colton, C.A. (1994) The neurobiology of NO· and ·OH. *Ann. New York Acad. Sci.*, 738: 1–471.

Chrousos, G.P., McCarty, R., Pacak, K.G., Sternberg E., Gold, P.W. and Kvetnansky, R. (1995) Stress: Mechanisms and clinical implications. *Ann. New York Acad. Sci*, 771: 1–730.

Clasen, R.A., Prouty, R.R., Bingham, W.G., Martin, F.A. and Hass, G.M. (1957) Treatment of cerebral edema with intravenous hypertonic glucose, albumin and dextran. *Surg. Gynecol. Obstet.*, 104: 591–606.

Clasen, R.A., Cooke, P.M., Pandolfi, S. and Carnecki, G. (1963) The effects of focal freezing on the central nervous system. *Presbyterian St. Luke's Med. Bull.*, 2: 36–46.

Couraud, P. and Scherman, A. (1996) *Biology and Physiology of the Blood–Brain Barrier*, Plenum Press, New York, pp. 1–310.

Cournand, A., Riley, A., Bradley, R.L., Breed, E.S., Noble, R.P., Lauson, H.D., Gregersen, M.I. and Richards, D.W. (1943) Studies of the circulation in clinical shock. *Surgery*, 13: 964–995.

Davison, C. (1940) Disturbances of temperature regulation in man. *Res. Nerv. Ment. Dis. Proc.*, 20: 774–823.

Davson, H. (1967) *Physiology of the Cerebrospinal Fluid*, Churchill, London.

Dickson, J.A., Mackenzie, A. and McLeod, K. (1979) Temperature gradients in pigs during whole body hyperthermia at 42°C. *J. Appl. Physiol.*, 47: 712–717.

Driscoll, B.F., Kramer, A.J. and Kies, M.W. (1974) Myelin basic protein: Location of multiple independent antigenic regions. *Science*, 184: 73–75.

Dey, P.K. and Sharma, H.S. (1983) Ambient temperature and development of traumatic brain oedema in anaesthetized animals. *Indian J. Med. Res.*, 77: 554–563.

Dey, P.K. and Sharma, H.S. (1984) Influence of ambient temperature and drug treatments on brain oedema induced impact injury on skull in rat. *Indian J. Physiol. Pharmacol.*, 28: 177–186.

Dey, P.K., Sharma, H.S. and Kumar, A. (1988) Modification of plasma and brain 5-HT level, BBB permeability, brain oedema, rCBF and lung MAO activity under acute and chronic heat stress in rats. In: K.N. Sharma, W. Silvamurthy and N. Bhattacharya (Eds.), *Brain Psychophysiology of Stress*, Indian Council of Medical Research, New Delhi, pp. 38–47.

Dey, S., Dey, P.K. and Sharma, H.S. (1993) Regional metabolism of 5-hydroxytryptamine in brain under acute and chronic heat stress. *Indian J. Physiol. Pharmacol.*, 37: 8–12.

Eakins, K.G. (1977) Prostaglandin and non-prostaglandin mediated breakdown of the blood-aqueous barrier. *Exp. Eye Res.*, 25: 483–489.

Edvinsson, E. and McKenzie, E.T. (1977) Amine mechanisms in the cerebral circulation. *Pharmacol. Rev.*, 28: 275–348.

Elliott, K.A.C. and Jasper, H. (1949) Measurement of experimentally induced brain swelling and shrinkage. *Am. J. Physiol.*, 157: 122–128.

Eshel, G., Safar, P., Sassano, J. and Stezoski, W. (1990) Hyperthermia-induced cardiac arrest in monkeys. *Resuscitation*, 20: 129–143.

Essman, W. (1978) *Serotonin in Health and Disease*, Vols. I–V, Spectrum, New York.

Faden, A.I. and Salzman, S. (1992) Pharmacological strategies in CNS trauma. *Trends Pharmacol. Sci.*, 13: 29–35.

Fernstrom, J.D. and Wurtman, R.J. (1971) Brain serotonin content: Physiological dependence on plasma tryptophan levels. *Science*, 173: 149–152.

Fike, J.R., Gobbel, G.T., Satoh, T. and Stauffer, P.R. (1991) Normal brain response after interstitial microwave hyperthermia. *Int. J. Hyperthermia*, 7: 795–808.

Freeman, W. and Dumoff, E. (1944) Cerebellar syndrome following heat stroke. *Arch. Neurol. Psychiatry*, 51: 67–72.

Friedman, A., Kaufer, D., Shemer, J., Hendler, I., Soreq, H. and Tur-Kapsa, I. (1996) Pyridostigmine brain penetration under stress enhances neuronal excitability and induces early immediate transcriptional response. *Nature Med.*, 2: 1382–1385.

Froese, G., Das, R.M. and Dunscombe, P.B. (1991) The sensitivity of the thoracolumbar spinal cord in the mouse to hyperthermia. *Radiat. Res.*, 125: 173–180.

Gauss, H. and Meyer, K.A. (1917) Heat stroke: report of one hundred and fifty-eight cases from Cook County Hospital, Chicago. *Am. J. Med. Sci.*, 154: 554–564.

Go, K.G. and Baethmann, A. (1984) *Recent Progress in the Study and Therapy of Brain Edema*, Plenum Press, New York, pp. 1–480.

Goehlert, U.G., Ng Ying Kin, N.M.K. and Wolfe, L.S. (1981) Biosynthesis of prostaglandin in rat cerebral microvessels and the choroid plexus. *J. Neurochem.*, 36: 1192–1201.

Goffinet, D.R., Choit, K.Y. and Brown, J.M. (1977) The combined effects of hyperthermia and ionising radiation of the adult mouse spinal cord. *Radiat. Res.*, 72: 238–245.

Guyton, A.C. (1963) A concept of negative interstitial pressure based on pressures in implanted perforated capsules. *Circ. Res.*, 12: 399–412.

Haefely, W., Pieri, L., Polc, P. and Schaffner, R. (1981) General pharmacology and neuropharmacology of benzodiazepine derivatives. *Handbook Exp. Pharmacol.*, 55: 114–152.

Hagen, A.A., White, R.P. and Robertson, J.T. (1979) Synthesis of prostaglandin and thromboxane B2 by cerebral arteries. *Stroke*, 10: 306–309.

Hahn, G.M. (1982) *Hyperthermia and Cancer*, Plenum Press, New York.

Hall, W.W. and Wakefield, F.G. (1927) A study of experimental heatstroke. *J. Am. Med. Assoc.*, 89: 177–182.

Hanin, I. (1996) The Gulf War, stress and a leaky blood–brain barrier (News & Views). *Nature Med.*, 2: 1307–1308.

Hanukoglu, I. (1977) Prostaglandins as first mediators of stress. *New Engl. J. Med.*, 296: 1414–1415.

Harris, A.B., Erickson, L., Kendig, J.H., Mugrino, S. and Goldring, S. (1962) Observations on selective brain heating in dogs. *J. Neurosurg.*, 19: 514–521.

Hart, G.R., Anderson, R.J., Crumpler, C.P., Shulkin, A., Reed, G. and Knochel, J.P. (1982) Epidemic classical heat stroke: clinical characteristics and course of 28 patients. *Medicine*, 61: 189–197.

Hartman, F.W. and Major, R.C. (1935) Pathological changes resulting from accurately controlled artificial fever. *Am. J. Clin. Pathol.*, 5: 392–410.

Haubbard, R.W., Bowers, W.D., Mather, W.T., Curtis, F.C., Criss, R.E.L., Sheldon, G.M. and Ratteree, J.W.J. (1977) Rat model of acute heat stroke mortality. *J. Appl. Physiol.*, 42: 807–816.

Haubrich, D.R., Perez-Cruet, J. and Reid, W.D. (1973) Prostaglandin E1 causes sedation and increases 5-HT turnover in rat brain. *Br. J. Pharmacol.*, 48: 80–87.

Heilman, M.W. and Montgomery, E.S. (1936) Heat disease. *J. Ind. Hyg. Toxicol.*, 18: 651–667.

Hirano, A. (1971) Edema damage. *Neurosci. Res. Prog. Bull.*, 9: 493–496.

Hirano, A., Levine, S. and Zimmerman, H.M. (1967) Experimental cyanide encephalopathy: Electron microscopic observations of early lesions in white matter. *J. Neuropathol. Exp. Neurol.*, 26: 200–213.

Hoyer, D. and Martin, G.R. (1996) Classification and nomenclature of 5-HT receptors: A comment on current issues. *Behav. Brain Res.*, 73: 263–268.

Hökfelt, T., Elde, R., Johansson, O., Ljungdahl, Å., Schultzberg, M., Fuxe, K., Goldstein, M., Nilsson, G., Pernow, B., Terenius, L., Ganten, D., Jeffocate, S.L., Rehfeld, J. and Said, S. (1978) Distribution of peptide containing neurons. In: M.A. Lipton, A. DiMascio and K.F. Killam (Eds.), *Psychopharmacology: A Generation of Progress*, Raven Press, New York, pp. 39–66.

Ito, U., Baethmann, A., Hossmann, K-A., Kuroiwa, T., Marmarou, A. and Takakura, K. (1994) Brain Edema IX. *Acta Neurochir. (Wien)*, Suppl. 60: 1–485.

James, H.E., Baethmann, A., Marmarou, A., Marshall, L.F. and Reulen, H.-J. (1997) Brain Edema, X. *Acta Neurochir. (Wien)* Suppl., pp. 1–298.

Johansson, B.B., Owman, Ch. and Widner, H. (1990) Pathophysiology of the blood–brain barrier. Fernström Foundation Series 14, Elsevier, Amsterdam, pp. 1–340.

Joó, F., Rakonczay, Z. and Wollemann, M. (1975) cAMP-mediated regulation of the permeability in the brain capillaries. *Experientia*, 31: 582–584.

Joó, F. (1985) The blood–brain barrier *in vitro*: Ten years of research on microvessels isolated from the brain. *Neurochem. Int.*, 7: 1–25.

Joó, F. (1987) A unifying concept on the pathogenesis of brain oedemas. *Neuropathol. Appl. Neurobiol.*, 13: 161–167.

Klatzo, I. (1967) Presidential address — Neuropathological aspects of brain edema. *J. Neuropathol. Exp. Neurol.*, 26: 1–14.

Klatzo, I. (1972) Pathophysiological aspects of brain edema. In: H.-J. Reulen and K. Schurmann (Eds.), *Steroids and Brain Edema*, Springer, Berlin, pp. 1–8.

Klatzo, I. (1987) Pathophysiological aspects of brain edema. *Acta Neuropathol. (Berlin)*, 72: 236–239.

Klatzo, I. and Seitelberger, F. (1967) *Brain Edema*, Springer, Berlin, pp. 1–350.

Klatzo, I., Piraux, A. and Laskowski, E.J. (1958) The relationship between edema, blood–brain barrier and tissue elements in local brain injury. *J. Neuropathol. Exp. Neurol.*, 17: 548–564.

Klatzo, I., Wísniewski, H. and Smith, D.E. (1965) Observation on penetration of serum proteins into the central nervous system. *Prog. Brain Res.*, 15: 73–88.

Knochel, J.P. (1974) Environmental heat illness. An eclectic review. *Arch Intern. Med.*, 133: 841–864.

Kopp, I. and Solomon, H.C. (1937) Shock syndrome in therapeutic hyperpyrexia. *Arch. Int. Med.*, 60: 597–622.

Larsson, B., Skarby, T., Edvinsson, L., Hardebo, J.E. and Owman, Ch. (1980) Vincristine reduces damage of the blood–brain barrier induced by high intravascular pressure. *Neurosci. Lett.*, 17: 155–159.

Leaf, A. (1973) Cell swelling: A factor in ischemic tissue injury. *Circulation*, 48: 455–458.

Lee, D.H.K. (1964) Terrestrial animals in dry heat. In: D.B. Dill, E.F. Adolph and C.G. Wilber (Eds.), *Handbook Physiol., Section IV, Adaptation to the Environment*, American Physiological Society, Washington, DC, pp. 55–72.

Lieb, W.R. and Stein, W.D. (1971) The molecular basis of simple diffusion within biological membranes. *Curr. Top. Membr. Transp.*, 2: 1–39.

Lo, Y.C. (1989) The effects of ionizing radiation and hyperthermia on mouse spinal cord. Thesis, University of California, Los Angles, UMI MN, USA.

Lyons, B.E., Obana, W.G. and Borchich, J.K. et al. (1986) Chronic histological effects of ultrasonic hyperthermia on normal feline brain tissue. *Radiat. Res.*, 106: 234–251.

Macy, D.W., Macy, C.A., Scott, R.J., Gilette, E.L. and Speer, J.F. (1985) Physiological studies of whole-body hyperthermia in dogs. *Cancer Res.*, 45: 2769–2773.

Malamud, N., Haymaker, W. and Custer, R.P. (1946) Heat stroke. clinicopathological study of 125 fatal cases. *Milit. Surg.*, 99: 397–449.

Marsh, F. (1930) The etiology of heat stroke and sun traumatism. *Trans. R. Soc. Trop. Med. Hyg.*, 24: 257–288.

Marsh, R.R., Yamane, H. and Potsic, W.P. (1984) Auditory brain-stem response and temperature. Relationship in the guinea pig. *Electroencephalogr. Clin. Neurophysiol.*, 57: 289–293.

McKendrick, J.G. (1868) A case of meningo-cerebritis, caused probably by exposure to the sun. *Edinburgh Med. J.*, 14: 517–522.

McKenzie, P. and LeCount, E.R. (1918) Heat stroke. *J. Am. Med. Assoc.*, 71: 260–263.

Mellergard, P. and Nordström, C.H. (1990) Epidural temperature and possible intracerebral temperature gradients in man. *Br. J. Neurosurg.*, 4: 31–38.

Messiter, A.F. (1897) A case of insolation accompanied by hemiplegia. *Lancet*, 1: 1741–1742.

Miller, J.D. (1976) Pressure-volume response — clinical aspects. In: R. McLaurin (Ed.), *Chicago Conference on Neural Trauma*, Grunne and Stratton, New York, pp. 35–46.

Milton, A.S. (1994) *Physiology of Thermoregulation*, Birkhauser, Basel, pp. 1–405.

Mohanty, S., Dey, P.K., Sharma, H.S. and Ray, A.K. (1985) Experimental brain edema: Role of 5-HT. In: S. Mohanty and P.K. Dey (Eds.), *Brain Edema*, Banaras Hindu University, Bhargava Bhushan Press, Varanasi, India, pp. 19–27.

Mohanty, S., Dey, P.K., Sharma, H.S., Singh, S., Chansouria, J.P.N. and Olsson, Y. (1989) Role of histamine in traumatic brain edema. An experimental study in the rat. *J. Neurol. Sci.*, 90: 87–97.

Morgan, L.O. (1938) Cell changes in some of the hypothalamic nuclei in experimental fever. *J. Neurophysiol.*, 1: 281–285.

Morgan, L.O. and Vonderahe, A.R. (1939) The hypothalamic nuclei in heat stroke. *Arch. Neurol. Psychiatry*, 42: 83–91.

Mustafa, A., Sharma, H.S., Olsson, Y., Gordh, T., Thóren, P.,Sjöquist, P.-O., Roos, P., Adem, A. and Nyberg, F. (1995) Vascular permeability to growth hormone in the rat central nervous system after focal spinal cord injury. Influence of a new antioxidant compound H 290/51 and age. *Neurosci. Res.*, 23: 185–194.

Olesen, S.P. (1989) An electrophysiological study of microvascular permeability and its modulation by chemical mediators. *Acta Physiol. Scand.*, 136 (Suppl. 579): 1–28.

Pappius, H.M. (1970) The chemistry and fine structure in various types of cerebral edema. *Riv. Patol. Nerv. Ment.*, 91: 311–322.

Petrovich, Z., Langholz, B., Gibbs, F.A., Sapozink, M.D., Kapp, D., Stewart, R.J., Emami, B., Olesen, J., Senzer, N., Slater, J. and Astrahan, M. (1989) Regional hyperthermia for advanced tumors: a clinical study of 535 patients. *Int. J. Radiat. Oncol. (Biol. Phys.)*, 16: 601–607.

Plum, F., Posner, J.B. and Troy, B. (1963) Edema and necrosis in experimental cerebral infarction. *Arch. Neurol.*, 9: 563–570.

Prosser, C.L. (1964) Perspectives of adaptation: Theoretical aspects. In: D.B. Dill, E.F. Adolph and C.G. Wilber (Eds.), *Handbook Physiol., Section IV, Adaptation to the Environment*, American Physiological Society, Washington, pp. 11–25.

Rapoport, S.I. (1976) *Blood-Brain Barrier in Physiology and Medicine*, Raven Press, New York, pp. 1–380.

Reulen, H.-J. and Kreysch, H.G. (1973) Measurement of brain tissue pressure in cold induced cerebral oedema. *Acta Neurochir. (Wien)*, 29: 29–40.

Reulen, H-J., Baethmann, A., Fenstermacher, J., Marmarou, A. and Spatz, M. (1990) Brain Edema VIII, *Acta Neurochir. (Wien)*, Suppl. 51: 1–414.

Rosomoff, H.L. and Zugibe, F.T. (1963) Distribution of intracranial contents in experimental edema. *Arch. Neurol.*, 9: 26–34.

Ryan, U.S. (1982) Structural bases for metabolic activity. *Annu. Rev. Physiol.*, 44: 233–239.

Rymer, M.M. and Fishman, R.A. (1973) Protective adaptation of brain to water intoxication. *Arch. Neurol.*, 28: 49–54.

Salzman, S.K. (1990) *Neural Monitoring. The Prevention of Intraoperative Injury*, Humanna Press, New Jersey.

Samaras, G.M., Salcman, M., Cheung, A.Y., Abdo, H.S. and Schepp, R.S. (1982) Microwave-induced hyperthermia: an experimental adjunct for brain tumour therapy. *Natl. Cancer Inst. Monogr.*, 61: 477–482.

Sasaki, M. and Ide, C. (1989) Demyelination and remyelination in the dorsal funiculus of the rat spinal cord after heat injury. *J. Neurocytol.*, 18: 225–239.

Schickele, E. (1946) Environment in fatal heat stroke. An analysis of 157 cases occurring in the Armed Forces in theUnited States during World War II. *Milit. Surg.*, Dec. 1946.

Selye, H. (1976) *Stress in Health and Disease*, Butterworths, London.

Sharabi, Y., Danon, Y.L., Berkenstadt, H., Almog, S., Mimouni-Bloch, A., Zisman, A., Dani, S. and Atsmon, J. (1991) Survey of symptoms following intake of pyridostigmine during Persian Gulf War. *Isr. J. Med. Sci.*, 27: 656–658.

Sharma, H.S. (1982) *Blood-Brain Barrier in Stress*, Ph.D. thesis, Banaras Hindu University, Varanasi, India.

Sharma, H.S. (1987) Effect of captopril (a converting enzyme inhibitor) on blood–brain barrier permeability and cerebral blood flow in normotensive rats. *Neuropharmacology*, 26: 85–92.

Sharma, H.S. and Dey, P.K. (1978) Influence of heat and immobilization stressors on the permeability of blood–brain and blood-CSF barriers. *Indian J. Physiol. Pharmacol.*, 22 Suppl. II: 59–60.

Sharma, H.S. and Dey, P.K. (1981) Impairment of blood–brain barrier by immobilization stress: role of serotonin. *Indian J. Physiol. Pharmacol.*, 25: 111–122.

Sharma, H.S. and Dey, P.K. (1984) Role of 5-HT on increased permeability of blood–brain barrier under heat stress. *Indian J. Physiol. Pharmacol.*, 28: 259–267.

Sharma, H.S. and Dey, P.K. (1986a) Probable involvement of 5-hydroxytryptamine in increased permeability of blood–brain barrier under heat stress. *Neuropharmacology*, 25: 161–167.

Sharma, H.S. and Dey, P.K. (1986b) Influence of long-term immobilization stress on regional blood–brain barrier permeability, cerebral blood flow and 5-HT level in conscious normotensive young rats. *J. Neurol. Sci.*, 72: 61–76.

Sharma, H.S., Dey, P.K. and Ashok Kumar (1986) Role of circulating 5-HT and lung MAO activity in physiological processes of heat adaptation in conscious young rats. *Biomedicine*, 6: 31–40.

Sharma, H.S. and Dey, P.K. (1987) Influence of long-term acute heat exposure on regional blood–brain barrier permeability, cerebral blood flow and 5-HT level in conscious normotensive young rats. *Brain Res.*, 424: 153–162.

Sharma, H.S. and Dey, P.K. (1988) EEG changes following increased blood–brain barrier permeability under long-term immobilization stress in young rats. *Neurosci. Res.*, 5: 224–239.

Sharma, H.S. and Olsson, Y. (1990) Edema formation and cellular alterations following spinal cord injury in rat and their modification with p-chlorophenylalanine. *Acta Neuropathol. (Berlin)*, 79: 604–610.

Sharma, H.S. and Cervós-Navarro, J. (1990a) Brain oedema and cellular changes induced by acute heat stress in young rats. *Acta Neurochir.* (Wien), Suppl. 51: 383–386.

Sharma, H.S. and Cervós-Navarro, J. (1990b) Nimodipine improves cerebral blood flow and reduces brain edema, cellular damage and blood–brain barrier permeability following heat stress in young rats. In: J. Krieglstein and H. Oberpichler (Eds.), *Pharmacology of Cerebral Ischemia*, CRC Press, Boca Raton, FL, pp. 303–310.

Sharma, H.S. and Cervós-Navarro, J. (1990c) Pathophysiology of blood–brain barrier in stress. *Clin. Neuropathol.*, 9: 111.

Sharma, H.S., Olsson, Y. and Dey, P.K. (1990) Changes in blood–brain barrier and cerebral blood flow following elevation of circulating serotonin level in anaesthetized rats. *Brain Res.*, 517: 215–223.

Sharma, H.S. and Cervós-Navarro, J. (1991) Role of histamine in the pathophysiology of heat stress. In: H. Timmermann and van der Groot (Eds.), *Recent Perspectives in Histamine Research, Agents Actions* Suppl. 33: 97–102.

Sharma, H.S., Zimmer, C. and Cervós-Navarro, J. (1991a) Neuropathological aspects of acute heat exposure in young rats. *Clin. Neuropathol.*, 10: 315.

Sharma, H.S., Cervós-Navarro, J. and Dey, P.K. (1991b) Acute heat exposure causes cellular alteration in cerebral cortex of young rats. *NeuroReport*, 2: 155–158.

Sharma, H.S., Cervós-Navarro, J. and Dey, P.K. (1991c) Rearing at high ambient temperature during later phase of the brain development enhances functional plasticity of the CNS and induces tolerance to heat stress. An experimental study in the conscious normotensive young rats. *Brain Dysfunction*, 4: 104–124.

Sharma, H.S., Cervós-Navarro, J., Gosztonyi, G. and Dey, P.K. (1992a) Role of serotonin in traumatic brain injury. An experimental study in the rat. In: M. Globus and W.D. Dietrich (Eds.), *The Role of Neurotransmitters in Brain Injury*, Plenum Press, New York, pp. 147–152.

Sharma, H.S., Zimmer, C., Westman, J. and Cervós-Navarro, J. (1992b) Acute systemic heat stress increases glial fibrillary acidic protein immunoreactivity in brain. An experimental study in the conscious normotensive young rats. *Neuroscience*, 48: 889–901.

Sharma, H.S., Nyberg, F., Cervós-Navarro, J. and Dey, P.K. (1992c) Histamine modulates heat stress induced changes in blood–brain barrier permeability, cerebral blood flow, brain oedema and serotonin levels: An experimental study in conscious young rats. *Neuroscience*, 50: 445–454.

Sharma, H.S., Kretzschmar, R., Cervós-Navarro, J., Ermisch, A., Rühle, H-J. and Dey, P.K. (1992d) Age-related pathophysiology of the blood-brain barrier in heat stress. *Progress in Brain Res.*, 91: 189–196.

Sharma, H.S., Westman, J., Nyberg, F., Cervós-Navarro, J. and Dey, P.K. (1992e) Role of serotonin in heat adaptation: An experimental study in the conscious young rat. *Endocr. Regul.*, 26: 133–142.

Sharma, H.S., Westman, J., Cervós-Navarro, J. and Gosztonyi, G. (1992f) Acute systemic heat exposure increases heat shock protein (HSP-70 kD) immunoreactivity in the brain and spinal cord of young rats. *Clin. Neuropathol.*, 11: 174–175.

Sharma, H.S., Nyberg, F., Cervós-Navarro, J. and Dey, P.K. (1992g) Role of catecholamines in the pathophysiology of heat stress. In: *Proc. Int. Catechol. Symp.*, p. 287, June 22–26, Amsterdam.

Sharma, H.S., Olsson, Y., Nyberg, F. and Dey, P.K. (1993a) Prostaglandins modulate alterations of microvascular permeability, blood flow, edema and serotonin levels following spinal cord injury. An experimental study in the rat. *Neuroscience*, 57: 443–449.

Sharma, H.S., Olsson, Y. and Cervós-Navarro, J. (1993b) P-Chlorophenylalanine, a serotonin synthesis inhibitor, reduces the response of glial fibrillary acidic protein induced by trauma to the spinal cord. *Acta Neuropathol. (Berlin)* 86: 422–427.

Sharma, H.S., Westman, J., Nyberg, F., Cervós-Navarro, J. and Dey, P.K. (1994a) Role of serotonin and prostaglandins in brain edema induced by heat stress. An experimental study in the rat. *Acta Neurochir.*, Suppl. 60: 65–70.

Sharma, H.S., Westman, J., Nyberg, F., Cervós-Navarro, J. and Dey, P.K. (1994b) Role of neurochemicals in the blood–brain barrier permeability, cerebral blood flow, vasogenic oedema and cell changes in heat stress. Experimental observations in the rat. *J. Physiol. (Lond.)*, 480: 12.

Sharma, H.S., Westman, J., Nyberg, F., Zimmer, C., Cervós-Navarro, J. and Dey, P.K. (1994c) Selective vulnerability of rat hippocampus in heat stress. In: A.S. Milton (Ed.), *Temperature Regulation*, Adv. Pharmacol. Sci., Birkhauser, Basel, pp. 267–272.

Sharma, H.S., Westman, J., Nyberg, F., Cervós-Navarro, J. and Dey, P.K. (1994d) Neuroprotective effects of an extract of Gingko biloba (EGB-761) in heat stress induced brain damage in the rat. In: E. Zeisberger, E. Schönbaum and P. Lomax (Eds.), *Thermal Balance in Health and Disease, Recent Basic Research and Clinical Progress*, Adv. Pharmacol. Sci., Birkhauser, Basel, pp. 461–468.

Sharma, H.S., Olsson, Y. and Nyberg, F. (1995a) Influence of dynorphin-A antibodies on the formation of edema and cell changes in spinal cord trauma. In: F. Nyberg, H.S. Sharma and Z. Wissenfeld-Halin (Eds.), *Progress in Brain Res.*, Vol. 104, Elsevier, Amsterdam, pp. 401–416.

Sharma, H.S., Olsson, Y., Pearsson, S. and Nyberg, F. (1995b) Trauma induced opening of the blood-spinal cord barrier is reduced by indomethacin, an inhibitor of prostaglandin synthesis. Experimental observations in the rat using ^{131}I-sodium, Evans blue and lanthanum as tracers. *Restor. Neurol. Neurosci.*, 7: 207–215.

Sharma, H.S., Olsson, Y. and Dey, P.K. (1995c) Serotonin as a mediator of increased microvascular permeability of the brain and spinal cord. Experimental observations in anaesthetised rats and mice. In: J. Greenwood, D. Begley, M. Segal and S. Lightman (Eds.), *New Concepts of a Blood-Brain Barrier*, Plenum Press, New York, pp. 75–80.

Sharma, H.S., Olsson, Y. and Westman, J. (1995d) A serotonin synthesis inhibitor, *p*-chlorophenylalanine reduces the heat shock protein response following trauma to the spinal cord. An immunohistochemical and ultrastructural study in the rat. *Neurosci. Res.*, 21: 241–249.

Sharma, H.S., Westman, J., Cervós-Navarro, J., Dey, P.K. and Nyberg, F. (1995e) Alterations of amino acid neurotransmitters following heat stress. *Amino Acids*, 6: 33.

Sharma, H.S., Westman, J., Olsson, Y. and Alm, P. (1996a) Involvement of nitric oxide in acute spinal cord injury: an immunohistochemical study using light and electron microscopy in the rat. *Neurosci. Res.*, 24: 373–384.

Sharma, H.S., Westman, J., Cervós-Navarro, J., Dey, P.K. and Nyberg, F. (1996b) Probable involvement of serotonin in the increased permeability of the blood–brain barrier by forced swimming. An experimental study using Evans blue and ^{131}I-sodium tracers in the rat. *Behav. Brain Res.*, 72: 189–196.

Sharma, H.S., Westman, J., Cervós-Navarro, J. and Nyberg, F. (1996c) A 5-HT$_2$ receptor mediated breakdown of the blood–brain barrier permeability and brain pathology in heat stress. An experimental study using cyproheptadine and ketanserin in young rats. In: P. Couraud and A. Scherman (Eds.), *Biology and Physiology of the Blood–Brain Barrier*, Plenum Press, New York, pp. 117–124.

Sharma, H.S., Westman, J., Cervós-Navarro, J., Dey, P.K. and Nyberg, F. (1997a) Blood–brain barrier in stress: a gateway to various brain diseases. In: R. de Kloet, D. Ben-Nathan and R. Levy (Eds.), *New Frontiers of Stress: Modulation of Brain Function*, Harwood, Amsterdam.

Sharma, H.S., Westman, J., Alm, P., Sjöquist, P.-Ö., Cervós-Navarro, J. and Nyberg, F. (1997b) Involvement of nitric oxide in the pathophysiology of acute heat stress in the rat. influence of a new antioxidant compound h 290/51. *Ann. New York Acad. Sci.*, 813: 581–590.

Sharma, H.S., Westman, J., Cervós-Navarro, J., Dey, P.K. and Nyberg, F. (1997c) Opioid receptor antagonists attenuate heat stress induced reduction in cerebral blood flow, increased blood–brain barrier permeability, vasogenic edema and cell changes in the rat. *Ann. New York Acad. Sci.*, 813: 559–571.

Siesjö, B.K. (1978) *Brain Energy Metabolism*, Wiley, Chicester.

Sminia, P., Troost, D. and Haveman, J. (1989) Histopathological changes after 434 MHz microwave hyperthermia in the region of the rat cervical spinal cord. *Int. J. Hyperthermia*, 5: 85–98.

Sminia, P., van der Zee, J., Wondergem, J. and Haveman, J. (1994) Effect of hyperthermia on the central nervous system: a review. *Int. J. Hyperthermia*, 10: 1–30.

Sneed, P.K., Matsumoto, K., Stauffer, P.R., Fike, J.R., Smith, V. and Gutin, P.H. (1986) Interstitial microwave hyperthermia in a canine brain model. *Int. J. Radiat. Oncol. (Biol. Phys.)*, 12: 1887–1897.

Sneed, P.K., Stauffer, P.R., Gutin, P.H., Phillips, T.L., Suen, S., Weaver, K.A., Lamb, S.A., Ham, B., Prados, M.D., Larson, D.A. and Wara, W.M. (1991) Interstitial irradiation and hyperthermia for the treatment of recurrent malignant brain tumors. *Neurosurgery*, 28: 206–215.

Snyder, S.H., Axelrod, J. and Zweig, M. (1965) A sensitive and specific fluorescence assay for tissue serotonin. *Biochem. Pharmacol.*, 14: 831–835.

Starling, E.H. (1896) On the absorption of fluids from the connective tissue spaces. *J. Physiol. (Lond.)*, 19: 312–326.

Staub, N.C. (1974) Pulmonary edema. *Physiol. Rev.*, 54: 678–811.

Stein, L., Wise, C.D. and Berger, B.D. (1973) Antianxiety action of benzodiazepines: decrease in activity of serotonergic neurones in the punishment system. In: S. Grattini, E. Mussini and L.O. Rindall (Eds.), *The Benzodiazepines*, Raven Press, New York, pp. 299–326.

Stern, J.R., Eggleston, L.V., Hems, R. and Krebs, H.A. (1949) Accumulation of glutamic acid in isolated brain tissue. *Biochem. J.*, 44: 410–418.

Stern, W.E. (1959) Studies in experimental brain swelling and brain compression. *J. Neurosurg.*, 16: 676–704.

Sterner, S. (1990) Summer heat illness. *Postgrad. Med.*, 87: 67–73.

Tanaka, R., Kim, C.H., Yamada, N. and Saito, Y. (1987) Radiofrequency hyperthermia for malignant brain tumors: preliminary results of clinical trials. *Neurosurgery*, 21: 478–483.

Thrall, D.E., Prescott, D.M., Samulski, T.V., Dewhirst, M.W., Cline, J.M., Lee, J., Page, R.L. and Oleson, J.R. (1992) Serious toxicity associated with annular microwave array induction of whole-body hyperthermia in normal dogs. *Int. J. Hyperthermia*, 8: 23–32.

Toh, C.C. (1960) Effect of temperature on the 5-hydroxytryptamine content of tissues. *J. Physiol. (Lond.)*, 151: 410–415.

Van der Zee, J. (1987) Whole body hyperthermia. The development of and experience with a clinical method. Thesis, Erasmus University, Rotterdam, The Netherlands.

Van Harreveld, A. and Dubrovsky, B.O. (1967) Water and electrolytes in hydrated grey and white matter. *Brain Res.*, 4: 81–86.

Wahl, M., Unterberg, A., Baethmann, A. and Schilling, L. (1988) Mediators of blood–brain barrier dysfunction and formation of vasogenic brain edema. *J. Cereb. Blood Flow Metab.*, 8: 621–634.

Wallace, A.W. (1943) Heat exhaustion. *Milit. Surg.*, 93: 140–146.

Weiner, J.C. (1938) Experimental study of heat collapse. *J. Ind. Hyg. Toxicol.*, 20: 389–400.

Weisenburg, T.H. (1912) Nervous symptoms following sunstroke. *J. Am. Med. Assoc.*, 58: 2015–2017.

Westergaard, E. (1980) Ultrastructural permeability properties of cerebral microvasculature under normal and experimen-

412

tal conditions after application of tracers. *Adv. Neurol.*, 28: 55–74.

Wiederhielm, C.A. (1968) Dynamics of transcapillary fluid exchange. *J. Gen. Physiol.*, 52: 29S–63S.

Wilcox, W.H. (1920) The nature, prevention and treatment of heat hyperpyrexia; the clinical aspect. *Br. Med. J.*, 1: 392–397.

Wilson, G. (1940) The cardiopathology of heat-stroke. *J. Am. Med. Assoc.*, 114: 557–558.

Wilson, S.J. and Doan, C.A. (1939) The pathogenesis of hemorrhage in artificially induced fever. *Ann. Inter. Med.*, 13: 1214–1229.

Winter, A., Laing, J., Paglione, R. and Sterzer, F. (1985) Microwave hyperthermia for brain tumors. *Neurosurgery*, 17: 387–399.

Youdim, M.B.H. and Holzbauer, M. (1980) Physiological aspects of the oxidative deamination of monoamines. *Ciba Found. Symp. (New York)*, 78: 129–134.

Youdim, M.B.H., Bakhle, Y.S. and Ben Harari, R.R. (1980) Inactivation of monoamines by the lung. In: *Metabolic Activities of the Lung, Ciba Found. Symp.* (new series), 78: 105–134.

Zeisburger, E., Schönbaum, E. and Lomax, P. (1994) *Thermal Balance in Health and Diseases. Recent Basic Research and Clinical Progress*, Adv. Pharmacol. Sci., Birkhauser, Basel.

Zimmerman, H.M. (1940) Temperature disturbances and the hypothalamus. *Res. Nerv. Ment. Dis. Proc.*, 20: 824–840.

H.S. Sharma and J. Westman (Eds.)
Progress in Brain Research, Vol 115
© 1998 Elsevier Science BV. All rights reserved.

CHAPTER 19

Blood–brain barrier permeability during hyperthermia

Richard R. Shivers* and John A. Wijsman

Department of Zoology, University of Western Ontario, London, Ontario N6A 5B7, Canada

Introduction

The blood–brain barrier has been defined as a selectively permeable interface between the vascular system and the extracellular milieu of the central nervous system (Rapoport, 1975b). The anatomical basis of the barrier was clearly shown by Brightman and Reese (1969) and Brightman et al. (1970) to be the tight junctions between endothelial cells that line brain microvessels. When the junction-sealed cells are intact, the interface (barrier) between blood and tissue fluid can be breached only by a highly selective molecular transport system (Rapoport, 1975b). Following the primary elucidation of barrier structure, numerous investigators added support to the tight junction of the endothelial cell as the main element of the barrier (Brightman et al., 1973; Shivers, 1979a; Shivers et al., 1984a). In fact, one study demonstrated that the tight junctions of isolated rat brain microvessels could withstand substantial abuse during isolation and subsequent storage, without losing the precise ultrastructural morphology associated with intact junctions (Gonzalez-Mariscal et al., 1984; Shivers et al., 1984a).

Intense studies of the barrier under both normal, as well as pathological conditions, have subsequently provided evidence for a second component to the blood–brain barrier, the transendothelial channel/vesicular system (Joo, 1971; Westergaard et al., 1976, 1977, 1978; Westergaard, 1977; Shivers, 1979b; Shinowara et al., 1982; Lossinsky et al., 1983; Farrell and Shivers, 1984; Shivers and Harris, 1984b; Lossinsky et al., 1986, 1989; Wijsman and Shivers, 1993). There is exceptionally strong support, provided mainly by electron microscope studies, for this dynamic alternate route for extravasation of tracer molecules as well as substances present in blood, to the brain parenchyma.

The blood–brain barrier is remarkably sensitive to a broad spectrum of physiological and invasive insults, that are manifest as detectable leaks of molecules from the blood into the extracellular compartment of the central nervous system (Rapoport, 1975a, 1976; Sterrett et al., 1976; Westergaard et al., 1976, 1977, 1978; Hedley-Whyte et al., 1977; Johansson and Nilsson, 1977; Shivers, 1979b; Cervos-Navarro et al., 1983; Lossinsky et al., 1983, 1989; Neuwelt et al., 1983; Farrell and Shivers, 1984; Shivers and Harris, 1984b; Rosenblum, 1986; Urakawa et al., 1995). In many instances, including those not cited here, the consequences of increased barrier permeability include accumulation of unwanted molecules in the brain with a concomitant disturbance in normal brain function. Many studies are currently under way which intend to describe the detailed

---

*Corresponding author. Tel: +1 519 6613133; fax: +1 519 6612014; e-mail: rshivers@julian.uwo.ca

mechanisms whereby the blood–brain interface is breached and, more importantly, how these events can be reversed, or prevented. For example, the possibility of reversible opening of the blood–brain barrier in order to deliver anti-tumor drugs, which are normally excluded by the barrier, has been supported by numerous feasibility studies (Rapoport, 1975b; Neuwelt et al., 1981, 1983, 1984; Bodor and Brewster, 1983). Certainly, manipulation of the blood–brain interface for the purpose of clinical management of brain disorders is today, a workable reality.

The tremendous assortment of physiological and physical insults that result in dysfunction of the blood–brain barrier is overwhelming. One of these, hyperthermia, is of particular interest and importance due to its deleterious effects on the blood–brain barrier. Fluctuations in environmental conditions of temperature constitute one source of potentially harmful stresses on the nervous system (Emami et al., 1980; Song, 1984; Miller et al., 1987; Leigh, 1988; Shivers et al., 1988; Moriyama et al., 1991; Wijsman and Shivers, 1993; Fahim and El-Sabban, 1995; Urakawa et al., 1995). A second source of variation in temperature could come from failure of an organism's thermoregulatory system; an event which could cause malfunction of the barrier (Del Maestro et al., 1979; Satoh et al., 1989; Dietrich et al., 1990; Moriyama, 1990; Lee et al., 1992; Koga et al., 1993; Urakawa et al., 1995). Finally, mechanical devices such as microwave ovens, magnetic resonance imaging equipment and other such types of apparatus, which are a source of heat-generating radiation, can have serious consequences on brain blood vessel endothelial cells (Oscar and Hawkins, 1977; Lin and Lin, 1982; Shivers et al., 1987; Tanaka et al., 1987; Prato et al., 1990, 1994).

It is the concept of hyperthermic stress on brain microvessel endothelial cells, i.e. the blood–brain barrier, that will be discussed in this review. The survey will document the current state of knowledge regarding thermal manipulation of the brain microvessel wall and its permeability, and consider the validity of parameters that are currently used as indicators of barrier function/dysfunction. Finally, this essay will examine the influence of stress and subsequent heat shock protein synthesis on cells of the barrier. Are brain microvessel endothelial cells heat-conditioned by initial exposures to heat shock or stress situations? What consequence does conditioning play on the outcome of hyperthermic studies of microvessels? These questions have great relevance for correct interpretation of results of experimental manipulation of temperature in brain microvessels or interpretation of events resulting from episodes of stress on brain microvessels.

Electron microscopy of heat damaged barrier

The most common approach to the study of the blood–brain barrier is to employ a protein tracer which will leak from brain microvessels when the vessel permeability is compromised (Brightman et al., 1973; Westergaard, 1977; Shivers, 1979a,b; Cervos-Navarro et al., 1983; Farrell and Shivers, 1984; Shivers and Harris, 1984b; Lossinsky et al., 1986; Wijsman and Shivers, 1993). The ability of this procedure to detect changes in vessel permeability depends on the ability of the electron microscopist to visualize (recognize) tracer reaction products in thin sections of plastic-embedded tissue (Shinowara et al., 1982) (Fig. 1). The greater the amount of tracer, the easier it is to see in the electron microscope and consequently, the greater the amount of tracer visible, the greater the damage and resultant leak to the endothelium (Fig. 2). The concern that must be expressed here is that this sort of detection system is not capable of resolving small amounts of extravasated tracer; for example, if 1/10th of the tracer shown in Figs. 1 and 2, 4a and 4b, and 5b of Wijsman and Shivers (1993) was all that was extravasated from a damaged microvessel, it would likely not be recognized by a microscopist. It is essential to establish practical limits on the resolution of horseradish peroxidase as an indicator of blood–brain microvessel permeability or, integrity.

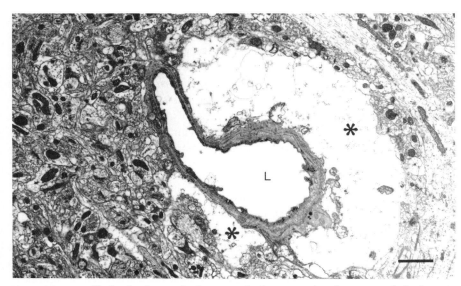

Fig. 1. Many capillaries in the cerebral cortex of mice exposed to heat stress (colonic temperature of 40°C, 60–135 min) are surrounded by a perivascular edema. This is seen in electron micrographs as grossly swollen astrocytic foot processes (asterisks) surrounding capillaries that often are compressed. Although there is evidence of horseradish peroxidase tracer within vesicles and tubulo-vesicle complexes in the endothelial cells, there is often no evidence of tracer extravasation from the capillary. Obviously in these capillaries there has been a substantial blood–brain barrier leak that is not discernable by high molecular weight tracers such as horseradish peroxidase. L = capillary lumen. Bar = 2.5 μm.

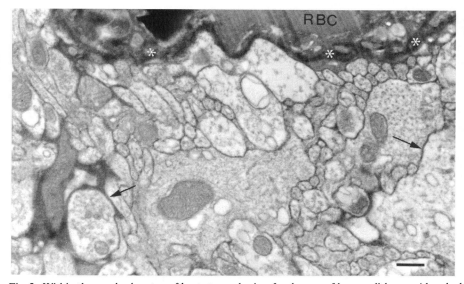

Fig. 2. Within the cerebral cortex of heat-stressed mice, focal areas of horseradish peroxidase leakage are seen by light microscopy. Examination of these areas by electron microscopy reveals horseradish peroxidase tracer within the endothelial cells, often completely permeating the basal lamina (asterisks) and extensive extravasation into the surrounding neuropil. Tracer can be seen surrounding the perivascular cells and astrocyte foot processes (arrows). Swollen astrocyte foot processes are also visible. RBC = red blood cell. Bar = 0.5 μm.

Other investigators have employed freeze-fracture, to study the blood−brain barrier (Shivers and Brightman, 1976; Shivers, 1979a,b; Farrell and Shivers, 1984; Shivers et al., 1984a, 1987, 1988; Kato et al., 1992). Examination of elements of tight junctions exposed during freeze-fracture can serve as a relatively reliable method for assessing intactness of the junctions (Shivers, 1979b; Shivers et al., 1984a, 1985, 1987; Wijsman and Shivers, 1993) (Figs. 3 and 4). Although in some respects, freeze-fracture analysis of blood−brain barrier tight junction integrity may be reliable (Fig. 4), the technique does suffer a severe sampling deficiency. Vast expanses of intramembrane surface must be scanned at moderately high magnification (10 000−15 000 diameters) in the electron microscope to even detect the presence of junctions. Often, junction structure is minimally displayed so that accurate conclusions about junction structure are not possible (to formulate) (Fig. 3). The preceding comments on analytical paradigms which are currently used in morphological assessments of the blood−brain barrier suggest they are severely limited in their ease of use and accuracy. As measures of barrier structure they have essentially poor resolution (sensitivity). This assessment of the technical features of barrier detection is necessary in order to properly approach a consideration of the effects of hyperthermia on brain microvessel endothelial cells and ways in which these effects can be detected and analysed. Recent advances in analytical and quantitative freeze-fracture cytochemistry (Severs and Robenek, 1983; Fugimoto, 1995) will ensure the future usefulness of freeze-fracture as a tool to measure the blood−brain barrier.

Physiological studies of heat-damaged barrier

Physiological manipulation studies have been carried out on the blood−brain barrier by many investigators (Rapoport, 1975a for example). In particular, hyperthermia has been used as a primary effector of changes in the permeability of brain microvessel endothelium (Sharma et al., 1992; Dey et al., 1993; Fajardo and Prionas, 1994; Ikeda et al., 1994; Ohmoto et al., 1996). These studies which serve as good examples of heat manipulation of the barrier have employed Evans Blue (either a visual assay or spectrophotometric analysis), fluorescent dextran, and various radiolabelled tracers to indicate leaks in the barrier.

A primary problem with such studies has been the difficulty in establishing exactly what conditions are necessary to open the barrier. Sharma et al. (1992) used 38°C on adult animals and failed to measure any tracer extravasation. In addition, they failed to define the practical limits of resolution of their study, so that if a particularly sensitive tracer had been used, barrier leakage might have been detected. Furthermore, most studies employing heat shock have used temperatures of at least 41°C up to 45°C to elicit blood−brain barrier defects (Shivers et al., 1988; Wijsman and Shivers, 1993; Ikeda et al., 1994).

Two of the best studies using hyperthermia to stress the blood−brain barrier have been done by Ohmoto et al. (1996) and Ikeda et al. (1994). The conditions for heat shock were carefully documented and in addition, several mechanisms for hyperthermia-induced brain injury were recognized. Included in these were cerebral ischemia, membrane permeability increases, and release of various neurochemicals which could cause brain damage (Sharma et al., 1991). Other problems that can be encountered with analyses of hyperthermic effects on blood−brain barrier integrity include cerebral capillary flow dynamics and consequent variability in flushing of capillaries (not 100%). Extravasation of Evans Blue as described in Ohmoto et al. (1996) signifies a massive breakdown of barrier permeability. Observation of Evans Blue on a macroscopic level and on a light microscopic level surely must reflect saturation of brain extracellular milieu in the neighbourhood of the compromised capillary(ies). Leaks of tracer of this magnitude are indicative of irreversible damage to microvessel endothelial cells; not a subtle opening of the blood−brain barrier (Nakajima et al., 1993).

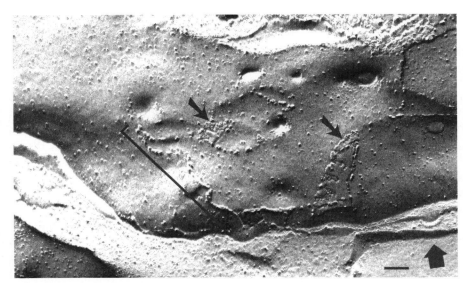

Fig. 3. A freeze-fracture replica of brain microvascular endothelial cells from heat-stressed mice presents a loss of tight junction complexity and organization. The normal tight junction structure of many anastamosing strands of intramembrane particles (IMPs) is not seen; in its place is a collection of IMPs that is suggestive of strands but are not tightly associated (brackets) and several aggregations of IMPs (arrows) with no evidence of strand structure. The lack of tight junction integrity in this capillary suggests that interendothelial cell leakage may have occurred at this site. Large arrow = direction of shadowing. Bar = 0.2 μm.

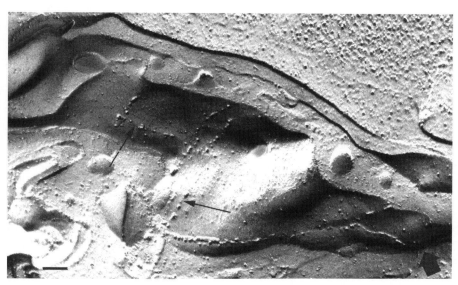

Fig. 4. This platinum replica of a heat-stressed mouse brain microvascular endothelial cell contains a tight junctional area with more retained structure than Fig. 3. Although the complex parallel and anastomosing strand structure is still visible, there are large spaces (greater than a single IMP) (arrows) within these strands indicating a loss of tight junction integrity. This loss of tight junction structure may be due to a reduction in production of IMPs by the cell, a reduction in the translocation of IMPs to the plasma membrane, increased destruction of IMPs, changes in membrane fluidity due to increased temperatures or other factors. Bar = 0.2 μm.

Discussion

Hyperthermia affects microvessel endothelial cells of the central nervous system (Oscar and Hawkins, 1977; Del Maestro et al., 1979; Preston et al., 1979; White, 1980a,c; Inasi and Brown, 1982; Lin and Lin, 1982; Shivers et al., 1988; Satoh et al., 1989; Dietrich et al., 1990; Moriyama, 1990; Moriyama et al., 1991; Lee et al., 1992; Wijsman and Shivers, 1993; Fahim and El-Sabban, 1995; Gobbel et al., 1995; Urakawa et al., 1995). Most studies report the consequences of sublethal hyperthermia on brain vasculature, to include an increased permeability of the barrier (Laszlo, 1992; Nakajima et al., 1993; and previous refs.). In addition to brain microvessels, hyperthermia also affects non-vascular cells of the brain. Glial cells such as astrocytes readily respond to elevation in temperature (Emami et al., 1980; Harper et al., 1990; Koga et al., 1993; Lee et al., 1992; Miller et al., 1987; Overgaard, 1977; Raaphorst et al., 1995; Salcman and Sammaras, 1981; Song et al., 1991; Tanaka et al., 1990). Responses of brain microvessels, glial cells, and selected brain tumors to hyperthermia, range from increased permeability of vessel endothelium (Wijsman and Shivers, 1993) to alterations in patterns of protein synthesis.

A universal response of cells to hyperthermia is a redirection of protein synthesis activity to produce a 'new' group of heat-shock proteins (Ashburner, 1982; Ashburner and Bonner, 1979; Atkinson and Walden, 1985; Gobbel et al., 1995; Inasi and Brown, 1982; Lee et al., 1992; Li and Laszlo, 1985; Rodenhiser et al., 1985; Shivers et al., 1988; White, 1980a,b,c, 1981a,b; White and Currie, 1982). It is generally accepted that similar or identical 'stress' proteins are made by cells in response to a wide variety of stress situations (Ashburner, 1982; Rodenhiser et al., 1985; White, 1980b; White and Currie, 1982; Wolffe et al., 1984), including for example, slicing fresh brain tissue for *in vitro* studies (White, 1981a). A broad range of parameters have been examined and deemed reflective of the heat-shock condition. Included in these features are increased membrane fluidity (Cossins, 1983; Cossins and Prosser, 1982; Dynlacht and Fox, 1992a, 1992b; Harper et al., 1990; Laszlo, 1992; Martin et al., 1976; Rice et al., 1986; Shivers et al., 1988; White, 1980b), synthesis of heat shock proteins (all references above), and various changes to vesicular and tubular components of microvascular endothelial cells (Lossinsky et al., 1989; Preston et al., 1979; Shinowara et al., 1982; Shivers and Harris, 1984b; Westergaard et al., 1976, 1977; Wijsman and Shivers, 1993). Numerous reviews are available for discussion of details of the heat-shock response by cells and tissues (e.g. Atkinson and Walden, 1985; Rodenhiser et al., 1985). The important point to note in this discussion is that all cells examined, redirect their protein synthetic activities to produce a new set of proteins (heat shock; stress) in response to hyperthermia and other stress conditions.

Brain microvessel endothelial cells, glial cells, brain tumor cells, as well as many other cells tested following exposure to hyperthermia conditions, display a conditioning phenomenon that renders them heat-acclimated (Cossins, 1977, 1981, 1983; Cossins and Prosser, 1982; Gobbel et al., 1995; Harper et al., 1990; Lee et al., 1992; Li and Laszlo, 1985; Macdonald, 1990; Martin et al., 1976; Neuwelt et al., 1983; Raaphorst et al., 1995; Rice et al., 1986; Song et al., 1991). Adaptation to hyperthermia has been thoroughly studied by Andrew Cossins and colleagues (1981). These studies have culminated in a theory of homeoviscous adaptation (Cossins, 1977, 1981, 1983; Macdonald, 1990), which simply stated, suggests that upon exposure to high temperatures, cells synthesize a special set of proteins which are involved in stabilizing cell structures in order that cell function may continue. For example, membrane fluid properties change with increased temperature and these changes can be offset by stabilization of the membrane by newly-made heat shock proteins (Cossins, 1977, 1981, 1983; Macdonald, 1990; Shivers et al., 1988). The attainment of thermotolerance then, will insure membrane and cell functioning in spite of heat- or stress-induced deleterious changes to the cell. In general, sublethal hyperthermia elicits a conditioning response that imparts to the cell, thermotolerance (Cossins and Prosser, 1982; Gobbel et al., 1995; Shivers et al., 1988).

Thermotolerant cells or tissues, when challenged with repeated episodes of hyperthermia, will be much more resistant to the damaging effects of high temperature than if they had received no prior treatment (Cossins and Prosser, 1982; Gobbel et al., 1995; Lee et al., 1992; Raaphorst et al., 1995; Song et al., 1991). Support in the research literature is overwhelmingly in favour of an initial beneficial alteration to cells by sub-lethal hyperthermia that will subsequently condition the cells to damage from further exposures.

The likelihood that all or part of an experimental paradigm to insult cells, microvessels, or tissues with sublethal doses of hyperthermia, may in reality, impart some degree of protection (conditioning) to the cells, etc. is fairly certain. This conditioning will enable tissues to behave essentially in a normal fashion (Cossins, 1977; Cossins and Prosser, 1982; Harper et al., 1990; Rice et al., 1986). If this notion is valid, then studies attempting to look at effects of high temperature or heat shock on, for example, brain microvessels, will be dealing with heat acclimated tissue (Wijsman and Shivers, 1993). Application of standard protocols for blood−brain barrier measurement with electron microscopy, will likely fail to show definitive changes to the 'heat-conditioned' barrier.

Two levels of hyperthermia-induced cell membrane/cell structure permutations can be predicted on the basis of the foregoing discussion: (a) a conditioning effect which imparts to the cell (and cell structures) a protective status that permits normal function and (b) a true hyperthermia influence which will elicit a response beyond and in addition to the conditioning in (a). Experiments designed to investigate the influence of hyperthermia on brain microvessels, cultured cells (cultured brain endothelial cells), brain tumors, and other tissues must be designed to have two control samples: (1) one unstimulated by heat and (2) one stimulated by hyperthermia at a level

below that used in the planned experiments. A third sample, the experimental, will be stimulated by an experimental level hyperthermia. It must be acknowledged that effects of the experimental hyperthermia are less than in the initial or control exposure. Careful attention must be given to avoid careless exposure of tissues to heat conditions, or stress situations, before experimental protocols are employed. The more stress, of any sort, that is applied to the tissue to be studied experimentally, before the experiment begins, the greater the chance of getting inaccurate or misleading results once experimental hyperthermia commences.

Studies of blood−brain barrier properties during various insults, including cold (Mitchell et al., 1979), heat, tumors, diseases of the central nervous system and other assorted conditions, must adopt new parameters for testing effects of barrier-compromising paradigms. Immunochemicals and procedures, available at both light, confocal and electron microscope levels, represent powerful tools to examine the functional blood−brain barrier at high resolution (Brackenhoff et al., 1979; Sheppard and Choudry, 1977). If experimental tissues can be assayed for barrier-specific compounds as CD-34 (Fina et al., 1990), ZO-1 (Stevenson et al., 1986), ZO-2 (Gumbiner et al., 1991), cingulin (Citi et al., 1988), 7H6 antibody (Zhong et al., 1993), $Na+$, $K+$-ATPase (Nag, 1990; Tontsch and Bauer, 1991), carbonic anhydrase (Ghandour et al., 1992), gamma glutamyl transpeptidase (DeBault and Cancilla, 1980; Tontsch and Bauer, 1991), monoamine oxidase (Meresse et al., 1989), occludin (McCarthy et al., 1996), and even the glucose transporter (Dick et al., 1984; Farrell and Pardridge, 1991; Pappius et al., 1979), accurate, reproducible and meaningful information regarding the blood−brain barrier can be obtained. Of primary importance is the requirement that all future studies on the blood−brain barrier that will employ hyperthermia, must do a thorough profile of heat shock protein synthesis by the tissue in question, so that the exact state of microvessel endothelium can be determined before experimentation begins. Hyperthermia induced changes in brain microvessel endothelium can be determined then against the background of a conditioned endothelium and a much more realistic and accurate measurement can be made of microvessel endothelial cell responses to hyperthermia.

Hyperthermic opening of the barrier for therapeutic procedures

Current attempts to open and close the blood–brain barrier in a controlled manner in order that drug delivery to the central nervous system (Bodor and Brewster, 1983) can be effected involve subjecting brain microvasculature to stress. Among various protocols for barrier opening, treatment with hyperthermia has shown promise as an effective means to selectively treat brain tumors (Bodor and Brewster, 1983; Cervos-Navarro et al., 1983; Emami et al., 1980; Koga et al., 1993; Lee et al., 1992; Neuwelt et al., 1981, 1983; Overgaard, 1977; Raaphorst et al., 1995; Salcman and Sammaras, 1981; Satoh et al., 1989; Schopman et al., 1995; Song et al., 1991; Tanaka et al., 1987). As the above discussion has pointed out, studies employing hyperthermia to open the blood–brain barrier must always account for any heat/stress conditioning that takes place during the study. Much more sensitive and accurate manipulations of the blood–brain barrier will then be possible.

Projected future research using heat-treated barrier

Future studies of hyperthermic manipulation of the blood–brain barrier will focus on the fact that tumour cells are more sensitive to heat (Fajardo and Prionas, 1994), and therefore can be targeted for heat treatment. Tumour blood vessels are also more sensitive to heat and are thus obvious candidates for thermal treatment.

Early exploration on combining hyperthermia with various classes of compounds to form an especially potent tool for tumour eradication has shown this approach to have merit. Lin et al. (1992) have for example, shown that dual application of hyperthermia (43°C for 60 min) and tumour necrosis factor (TNF) affects tumour blood flow, vascular permeability, the cytoskeleton and cytoskeleton-dependent cellular functions. Song et al. (1996) have also shown an increased oxygenation of tumours that have been subjected to heat, thereby rendering them more treatable.

Future studies on the blood–brain barrier during hyperthermia must carefully consider the role of pre-conditioning of microvessels by exposure to heat and the effect this will have on barrier responses to additional heat treatment. Heat shock or stress conditions experienced by cells and tissues will surely alter cell structure and function in a homeoviscotic manner and render them more resistant to further stress. High resolution studies of the blood–brain barrier must first precisely define the condition of heat shock and cell conditioning to heat before attempting to assay the barrier for permeability disruptions. Quantitative studies on the barrier must use sophisticated procedures such as immunochemistry of blood–brain barrier-specific proteins as sensitive indicators of barrier disturbance which can be correlated with carefully controlled tracer studies. Simple, crude stimulation of the barrier followed by analysis of tracers such as horseradish peroxidase is no longer acceptable as the primary quantitative analytical tool for experimental study of the blood–brain barrier.

Acknowledgements

This study was supported by the Natural Science and Engineering Research Council of Canada.

References

Ashburner, A. (1982) The effects of heat shock and other stresses on gene activity: an introduction. In: M.J. Schlessinger, M. Ashburner and A. Tissieres (Eds.), *Heat Shock from Bacteria to Man*, Cold Spring Harbor Laboratory, New York.

Ashburner, M. and Bonner, J.J. (1979) The induction of gene activity in *Drosophila* by heat shock. *Cell*, 18: 241–254.

Atkinson, B.G. and Walden, D.B. (1985) *Changes in Gene Expression in Response to Environmental Stress*, Academic Press, New York.

Bodor, N. and Brewster, M.E. (1983) Problems of delivery of drugs to the brain. *Pharmacol. Ther.*, 19: 337–386.

Brackenhoff, G.J., Blom, P. and Barends, P. (1979) Confocal scanning light microscopy with high aperture immersion lenses. *J. Microsc.*, 117(2): 219–232.

Brightman, M.W. and Reese, T.S. (1969) Junctions between intimately apposed cell membranes in the vertebrate brain. *J. Cell Biol.*, 40: 648–677.

Brightman, M.W., Klatzo, I., Olsson, Y. and Reese, T.S. (1970) The blood–brain barrier to proteins under normal and pathological conditions. *J. Neurol. Sci.*, 10: 215–239.

Brightman, M.W., Hori, M., Rapoport, S.I., Reese, T.S. and Westergaard, E. (1973) Osmotic opening of tight junctions in cerebral endothelium. *J. Comp. Neurol.*, 152: 317–326.

Cervos-Navarro, J., Artigas, J. and Mrsulja, B.J. (1983) Morphofunctional aspects of the normal and pathological blood–brain barrier. *Acta Neuropathol.*, Suppl. VIII: 1–19.

Citi, S., Sabany, H., Jakes, R., Geiger, B. and Kendrick-Jones, J. (1988) Cingulin, a new peripheral component of tight junctions. *Nature (Lond.)*, 333: 272–276.

Cossins, A.R. (1977) Adaptation of biological membranes to temperature. The effect of temperature acclimation of goldfish upon the viscosity of synaptosomal membranes. *Biochim. Biophys. Acta*, 470: 395–411.

Cossins, A.R. (1981) The adaptation of membrane dynamic structure to temperature. In: G.J. Morris and A. Clarke (Eds.), *Effects of Low Temperatures on Biological Membranes*, Academic Press, New York, pp. 83–106.

Cossins, A.R. (1983) The adaptation of membrane structure and function to changes in temperature. In: A.R. Cossins and P. Sheterline (Eds.), *Cellular Acclimatization to Environmental Changes*, Cambridge University Press, Cambridge, pp. 3–32.

Cossins, A.R. and Prosser, C.L. (1982) Variable homeoviscous responses of different brain membranes of thermally-acclimated gold fish. *Biochim. Biophys. Acta*, 687: 303–309.

DeBault, L.E. and Cancilla, P.A. (1980) Gamma glutamyl transpeptidase in isolated brain endothelial cells: induction by glial cells *in vitro*. *Science*, 207: 653–655.

Del Maestro, R.F., Arfors, K.E. and McKenzie, F.N. (1979) The effect of infusion solution temperature on albumin permeability through the intact and damaged blood–brain barrier. *Bibl. Anat.*, 18: 229–232.

Dey, S., Dey, P.K. and Sharma, H.S. (1993) Regional metabolism of 5-hydroxytryptamine in brain under acute and chronic heat stress. *Indian J. Physiol. Pharmacol.*, 37: 8–12.

Dick, A.P., Harik, S.I., Klip, A. and Walker, D.M. (1984) Identification and characterization of the glucose transporter of the blood–brain barrier by cytochalasin B binding and immunological reactivity. *Proc. Natl. Acad. Sci. USA*, 81: 7233–7237.

Dietrich, W.D., Busto, R., Halley, M. and Valdes, I.. (1990) The importance of brain temperature in alterations of the blood–brain barrier following cerebral ischemia. *J. Neuropathol. Exp. Neurol.*, 49: 486–497.

Dynlacht, J.R. and Fox, M.H. (1992a) Heat-induced changes in the membrane fluidity of Chinese hamster ovary cells measured by flow cytometry. *Radiat. Res.*, 130: 48–54.

Dynlacht, J.R. and Fox, M.H. (1992b) The effect of 45°C hyperthermia on the membrane fluidity of cells of several lines. *Radiat. Res.*, 130: 55–60.

Emami, B., Nussbaum, G.H., TenHaken, R.K. and Hughes, W.L. (1980) Physiological effect of hyperthermia: response of capillary blood flow and structure to local tumor heating. *Radiology*, 137: 805–809.

Fahim, M.A. and El-Sabban, F. (1995) Hyperthermia induces ultrastructural changes in mouse pial microvessels. *Anat. Rec.*, 242: 77–82.

Fajardo, L.F. and Prionas, S.D. (1994) Endothelial cells and hyperthermia (review). *Int. J. Hyperthermia*, 10: 347–353.

Farrell, C.L. and Shivers, R.R. (1984) Capillary junctions of the rat are not affected by osmotic opening of the blood–brain barrier. *Acta Neuropathol.*, 63: 179–189.

Farrell, C.L. and Pardridge, W.M. (1991) Blood–brain barrier glucose transporter is asymmetrically distributed on brain capillary endothelial lumenal and ablumenal membranes: an electron microscopic immunogold study. *Proc. Natl. Acad. Sci. USA*, 88: 5779–5783.

Fina, L., Molgaard, H.V., Robertson, D., Bradley, N.J., Monaghan, P., Delia, D., Sutherland, R.S., Baker, M.A. and Greaves, M.F. (1990) Expression of the CD-34 gene in vascular endothelial cells. *Blood*, 75: 2417–2426.

Fugimoto, K. (1995) Freeze-fracture replica electron microscopy combined withS.D.S digestion for cytochemical labelling of intercellular junctional complexes. *J. Cell Sci.*, 108: 3443–3449.

Gobbel, G.T., Chan, T.Y-Y. and Chan, P.H. (1995) Amelioration of hypoxic and hypoglycemic damage to cerebral endothelial cells. Effects of heat shock pretreatment. *Mol. Chem. Neuropathol.*, 24: 107–120.

Ghandour, M.S., Langley, O.K., Zhu, X.L., Waheed, A. and Sly, W.S. (1992) Carbonic anhydrase IV on brain capillary endothelial cells: a marker associated with the blood–brain barrier. *Proc. Natl. Acad. Sci. USA*, 89: 6823–6827.

Gonzalez-Mariscal, L., Chavez-Ramirez, B. and Cereijido, M. (1984) Effect of temperature on the occluding junctions of monolayers of epithelioid cells (MDCK). *J. Membr. Biol.*, 79: 175–184.

Gumbiner, B., Lowenkopf, T. and Apatira, D. (1991) Identification of a 160 kDa polypeptide that binds to the tight junction protein ZO-1. *Proc. Natl. Acad. Sci. USA*, 88: 3460–3464.

Harper, A.A., Watt, P.W., Hancock, N.A. and Macdonald, A.G. (1990) Temperature acclimation effects on carp nerve: a comparison of nerve conduction, membrane fluidity and lipid composition. *J. Exp. Biol.*, 154: 305–320.

Hedley-Whyte, E.T., Lorenzo, A.V. and Hsu, D.W. (1977) Protein transport across cerebral vessels during metrazole-induced convulsions. *Am. J. Physiol.*, 233: C74–C85.

Ikeda, N., Hayashida, O., Kameda, H., Ito, H. and Matsuda, T. (1994) Experimental study on thermal damage to dog normal brain. *Int. J. Hyperthermia*, 10: 553–561.

Inasi, B.S. and Brown, I.R. (1982) Synthesis of a heat shock protein in the microvascular system of the rabbit brain following elevation in body temperature. *Biochem. Biophys. Res. Commun.*, 106: 881–887.

Johansson, B. and Nilsson, B. (1977) The pathophysiology of the blood–brain barrier dysfunction induced by severe hypercapnia and by epileptic brain activity. *Acta Neuropathol.*, 38: 153–158.

Joó, F. (1971) Increased production of coated vesicles in the brain capillaries during enhanced permeability of the blood–brain barrier. *Br. J. Exp. Pathol.*, 52: 646–649.

Kato, M., Herz, F., Kato, S. and Hirano, A. (1992) Expression of stress-response (heat shock) protein 27 in human brain tumors: an immunohistochemical study. *Acta Neuropathol.*, 83: 420–422.

Koga, H., Mori, K. and Tokuda, Y. (1993) Interstitial radiofrequency hyperthermia for brain tumors — preliminary laboratory studies and clinical application. *Neurol. Med.-Chir. (Tokyo)*, 33: 290–294.

Laszlo, A. (1992) The effects of hyperthermia on mammalian cell structure and function. *Cell Prolif.*, 25: 59–87.

Lee, W.-C., Liu, H.-C., Pan, D.H.C.P., Jou, T.-C. and Lai, Y.K. (1992) Cell survival and heat shock protein synthesis of normal and malignant rat brain cells during and after hyperthermia. *J. Therm. Biol.*, 17: 33–41.

Leigh, K. (1988) The effect of heat shock on the blood–brain barrier of the rat. Honors Zoology 450/451 Research Project. University of Western Ontario, London, Ontario.

Li, G. and Laszlo, A. (1985) Thermotolerance in mammalian cells: a possible role for heat shock proteins. In: B.G. Atkinson and D.B. Walden (Eds.), *Changes in Eukaryotic Gene Expression in Response to Environmental Stress*, Academic Press, New York, pp. 227–254.

Lin, J.C. and Lin, M.F. (1982) Microwave hyperthermia-induced blood brain barrier alterations. *Radiat. Res.*, 89: 77–87.

Lin, P.S., Ho, K.C., Sung, S.J. and Gladding, J. (1992) Effect of tumour necrosis factor, heat and radiation on the viability and microfilament organization in cultured endothelial cells. *Int. J. Hyperthermia*, 8: 667–677.

Lossinsky, A.S., Vorbrodt, A.W. and Wisniewski, H.M. (1983) Ultracytochemical studies of vesicular and canalicular transport structures in the injured mammalian blood–brain barrier. *Acta Neuropathol.*, 61: 239–245.

Lossinsky, A.L., Vorbrodt, A.W. and Wisniewski, H.M. (1986) Characterization of endothelial cell transport in the developing mouse blood–brain barrier. *Dev. Neurosci.*, 8: 61–75.

Lossinsky, A.S., Song, M.J. and Wisniewski, H.M. (1989) High voltage electron microscopic studies of endothelial cell tubular structures in the mouse blood–brain barrier following brain trauma. *Acta Neuropathol.*, 77: 480–488.

Macdonald, A.G. (1990) The homeoviscous theory of adaptation applied to excitable membranes: a critical evaluation. *Biochim. Biophys. Acta*, 1031: 291–310.

Martin, C.E., Hiramitsu, K., Kitajama, Y., Nozawa, Y., Skriver, L. and Thompson, G.A. (1976) Molecular control of membrane properties during temperature acclimation. Fatty acid desaturase regulation of membrane fluidity in acclimating Tetrahymena cells. *Biochemistry*, 15: 5218–5227.

McCarthy, K.M., Skare, I.B., Stankewich, M.C., Furuse, M., Tsukita, S., Rogers, R.A., Lynch, R.D. and Schneeberger, E.E. (1996) Occludin is a functional component of the tight junction. *J. Cell Sci.*, 109: 2287–2298.

Meresse, S., Dehouck, M.-P., Delorme, P., Bensaid, M., Tauber, J.-P., Delbart, C., Fruchart, J.-C. and Cecchelli, R. (1989) Bovine brain endothelial cells express tight junctions and monoamine oxidase activity in long-term culture. *J. Neurochem.*, 53: 1363–1371.

Miller, D.B., Blackman, C.F. and O'Callaghan, J.P. (1987) An increase in glial fibrillary acidic protein follows brain hyperthermia in rats. *Brain Res.*, 415: 371–374.

Mitchell, J., Weller, R.O. and Evans, H. (1979) Reestablishment of the blood–brain barrier to peroxidase following cold injury to mouse cortex. *Acta Neuropathol.*, 46: 45–49.

Moriyama, E. (1990) Cerebral blood flow changes during localized hyperthermia. *Neurol. Med.-Chir. (Tokyo)*, 30: 923–929.

Moriyama, E., Salcman, M. and Broadwell, R.D. (1991) Blood–brain barrier alteration after microwave-induced hyperthermia is purely a thermal effect. I. Temperature and power measurements. *Surg. Neurol.*, 35: 177–182.

Nag, S. (1990) Ultracytochemical localization of Na+, K+-ATPase in cerebral endothelium in acute hypertension. *Acta Neuropathol.*, 80: 7–11.

Nakajima, T., Roberts, D.W., Ryan, T.P., Hoopes, P.J., Coughlin, C.T., Trembly, B.S. and Strohbehn, J.W. (1993) Pattern of response to interstitial hyperthermia and brachytherapy for malignant intracardial tumour: a CT analysis. *Int. J. Hyperthermia*, 9: 491–502.

Neuwelt, E.A., Barranger, J.A., Brady, R.O., Pagel, M., Furbish, F.S., Quirk, J.M., Mook, G.E. and Frenkel, E. (1981) Delivery of hexosaminidase A to the cerebrum after osmotic modification of the blood–brain barrier. *Proc. Natl. Acad. Sci. USA*, 78: 5838–5841.

Neuwelt, E.A., Glasberg, M., Frenkel, E. and Barnett, P. (1983) Neurotoxicity of chemotherapeutic agents after blood–brain barrier modification: neuropathological studies. *Ann. Neurol.*, 14: 316–324.

Neuwelt, E.A., Hill, S.A. and Frenkel, S.A. (1984) Osmotic blood–brain barrier modification and combination chemotherapy: concurrent tumor regression in areas of barrier opening and progression in brain regions distant to barrier opening. *Neurosurgery*, 15: 362–366.

Ohmoto, Y., Fujisawa, H., Ishikawa, T., Koisumi, H., Matsuda, T. and Ito, H. (1996) Sequential changes in cerebral blood flow, early neuropathological consequences and blood–brain barrier disruption following radiofrequency-induced localized hyperthermia in the rat. *Int. J. Hyperthermia*, 12: 321–334.

Oscar, K.J. and Hawkins, T.D. (1977) Microwave alteration of the blood–brain barrier system of rats. *Brain Res.*, 126: 281–293.

Overgaard, J. (1977) Effect of hyperthermia on malignant cells *in vivo*. A review and a hypothesis. *Cancer*, 39: 2637–2646.

Pappius, H.M., Savaki, H.E., Fieschi, C., Rapoport, S.I. and Sokoloff, L. (1979) Osmotic opening of the blood–brain barrier and local glucose utilization. *Ann. Neurol.*, 5: 211–219.

Prato, F.S., Frappier, J.R.H., Shivers, R.R., Kavaliers, M., Zabel, P.M., Drost, D. and Lee, T.-Y. (1990) Magnetic resonance imaging increases the blood–brain barrier permeability to 153-gadolinium diethylenetriaminepentaacetic acid in rats. *Brain Res.*, 523: 301–304.

Prato, F.S., Willis, J.M., Frappier, J.R.H., Drost, D.J., Lee, T.-Y., Shivers, R.R. and Zabel, P. (1994) Blood–brain barrier permeability in rats is altered by exposure to magnetic fields associated with magnetic resonance imaging at 1.5 T. *Microsc. Res. Tech.*, 27: 528–534.

Preston, E., Vavasour, E.J. and Assenheim, H.M. (1979) Permeability of the blood–brain barrier to mannitol in the rat following 2450 MHz microwave irradiation. *Brain Res.*, 174: 109–117.

Raaphorst, G.P., Mao, J. and Ng, C.E. (1995) Thermotolerance in human glioma cells. *Int. J. Hyperthermia*, 11: 523–529.

Rapoport, S.I. (1975a) Experimental modification of blood–brain barrier permeability by hypertonic solutions, convulsions, hypercapnia and acute hypertension. In: H.F. Cserr, J.D. Fenstermacher and V. Fencl (Eds.), *Fluid Environment of the Brain*, Academic Press, New York.

Rapoport, S.I. (1975b) *The Blood-Brain Barrier in Physiology and Medicine*, Raven Press, New York.

Rapoport, S.I. (1976) Opening the blood–brain barrier by acute hypertension. *Exp. Zool.*, 52: 467–479.

Rice, G., Laszlo, A., Li, G., Gray, J. and Dewey, W. (1986) Heat shock proteins within the mammalian cell cycle: relationship to thermal sensitivity, thermal tolerance and cell cycle progression. *J. Cell. Physiol.*, 126: 291–297.

Richmon, J.D., Fukuda, K., Sharp, F.R. and Noble, L.J. (1995) Induction of HSP-70 after hyperosmotic opening of the blood–brain barrier in the rat. *Neurosci. Lett.*, 202: 1–4.

Rodenhiser, D., Jung, J.H. and Atkinson, B.G. (1985) Mammalian lymphocytes: stress-induced synthesis of heat-shock protein in vitro and *in vivo*. *Can. J. Biochem. Cell Biol.*, 63: 711–722.

Rosenblum, W.I. (1986) Biology of disease. Aspects of endothelial malfunction and function in cerebral microvessels. *Lab. Invest.*, 55: 252–268.

Salcman, M. and Sammaras, G.M. (1981) Hyperthermia for brain tumor: biophysical rationale. *Neurosurgery*, 9: 327–335.

Satoh, T., Nakasone, S. and Nishimoto, A. (1989) Cerebral blood flow response to the tissue temperature in tumor and brain tissues. *Int. J. Hyperthermia*, 5: 683–696.

Schopman, E.M., Van Bree, C., Kipp, J.B.A. and Barendsen, G.W. (1995) Enhancement of the effectiveness of methotrexate for the treatment of solid tumors by application of local hyperthermia. *Int. J. Hyperthermia*, 11: 561–573.

Sharma, H.S., Cervos-Navarro, J. and Dey, P.K. (1991) Acute heat exposure causes cellular alteration in cerebral cortex of young rats. *Neuroreport*, 2: 155–158.

Sharma, H.S., Kretzschman, R., Cervos-Navarro, J., Ermisch, A., Ruhle, H.J. and Dey, P.K. (1992) Age-related pathophysiology of the blood–brain barrier in heat stress. *Prog. Brain Res.*, 91: 189–196.

Sheppard, C.J.R. and Choudry, A. (1977) Image formation in the scanning microscope. *Optica*, 24: 1051.

Severs, N.J. and Robenek, H. (1983) Detection of microdomains in biomembranes. An appraisal of recent developments in freeze-fracture cytochemistry. *Biochim. Biophys. Acta*, 737: 373–408.

Shinowara, N.L., Michel, M.E. and Rapoport, S.I. (1982) Morphological correlates of permeability in the frog perineurium: vesicles and 'transcellular channels'. *Cell Tissue Res.*, 227: 11–22.

Shivers, R.R. and Brightman, M.W. (1976) *trans*-glial channels of crayfish ventral nerve roots in freeze-fracture. *J. Comp. Neurol.*, 167: 1–26.

Shivers, R.R. (1979a) The blood–brain barrier of a reptile, *Anolis carolinensis*. A freeze-fracture study. *Brain Res.*, 169: 221–230.

Shivers, R.R. (1979b) The effect of hyperglycemia on brain capillary permeability in the lizard, *Anolis carolinensis*: a freeze-fracture analysis of blood–brain barrier pathology. *Brain Res.*, 170: 509–522.

Shivers, R.R., Betz, A.L. and Goldstein, G.W. (1984a) Isolated rat brain capillaries possess intact, structurally complex, interendothelial tight junctions: freeze-fracture verification of tight junction integrity. *Brain Res.*, 324: 313–322.

Shivers, R.R. and Harris, R.J. (1984b) Opening of the blood–brain barrier in *Anolis carolinensis*. A high voltage electron microscope protein tracer study. *Neuropathol. Appl. Neurobiol.*, 10: 343–356.

Shivers, R.R., Bowman, P.D. and Martin, K. (1985) A model for de novo synthesis and assembly of tight intercellular junctions. Ultrastructural correlates and experimental verification of the model revealed by freeze-fracture. *Tissue Cell*, 17: 417–440.

Shivers, R.R., Kavaliers, M., Teskey, G.C., Prato, F.S. and Pelletier, R.-M. (1987) Magnetic resonance imaging temporarily alters blood–brain barrier permeability in the rat. *Neurosci. Lett.*, 76: 25–31.

424

Shivers, R.R., Pollock, M., Bowman, P.D. and Atkinson, B.G. (1988) The effect of heat shock on primary cultures of brain capillary endothelium: inhibition of assembly of zonulae occludentes and the synthesis of heat-shock proteins. *Eur. J. Cell Biol.*, 46: 181–195.

Song, C.W. (1984) Effect of local hyperthermia on blood flow and microenvironment: a review. *Cancer Res.*, 44: 4721s–4730s.

Song, C.W., Lin, J.-C., Chelstrom, L.M. and Sahu, S.K. (1991) Induction of thermoresistance in tumor blood vessels. *Int. J. Radiat. Biol.*, 60: 355–361.

Song, C.W., Shakil, A., Osborn, J.L. and Iwata, K. (1996) Tumour oxygenation is increased by hyperthermia at mild temperatures. *Int. J. Hyperthermia*, 12: 367–373.

Sterrett, P.R., Bradley, I.M., Kitten, G.T., Janssen, H.F. and Holloway, L.S. (1976) Cerebrovascular permeability changes following experimental angiography. *J. Neurol. Sci.*, 30: 385–403.

Stevenson, B.R., Siliciano, J.D., Mooseker, M.S. and Goodenough, D.A. (1986) Identification of ZO-1: a high molecular weight polypeptide associated with the tight junctions (zonula occludentes) in a variety of epithelia. *J. Cell Biol.*, 103: 755–766.

Tanaka, R., Kim, C.H., Yamada, N. and Saito, Y. (1987) Radiofrequency hyperthermia for malignant brain tumors: preliminary results of clinical trials. *Neurosurgery*, 21: 478–483.

Tontsch, U. and Bauer, H.-C. (1991) Cells and neurons induce blood–brain barrier related enzymes in cultured cerebral endothelial cells. *Brain Res.*, 539: 247–253.

Urakawa, M., Yamaguchi, K., Tsuchida, E., Kashiwagi, S., Ito, H. and Matsuda, T. (1995) Blood–brain barrier disturbance following localized hyperthermia in rats. *Int. J. Hyperthermia*, 11: 709–718.

Westergaard, E. (1977) The blood–brain barrier to horseradish peroxidase under normal and experimental conditions. *Acta Neuropathol.*, 39: 181–187.

Westergaard, E., Go, G., Klatzo, I. and Spatz, M. (1976) Increased permeability of cerebral vessels to horseradish peroxidase induced by ischemia in Mongolian gerbils. *Acta Neuropathol. (Berlin)*, 35: 307–325.

Westergaard, E., Van Deurs, B. and Bronsted, H.E. (1977) Increased vesicular transfer of horseradish peroxidase across cerebral endothelium evoked by acute hypertension. *Acta Neuropathol.*, 37: 141–152.

Westergaard, E., Hertz, M.M. and Bolwig, T.G. (1978) Increased permeability to horseradish peroxidase across cerebral vessels, evoked by electrically induced seizures in the rat. *Acta Neuropathol.*, 41: 73–80.

White, F.P. (1980a) The synthesis and possible transport of specific proteins by cells associated with brain capillaries. *J. Neurochem.*, 35: 88–94.

White, F.P. (1980b) Protein synthesis in rat telencephalon slices: high amounts of newly synthesized protein found in association with brain capillaries. *Neuroscience*, 5: 173–178.

White, F.P. (1980c) Differences in protein synthesized *in vivo* and *in vitro* by cells associated with the cerebral vasculature. A protein synthesized in response to trauma? *Neuroscience*, 5: 1793–1799.

White, F.P. (1981a) The induction of 'stress' proteins in organ slices from brain, heart and lung as a function of postnatal development. *J. Neurosci.*, 1: 1312–1319.

White, F.P. (1981b) Protein and RNA synthesis in cerebral microvessels: a radioautographic study. *Brain Res.*, 229: 43–52.

White, F.P. and Currie, R.W. (1982) A mammalian response to trauma: the synthesis of a 71 kD protein. In: M. Schlessinger, M. Ashburner and A. Tissieres (Eds.), *Heat Shock from Bacteria to Man*, Cold Spring Harbor, New York, pp. 379–386.

Wijsman, J.A. and Shivers, R.R. (1993) Heat stress affects blood–brain barrier permeability to horseradish peroxidase in mice. *Acta Neuropathol.*, 86: 49–54.

Wolffe, A.P., Glover, J.F. and Tata, J.R. (1984) Culture shock. Synthesis of heat-shock-like proteins in fresh primary cell cultures. *Exp. Cell Res.*, 154: 581–590.

Yatvin, M.B. and Cramp, W.A. (1993) Role of cellular membranes in hyperthermia: some observations and theories reviewed. *Int. J. Hyperthermia*, 9: 165–185.

Zhong, Y., Saitoh, T., Minase, T., Sawada, N., Enomoto, K. and Mori, M. (1993) Monoclonal antibody 7H6 reacts with a novel tight junction-associated protein distinct from ZO-1, cingulin, and ZO-2. *J. Cell Biol.*, 120: 477–483.

H.S. Sharma and J. Westman (Eds.)
Progress in Brain Research, Vol 115

CHAPTER 20

Cytokines and blood–brain barrier permeability

A.G. de Boer* and D.D. Breimer

Division of Pharmacology, Leiden / Amsterdam Center for Drug Research, Leiden University, Sylvius Laboratories, P.O. Box 9503, 2300 RA Leiden, The Netherlands

Introduction

The BBB comprises the endothelial lineage of the microvessels in the brain and has special properties which distinguish it from peripheral endothelium (van Bree et al., 1992; de Boer and Breimer, 1994; Pardridge, 1991; Bradbury, 1979). It has narrow tight junctions, no intercellular clefts, minor pinocytotic activity, it is not fenestrated; it has a continuous basement membrane, many mitochondria (Reed, 1980) and a high electrical resistance (1500–2000 Ohm.cm^2) (Butt et al., 1990).

Current insights into the anatomical basis of the BBB clearly indicate that, in contrast to what has long been generally accepted, it is not a static homogeneous impermeable barrier. Its permeability is regulated dynamically with special features (its physical and metabolic barrier properties), like the presence of tight junctions and blood components like hormones. In addition, there are several other cells that may influence the BBB, comprising pericytes, microglia which have been shown to be immuno-competent cells (Frei and Fontana, 1989), and neurones, while there are also leukocytes, lymphocytes and monocytes and in surrounding larger vessels, perivascular macrophages and mast cells (Fig. 1). These features together with the various cells present at

the BBB including their regulatory systems, may provide the physiological basis to understand changed BBB permeability which may be used to enhance drug delivery to the CNS.

In addition to their role in numerous metabolic functions, endothelial cells play a role in coagulation and thrombolysis, the control of vasotonus and antigen presentation, and basement membrane and growth factor synthesis (Fajardo, 1989; Pearson, 1991). They present a very heterogenous cell population that varies in different organs but also in different vessel calibers within an organ (McCarthy et al., 1991; Bicknell, 1993). The endothelial and hematopoietic cells originate from a common precursor cell (Favaloro, 1993; Augustin et al., 1994; Schlossman et al., 1994) and the constitutive organ- and microenvironment-specific phenotype of endothelial cells controls internal body compartmentation regulating the trafficking of circulating cells via adhesion molecules (E-selectin, P-selectin, VCAM-1, ICAM-1) to distinct vascular beds (Springer, 1994). The activated cytokine inducible endothelial phenotype together with surface molecules play a key role in pathological conditions like inflammation, tumour angiogenesis and wound healing (Augustin et al., 1994).

The importance of endothelial cells as an interface between the blood compartment and various tissues is illustrated by its high degree of adaptability. Differentiation of the constitutive phenotype of endothelial cells is similar to that of

---

*Corresponding author.

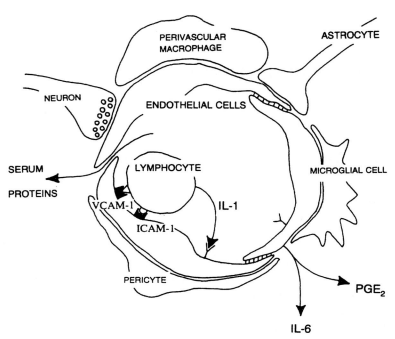

Fig. 1. The various cells presenting and influencing the blood–brain barrier. In addition, these cells may influence the functionality of the brain microvessel endothelial cells. In particular the interaction with lymphocytes is illustrated which is mediated via adhesion molecules like ICAM-1 (intercellular adhesion molecule) and VCAM-1 (vascular cellular adhesion molecule). Lymphocytes may release IL-1 (interleukin-1) which may induce endothelial cells to release IL-6 and PGE$_2$ (prostaglandin-E$_2$). This may result in opening of the blood–brain barrier (redrawn from de Vries, 1995).

hematopoietic cells; however, the differentiation of hematopoietic cells is unidirectional, while endothelial cells have the capacity to transdifferentiate in order to adapt best to local requirements to perform their complex structural and metabolic functions (Augustin et al., 1994). This may be illustrated by the fact that BBB cells transplanted into the periphery will lose their BBB characteristics while endothelium transplanted into the periphery and cultured together with astrocytes got BBB characteristics (Janzer and Raff, 1987).

Cells of the central nervous system and from the immune system including hormones from the systemic circulation, may influence the functionality of the BBB, thereby restoring or even disturbing the homeostasis of the brain following stress and cytokines play an increasingly important role in these processes. Cytokines are cellular hormones (Table 1) like neurotrophins, neuropoietic factors, interleukins, interferons, colony stimulating factors, chemokines, growth factors and thymic hormones which are released following stress. They present one way of communication between leukocytes and endothelial cells (Mantovani and Dejana, 1989) and the brain and the immune system, by signalling back to the higher centres in the brain via the systemic circulation (Carr and Weigert, 1990; Spellerberg et al., 1995), afferent neurons, etc. (Berkenbosch et al., 1987; Sapolsky et al., 1987; Tsagarakis et al., 1989; Ojeda et al., 1992; Watkins et al., 1995a, Watkins et al., 1995b). Recently another route of communication between the CNS and the immune system has been demonstrated which involves the outflow pathways from the brain across the arachnoid villi or along certain cranial nerves and spinal nerve roots to the lymphatics (Cserr et al., 1992).

One of the most common and frequently ap-

TABLE 1

Cytokine families, their members and their major activities and features

Neurotrophins	Growth and differentiation of neurones
NGF	Nerve growth factor
BDNF	Brain derived neurotrophic factor
NT-3,4,5,6	Neurotrophins 3, 4, 5, 6
GDNF	Glial-derived neurotropic factor
Neuropoietins	Cytokines acting on the nervous system, and acting via a related receptor complex
CDF/LIF	Cholinergic differentiation factor/leukaemia inhibiting factor
CNTF	Ciliary neurotrophic factor
ONC	Oncostatin M
GPA	Growth-promoting activity
MANS	Membrane-associated neurotransmitter-stimulating factor
SGF	Sweat gland factor
OM	Oncostatin M
Interleukins	Multiple tissue and immunoregulatory activities; no similarity of activity is implied by membership of this family
IL-1 α,β	Interleukin-1 α and β
IL-1ra	Interleukin-1 receptor antagonist
IL-2, 6, 11, 15	Interleukin-2, 6, 11 and 15
Growth factors	Cell growth and differentiation
EGF	Epidermal growth factor
FGF	Basic and acidic fibroblast growth factor
TGF-α,β	Transforming growth factors, α and β
TNF-α,β	Tumour necrosis factors, α and β
PDGF	Platelet-derived growth factor
ECGF	Endothelial cell growth factor
Colony stimulating factors	Colony cell formation in the bone marrow and activation of mature leukocyte functions
G-CSF	Granulocyte colony stimulating factor
M-CSF	Macrophage colony stimulating factor
GM-CSF	Granulocyte-macrophage colony stimulating factor
IL-3	Interleukin-3
Interferons	Inhibition of intracellular viral replication and cell growth regulation; IFN-γ is primarily immunoregulatory
IFN-α,β,γ	Interferon-α,β,γ
Chemokines	Leukocyte chemotaxis and cellular activation
IL-8/NAP-1	Interleukin-8/neutrophil activating protein 1
NAP-2	Neutrophil activating protein 2
MIP-1 α,β	Macrophage inflammatory protein α,β
MCAF/MCP-1	Monocyte chemotactic and activating factor/monocyte chemotactic protein 1
MGSA	Melanoma growth stimulatory activity
RANTES	Regulated upon activation normal expressed and secreted

Adapted from Patterson and Nawa, 1993; Hopkins and Rothwell, 1995.

plied stress stimulus is hyperthermia. It may be considered as a physical and physiological stressor and may have severe influences on the functionality of the BBB, directly or indirectly. It can be defined in physiological terms, as the condition of a temperature regulator (organism which regulates its body temperature) when core temperature is above its set range specified for the normal active state of the species (IUPS, 1987). Cytokines, bacterial products and viruses cause hyperthermia but also open field stress in rats (Watkins et al., 1995b) while it is also frequently applied in the treatment of (brain) tumours (Sminia et al., 1994; Issels, 1995).

In the following the possibilities of BBB permeability, the properties and effects of cytokines, the effects of hyperthermia on cytokines and the effects of cytokines on BBB permeability will be reviewed.

BBB permeability

The BBB comprises various cells types as stated earlier, which all contribute to the functional regulation of the BBB particularly with respect to its permeability. Apart from receptor- or carrier-mediated transport, BBB permeability may be increased by paracellular transport (tight-junctions), increased pinocytosis (Sharma et al., 1991, 1996; Black, 1995) or by pore formation as suggested by Juhler et al. (1985). In particular, the tightness of the microvascular endothelium in the brain prohibits the transport of hydrophilic and large molecules into the brain. Therefore, brain endothelium, including the BBB, presents more possibilities for the transport of particularly small molecules (mol. weight 400–600) compared to large ones (van Bree et al., 1988; Pardridge, 1995). BBB tightness is maintained by various intercellular junctions, e.g. tight junctions (Risau and Wolburg, 1990; Anderson et al., 1993; Gumbiner, 1993), adherence junctions (Rubin, 1992), gap junctions (Beyer, 1993) and syndesmos (Schmelz and Franke, 1993) from which the tight junctions seem to be the most important in restricting passive hydrophilic transport (see Fig. 2; Dejana et al., 1995). In addition, increased BBB permeability via the paracellular route is more or less size-dependent (van Bree et al., 1988), while tran-

scellular pinocytosis is relatively size independent (Black, 1995).

The interaction of endothelial cells with the extracellular matrix is important for establishing a tight layer of cells. This is facilitated by receptors for type I and IV collagen, laminin, fibronectin and vitronectin (van Mourik et al., 1990) and the cell attachment of these proteins is characterized by the amino acid sequence Arg-Gly-Asp (RGD; Hynes, 1987).

The endothelial cells play an important role in the exchange between blood and lymph, therefore the intercellular junctions need to be dynamically and functionally regulated. Since the endothelium is functionally different in various parts of the vascular tree, its barrier function may vary accordingly (Dejana et al., 1995; Wilting et al., 1995). This may explain the differential influences of various biological modulators of vascular permeability which seem to have differential effects on various endothelia (Hoek, 1992; Caveda et al., 1994). This is also supported by the differences seen in eicosanoid production following stimulation of confluent monolayers of brain microvascular and aortic endothelial cells where in particular the production of PGE_2 and 6-keto-$PGF_{1\alpha}$ differs considerably (see Fig. 3; de Vries et al., 1995a).

Intracellular systems, like second-messenger systems, also play an important role in endothelial permeability. It has been shown that thrombin increases intracellular Ca^{2+} and stimulates protein kinase C, that hypoxia decreases cyclic adenosine 5'-monophosphae levels, H_2O_2 activates protein kinase C and prostaglandin I_2 and prostaglandin E_1 increase cyclic adenosine 5'-monophosphate in endothelial cells (Dejana et al., 1995). However, opposite effects may occur in various endothelia. Therefore, environmental factors (see also the Introduction) may determine to a large extent the functionality and response of endothelium with respect to its permeability.

Cytokines

Cytokines are cellular hormones comprising solu-

429

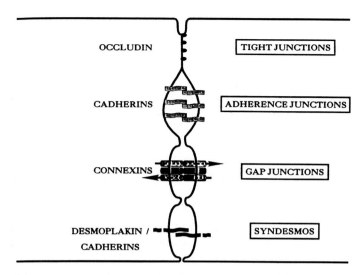

Fig. 2. Schematic representation of the four types of endothelial cell-to-cell junctions [redrawn from Dejana et al. (1995), reprinted with kind permission of *FASEB*, Bethesda, MD, USA].

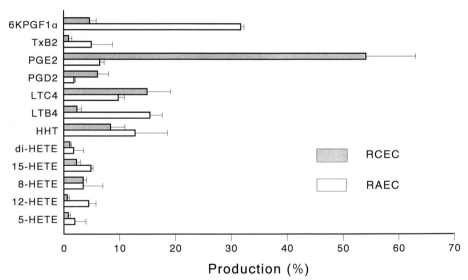

Fig. 3. Profile of eicosanoid production by rat brain capillary endothelial cells (RCEC) and rat aortic endothelial cells (RAEC). Primary cultures were exposed to traces of ^{14}C-labelled arachidonic acid (2.5 μCi) for 10 min, stimulated with Ca^{2+}-ionophore A23187 to determine the maximal capacity to form eicosanoids. Data are expressed as mean $\pm$ S.E.M.; $n = 3$) (redrawn from de Vries et al., 1995a).

ble polypeptide compounds. They control the growth, differentiation, and function of most cell types and play a particular role as mediators of inflammation (Balkwill, 1989). They take care of the coordination of processes between different cells and act in response to environmental stress

430

(Clemens, 1991). Cytokines regulate homeostasis in the tissue of origin, either via local actions or by recruitment of external systems that facilitate restoration of local homeostasis (Hopkins and Rothwell, 1995). In particular cytokines are active in embryonic development, fever, neuro-endocrine activation, changes in behaviour and mood, following brain trauma, regulation of the immune response to foreign antigens and the development of cellular and humoral immunity and inflammatory responses (Hopkins and Rothwell, 1995; Woodroofe, 1995), while cytokines may also play a role in circadian rhythms, long-term potentiation and synaptic plasticity (Patterson and Nawa, 1993; see Fig. 4).

Cytokines include neurotrophins, neuropoietins, interleukins, growth factors, colony stimulating factors, interferons and chemokines (Table 1) (Baron et al., 1991; Patterson and Nawa, 1993; Hopkins and Rothwell, 1995). Their immense range of activities overlaps considerably and many cells may produce several cytokines under various disease conditions (Table 2) while their action is mainly determined by their site of production, their nature, their systemic pharmacokinetics and where and if they enter the CNS.

The constitutive expression of cytokines under normal conditions in tissues is extremely low but under stress conditions this may increase con-siderably (Frei and Fontana, 1989; Hofman, 1989; Gadient et al., 1990; Minami et al., 1991; Fontana et al., 1993). Under such conditions cytokines may be produced by endothelial cells (IL-1, IL-6), neurons (IL-1), astrocytes (IL-1, IL-6, TNF-α, MM-CSF, GM-CSF, TGFβ_2, INF-α, IFN-β), microglia (IL-1, IL-6, TGF-β, TNF-α (IFN-γ)) and perivascular macrophages (via IFN-γ: IL-1, IL-6, TGF-β and TNF-α) (Table 2) (May et al., 1989; Cozzolino et al., 1990; Plata-Salam n, 1991; Morganti-Kossmann et al., 1992; Woodroofe, 1995). Glucocorticoids may influence cytokine gene expression since dexamethason has been shown to differentially affect the expression of nerve growth factor (NGF) in cultured neurons and astrocytes from the hippocampus (Lindholm et al., 1992). In addition, cortisol controls the IL-1/IL-1ra (IL-1 receptor antagonist) system in monocytes during inflammation or immune processes by regulating and counteracting IL-1ra synthesis mediated by the mineralo-corticoid receptor (MR) and glucocorticoid receptor (GR; Sauer et al., 1996).

Cytokines may have direct effects on the CNS (e.g. neurotransmitters, second messengers systems, neuronal differentiation and growth, synaptic plasticity, long-term potentiation), may produce effects via the CNS (e.g. HPA-axis) and may directly influence the peripheral nervous system (e.g. adrenal glands) (Rothwell, 1991; Rothwell

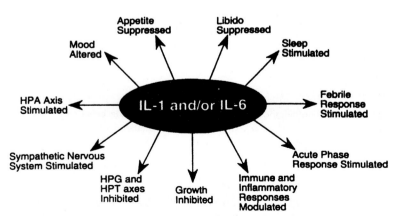

Fig. 4. The actions of IL-1 (interleukin-1) and IL-6 (interleukin-6) in the neuroendocrine-immune network [redrawn from Wilder (1995), reprinted with kind permission of Annual Reviews Inc., Palo Alto, CA, USA].

TABLE 2

Cytokines identified in the CNS and implicated in neuropathologies

Stimulus	Cytokine	Probable sources
Peripheral infection endotoxin	IL-1β, IL-6	Neurones?, microglia,
CNS infection: malaria, HIV, meningitis, cytomegalovirus	IL-1β, IL-6, TNF-α, TGF-β, IFN-γ, MIP-1, MIP-2	Microglia, astrocytes, macrophages
Brain injury	IL-1β, IL-2, IL-6, IL-8, LIF, NGF, FGF, PDGF, EGF, TGF-β	Microglia, neurones?, vastrocytes
Convulsants	IL-1β, IL-6, TNF-α, LIF	Neurones?
Ischaemia	IL-1β, IL-6, FGF, TGF-β	Microglia?, neurones, perivascular cells
Multiple sclerosis	IL-1β, IL-2, IL-6, TNF-α, TNF-β, IFN-γ	Microglia, T-lymphocytes astrocytes
Down's syndrome	IL-1β	Microglia
Alzheimer's disease	IL-1β, IL-2, IL-6 (FGF?), NGF	Microglia, macrophages, astrocytes
Newcastle disease virus	IFN-α,β	Astrocytes

HIV, human immunodeficiency virus; adapted from Morganti-Kossmann et al. (1992) and Hopkins and Rothwell (1995).

and Hopkins, 1995). In addition, cytokines may react in an autocrine, a paracrine and an endocrine manner and influence the various cells present at and surrounding the BBB establishing cell–cell contact and signal transduction (Plata-Salam n, 1991). Cytokines may signal in a peripherally directed (anterograde) and in a centrally directed (retrograde) way which underscores their functional role in the communication between central nervous system and the periphery (Patterson and Nawa, 1993). It has been suggested that a regulatory feedback exists between the nervous and the immune system via cytokines released by both systems. In addition, there is a strong interplay between hormones, cytokines and interferons (IFNs) (Baron et al., 1991; Patterson and Nawa, 1993). IFNs, like INF-α, IFN-β and IFN-γ may have direct effects on cells (e.g. antiproliferating effects and enhancement of cell lysis) but also indirect effects (e.g. increased expression of major-histocompatibility-complex II (MHC-II), and increase the expression of TNF-receptors, increase cell lysis, enhance the induction of antibodies to tumour cells and induce (tumour) toxicity of macrophages, T-cells and NK-cells. A very important effect of cytokines is the upregulation of CRF production in various regions of the brain, particularly in the hypothalamus (Wilder, 1995) which may turn on the whole cascade of the HPA-axis (Fig. 5). In addition, cytokines have been shown to reduce the affinity of the hippocampal mineralo-corticoid receptors (MR) in parallel with a prolonged and dramatic elevation of basal HPA-activity (Schöbitz et al., 1994).

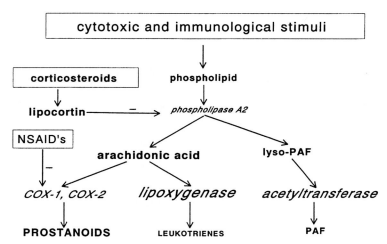

Fig. 5. Schematic representation of the production of eicosanoids and platelet activating factor (PAF) following a cytotoxic and immunological stress stimulus. COX = cyclooxygenase; NSAID = non-steroidal anti-inflammatory drug (redrawn from van Haeringen and Meijer, 1995).

Hormones and cytokines may modulate the effects of IFNs by having, e.g. a profound influence on their production. IL-1 produced by macrophages can induce T-cells to produce IL-2 which in turn induces IFN-γ or IFN-β (Le et al., 1986). NK-cell activity enhancement by IL-2 is partly due to IFN-γ production (Baron et al., 1987), while IFN-γ activates macrophages by inducing the production of TNF (Philip and Epstein, 1986). Interferons and cytokines (e.g. INF-α, INF-γ, TNF and IL-1) may also interfere with hypothalamic or pituitary functions (Barros et al., 1992) and IFN-α has been shown to inhibit the secretion of luteinizing hormone (LH) resulting in reduced secretion of oestradiol and progesteron in women (Kaupilla et al., 1982) and of testosterone in man (Orava et al., 1986).

Because of their physico-chemical characteristics (hydrophilicity, size), it is not likely that cytokines can easily pass the BBB. The only possibility for transport into the brain may exist in the circumventricular organs where the BBB is rather leaky (Gross et al., 1986) but where the ependyma and the choroid plexus present an epithelial (tight junctional and or metabolic) barrier. Therefore, it is not likely that passive transport from blood to

brain and/or from blood via the CSF to brain, may be sufficient to elicit a response to cytokine action in the brain since the concentrations may be too low, although secondary systems (whether or not via IL-receptors) may be involved that may result in BBB permeability. However, this may be different in disease state when BBB disruption has occurred. In addition, in mice active BBB transport systems have been described for the pro-inflammatory cytokines (TNF-α, IL-1α and IL-1β) (Banks et al., 1991; Gutierrez et al., 1993) while for the anti-inflammatory cytokines (TGF-β, IL-4 and IL-10) this is unknown. Cytokines may also indirectly influence BBB functionality. It has been shown that endothelial cells possess IL-1 receptors suggesting an autocrine regulation (May et al., 1989; Cozzolino et al., 1990) and recently it has been demonstrated that rat brain endothelial cells exhibit specific IL-1β binding sites which belong to the type I IL-1 receptor (van Dam et al., 1996). IL-1 receptors are particularly localized in specific areas of the brain: hypothalamus, the pyramidal cells of the hippocampus, and the granule cells of the dentate gyrus of the hippocampus, the frontal cortex and in vascular structures like vessels and the choroid plexus and in the adenohypophysis (Farrar et al., 1987; Ericsson et al., 1994; Haour et al., 1995). In addition, receptors for IFN-γ, IL-1, IL-6 and TNF-α were found in the pituitary (Carr and Weigert, 1990; Spellerberg et al., 1995). IL-1 receptors have also been found in the periphery of the body, e.g. the paraganglia in the rat liver hilus and hepatic vagus (Watkins et al., 1995b) which may implicate central effects via afferent nerves following peripheral stimulation by cytokine.

Induction of fever by cytokines

Fever can be induced by cytokines like IL-1α, IL-1β, IL-2, TNF-α, IL-6 and IFN-α,β,γ (Bendtzen, 1988; Dinarello et al., 1988; Tomasovic and Klosergaard, 1989) and there seems to be a negative feedback of temperature on the production of these cytokines (Kappel et al., 1991). Several of these cytokines (IL-1, TNF-α and IFN) act on temperature-sensitive neurons in the hypothalamus causing fever through their stimulatory effects on prostaglandin synthesis (Stitt, 1990; Kent et al., 1992). In addition, PGE_2 is a second mediator of IL-1 and possibly TNF-α and IL-6 (Dinarello et al., 1986). It is known to be a potent inducer of fever when administered in the organum vasculosum laminae terminalis (OVLT) in the CNS (Stitt, 1990) and is associated with the acute phase response to infection, inflammation, trauma and cancer (Chance and Fischer, 1991; Morganti-Kossmann et al., 1992; Woodroofe, 1995). TNF-α is also a potent inducer of fever. Its expression in particular in macrophages, is strongly regulated at the level of transcription, transcript stability and translation (Beutler, 1990) while there is a negative feedback via PGE_2 (Kunkel et al., 1988), glucocorticoids (Beutler, 1990) and fever (Klostergaard et al., 1989; Fouqueray et al., 1992).

Intraventricular IL-1β (Palmi et al., 1994) induces fever which is mediated by the release of Ca^{2+} into the CSF which in turn activates phospholipase A_2 (PLA_2). This membrane bound enzyme is Ca^{2+}-dependent and converts arachidonic acid into eicosanoids like PGE_2 which induces among others hyperthermia. These effects could be blocked by glucocorticoids which seem to induce Ca^{2+} uptake by the cells (Hayashi et al., 1991) and to inhibit the synthesis of IL-1β-mRNA and the posttranscriptional expression of PLA_2 and inhibits enzymatic activity by inducing the synthesis of lipocortins which possess anti-inflammatory and antipyretic activity (Solito and Parente, 1989; Davidson et al., 1991; Solito et al., 1991). In addition, other cytokines (IL-1, TNF-α, TGF-γ and PDGF) may induce the production of eicosanoids by inducing the transcription of synthetic enzymes like cyclooxygenase (COX) and PLA_2 (Rothwell and Hopkins, 1995) which ultimately may result in fever.

Production of cytokines and subsequently other compounds

The production of cytokines may be induced by various kinds of stress including bacterial products (e.g. endotoxins), viruses, temperature and other endogenous compounds (like bradykinin). In addition, subsequently various other compounds may be induced (like eicosanoids, PAF) which may influence BBB permeability.

Endotoxins, like LPS, and rabies virus can induce in the mouse the secretion of TNF-α and IL-1 and influence the HPA-axis and downregulate IL-1 binding in the hippocampus while binding at the receptors in the pituitary remained at the same level as in the control. However, restraint stress and dexamethasone did increase the IL-1 receptor density in the adenohypophysis but not in the hippocampus (Haour et al., 1995).

Viruses have been shown to induce the secretion of cytokines like IL-1 and TNF-α by macrophages which may damage myelin and or oligodendrocytes (Tyor et al., 1993) while other macrophage factors have been shown to cause neurotoxic effects (Guillian et al., 1990). In addition, endothelial cells in the brain of HIV-1 positive individuals do have a positive staining for IL-1, IL-6, IFN-γ and TNF-α (Tyor et al., 1992).

Temperature may also influence the release pattern of cytokines. It has been shown that LPS at 37°C induces the release of IL-6 and TNF-α in human monocyte derived macrophages while at 40°C there was only release of IL-6 (Ensor et al., 1994). In addition, it has been demonstrated that whole body hyperthermia (WBH) induces IL-1 *in vivo* (Neville and Sauder, 1988).

Many stress stimuli, including cytotoxic and immunological stimuli, induce the production of cytokines. Several of these cytokines (IL-1, TNF, TGF-β and PDGF) stimulate the synthetic enzymes (COX and PLA$_2$; see Fig. 5) to produce eicosanoids (Rothwell and Hopkins, 1995; see Fig. 5) like prostaglandins and leukotrienes and platelet activating factor (PAF) by endothelial cells, platelets, macrophages and neutrophils (Spellerberg and Tuomanen, 1994). *In vitro* studies have shown that eicosanoid production could be induced by LPS, IL-1 and IL-6 in confluent monolayers of rat brain microvessel endothelial cells and rat aortic endothelial cells but that the patterns of eicosanoids production were different. Particularly brain microvessel endothelial cells produced more PGE$_2$ while in aortic endothelial cells more 6-keto-PGF$_{1\alpha}$ (a stable metabolite of prostacyclin (PGI$_2$)) was produced (de Vries et al., 1995a) which indicates a difference in response between microvessel and larger vessel endothelium (Fig. 3). In addition, bradykinin may induce macrophages to release TNF-α, which in turn may induce the release of IL-1 and IL-6. Both may induce cyclooxygenase-2 (COX-2), in contrast to the constitutively expressed COX-1, in endothelial cells and result in the production of eicosanoids, which may result in increased BBB permeability. However, this production can also induced in neurones by IL-8 (Dray and Bevan, 1993). All these compounds have been shown to increase BBB permeability (Estrada et al., 1995, Rothwell and Hopkins, 1995).

Expression of adhesion molecules and major-histocompatibility-complex (MHC) at the BBB

Cytokines and endotoxins may induce the expression of several adhesion molecules at endothelial cells (see Table 3; Springer, 1990, 1994; Belivac-

qua et al., 1991; Carlos and Harlan, 1994; de Vries et al., 1994, 1996a; de Vries, 1995). These molecules can be categorized into three superfamilies: the selectins, the immunoglobulins and the integrins and play an important role in the recognition by binding at and migration of lymphocytes through the BBB (Osborn, 1990; Springer, 1990; Carlos and Harlan, 1994). In addition, the LFA-1/ICAM-1, the VLA-4/VCAM-1 and the E-selectin (ELAM-1) pathways are specifically involved in lymphocyte adhesion to stimulated brain endothelial cells (Table 3; Shimizu et al., 1991; Carlos and Harlan, 1994).

LPS, INF-γ, TNF-α and IL-1 may upregulate ICAM-1 *in vitro* at brain microvessel endothelial cells in a dose and time-dependent way (Fabry et al., 1992; Wong and Dorovini-Zis, 1992) while also upregulation of LFA-3 and VCAM-1 at the BBB has been demonstrated (Lassmann et al., 1991; Waight-Sharma et al., 1992).

It has been shown *in vitro* that following LPS, IL-1 and IL-6 stimulation, lymphocyte binding to bovine brain capillary endothelial cells could be inhibited by antibodies against LFA-1 and VLA-4 (81% and 96% respectively) which belong to the LFA-1/ICAM-1 and the VLA-4/VCAM-1 pathways while the effects of IL-6 could be almost completely blocked by co-incubation with IL-6 antibodies (de Vries et al., 1994). In addition, adhesion of lymphocytes to BBB endothelium *in vitro* was lower than to aortic endothelial cells, while in contrast, induction of lymphocyte-binding to BBB endothelium induced by cytokines was more rapid than to aortic endothelium which suggests a rapid accumulation of these cells during inflammatory reactions and immune responses (Male et al., 1990b).

Virus may also increase the expression of adhesion molecules at the BBB, since upregulation of specifically ICAM-1 has been reported in HIV-infected endothelial cells together with an increased binding of HIV-infected monocytes (Black and Sager, 1994).

The expression of major histocompatibility complex I (MHC-I) and MHC-II is also controlled by cytokines. MHC-1 can be induced on

TABLE 3

The adhesion molecule superfamilies and their corresponding ligands and the cells where these can be expressed

	Family	Ligand	Expressed on
CD11a/CD18 (LFA-1)	Integrins	ICAM-1, ICAM-1	All leukocytes
CD11b/CD18 (Mac-1)	Integrins	ICAM-1, fibrinogen	Monocytes, neutrophils, lymphocytes
CD11c/CD18 (p150,95)	Integrins	iC3b,	Monocytes, neutrophils
VLA-4 CD11a/CD18	Integrins	VCAM-1, fibrinogen	All leukocytes except neutrophils
ICAM-1	Ig-superfamily	CD11a/CD18, CD11b/CD18	Various, including endothelial cells
ICAM-2	Ig-superfamily	CD11a/CD18	Endothelial cells
VCAM-2	Ig-superfamily	VLA-4	Endothelial cells
E-selectin (ELAM-1)	Selectins	Sialyl-Lex	Activated endothelial cells
P-selectin (GMP-140)	Selectins	Carbohydrate	Degranulated endothelial cells and platelets
L-selectin (LAM-1)	Selectins	Carbohydrate	Monocytes, neutrophils, lymphocytes

Adapted from Springer, 1990; Belivacqua et al., 1991; Carlos and Harlan, 1994; de Vries, 1995.

all cells including the BBB, while MHC-II expression is restricted to monocytes, macrophages and dendritic cells and can be induced in endothelial cells, microglia and astrocytes in vitro by IFN-γ (Hirsch et al., 1983; Wong et al., 1984; Fierz et al., 1985). However, astrocytes may only express MHC-II following a relatively high dose of IFN-γ (Vass and Lassmann, 1990).

Cytokines and hyperthermia

Hyperthermia induced by intracerebroventricular administered IL-1β can be reduced by EDTA which is related to the binding of Ca^{2+} excreted by neurons upon IL-1β stimulation (Palmi et al., 1994; see *Induction of fever by cytokines*). Fever can be induced not only via a central action but also by a peripheral action. It has been shown

that transsection of the the subdiaphragmatic vagus inhibits hyperthermia induced by peripheral application of IL-1β (Watkins et al., 1995b). Afferent vagus neurons project into the nucleus tractus solitarius which can be strongly activated by IL-1. In addition, hyperthermia was longer lasting in rats stressed by exposure to IL-1β and handling, than when additionally an IL-1 receptor antagonist (IL-1ra) was given. These data indicate that peripherally administered endotoxin induces hyperthermia which could be inhibited by administration of IL-1ra but not hyperthermia-induced by stress like handling. This means that peripheral stress can induce hyperthermia via afferent neurons in the CNS which constitutes another route of immune-brain communication. In addition, fever induced by LPS in pigs by stimulation of the median preoptic, supraoptic and paraventricular nuclei, could be inhibited by indomethacin (Parrott et al., 1995).

Stress-induced hyperthermia may also possess an opioid component. It was shown in rats that sleep deprivation combined with low dose antigen challenge (sheep red blood cells) both in themselves nonpyrogenic, gave an opioid and not an IL-1 mediated rise in colonic temperature which could be inhibited by pretreatment with naloxon (Brown et al., 1992).

Hyperthermia has been shown to modulate the activity of monocytes, NK cells and lymphocytes and was associated with an increase of IFN-γ and IL-2 production but had no effect on TNF-α production by monocytes isolated from hyperthermic persons. In addition, hyperthermia (39.5°C) did not influence the production of cytokines (IL-1α, IL-1β, TNF-α and IFN-γ) from stimulated (phytohemagglutinin) human monocytes while indomethacin enhanced the ex vivo production of TNF-β by monocytes under hyperthermic and thermoneutral conditions. It was suggested that these results indicate the existence of a negative feedback of fever and that hyperthermia alters the sensitivity of monocytes to prostaglandins (Kappel et al., 1995).

Hyperthermia activates T-cells at 40°C but inhibits the activity of these cells at a temperature of 42°C (Shen et al., 1994). Similar results have been seen with NK cell activity which was associated with induced IFN-γ production (Fleischmann et al., 1986). In addition, LPS at 37°C induces the release of IL-6 and TNF-α in human monocyte derived macrophages while at 40°C there was only release of IL-6, a 75-fold increase of HSP72-mRNA and a 56% inhibition of protein synthesis while cell viability was unaffected (Ensor et al., 1994). Therefore heat shock seems to reduce the release of TNF-α but also of IL-1 (Klostergaard et al., 1989; Fouqueray et al., 1992). Increased levels of IL-1β and granulocyte-colony stimulating factor (G-CSF) were found following WBH applied in patients for 1 h at 41.8°C while in 2 of 9 patients increased levels of tumour necrosis factor (TNF) were found (d'Oleire et al., 1993).

It may be concluded from these data that hyperthermia may have consequences for the production of cytokines by various cells at the level of the BBB during inflammatory processes in the brain. However, little is known about the effects of hyperthermia on the production of cytokines by BBB endothelial cells. In addition, hyperthermia increases hsp release and production and therefore induces thermotolerance which protects cells against damage.

Cytokines and BBB permeability

Cytokines play an important role in many (CNS)-diseases. They may directly or indirectly change BBB functionality and permeability in many diseases with an inflammatory component, e.g. bacterial meningitis increases BBB permeability, in particular at the arachnoidal membrane, choroid plexus epithelium and the cerebral microvascular endothelium (Tunkel and Scheld, 1993). Cytokines are soon present in the CSF following a challenge by bacteria or bacterial products (Spellerberg and Tuomanen, 1994). One to three hours following intracisternal challenge with life bacteria or bacterial components, peak levels of TNF-α, IL-1β, and IL-6 can be measured in the CSF. Several of these cytokines, produced by astrocytes (Chung and Benveniste, 1990), macrophages (Sminia et al., 1986), monocytes, microglia and endothelial cells (see also Cytokines), may cause increased BBB permeability, decreased (regional) cerebral bloodflow (CBF) and increased intra-cranial pressure (ICP) and recruitment of leukocytes (via upregulated adhesion molecules) (Dinarello, 1989; Spellerberg and Tuomanen, 1994). Some cytokines, like TNF-α, IFN-γ and IL-1 may cause functional changes in BBB permeability, BBB endothelial damage and oligodendrocyte death (Sharief and Thompson, 1992; Vartanian et al., 1995), while others, like TFG-β and IL-10, may play a neuroprotective role probably by damping the inflammatory response in the brain (Chao et al., 1993).

In vivo, 4 h following intracisternal inoculation of LPS, a maximal increase in BBB permeability was found by measuring intravenously administered ^{125}I-labelled albumin in the CSF (Tunkel and Scheld, 1993). A similar observation was made in Lewis rats following induction of EAE (experimental allergic encephalomyelitis). Increased CSF concentrations of intravenous administration of fluorescein were observed which could be explained by an increased BBB permeability and/or decreased brain elimination of fluorescein (Fig. 6a, de Vries et al., 1995b). In addition, when LPS was given intravenously to rats, increased BBB transport of the intravenously administered hydrophilic marker fluorescein was found, which could be completely explained by the changed plasma pharmacokinetics of fluorescein under LPS conditions (Fig. 6b) suggesting that BBB permeability had not changed. However, the opening of the BBB following systemic administration of LPS may be dose-dependent and higher doses, which may occur during sepsis, may open the BBB. In rats IL-2 and IL-6 have been shown to increase BBB permeability (^{14}C-AIB) in several tissues and to decrease regional cerebral blood flow, which seems to correspond to the presence of a high number of specific IL-2 binding sites in the cerebral cortex, the hippocampus

and the hypothalamus (Saija et al., 1995). However, apart from IL-6 (de Vries et al., 1994), there is no evidence that IL-2 acts directly upon endothelial cells and it is likely that the effect on BBB permeability is mediated by a stimulated release of vasoactive substances like platelet activating factor (PAF; Greenwood, 1992). In rats, intra-carotic administration of IL-1β did not have any effect, while TNF-α decreased BBB permeability and increased regional CBF. The increased regional CBF could be caused by the effect of TNF-α on endothelial cells by affecting the synthesis and release of vasodilator agents like PGI$_2$, PAF and the formation of NO (nitric oxide); (Estrada et al., 1995; Saija et al., 1995) causing hypotension (Tracey et al., 1986). However, also vasoconstrictive agents like PDGF (Saija et al., 1995) and endothelin-1 (ET-1) (Estrada et al., 1995) may be released too by endothelium. PAF, which is a mediator of inflammation, is mainly produced by endothelial cells, macrophages, neutrophils and platelets following injury and increases BBB permeability (Issekutz and Szpejda, 1986; Wissner et al., 1986). It may cause vasogenic oedema (Niemoller and Tauber, 1989), particular in the white matter, which results in in-

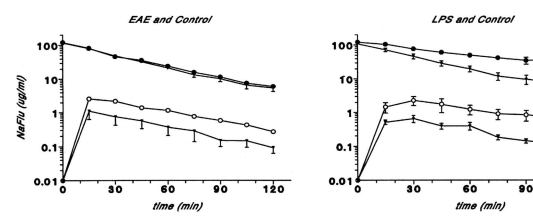

Fig. 6. (a) (left) Concentrations of sodium fluorescein (NaFlu) in plasma (solid symbols) and cerebro-spinal fluid (CSF; open symbols) in control animals (triangles) and in animals with experimental allergic encephalomyelitis (EAE; circles) following intravenous infusion of 10 mg NaFlu (de Vries et al., 1995b); (b) (right) Concentrations of sodium fluorescein (NaFlu) in plasma (solid symbols) and cerebro-spinal fluid (CSF; open symbols) in control animals (triangles) and in animals pretreated with lipopolysaccharide (LPS; 2 mg/kg; circles) following intravenous infusion of 10 mg NaFlu [from de Vries et al. (1995b), reprinted with kind permission of Plenum Publishing Corp., New York, NY, USA].

creased endothelial permeability, in cytotoxic oedema (Tauber et al., 1993), in the swelling of glia, neurons and endothelial cells caused by toxins, and in interstitial oedema (Scheld et al., 1980), as a result of impaired CSF outflow via the arachnoids. This all may subsequently contribute to increased BBB permeability, reduced CBF and increased ICP.

Opposing results are sometimes seen following *in vitro* and in vivo experiments. It was shown that TNF-α may decrease *in vivo* BBB permeability (Saija et al., 1995) while others showed increased capillary permeability (Estrada et al., 1995). In addition, *in vitro* a delayed permeability for sucrose and inulin was induced after 16 h and a reorganization of F-actin filaments into stress fibers following TNF-α exposure for 1 h to bovine brain endothelial cells (Deli et al., 1995a).

TNF-α, which may also cause angiogenesis (Fràter-Schröder et al., 1987), may not only induce NO production by bovine cerebral endothelial cells but also by bovine cerebral smooth muscle cells which may lead to a cytotoxic effect on the endothelial cells and to changes in BBB permeability and brain edema (Estrada et al., 1995). Under physiological conditions the BBB lacks the constitutive expression of nitric-oxide synthase (NOS) (Shukla et al., 1995). However, inflammatory mediators including inactivated *Escherischia coli* (comparable to lipopolysaccharide) or poly(I:C) (an inducer of α-, β- and γ-interferon) may induce the expression of NOS in brain (Koprowski et al., 1993), macrophages (Drapier et al., 1988) and endothelial cells (Palmer et al., 1992). These effects were potentiated by L-arginine, which is a substrate for NOS, and not by D-arginine. In addition, the effects could be inhibited by N-nitro L-arginine methyl ester, an inhibitor of NOS and by dexamethasone, an inhibitor of NOS induction, indicating that NOS can be induced at the BBB which may result in increased NO release and increased BBB permeability.

BBB permeability may also be induced by TNF-α via another pathway. It has been shown that TNF-α, which is produced under many neurological conditions, can induce the production of

matrix metalloproteinase in particular gelatinase B (Rosenberg et al., 1995). Gelatinases attack, in concert with urokinase-type plasminogen activator (uPA) (Reich et al., 1988), the basal lamina macromolecules like type IV collagen surrounding the brain microvessels resulting in an increased sucrose permeability after 24 h. In particular, gelatinase B is increased during inflammatory processes while gelatinase A is associated with tumour invasion and angiogenesis (Hibbs et al., 1985). In addition, microglial cells, foetal astrocytes, glioma cells and endothelial cells produce metalloproteinases in culture (Herron et al., 1986a,b; Apodaca et al., 1990; Colton et al., 1993). These data indicate that in rats there seems to be a link between increased TNF-α production following injury and endothelial capillary permeability mediated via induced expression of metalloproteinases like gelatinase B. In addition, it was shown that an intracerebral injection of gelatinase A also opens the BBB (Rosenberg et al., 1992).

In vitro experiments with LPS enhanced BBB permeability of fluorescein in confluent monolayers of BMEC (Fig. 7a,b; de Vries et al., 1996b), and similar effects were found following stimulation of rat BMEC with TNF-α, IL-1β and IL-6 (de Vries et al., 1996b). In addition, the increased permeability as measured by reduced TEER (transendothelial electrical resistance), could be blocked with indomethacin while the effect of IL-1β could be blocked with IL-1 receptor antagonist (Fig. 8a,b). In these experiments it is interesting to note that TEER following incubation with TNF-α and IL-1β recovered to control values after about 200 min while following incubation with IL-6, TEER did not recover but was still slowly decreasing. Enhanced permeability of monolayers of brain microvessel endothelial cells (BMEC) has been shown following stimulation with IFN-γ and TNF-α (Hughes et al., 1988; Male et al., 1990a; Huynh and Dorovini-Zis, 1993). Similar effects have been shown following stimulation of bovine BMEC with LPS where the TEER decreased and transport of the hydrophilic paracellular marker fluorescein increased (de Vries et

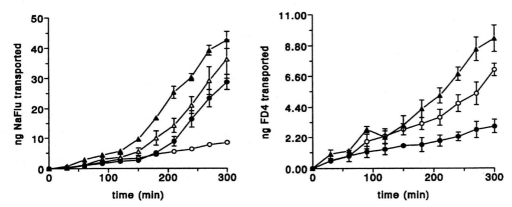

Fig. 7. (a) (left) Transport of sodium fluorescein across confluent monolayers of bovine brain microvessel endothelial cells (BMEC) after treatment with lipopolysaccharide (LPS). Sodium fluorescein (1 μg/ml) was administered at the luminal site of the monolayers and transport across monolayers of BMEC treated with 0 (○), 10 (●), 50 (△) and 100 (▲) ng of LPS was measured (redrawn from de Vries et al., 1996b); (b) (right) Transport of fluorescein dextran (FD4; mol. weight 4000) across confluent monolayers of bovine brain microvessel endothelial cells (BMEC) after treatment with lipopolysaccharide (LPS). FD4 (1 μg/ml) was administered at the luminal site of the monolayers and transport across monolayers of BMEC treated with 0 (●), 10 (○), and 100 (▲) ng of LPS was measured (redrawn from de Vries et al., 1996b).

al., 1996b). In addition, the decrease in TEER could be blocked to control levels when the monolayers were pretreated with indomethacin (Fig. 8c) which indicates a role for eicosanoids in BBB permeability (Fig. 3 and Fig. 5). In this respect it is important to note that macrophages may also contribute to increased BBB permeability since they may release eicosanoids but also quinolinate, proteinases and ROS (radical oxygen species), while they also express MHC-II (antigen presentation) and Fc-receptors (phagocytosis) upon induction by IFN-γ (Black, 1995; Woodroofe, 1995).

Interleukins too, particularly IL-1 and IL-6, may induce COX-2, in endothelial cells and result in the production of eicosanoids, which may result in increased BBB permeability (see Fig. 5, Dray and Bevan, 1993).

Cytokines may also induce microglia to produce ROS which may damage membranes (Selmaj and Raine, 1988; Loughlin et al., 1992) and add to increased BBB permeability. In addition, LPS increases the production of several free radicals like hydrogen peroxide, singlet oxygen, superoxide anion and hydroxyl radicals in macrophages

(Nathan, 1982). However, protecting systems like Cu/Zn superoxide dismutase (SOD) which catalyses superoxide radical to oxygen and hydrogen peroxide (Hass and Massaro, 1988; Lagrange et al., 1994), are present at the BBB for scavenging ROS products. Hyperthermia and LPS have been shown to induce Mn-SOD in HT-29 epithelial cells and in the pancreas respectively (Wong et al., 1989; Lee et al., 1993; Abe et al., 1995) but it is not evident from the literature if this also occurs at the level of the BBB.

Surface molecules and BBB permeability

Although during inflammation, BBB destruction rarely occurs in vivo, increased migration of cells into the CNS may occur (Lassmann, 1983). Activated T-cells may migrate into the brain via the BBB recognizing antigens which are beyond the BBB and play, irrespective of their antigen specificity, an important role in immune-surveillance of the brain (Wekerle et al., 1991). Cytokines are in particular involved in the upregulation of adhesion molecules and MHC II at the BBB which may lead to increased lymphocyte migration. In

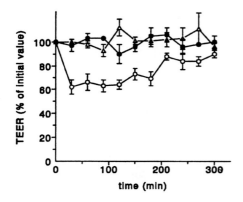

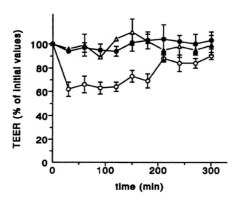

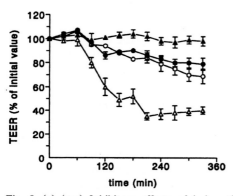

particular the LFA-1/ICAM-1, the VLA-4/VCAM-1 and the E-selectin (ELAM-1) pathways are involved in lymphocyte adhesion to stimulated brain endothelial cells (Shimizu et al., 1991; de Vries et al., 1994).

It has been shown that increased endothelial permeability in vitro coincided with increased expression of MHC II following stimulation with IFN-γ and TNF-α (Hughes et al., 1988; Male et al., 1990a; Huynh and Dorovini-Zis, 1993). In addition, in vitro it was observed that TNF-α induced the expression of ELAM-1 and VCAM-1 and also the constitutive expression of ICAM-1 and MHC-I in human-umbilical vein endothelial cells (HUVEC); however hyperthermia combined with TNF-α failed to induce the expression of ELAM-1 and VCAM-1 while the constitutive expression of ICAM-1 and MHC-I was not affected by heat but upregulation was inhibited (Waight-Sharma et al., 1992). It is not known if these effects do also occur at the level of the BBB, since literature date are not available.

Fig. 8. (a) (top) Inhibitory effects of indomethacin on the IL-1β-induced effects. Confluent monolayers from rat brain microvessel endothelial cells were pretreated with indomethacin (1 μM), a cyclooxygenase inhibitor, for 30 min ($\triangle$) and subsequently 100 ng of IL-1β/ml ($\bullet$) was administered. Incubation of the monolayers with 100 ng of IL-1β ($\bigcirc$) caused a decrease in *trans*-endothelial electrical resistance (TEER) compared to untreated monolayers (redrawn from de Vries et al., 1996a); (b) (middle) Inhibitory effects of indomethacin on the IL-1 receptor antagonist on the IL-1β-induced effects. Confluent monolayers from rat brain microvessel endothelial cells were pretreated with IL-1 receptor antagonist (10^{-7} M) for 30 min ($\triangle$) and subsequently 100 ng of IL-1β/ml ($\bullet$) was administered. Incubation of the monolayers with 100 ng of IL-1β ($\bigcirc$) caused a decrease in *trans*-endothelial electrical resistance (TEER) compared to untreated monolayers. Data are expressed as % of the initial (t = 0) value of the same monolayer and as mean $\pm$ S.E.M. ($n = 5$) (redrawn from de Vries et al., 1996a); (c) (bottom) Inhibitory effects of indomethacin on the LPS-induced effects. Confluent monolayers of bovine brain microvessel endothelial cells (BMEC) were pretreated with indomethacin (1 μM), a cyclooxygenase inhibitor, for 30 min ($\bullet$) and subsequently 100 ng of LPS/ml ($\bigcirc$) was administered. Incubation of the BMEC with 100 ng of LPS/ml ($\triangle$) caused a decrease in transendothelial electrical resistance (TEER), compared to the TEER across untreated monolayers ($\blacktriangle$). Data are expressed as percentage of the initial (t = 0) value of the same monolayer and as mean $\pm$ S.E.M. ($n = 5$). For this experiment, initial control values (285 $\pm$ 8 ohm/cm^2; $n = 5$; mean $\pm$ S.E.M.) were taken as 100% value (redrawn from de Vries et al., 1996b).

Hyperthermia and BBB permeability

Heat stress particularly in young but not old rats caused increased *BBB permeability* for Evans blue (up to 464%) and ^{131}I-sodium (515%) (Sharma et al., 1992, 1994) and serotonin concentrations in plasma and brain increased 687 and 267%, respectively. It was suggested that serotonin was bound to $5HT_2$-receptors which did increase the production of prostaglandins thereby elevating cAMP levels which caused increased vesicular (pinocytotic) transport (Sharma et al., 1996).

Hyperthermia also induces various *stimulating activities*. It may activate various cells, from which it is known that they may damage the BBB. Temperatures up to 40°C increase significantly the T-cell proliferative capacity, the lectin-dependent cell cytotoxicity and LAK cell cytotoxicity (Shen et al., 1994), while it also increases the NK cell activity associated with induced IFN-γ production (Fleischmann et al., 1986; Downing et al., 1987). However, at 42°C, these enhancements were considerably reduced (Shen et al., 1994).

Hyperthermia also increases the release and synthesis of hsps which provide protection against the effects of various stress stimuli. Upregulation of hsp70 in various cells, e.g. glia, neurons and endothelial cells has been demonstrated. In addition, it was suggested that hsps may amplify the local immune response or play a protective role against stress stimuli maybe via the induction of immune tolerance, while heat shock may also modulate the production of cytokines and inhibit in neutrophils the release of inflammatory mediators (ROS, leukotrienes) that are involved in acute inflammation and allergy (Polla and Kantengwa, 1991).

It has been shown that steroids may modulate the heat shock response in human macrophages-monocytes (Polla et al., 1993) and also in T-lymphocytes (Norton and Latchman, 1989) and fibroblastic cell lines (Kasambalides and Lanks, 1983) by interference with hsp synthesis. However, hyperthermia may also influence steroid receptor binding since this seems to be very heat sensitive although it may recover quickly (Anderson et al., 1991). This may have consequences for the effects particularly of glucocorticoids during hyperthermia, since high dose dexamethasone has been shown to prevent BBB permeability of albumin in normothermic rats (Paul and Bolton, 1995).

Hyperthermia may also induce the release and production of cytokines. WBH in mice (20 min at 42°C) induced threefold increased plasma IL-1α concentrations and TNF-α concentrations were unchanged; however, no data were shown on BBB permeability (Blake et al., 1994). In addition, it has been shown that heat shock and LPS may decrease the release of IL-1 and TNF-α and induce an hsp response (Hall, 1994). Cytokines (IL-1, IL-2, IFN's, TNF-α) generally do not induce but modulate hsps directly or indirectly via their pyrogenic activity (Polla and Kantengwa, 1991). However, induction of hsp70 has been shown in IL-2 receptor bearing T-lymphocytes and of metallothioneins by IL-6 in hepatocytes. Effects of IL-1, TNF-α, IFN-α,β,γ have been shown on hsps and oxidation specific stress proteins but only in peripheral tissues and cells and no data are available for the effects of cytokines on hsps in CNS-tissues (Polla et al., 1993).

Various other effects of hyperthermia that may influence endothelial cells

The expression of *adhesion molecules* requires protein synthesis and it is known that environmental stress like hyperthermia (41–43°C) can reduce protein synthesis considerably (Hurst, 1990). Hyperthermia indeed inhibited the de novo synthesis of ELAM-1 and VECAM-1 in HUVEC but upregulated the expression of ICAM-1 and MHC-I by TNF-α (Polla, 1988); however it is not known if this also happens at the level of the BBB. In addition, all kinds of intracellular processes may be hampered that are needed to maintain homeostasis of the BBB while, in contrast, hsps may be released and induced.

Hyperthermia may also influence *blood clotting* since it increased plasminogen activator-inhibitor type 1 (PAI-1) and decreased tissue-type plasminogen activator (tPA) (Wojta et al., 1991).

Metabolism may be influenced by hyperthermia which may lead to reduced hepatic elimination. WBH together with IL-1 and to a lesser extent WBH alone, decreases N-demethylation in the liver in mice but did not have an effect on cytochrome P_{450} (cyt-P_{450}) and b_5 (Neville and Sing, 1990). In addition, it was shown that LPS inhibited microsomal P_{450} metabolism (Gorodischer et al., 1976) in the liver while also IL-1 (Ghezzi et al., 1986a) and TNF (Ghezzi et al., 1986b) were shown to inhibit hepatic drug metabolism. It has been shown that the BBB presents cyt-P_{450} (Minn et al., 1991) but based on the results at the level of the liver, it is not likely that hyperthermia may affect cyt-P_{450}-mediated metabolism. Nevertheless, several other enzymes have been shown to be present at the BBB which may be affected by hyperthermia, but the effect of hyperthermia on the functionality of these enzymes at the level of the BBB is not known.

Systemic hyperthermia may also induce the release of *nitric oxide* (NO) by endothelial cells, which causes vasodilatation and decreases platelet aggregation (Fajardo and Prionas, 1994) and increases BBB permeability (Estrada et al., 1995).

Heat shock has been shown to upregulate the expression of *HIV* in U1 (promonocytic) and ACH-2 (T-lymphocyte) cells which were chronically infected with HIV (Stanley et al., 1990) and similar effects have been shown by stimulation with phorbol esters like PMA (Folks et al., 1988), cytokines (TNF-α, and TNF-β) (Poli et al., 1989), GM-CSF (Folks et al., 1987) and IL-6 (Poli et al., 1990). It was concluded that although physiologic levels of heat were not sufficient to induce virus expression, combined treatment with cytokines was, which may suggest that hyperthermia associated with opportunistic infections may play a role in the induction of virus in infected cells. This may have consequences for HIV present in the brain since BBB endothelial cells may be directly infected by HIV (Poland et al., 1995).

It was shown that *psychological stress* causes a rapid rise in body temperature in rats, rabbits and humans (Long et al., 1990). In rats, increases in temperature caused by exposure to a novel environment could be partly (up to 77%) blocked by salicylate (Singer et al., 1986) or indomethacin (Kluger et al., 1987). Support for the hypothesis that stress-induced hyperthermia is a true fever, was obtained from experiments in rats pretreated with antiserum against TNF (Long et al., 1990). In these animals a significantly ($P < 0.002$) greater hyperthermia was observed than in control serum injected rats (1.38 $\pm$ 0.11 vs.. 0.79 $\pm$ 0.14°C). Similar results were obtained after cage-switching stress and in animals injected with LPS and pretreated with antiserum against TNF. Although TNF could not be detected in plasma nor the CSF following exposure to open-field stress, TNF seems to play an antipyretic role in these stress responses and the apparent involvement of TNF in modulating the stress response is consistent with the concept that acute psychological stress activates the immune system; however it is not known if BBB permeability is increased under these conditions.

Mild exercise, which results in hyperthermia, causes increased IL-6 concentrations in plasma while IL-1α, IL-1β and TNF-α could not be reliably detected during exercise (Pedersen and Ullum, 1994). Since it has been shown *in vitro* that IL-6 may open the BBB, exercise may be able to change *in vivo* BBB permeability. During exercise, NK cells with a high IL-2 response capacity were recruited to the blood. This stimulation of the immune system was probably mediated by increased WBH, cytokines (IL-1, IL-6 and TNF-α) or stress hormones (adrenaline, growth hormone, beta-endorphins, cortisol) induced by exercise. In addition, it was shown that severe exercise decreased NK-activity and IL-1 concentrations in plasma and increased therefore the chance of infections.

The combination of psychological and exercise-induced stress on BBB permeability could be an explanation for the results observed following forced swimming. Particularly in young rats (8–9 weeks) and not in old rats (24–32 weeks) this resulted in increased serotonin concentrations in plasma (180%) and brain (250%) and an increased BBB permeability to ^{131}I-sodium and Evans blue (Sharma et al., 1991, 1996). Both effects could be prevented by pretreatment with a 5-HT$_2$-receptor antagonist. In addition, vinblastine which inhibits vesicular transport by inhibiting the formation of microtubuli, prevented extravasation of the tracers.

Other secondary mediators that may influence BBB permeability

In vitro a selective induction of albumin permeation through confluent monolayers of bovine brain endothelial cells has been shown following histamine exposure (Deli et al., 1995b) while cyclic adenosine 3′,5′-monophosphate decreased the paracellular transport of sucrose and inuline (Deli et al., 1995c).

Several other compounds that may be produced following various kinds of stress (LPS, IL-1, heat stress, forced swimming) like arachidonic acid, prostaglandins and leukotrienes as mentioned before, but also bradykinin, serotonin and polyamines, may increase BBB permeability, some in particular in brain tumours (like leukotrienes, bradykinin analogues, histamine) (Black, 1995; Cloughesy and Black, 1995). Due to the low expression of γ-glutamyl transpeptidase in tumour endothelial cells, leukotrienes are metabolized to a lesser extent (LTC4 to LTD4) and may increase the vascular permeability in tumours, particularly for small molecules. In addition, histamine may change the bloodflow and permeability in systemic and cerebral vessels (Shiling et al., 1987, 1993) probably via H$_2$-receptors (Boertje et al., 1992).

Bradykinin is a peptide formed from high molecular weight kininogen by kallikrein. In low doses it is able to selectively increase the permeability of abnormal (tumour) capillaries to low and high molecular weight agents (Inamura and Black, 1994). Serotonine is one of the components that may be found in plasma following stress (Sharma et al., 1991, 1996). It may also open the BBB as shown in experiments in anes-

thetized rats where extravasation of Evans Blue and increased amounts of ^{131}I-sodium were found in whole brain (Sharma et al., 1990). The permeability for the latter compound was increased in the cerebral cortex, hippocampus, caudate nucleus, hypothalamus, colliculus and the cerebellum but not in the pons and the medulla oblongata. These effects could be inhibited by cyproheptadine, a 5HT$_2$-antagonist and indomethacine, a COX inhibitor. These data correspond well with *in vitro* data on BBB permeability following LPS treatment of confluent monolayers of bovine microvessel endothelial cells where the increased permeability could be blocked to control levels by pretreatment with indomethacin (de Vries et al., 1996b). Polyamines, which are produced following brain injury, may increase pinocytotic activity at the BBB (Trout et al., 1986) and therefore increase BBB permeability. In addition, polyamines and NO seem to be increased in CNS-vessels at the onset of EAE, supporting a role for these compounds in loss of BBB integrity (Bolton et al., 1994).

An interesting observation is that some of these compounds may increase paracellular permeability which is characterized by being more or less size-dependent (van Bree et al., 1988), transcellular pinocytosis which is relatively size-independent, or both (Black, 1995).

Conclusions

It may be concluded that cytokines change BBB functionality and permeability in various ways. Several cascades of effects may occur and many mediators may play a role in what may ultimately lead to effects at the level of the BBB. Several of these effects caused by cytokines have been studied separately and few in a comprehensive way. The data in the literature on BBB permeability are rather diffuse and the results are influenced by many variations like species, dose, time, site, cells involved, stress stimuli, etc., which make comparison difficult. To complete the whole picture may be a difficult task because it may be only accomplished following an integrated approach by various collabourating groups with different and complementary expertise. Nevertheless, this knowledge is necessary to understand the functionality of the BBB particularly in disease state and to be used to treat CNS diseases.

Acknowledgements

The help and suggestions of W. Sutanto and P.J. Gaillard to improve the manuscript are very much appreciated.

References

Abe, R., Shimosegawa, T., Morrizumi, S., Kikuchi, Y., Kimura, K., Satoh, A., Koizumi, M. and Toyota, T. (1995) Lipopolysaccharide induces manganese superoxide dismutase in the rat pancreas: its role in caerulein pancreatitis. *Biochem. Biophys. Res. Commun.*, 217: 1216–1222.

Anderson, R.L., Kraft, P.E., Bensaude, O. and Hahn, G. (1991) Binding activity of glucocorticoid receptors after heat shock. *Exp. Cell Res.*, 197: 100–106.

Anderson, J.M., Balda, M.S. and Fanning, A.S. (1993) The structure and regulation of tight junctions. *Curr. Opin. Cell Biol.*, 5: 772–778.

Apodaca, G., Rutka, J.T., Bopuhana, K., Berens, M.E., Giblin, J.R., Rosenblum, M.L., McKerrow, J.H. and Banda, M.J. (1990) Expression of metalloproteinases and metalloproteinase inhibitors by foetal astrocytes and glioma cells. *Cancer Res.*, 50: 2322–2329.

Augustin, H.G., Kozian, D.H. and Johnson, R.C. (1994) Differentiation of endothelial cells: analysis of the constitutive and activated endothelial cell phenotypes. *BioEssays*, 16 (12): 901–906.

Balkwill, F. (1989) *Cytokines and Cancer Therapy*, Oxford University Press, London.

Banks, W.A., Ortiz, L., Plotkin, S.R. and Kastin, A.J. (1991) Human IL-1 and murine IL-1 are transported from blood to brain in the mouse by a shared saturable mechanism. *J. Pharmacol. Exp. Ther.*, 259: 988–996.

Baron, S., Danzani, F., Stanton, G.J. and Fleischmann, W.R. Jr.. eds. (1987) *The Interferon System: A Current Review*, University of Texas, Austin.

Baron, S., Tyring, S.K., Fleischmann, W.R. Jr, Coppenhaver, D.H., Niesel, D.W., Klimpel, G.R., Stanton, G.J. and Hughes, T.K. (1991) The interferons: mechanisms of action and clinical applications. *J. Am. Med. Assoc.*, 266(10): 1375–1383.

Barros, C.M., Betts, J.G., Thatcher, W.W. and Hansen, P.J. (1992) Possible mechanisms for reduction of circulating concentrations of progesterone by interferons in cows: effects on hyperthermia, lueal cells, metabolism of progesterone and secretion of LH. *J. Endocrinol.*, 133: 175–182.

Belivacqua, M.E., Butcher, E., Furie, B., Gallatin, M., Gimbrone, M., Harlan, J., Kishimoto, K., Lasky, L., McEver, R., Paulson, J., Rosen, S., Seed, B., Siegelman, M., Springer, T., Stoolman, L., Tedder, T., Varki, A., Wagner, D. and Zimmerman, G. (1991) Selectins: a family of adhesion receptors *Cell*, 67: 233.

Bendtzen, K. (1988) Interleukin 1, interleukin 6 and tumor necrosis factor in infection, inflammation and immunity. *Immunol. Lett.*, 19: 183–191.

Berkenbosch, F., van Oers, J., del Rey, A., Tilders, F. and Besedovsky, H. (1987) Corticotropin-releasing factor producing neurons in the rat activated by interleukin-1. *Science*, 238: 524–526.

Beutler, B. (1990) The complex regulation and biology of TNF. *Oncogenesis*, 2: 9–18.

Beyer, E.C. (1993) Gap junctions. *Int. Rev. Cytol.*, 137C: 1–37.

Bicknell, R. (1993) Heterogeneity of the endothelial cell. *Behring Inst. Mitt.*, 92: 1–7.

Black, K.L. (1995) Biochemical opening of the blood–brain barrier. *Adv. Drug Deliv. Rev.*, 15: 37–52.

Black, R. and Sager, P. (1994) Summary of workshop contributions. *Adv. Neuroimmunol.*, 4: 149–156.

Blake, D., Bessey, P., Karl, I., Nunnally, I. and Hotchkiss, R. (1994) Hyperthermia induces IL-1α but does not decrease release of IL-1α or TNF-α after endotoxin. *Lymphokine Cytokine Res.*, 13(5): 271–275.

Boertje, S.B., Ward, S. and Robinson, A. (1992) H_2-receptors mediate histamine-induced variations in the permeability of the blood–brain barrier of rats. *Res. Commun. Chem. Pathol. Pharmacol.*, 76: 143–154.

Bolton, C., Lees, P., Paul, C., Scott, G.S., Williams, K.I. and Woodyer, P. (1994) Aspects of the biochemical pharmacology of neurovascular disruption in experimental allergic encephalomyelitis (EAE). *J. Neuroimmunol.*, 52: 113–115.

Bradbury, M. (1979) In: *The concepts of the blood–brain barrier*, Wiley, Chichester, p. 32.

Brown, R., King, M.G. and Husband, A.J. (1992) Sleep deprivation-induced hyperthermia following antigen challenge due to opioid but not interleukin-1 involvement. *Physiol. Behav.*, 51: 767–770.

Butt, A.M., Jones, H.C. and Abbott, N.J. (1990) Electrical resistance across the blood–brain barrier in anaesthetized rats: a developmental study. *J. Physiol.*, 429: 47–62.

Carlos, R.M. and Harlan, J.M. (1994) Leukocyte-endothelial adhesion molecules. *Blood*, 84(7): 2068–2101.

Carr, D.J.J. and Weigert, D.A. (1990) Neuropeptides and immunopeptides: messengers in a neuroimmune axis. *Prog. Neuroendocrinimmunol.*, 3: 61–66.

Caveda, L., Corada., M, Martin-Padura, I., Del Maschio, A., Breviario, F., Lampugnani, M.G. and Dejana, E. (1994) Structural characteristics and functional role of endothelial cell to cell junctions. *Endothelium*, 2: 1–10.

Chance, W.T. and Fischer, J.E. (1991) Aphagic and adipsic effects of interleukin-1. *Brain Res.*, 568: 261–264.

Chao, C.C., Molitor, T.W. and Hu, S. (1993) Neuroprotective role of IL-4 against activated microglia. *J. Immunol.*, 151: 1473–1481.

Chung, I.Y. and Benveniste, E.N. (1990) Tumor necrosis factor-α production by astrocytes. Induction by lipopolysaccharide, IFN-gamma and IL-1β. *J. Immunol.*, 144: 2999–3007.

Clemens, M.J. (1991) *Cytokines*, A.P. Read and T. Brown (Eds.), Medical Perspectives Series, Bios Scientific Publishers, Oxford.

Cloughesy, T.F. and Black, K.L. (1995) Pharmacological blood–brain modification for selective drug delivlery. *Neuro-Oncology*, 26: 125–132.

Colton, C.A., Keri, J.E., Chen, W.T. and Monsky, W.L. (1993) Protease production by cultured microglia: substrate gel analysis and immobilized matrix degradation. *J. Neurosci. Res.*, 35: 297–304.

Cozzolino, F., Torcia, M., Aldinucci, D., Ziche, M., Almerigogna, F., Bani, D. and Stern, D.M. (1990) Interleukin-1 is an autocrine regulator of human endothelia. *Proc. Natl. Acad. Sci. USA*, 87: 6487–6491.

Cserr, H.F., Harling-Berg, C.J. and Knopf, P.M. (1992) Drainage of brain extracellular fluid into blood and deep cervical lymphand its immunological significance. *Brain Pathol.*, 2: 269–276.

d'Oleire, F., Schmitt, C.L., Robins, H.I., Cohen, J.D. and Spriggs, D. (1993) Cytokine induction in humans by 41.8°C whole body hyperthermia. *J. Natl. Cancer Inst.*, 85(10): 833–834.

Davidson, J., Flower, R.J., Milton, A.S., Peers, S.H. and Rotondo, D. (1991) antipyretic action of humans recombinant lipocortin-1. *Br. J. Pharmacol.*, 102: 7–9.

de Boer, A.G. and Breimer, D.D. (1994) The blood–brain barrier (BBB): clinical implications for drug delivery to the brain. *J. R. Soc. Phys. Lond.*, 28(6): 1–9.

de Vries, H.E., Moor, A.C.E., Blom-Roosemalen, M.C.M., de Boer, A.G., Breimer, D.D., van Berkel, Th.J.C. and Kuiper, J. (1994) Lymphocyte adhesion to brain capillary endothelial cells in vitro. *J. Neuroimmunol.*, 52: 1–8.

de Vries, H.E. (1995) Characteristics of blood–brain barrier endothelial cells in response to inflammatory stimuli. Ph.D. thesis, University of Leiden, The Netherlands.

de Vries, H.E., Hoogendoorn, K.H., van Dijk, J.J., Zijlstra, F.J., van Dam, A-M., Breimer, D.D., van Berkel, Th.J.C., de Boer, A.G. and Kuiper, J. (1995a) Eicosanoid production by rat cerebral endothelial cells, stimulation by lipopolysaccharide, interleukin-1 and interleukin-6. *J. Neuroimmunol.*, 59: 1–8.

de Vries, H.E., Eppens, E.F., Prins, M., Kuiper, J., van Berkel, Th.J.C., de Boer, A.G. and Breimer, D.D. (1995b) Blood–brain barrier permeability during experimental allergic encephalomyelitis and acute septic shock. *Pharm. Res.*, 12(12): 1932–1936.

de Vries, H.E., Blom-Roosemalen, M.C.M., de Boer, A.G., van Berkel, Th.J.C., Breimer, D.D. and Kuiper, J. (1996a) The influence of cytokines on the integrity of the blood–brain barrier *in vitro*. *J. Neuroimmunol.*, 64: 37–43.

de Vries, H.E., Blom-Roosemalen, C.M., de Boer, A.G., Breimer, D.D., van Berkel, Th.J.C. and Kuiper, J. (1996b) Effect of endotoxin on the permeability of bovine cerebral endothelial cell layers *in vitro*. *J. Pharmacol. Exp. Ther.*, 277(3): 1418–1423.

Dejana, E., Corada, M. and Lampugnani, M.G. (1995) Endothelial cell-to-cell junctions. *FASEB J.*, 9: 910–918.

Deli, M.A., Descamps, L., Dehouck, M-P., Cecchelli, R., Joó, F., Abrah m, C.S. and Torpier, G. (1995a) Exposure of TNF-α to luminal membrane of bovine brain capillary endothelial cells cocultured with astrocytes induces a delayed increase of permeability and cytoplasmic stress fiber formation of actin. *J. Neurosci. Res.*, 41: 717–726.

Deli, M.A., Dehouck, M-P., Cecchelli, R., Abrah m, C.S. and Joó, F. (1995b) Histamine induces a selective albumin permeation through the blood–brain barrier *in vitro*. *Inflamm. Res.*, 44(suppl. 1): S56–S57.

Deli, M.A., Dehouck, M-P., Abrah m, S., Cecchelli, R. and Joó, F. (1995c) Penetration of small molecular weight substances through cultured bovine brain capillary endothelial cell monolayers: the early effects of cyclic adenosine 3′,5′-monophosphate. *Exp. Physiol.*, 80: 675–678.

Dinarello, C.A., Dempsey, R.A., Allegretta, M., Lopreste, G., Dainiak, N., Parkinson, D.R. and Mier, J.W. (1986) Inhibitory effects of elevated temperature on human cytokine production and natural killer cell activity. *Cancer Res.*, 46: 6236–6241.

Dinarello, C.A., Cannon, J.G. and Wolff, S.M. (1988) New concepts on the pathogenis of fever. *Rev. Infect. Dis.*, 10: 168–189.

Dinarello, C.A. (1989) Interleukin-1 and its biologically related cytokines *Adv. Immunol.*, 44: 153–205.

Downing, J.F., Taylor, M.W., Wei, K.M. and Elizondo, R.S. (1987) *In vivo* hyperthermia enhances plasma antiviral activity and stimulates peripheral lymphocytes for increased synthesis of interferon. *J. Interferon Res.*, 7: 185–193.

Drapier, J.C., Witzerbin, J. and Hibbs, J.B. (1988) Interferon-gamma and tumor necrosis factor induce the L-arginine-dependent cytotoxic effector mechanism in murine macrophages. *Eur. J. Immunol.*, 18: 1587–1592.

Dray, A. and Bevan, S. (1993) Inflammation and hyperalgesia: highlighting the team effort. *Trends Pharmacol. Sci.*, 14: 287–290.

Ensor, J.F., Wiener, S.M., McCrea, K.A., Viscardi, R.M., Crawford, E.K. and Haskay, J.D. (1994) Differential effects of hyperthermia on macrophage interleukin-6 and tumor necrosis factor-α expression. *Am. J. Physiol.*, 266: C974–C976.

446

Ericsson, A., Kovacs, K.J. and Sawchenko, P.E. (1994) A functional anatomical analysis of central pathways subserving the effects of interleukin-1 on stress-related neuroendocrine neurons. *J. Neurosci.*, 14: 897–913.

Estrada, C., Gmez, C. and Mart-n, C. (1995) Effects of TNF-α on the production of vasoactive substances by cerebral endothelial and smooth muscle cells in culture. *J. Cereb. Blood Flow Metab.*, 15: 920–928.

Fabry, Z., Waldschmidt, M.M., Hendrickson, D., Keiner, J., Love-Homan, L., Takei, F. and Hart, M.N. (1992) Adhesion molecules on murine brain microvascular endothelial cells: expression and regulation of ICAM-1 and Lgp55. *J. Neuroimmunol.*, 36: 1–11.

Fajardo, L.F. (1989) The complexity of endothelial cells, *Am. J. Clin. Pathol.*, 92: 241–250.

Fajardo, L.F. and Prionas, S.D. (1994) Endothelial cells and hyperthermia. *Int. J. Hyperthermia*, 10: 347–353.

Farrar, W.L., Kilian, P.L., Ruff, M.R. et al. (1987) Visualization and characteriztion of IL-1 receptors in brain. *J. Immunol.*, 139: 459–463.

Favaloro, E.J. (1993) Differential expression of surface antigens on activated endothelium. *Immunol. Cell Biol.*, 71: 571–581.

Fierz, W., Endler, B., Reske, K., Wekerle, H. and Fontana, A. (1985) Astrocytes as antigen presenting cells: Induction of Ia antigen expression on astrocytes by T-cells via immune interferon and its effects on antigen presentation. *J. Immunol.*, 134: 3785–3793.

Fleischmann, W.R. Jr., Fleischmann, C.M. and Gindhart, T.D. (1986) Effect of hyperthermia and antiproliferative activities of murine α-, β- and γ-interferon; differential enhancement of murine-interferon. *Cancer Res.*, 46: 8–13.

Folks, T.M., Justement, J., Kinter, A., Dinarello, A. and Fauci, A.S. (1987) Cytokine-induced expression of HIV-1 in a chronically infected promonocytic cell line. *Science*, 238: 800.

Folks, T.M., Justement, J.S., Kinter, A., Schnittman, S., Orenstein, J., Poli, G. and Fauci, A.S. (1988) Characterization of a promonocytic clone chronically infected with HIV and inducible by 13-phorbol-12-myristate acetate. *J. Immunol.*, 140: 1117–1122.

Fontana, A. et al. (1993) *Clinical Applications of Cytokines: Role in Pathogenesis, Diagnosis and Therapy.* J.J. Oppenheim, J.L. Rossio and A.J.H. Gearing (Eds.), Oxford University Press, London, pp. 357–366.

Fouqueray, B., Philippe, C., Amrani, A., Perez, J. and Baud, L. (1992) Heat shock prevents LPS-induced TNF-α synthesis by rat mononuclear phagocytes. *Eur. J. Immunol.*, 22: 2983–2987.

Fràter-Schröder, M., Risau, W., Hallmann, R., Gautschi, P. and Böhlen, P. (1987) Tumor necrosis factor type α, a potent inhibitor of endothelial cell growth *in vitro* is angiogenic in vivo. *Proc. Natl. Acad. Sci. USA*, 84: 5277–5281.

Frei, K. and Fontana, A. (1989) *Neuroimmune Networks: Physiology and Diseases*, Alan R. Liss, New York, pp. 127–132.

Gadient, R.A., Cron, K.C. and Otten, U. (1990) Interleukin 1 beta and tumor necrosis factor alpha synergistically stimulate nerve growth factor (NGF) release from cultured astrocytes. *Neurosci. Lett.*, 117: 335–340.

Ghezzi, P., Saccardo, B., Villa, P., Rossi, V., Bianchi, M. and Dinarello, C.A. (1986a) Role of interleukin-1 in the depression of liver drug metabolism by endotoxin. *Infect. Immun.*, 54: 837–840.

Ghezzi, P., Saccardo, B. and Bianchi, M. (1986b) Recombinant tumor necrosis factor depresses cytochrome P_{450}-dependent microsomal drug metabolism in mice. *Biochem. Biophys. Res. Commun.*, 136: 316–321.

Gorodischer, R., Krasner, J.J., McDevitt, J., Nolan, P. and Yaffe, S.J. (1976) Hepatic microsomal drug metabolism after administration of endotoxin in rats. *Biochem. Pharmacol.*, 25: 351.

Greenwood, J. (1992) *Physiology and Pharmacology of the Blood–brain Barrier*, M.W.B. Bradbury (Ed.), Springer, Berlin, pp. 459–486.

Gross, P.M., Sposito, N.M., Pettersen, S.E. and Fenstermacher, J.D. (1986) Differences in function and structure of the capillary endothelium in grey matter, white matter and a circumventricular organ of rat brain. *Blood Vessels*, 23: 261–270.

Guillian, D., Vaca, K. and Noonan, C.A. (1990) Secretion of neurotoxins by mononuclear phagocytes infected with HIV-1. *Science*, 250: 1593–159.

Gumbiner, B.M. (1993) Breaking through the tight junction barrier. *J. Cell Biol.*, 123: 1631–1633. Gutierrez, E.G., Banks, W.A. and Kastin, A.J. (1993) Murine tumor necrosis factor alpha is transported from blood to brain in the mouse. *J. Neuroimmunol.*, 47: 169–176.

Hall, T.J. (1994) Role of hsp70 in cytokine production. *Experientia*, 50: 1048–1053.

Haour, F., Marquette, C., Ban, E., Crumeyrolle-Arias, M., Rostene, W., Tsiang, H. and Fillion, G. (1995) Receptors for IL-1 in the central nervous and neuroendocrine systems. *Annales d'Endocrinologie (Paris)*, 56: 173–179.

Hass, M.A. and Massaro, D. (1988) Regulation of the synthesis of superoxide dismutases in rat lungs during oxidant and hyperthermic stresses. *J. Biol. Chem.*, 263: 776–781.

Hayashi, T., Nakai, T. and Miyabo, S. (1991) Glucocorticoids increase Ca^{2+} uptake and ^3H-dihydropyridine binding in A7r5 vascular smooth muscle cells. *Am. J. Physiol.*, 261: C106–C114.

Herron, G.S., Werb, Z., Dwyer, K. and Banda, M.J. (1986a) Secretion of metalloproteinases by stimulated capillary endothelial cells. I. Production of procollagenase and stromelysin exceeds expression of proteolytic activity. *J. Biol. Chem.*, 261: 2810–2813.

Herron, G.S., Banda, M.J., Clark, E.J., Gavrilovic, J. and Werb, Z. (1986b) Secretion of metalloproteinases by stimulated capillary endothelial cells. II. Expression of collagenase and stromelysin activities is regulated by endogenous inhibitors. *J. Biol. Chem.*, 261: 2814–2818.

Hibbs, M.S., Hasty, K.A., Seyer, J.M., Kang, A.H. and Mainardi, C.L. (1985) Biochemical and immunological characterization of the secreted forms of human neutrophil gelatinase. *J. Biol. Chem.*, 260: 2493–2500.

Hirsch, M.R., Wietzerbin, J., Pierres, M. and Goridis, C. (1983) Expression of I1 antigens by cultured astrocytes treated with gamma interferon. *Neurosci. Lett.*, 41: 199–204.

Hoek, J.B. (1992) Intracellular signal transduction and the control of endothelial permeability. *Lab. Invest.*, 67: 1–3.

Hofman, F. (1989) In: *Neuroimmune Networks: Physiology and Diseases*, Alan R. Liss, New York, pp. 64–71.

Hopkins, S.J. and Rothwell, N.J. (1995) Cytokines and the nervous system I: expression and recognition. *Trends Neurosci.*, 18(2): 83–88.

Hughes, C.C.W., Male, D.K. and Lantos, P.L. (1988) Adhesion of lymphocytes to cerebral microvascular cells: effects of interferon-gamma, tumor necrosis factor and interleukin-1. *Immunology*, 64: 677–681.

Hurst, N.P. (1990) Stress (heat shock) proteins and rheumatic disease. *Rheumatol. Int.*, 9: 271–276.

Huynh, H.K. and Dorovini-Zis, K. (1993) Effects of interferon-gamma on primary cultures of human brain microvessel endothelial cells. *Am. J. Pathol.*, 142: 1265–1278.

Hynes, R. (1987) Integrins: a family of cell surface receptors. *Cell*, 48: 549–554.

Inamura, T. and Black, K.L. (1994) Bradykinin selectively opens blood-tumor barrier in experimental brain tumors. *J. Cerebr. Blood Flow. Metab.*, 14: 862–870.

Issekutz, A.C. and Szpejda, M. (1986) Evidence that platelet activating factor may mediate some acute inflammatory responses. *Lab. Invest.*, 54: 275–281.

Issels, R.D. (1995) Regional hyperthemia combined with systemic chemotherapy of locally advanced sarcoma: preclinical aspects and clinical results. *Recent Results Cancer Res.*, 138: 81–90.

IUPS Thermal Commission (1987) Glossary of terms for thermal physiology. *Pfl – g. Arch.*, 410: 567–587.

Janzer, R.C. and Raff, M.C. (1987) Astrocytes induce blood–brain barrier properties in endothelial cells. *Nature*, 325: 253–257.

Juhler, M., Blasberg, R.G., Fenstermacher, J.D., Patlak, C.S. and Paulson, O.B. (1985) A spatial analysis of the blood–brain barrier damage in experimental allergic encephalomyelitis. *J. Cereb. Blood Flow Metab.*, 5: 545–553.

Kappel, M., Diamant, M., Hansen, M.B., Klokker, M. and Pedersen, B.K. (1991) Effects of *in vitro* hyperthermia on the proliferative response of blood mononuclear cell subsets and detection of interleukins 1 and 6, tumor necrosis factor-α and interferon-gamma. *Immunology*, 73: 304–308.

Kappel, M., Tvede, N., Hansen, M.B., Stadeager, C. and Pedersen, B.K. (1995) Cytokine production ex vivo: effect of raised body temperature. *Int. J. Hyperthermia*, 11(3): 329–335.

Kasambalides, E.J. and Lanks, K.W. (1983) Dexamethasone can modulate glucose-regulated heat shock protein synthesis. *J. Cell. Physiol.*, 114: 93–98.

Kaupilla, A., Cantell, K., Janne, O., Kokko, E. and Vihki, R. (1982) Serum sex steroid and peptide hormone concentration, and endometrial estrogen and progestin receptor levels during administration of leukocyte interferon. *Int. J. Cancer*, 29: 291–294.

Kent, S., Bluth,, R.-M., Kelly, K.W. and Dantzer, R. (1992) Sickness behaviour as a new target for drug development. *Trends Pharmacol. Sci.*, 13: 24–28.

Klostergaard, J., Barta, M. and Tomasovic, S.P. (1989) Hyperthermic modulation of tumor necrosis factor dependent monocyte/macrophage tumor cytotoxicity *in vitro*. *J. Biol. Response Modif.*, 8: 262–277.

Kluger, M.J., O'Reilly, B., Shope, T.R. and Vander, A.J. (1987) Further evidence that stress hyperthermia is a fever, *Physiol. Behav.*, 39: 763–766.

Koprowski, H., Zeng, Y.M., Katz, E.H., Fraser, N., Rorke, L., Fu, Z.F., Hanlon, D. and Dietzschold, B. (1993) *In vivo* expression of inducible nitric oxide synthase in experimentally induced neurologic diseases. *Proc. Natl. Acad. Sci. USA*, 90: 3024–3027.

Kunkel, S.L., Spengler, M., May, M.A., Spengler, R., Larrick, J. and Remick, D. (1988) Prostaglandin E_2 regulates macrophage-derived tumor necrosis factor gene expression. *J. Biol. Chem.*, 263: 5380–5384.

Lagrange, P., Livertoux, M-H., Grassiot, M-C. and Minn, A. (1994) Superoxide anion production during monoelectronic reduction of xenobiotics by preparations of rat brain cortex, microvessels and choroid plexus. *Free Radic. Biol. Med.*, 17(4): 355–359.

Lassmann, H. (1983) *Comparative neuropathology of chronic experimental allergic encephalomyelitis and multiple sclerosis*, Springer, Berlin.

Lassmann, H., R ssler, K., Zimprich, F. and Vass, K. (1991) Expression of adhesion molecules and histocompatibility antigens at the blood–brain barrier. *Brain Pathol.*, 1: 115–123.

Le, J., Lin, J.X., Henriksen-DeStefano, D. and Vilcek, J. (1986) Bacterial Lipopolysaccharide-induced IFN gamma production: roles of IL-1 and IL-2. *J. Immunol.*, 136: 4525–4531.

Lee, Y.J., Hou, Z., Curetty, L., Cho, J.M. and Corry, P.M. (1993) Synergistic effects of cytokine and hyperthermia on cytotoxicity in HT-29 cells are not mediated by alteration of induced protein levels *J. Cell. Physiol.*, 155: 27–35.

Lindholm, D., Castr,n, E., Hengerer, B., Zafra, F., Berninger, B.B. and Thoenen, H. (1992) Differential regulation of nerve growth factor (NGF) synthesis in neurons and astrocytes by glucocorticoid hormones. *Eur. J. Neurosci.*, 4: 404–410.

Long, N.C., Vander, A.J., Kunkel, S.L. and Kluger, M.J. (1990) Antiserum against tumor necrosis factor increases stress hyperthermia in rats. *Am. J. Physiol.*, 258: R591–R595.

Loughlin, A.J., Woodroofe, M.N. and Cuzner, M.L. (1992) Regulation of Fc receptor and major histocompatibility complex antigen expression on isolated rat microglia by tumor necrosis factor, interleukin-1 and lipopolysaccharide: effects on interferon-gamma induced activation. *Immunology*, 75: 170–175.

Male, D., Pryce, G. and Rahman, J. (1990a) Comparison of the immunological properties of rat cerebral and aortic endothelium. *J. Neuroimmunol.*, 30: 161–168.

Male, D., Pyrce, G., Hughes, C. and Lantos, P. (1990b) Lymphocyte migration into brain modelled *in vitro*: control by lumphocyte activation, cytokines and antigen. *Cell Immunol.*, 127: 1–11.

Mantovani, A. and Dejana, E. (1989) Cytokines as communication signals between leukocytes and endothelial cells. *Immunol. Today*, 10(11): 370–375.

May, L.T., Torcia, G., Cozzolino, F., Ray, A., Tatter, S.B., Santhanam, U. and Sehgal, P.B. (1989) Interleukin-6 gene expression in human endothelial cells RNA start sites, multiple IL-6 proteins and inhibition of proliferation. *Biochem. Biophys. Res. Commun.*, 169: 991–999.

McCarthy, S.A., Kuzu, I., Gatter, K.C. and Bicknell, R. (1991) Heterogeneity of the endothelial cell and its role in organ preference of tumour metastasis. *Trends Pharmacol. Sci.*, 12: 462–467.

Minami, M., Kuraishi, Y. and Satoh, M. (1991) Effects of kainic acid on messenger RNA levels of IL-1beta, IL-6, TNF-α and LIF in the rat brain. *Biochem. Biophys. Res. Commun.*, 176: 593–598.

Minn, A., Ghersi-Egea, J-F., Perrin, R., Leinigner, B. and Siest, G. (1991) Drug metabolizing enzyme in the brain and cerebral microvessels. *Brain Res. Rev.*, 16: 65–82.

Morganti-Kossmann, M.C., Kossmann, T. and Wahl, S.M. (1992) Cytokines and neuropathology. *Trends Pharmacol. Sci.*, 13: 286–291.

Nathan, C.F. (1982) Secretion of oxygen intermediates: role in effector functions of activated macrophages. *Fed. Proc.*, 41: 2206–2211.

Neville, A.J. and Sauder, D.N. (1988) Whole body hyperthermia (41–42°C) induces interleukin-1 *in vivo*. *Lymphokine Res.*, 7: 201–206.

Neville, A.J. and Sing, G. (1990) Effect of whole-body hyperthermia on cytochrome P450. *Cancer Chemother. Pharmacol.*, 25: 342–344.

Niemoller, M. and Tauber, M.G. (1989) Brain edema and increased intracranial pressure in the pathophysiology of bacterial meningitis. *J. Clin. Microbiol. Infect. Dis.*, 8: 109–117.

Norton, P.M. and Latchman, D.D. (1989) Levels of the 90 kD heat shock protein and resistance to glucocorticosteroid-mediated cell killing in a range of human and murine lymphocyte cell lines. *J. Steroid Biochem.*, 33: 149–154.

Ojeda, S.R., Dissen, G.A. and Junier, M.-P. (1992) Neurotrophic factors and female sexual development. *Front. Neuroendocrinol.*, 13: 120–162.

Orava, M., Cantell, K. and Vihko, R. (1986) Treatment with preparations of human leukocyte interferon decreases serum testosterone concentrations in man. *Int. J. Cancer*, 38: 295–296.

Osborn, L. (1990) Leukocyte adhesion to endothelium in inflammation. *Cell*, 62: 3–6.

Palmer, R.M.J., Bridje, L., Foxwell, N.A. and Moncada, S. (1992) The role nitric oxide in endothelial damage and its inhibition by glucocorticoids. *Br. J. Pharmacol.*, 105: 11–12.

Palmi, M., Frosini, M., Becherucci, C., Sgargli, G.P. and Parente, L. (1994) Increase of extracellular brain calcium involved in interleukin-1 β-induced pyresis in the rabbit: antagonism by dexamethasone. *Br. J. Pharmacol.*, 112: 449–452.

Pardridge, W.M. (1995) Transport of small molecules through the blood–brain barrier: biology and methodology. *Adv. Drug Deliv. Rev.*, 15: 5–36.

Pardridge, W.M. (1991) *Peptide Drug Delivery to the Brain*, Raven Press, New York.

Parrott, R.F., Vellucci, S.V., Goode, J.A., Lloyd, D.M. and Forsling, M.L. (1995) Cyclo-oxygenase mediation of endotoxin-induced fever, anterior and posterior pituitary hormone release, and hypothalamic c-Fos expression in the prepubertal pig. *Exp. Physiol.*, 80: 663–674.

Patterson, P.H. and Nawa, H. (1993) Neuronal differentiation factors/cytokines and synaptic plasticity. *Cell*, 72/Neuron, Vol. 10 (Suppl.): 123–137.

Paul, C. and Bolton, C. (1995) Inhibition of blood–brain barrier disruption in experimental allergic encephalomyelitis by short-term therapy with dexamethasone or cyclosporin-A. *Int. J. Immunopharmacol.*, 17(6): 497–503.

Pearson, J.D. (1991) Endothelial cell biology. *Radiology*, 179: 9–14.

Pedersen, B.K. and Ullum, H. (1994) NK cell response to physical activity: possible mechanisms of action. *Med. Sci. Sports Exerc.*, 26(2): 140–146.

Philip, R. and Epstein, L.B. (1986) Tumor necrosis factor as immunomodulator and mediator of monocyte cytotoxicity induced by itself, gamma-IFN and IL-1. *Nature*, 323: 86–89.

Plata-Salam n, C.R. (1991) Immunoregulators in the nervous system. *Neurosci. Biobehav. Rev.*, 15: 185–215.

Poland, S.D., Rice, G.P.A. and Dekaban, G.A. (1995) HIV-1 Infection of human brain-derived microvascualr endothelial cells *in vitro*. *J. Acquired Immune Deficiency Syndromes Hum. Retrovirol.*, 8: 437–445.

Poli, G., Bressler, P., Kinter, A., Duh, E., Timmer, W.C., Rabson, A., Justement, J.S., Stanley, S. and Fauci, A.S. (1990) Interleukin-6 induces human immunodeficiency virus expression in infected monocytic cells alone and a synergy with tumor necrosis factor-α by transcriptional and post-transcriptional mechanisms. *J. Exp. Med.*, 172: 151–158.

Poli, G., Kinter, A., Justement, J.S., Kehrl, J.H., Bressler, P., Stanley, S. and Fauci, A.S. (1989) Tumor necrosis factor-alpha functions in an autocrine manner in the induction of HIV expression. *Proc. Natl. Acad. Sci. USA*, 87: 782–785.

Polla, B. (1988) A role for heat shock proteins in inflammation? *Immunol. Today*, 9: 134–137.

Polla, B.S. and Kantengwa, S. (1991) Heat shock proteins and inflammation. In: S.H.E. Kaufman (Ed.), *Current Topics in Microbiology and Immunology*, Vol. 167, Springer, Berlin, pp. 93–108.

Polla, B.S., Perin, M. and Pizurki, L. (1993) Regulation and functions of stress proteins in allergy and inflammation, *Clin. Exp. Allergy*, 23: 548–556.

Reed, D.J. (1980) Drug transport into the central nervous system. In: G.H. Glaser, J.K. Pentry and D.M. Woodbury (Eds.), *Antiepileptic Drugs: Mechanisms of Action*, Raven Press, New York, pp. 199–205.

Reich, R., Thompson, E.W., Iwamoto, Y., Martin, G.R., Deason, J.R., Fuller, G.C. and Miskin, R. (1988) Effects of inhibitors of plasminogen activator, serine proteinases, and collagenase IV on the invasion of basement membranes by metastatic cells. *Cancer Res.*, 48: 3307–3312.

Risau, W. and Wolburg, H. (1990) Development of the blood–brain barrier. *Trends Neurosci.*, 13: 174–178.

Rosenberg, G.A., Kornfeld, M., Estrada, E., Kelley, R.O., Liotta, L.A. and Stetler-Stevenson, W.G. (1992) TIMP-2 reduces proteolytic opening of blood–brain barrier by type IV collagenase. *Brain Res.*, 576: 203–207.

Rosenberg, G.A., Estrada, E.Y., Dencoff, J.E. and Stetler-Stevenson, W.G. (1995) Tumor necrosis factor-α-induced gelatinase B causes delayed opening of the blood–brain barrier: an expanded therapeutic window. *Brain Res.*, 703: 151–155.

Rothwell, N.J. and Hopkins, S.J. (1995) Cytokines and the nervous system II: actions and mechanisms of action. *Trends Neurosci.*, 18(3): 130–136.

Rothwell, N.J. (1991) Functions and mechanisms of interleukin-1 in the brain. *Trends Pharmacol. Sci.*, 12: 430–436.

Rubin, L.L. (1992) Endothelial cells: adhesion and tight junctions. *Curr. Opin. Cell Biol.*, 4: 830–833.

Saija, A., Princi, P., Lanza, M., Scalese, M., Aramnejad, E. and De Sarro, A. (1995) Systemic cytokine administration can affect blood–brain barrier permeability in the rat. *Life Sci.*, 56(10): 775–784.

Sapolsky, R., Rivier, C., Yamamoto, G., Plotsky, P. and Vale, W.. (1987) Interleukin-1 stimulates the secretion of hypothalamic corticotropin-releasing factor. *Science*, 238: 522–524.

Sauer, J., Castren, M., Hopfner, U., Holsboer, F., Stalla, G.K. and Arzt, E. (1996) Inhibition of lipopolysaccharide-induced monocyte interluekin-1 receptor antagonist synthesis by cortisol: involvement of the mineralocorticoid receptor. *J. Clin. Endocrinol. Metab.*, 81: 73–79.

Scheld, W.M., Dacey, R.G. and Winn, H.R. (1980) Cerebrospinal outflow resistance in rabbits with experimental meningitis, Alterations with penicillin and methylprednisolon. *J. Clin. Invest.*, 66: 243–253.

Schlossman, S.F., Boumsell, L., Gilks, W., Harlan, J.M., Kishimoto, T., Morimoto, C., Ritz, J., Shaw, S., Silversetin, R.L., Springer, T.A., Tedder, T.F. and Todd, R.F. (1994) CD antigens 1993. *Immunol. Today*, 15: 98–99.

Schmelz, M. and Franke, W.W. (1993) Complexus adhaerentes, a new group of desmoplakin-containing junctions in endothelial cells: the syndesmos connecting retothelial cells of lymph nodes. *Eur. J. Cell Biol.*, 61: 274–289.

Schöbitz, B., Sutanto, W., Carey, M.P., Holsboer, F. and de Kloet, E.R. (1994) Endotoxin and interleukin 1 decrease the affinity of hippocampal mineralocorticoid (type 1) receptor parallel to activation of the hypothalamic-pituitary-adrenal axis. *Neuroendocrinology*, 60: 124–133.

Selmaj, K. and Raine, C.S. (1988) Tumor necrosis factor mediates myelin and oligodendrocyte damage *in vitro*. *Ann. Neurol.*, 23: 339–346.

Sharief, M.K. and Thompson, E.J. (1992) *In vivo* relationship of tumor necrosis factor-α to blood–brain barrier damage in patients with active multiple sclerosis. *J. Neuroimmunol.*, 38: 27–34.

Sharma, H.S., Olsson, Y. and Dey, P.K. (1990) Changes in blood–brain barrier cerebral blood flow following elevation of circulation serotonin level in anesthetized rats. *Brain Res.*, 517(1–2): 215–223.

Sharma, H.S., Westman, J., Nyberg, F., Cervos-Navarro, J. and Dey, P.K. (1994) Role of serotonin and prostaglandins in brain edema induced by heat stress. An experimental study in the young rat. *Acta Neurochir. Suppl.*, 60: 65–70.

Sharma, H.S., Kretzschmar, R., Cervós-Navarro, J., Ermisch, A., Rühle, H.-J. and Dey, P.K. (1992) Age-related pathophysiology of the blood–brain barrier in heat stress. *Prog. Brain Res.*, 91: 189–196.

Sharma, H.S., Westman, J., Cervós Navarro, J., Dey, P.K. and Nyberg, F. (1996) Probable involvement of serotonin in the increased permeability of the blood–brain barrier by forced swimming. An experimental study using Evans blue and ^{131}I-sodium tracers in the rat. *Behav. Brain Res.*, 72: 189–196.

Sharma, H.S., Cervos-Navarro, J. and Dey, P.K. (1991) Increased blood–brain barrier permeability following acute short-term swimming exercise in conscious normotensive young rats. *Neurosci. Res.*, 10(3): 211–221.

Shen, R-N., Lu, L., Yong, P., Shidnia, H., Hornback, N.B. and Broxmeyer, H.E. (1994) Influence of elevated temperature on natural killer cell activity, lymphokine-activated killer cell activity and lectin-dependent cytotoxicity of human umbilical cord blood and adult blood cells. *Int. J. Radiat. Oncol. Biol. Phys.*, 29(4): 821–826.

Shiling, L., Ksoll, E. and Wahl, M. (1987) Vasomotor and permeability effects of histamine in cerebral vessels. *Int. J. Microcirc. Clin. Exp.*, 6: 70–71.

Shiling, L., Ksoll, E. and Wahl, M. (1993) Mediators of vascular and parenchymal mechanisms in secondary brain damage. *Acta Neurochir. Suppl.*, 57: 64–72.

Shimizu, Y., Newman, W., Gopal, T.V., Horgan, K.J., Graber, N., Beall, L.D., Van Seventer, G.A. and Shaw, S. (1991) Four molecular pathways of T-cell adhesion to endothelial cells: roles of LFA-1, VCAM-1 and ELAM-1 and changes in pathways hierarchy under different activation conditions. *J. Cell Biol.*, 113: 1203–1212.

Shukla, A., Dikshit, M. and Srimal, R.C. (1995) Nitric oxide modulates blood–brain barrier permeability during infections with an inactivated bacterium. *NeuroReport*, 6: 1629–1632.

Singer, R., Harker, C.T., Vander, A.J. and Kluger, M.J. (1986) Hyperthermia induced by open-field stress is blocked by salicylate. *Physiol. Behav.*, 36: 1179–1182.

Sminia, T., de Groot, C.J.A., Dijkstra, C.D., Koetsier, J.C. and Polman, C.H. (1986) Macrophages in the central nervous system of the rat. *Immunobiology*, 174: 43–50.

Sminia, P., van der Zee, J., Wondergem, J. and Haveman, J. (1994) A review on the effect of hyperthermia on the central nevous system. *Int. J. Hyperthermia*, 10: 1–30.

Solito, E., Raugei, G., Melli, M. and Parente, L. (1991) Dexamethasone induces the expression of mRNA of lipocortin 1 and 2 and the release of lipocrotin 1 and 5 in differentiated but not undifferentiated U-937 cells. *FEBS Lett.*, 291: 238–244.

Solito, E. and Parente, L. (1989) Modulation of phospholipase A_2 activity in human fibroblasts. *Br. J. Pharmacol.*, 96: 656–660.

Spellerberg, B. and Tuomanen, E.I. (1994) The pathophysiology of pneumococcal meningitis. *Trends Mol. Med., Ann. Med.*, 26: 411–418.

Spellerberg, B., Prasad, S., Cabellos, C., Burroughs, M., Cahill, F. and Tuomanen, E. (1995) Penetration of the blood–brain barrier: enhancement of drug delivery and imaging by bacterial glycopeptides. *J. Exp. Med.*, 182: 1037–1043.

Springer, T.A. (1994) Traffic signals for lymphocytes recirculation and leukocyte emigration: the multistep paradigm. *Cell*, 76: 301–314.

Springer, T.A. (1990) Adhesion receptors of the immune system. *Nature*, 346: 425–434.

Stanley, S.K., Bressler, P.B., Poli, G. and Fauci, A.S. (1990) Heat shock induction of HIV production from chronically infected promonocytic and T cell lines. *J. Immunol.*, 145: 1120–1126.

Stitt, J.T. (1990) Passage of immunomodulators across the blood–brain barrier. *Yale J. Biol. Med.*, 63: 121–131.

Tauber, M.G., Ferriero, D., Kennedy, S.L., Sheldon, R.A. and Guerra, R.L. (1993) Brain levels of neuropeptide Y in experimental pneumococcal meningitis. *Mol. Chem. Neuropathol.*, 18: 15–26.

Tomasovic, S.P. and Klosergaard, J. (1989) Hyperthermia modulation of macrophage-tumor cell interactions. *Cancer Metastasis Rev.*, 8: 215–229.

Tracey, K.J., Beutler, B., Lowry, S.F., Merryweather, J., Wolpe, S., Milsark, I.W., Hariri, R.J., Fahey, T.J. III, Zentella, A., Albert, J.D., Shires, G.T. and Cerami, A. (1986) Shock and tissue injury induced by recombinant human cachectin. *Science*, 234: 470–474.

Trout, J.J., Koenig, H., Goldstone, A.D. and Lu, C.Y. (1986) Blood-brain barrier breakdown by cold injury. Polyamine signals mediate acute stimulation of endocytosis, vesicular transport, and microvillus formation in rat cerebral capillaries. *Lab. Invest.*, 55: 622–631.

Tsagarakis, S., Gillies, G., Rees, L.H., Besser, M. and Grassman, A. (1989) Interleukin-1 directly stimulates the release of corticotropin releasing factor from rat hypothalamus. *Neuroendocrinology*, 49: 98–101.

Tunkel, A. and Scheld, W.M. (1993) Pathogenesis and pathophysiology of bacterial meningitis. *Annu. Rev. Med.*, 44: 103–120.

Tyor, W.R., Glass, J.D., Baumrind, N.et al. (1993) Cytokine expression of macrophages in HIV-1-associated vacuolar myelopathy. *Neurology*, 43: 1002–1009.

Tyor, W.R., Glass, J.D., Griffin, J.W.et al. (1992) Cytokine expression in the brain during the acquired immunodeficiency syndrome. *Ann. Neurol.*, 31: 349–360.

van Dam, A.M., de Vries, H.E., Kuiper, J., Zijlstra, F.J., de Boer, A.G., Tilders, F.J.G. and Berkenbosch, F. (1996) Interleukin-1 receptors on rat brain endothelial cells: a role in neuroimmune interaction? *FASEB J.*, 10: 351–356.

van Bree, J.B.M.M., de Boer, A.G., Danhof, M., Ginsel, L.A. and Breimer, D.D. (1988) Characterization of an *in vitro* blood–brain barrier: effects of molecular size and lipophilicity on cerebrovascular endothelial transport rates of drugs. *J. Pharmacol. Exp. Ther.*, 1247(3): 1233–1239.

van Bree, J.B.M.M., de Boer, A.G., Danhof, M. and Breimer, D.D. (1992) Drug transport across the blood–brain barrier: I. Anatomical and physiological aspects. *Pharm. Weekblad Sci. Ed.*, 14(5): 305–310.

van Haeringen, N.J. and Meijer, F. (1995) De toepassing van NSAID's in het oog. *Geneesmiddel Bull.*, 29(7): 72–75.

van Mourik, J.A., von dem Borne, A.E. and Giltay, J.G. (1990) Pathophysiological significance of integrin expression by vascular endothelial cells. *Biochem. Pharmacol.*, 39: 233–239.

Vartanian, T., Li, Y., Zhao, M. and Stefansson, K. (1995) Interferon-γ-induced oligodendrocyte cell death: implications for pathogenesis of multiple sclerosis. *Mol. Med.*, 1: 732–743.

Vass, K. and Lassmann, H. (1990) Intrathecal application of interferon-gamma: progressive appearance of MHC antigens within the rat nervous system. *Am. J. Pathol.*, 137(4): 789–800.

Waight-Sharma, A., Grooby, W., Betts, W.H. and Russ, G.R. (1992) Effects of *in vitro* hyperthermia on the expression of adhesion molecules in cytokine-stimulated human umbilical vein endothelial cells. *Transplant. Proc.*, 24 (5): 2319–2320.

Watkins, L.R., Mayer, S.T. and Goehler, L.E. (1995a) Cytokine-to-brain communication: a review and analysis of alternative mechanisms. *Life Sci.*, 56 (11): 1011–1026.

Watkins, L.R., Goehler, L.E., Relton, J.K., Tartaglia, N., Silvert, L., Margin, D. and Maier, S.F. (1995b) Blockade of interleukin-1 induced hyperthermia by subdiaphragmatic vagotomy: evidence for vagal mediation of immune-brain communication. *Neurosci. Lett.*, 183: 27–31.

Wekerle, H., Engelhardt, B., Risau, W. and Meyermann, R. (1991) Interaction with T-lymphocytes with cerebral endothelial cells *in vitro*. *Brain Pathol.*, 1: 107–114.

Wilder, R.L. (1995) Neuroendocrine-immune system interactions and autoimmunity. *Annu. Rev. Immunol.*, 13: 307–338.

Wilting, J., Brand-Saberi, B., Kurz, H. and Christ, B. (1995) Development of the embryonic vascular system. *Cell. Mol. Biol. Res.*, 41(4): 219–232.

Wissner, A., Schaub, R.E., Sum, P.E., Kohler, C.A. and Goldsein, B.M. (1986) Analogues of platelet activating factor 4. Some modifications of the phosphocholine moiety. *J. Med. Chem.*, 29: 328–333.

Wojta, J., Holzer, M., Hufnagl, P., Christ, G., Hoover, R.L. and Binder, B.R. (1991) Hyperthermia stimulates plasminogen activator inhibitor type 1 expression in human umbilical vein endothelial cells *in vitro*. *Am. J. Pathol.*, 139: 911–919.

Wong, G.H., Elwell, J.H., Oberley, L.W. and Goeddel, D.V. (1989) Manganous superoxide dismutase is essential for cellular resistance to cytotoxicity of tumor necrosis factor. *Cell*, 58: 923–931.

Wong, D. and Dorovini-Zis, K. (1992) Upregulation of intercellular adhesion molecule-1 (ICAM-1) expression in primary cultures of human brain microvessel endothelial cells by cytokines and lipopolysaccharide. *J. Neuroimmunol.*, 39: 11–22.

Wong, G.H., Bartlett, P.F., Clark-Lewis, I., Battye, F. and Schrader, J.W. (1984) Inducible expression of H-2 and Ia antigens on brain cells. *Nature*, 310: 688–691.

Woodroofe, M.N. (1995) Cytokine production in the central nervous system. *Neurology*, 45(6): S6–S10.

H.S. Sharma and J. Westman (Eds.)
Progress in Brain Research, Vol 115
© 1998 Elsevier Science BV. All rights reserved.

CHAPTER 21

Nerve thermal injury

C.D.P. Lynch and M. Pollock*

Department of Neurology, Department of Medicine, University of Otago Medical School, P.O. Box 913, Dunedin, New Zealand

Introduction

The clinical syndromes of nerve thermal injury have been described since the time of Hippocrates. They have commanded particular attention during military exercises including the Crusades, Napolean's Russian Campaign, the Crimean War, the First and Second World Wars, the Korean conflict and the Falklands War. Spurred on by clinicians, basic investigators have shown that nerve structure and function are critically dependent on ambient temperature and if nerve temperature falls outside a relatively narrow range, neural function becomes sub-optimal or fails.

There has been considerable research, both experimental and clinical, on nerve injury following cold exposure but by contrast that of heat injured nerve has been largely neglected. This is surprising given the clinical importance of hyperthermic nerve injury in a variety of specialties.

Pertinent to the subject of nerve thermal injury in general is the considerable body of evidence that suggests that important underlying pathogenetic mechanisms are a breakdown of the blood–nerve barrier and impairment of endothelial synthetic function. In addition, blood coagulation dynamics and platelet physiology show ther-

mal sensitivity. These factors culminate in focal angiopathy that is central to the genesis of nerve thermal injury.

Here we review the clinical aspects of nerve thermal injury and discuss the experimental studies that illuminate these conditions.

Nerve heat injury

Experience of nerve thermal injury in the peripheral nervous system is largely restricted to Emergency and Military Physicians and to those practitioners residing in environments with extremes of ambient temperature (Table 1) (Smith et al., 1915; Ungley and Blackwood, 1942; Malamud et al., 1946; Yaqub et al., 1986; Yaqub, 1987; Zhi-Cheng and Yi-Tang, 1991). However, Neurologists, Psychiatrists, Oncologists, Geriatricians, Paediatricians, and Sports Medicine doctors also need to be cognizant of these disabling and sometimes life threatening conditions (King et al., 1981; Gerad et al., 1984; Emami, 1991; Oshima et al., 1992; Marquez et al., 1993).

There have been significant advances in the pathogenesis and treatment of heat stroke and related disorders since they were reviewed by Stefanini (1975) and Goetz and Klawans (1979). In particular, research into malignant hyperthermia and neuroleptic syndrome has provided new insights into our understanding of thermogenesis and thermoregulation (Blatteis, 1992; Zeis-

---

*Corresponding author. Tel: +64 3 4740999; fax: +64 3 4747641; e-mail: jan.kettink@stonebow.otago.ac.nz

TABLE 1

Clinical syndromes of nerve thermal injury

Heat
   Hyperthermic syndromes
      1. Heat stroke
      2. Malignant hyperthermia
      3. Neuroleptic malignant syndrome

   Burns
   Whole body hyperthermia

Cold
   Trench foot
   Immersion limb
   Frost bite

---

berger and Merker, 1992; Kao et al., 1994; Lin et al., 1995; Parada et al., 1995).

Peripheral nerve injury is a rare complication of hyperthermic syndromes (Garvey et al., 1940; Bull et al., 1979; Adam et al., 1987) with cases of peripheral neuropathy falling into two groups: a Guillain-Barre, syndrome (Garvey et al., 1940; Wijesundene, 1992), and a multifocal sensorimotor polyradiculoneuropathy (Mehta and Baker, 1970; Dhopesh et al., 1976; Bouges et al., 1987). It is possible that the Guillain-Barre, syndrome is a consequence of antigens from heat damaged neural tissue initiating a secondary immunological injury.

Neuropathy in burn patients is more common, but frequently not diagnosed even in burns units (Henderson et al., 1971; Helm et al., 1977; Helm et al., 1985; Marquez et al., 1993). Most burn patients exhibit a mononeuritis multiplex (69%), but mononeuropathy, radiculopathy and generalised axonal polyneuropathy have all been described (Marquez et al., 1993). These axonal neuropathies have a predilection for burnt areas. Both burn thickness and total burn surface area correlate with the number of nerves affected. Long term follow up of burn patients has demonstrated that 75% have moderate to severe clinical and electrophysiological deficits relating to their neuropathy (Marquez et al., 1993). A small group

of burn patients have neuropathy in areas distant to the site of burn, unrelated to pressure areas or escharotomy sites. An unknown 'humoral' or toxic mediator has been proposed to explain these rare phenomena (Sepulchre et al., 1979; Bouges et al., 1987).

Occasionally neuropathies have been reported following whole body hyperthermia (WBH) for cancer treatment. Bull et al. (1979) described multifocal conduction block in four patients, three of whom presented within 24 h of exposure to 42.8°C. All patients recovered although two affected patients continued to have WBH. Gerad et al. (1984) documented transient paraesthesias in three of 11 patients and a further patient developed wrist drop. Adam et al. (1987) report a case of weakness, patchy sensory loss, and areflexia following three treatments of WBH at 41.8°C. Onset was rapid, progressed over 10 days and had incompletely resolved at 6 months. On investigation there was widespread sensorimotor conduction abnormalities with evidence of denervation.

The electrical response of large myelinated A-fibres to a 'low grade' hyperthermic injury (47°C) is preferentially abolished over 2 h (Lele, 1963; Klumpp and Zimmermann, 1980; Xu and Pollock, 1994) (Fig. 1). This correlates morphologically with a loss of myelinated fibres (Fig. 2), leaving the unmyelinated fibre population intact. Boykin et al. (1980) has provided evidence that platelet microthrombi are responsible for this post-heat injury. The subsequent loss of large medullated nerve fibres arises from their sensitivity to ischaemia and hypoxia (Dahlin et al., 1989; Fujimura et al., 1991; Xu and Pollock, 1994). The vulnerability of unmyelinated fibres to higher temperatures is revealed by an immediate, selective abolition of C-fibre potentials at 58°C with a corresponding degeneration of unmyelinated nerve fibres (Xu and Pollock, 1994) (Figs. 3 and 4).

Nerve cold injury

Peripheral nerve injury in hypothermic disorders is far more common than nerve heat injury. Cases

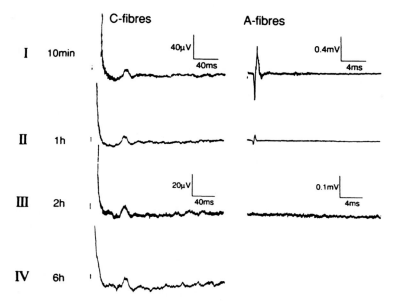

Fig. 1. Early changes in compound action potentials following low grade heating. The left and right columns show C- and A-fibre compound potentials. In I, II and III the cumulative time following nerve thermal injury is shown. IV shows a typical C-fibre compound potential, 6 h after abolition of the A-fibre compound action potential [from Xu and Pollock (1994), with kind permission of Oxford University Press].

of cold-induced neuropathy are not limited to military exercises (Smith et al., 1915; Ungley and Blackwood, 1942; Ungley et al., 1943) but may be seen in civilian practise. They are prevalent among mountaineers (Carter et al., 1988), arise as a complication of cryotherapy (Bassett et al., 1992), or open heart surgery (Efthimiou et al., 1991) and are familiar to seafarers (Semsarian, 1994).

If one uses the traditional nomenclature there is a continuum of severity in cold-induced neuropathy from Trench Foot to Cold Immersion Syndrome to Frostbite.

Trench Foot is characterised by paralysis, anaesthesia and swelling of the lower extremities (Smith et al., 1915). It usually begins in wet, non-freezing conditions, often associated with relative immobility and an upright posture. Initially numbness and tightness of the feet are noted, later pain, and weakness on walking. While sensory disturbances last for weeks, complete recovery is possible, though many have persistent paraesthesiae.

Cold Immersion Syndrome has a more acute onset, and is usually characterised by four stages; cold exposure, pre-hyperaemia (hours), hyperaemia (2–48 h) and post-hyperaemia. Within minutes of exposure to non-freezing sea water [0–8°C], numbness and weakness ensue. While severe neurological injury may result within 14 h, pain is rare, but cramps or tenderness are common. After removal from the water, such patients are unable to walk or use their hands due to a dense numbness. Within 2–5 h the limbs become hyperaemic and very painful. A burning, throbbing sensation peaks in intensity within 36 h but may continue for weeks. Mueller et al. (1993) suggest it is reperfusion that produces major nerve damage following hypothermia. Up to 10 days later, lancinating pains may occur, particularly with warmth, exertion or dependency. Sensory symptoms may abate over 6–14 weeks, but occasionally, they recur intermittently. Autonomic dysfunction is common, manifest by anhidrosis in anaesthetic areas and hyperhydrosis at the border

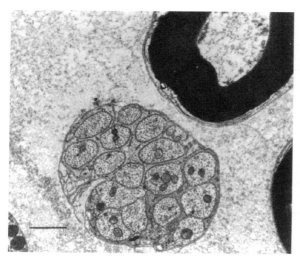

Fig. 2. An electron micrograph of a rat sciatic nerve, 2 days after low grade nerve heating, showing preserved unmyelinated fibres but degenerating myelinated fibres. Bar = 1 μm [from Xu and Pollock (1994) with kind permission of Oxford University Press].

Frost-bite results in freezing and necrosis of tissues. While tissues freeze at $-2.5°C$, seawater freezes at $-1.9°C$. It is therefore more likely that immersed body parts will not be 'frost bitten' unless a 'cold vasculopathy' is severe enough to cause infarction (Ungley and Blackwood, 1942). The spectrum of symptoms is similar to other cold syndromes but with more severe tissue loss. Sensorimotor changes, similar to the cold immersion syndrome are found proximal to gangrenous areas. Permanent sequelae always result from 'frost-bite'.

Conduction velocity in hypothermic nerve is progressively reduced as temperature falls (Basbaum, 1973) (Fig. 5). Myelinated fibres show a differential sensitivity, with Type 2 (Aβ) fibres failing first followed by type 3 (C) and then type 1 (Aα). These changes may be attributed to both energy dependent and physical factors. Physical changes in cell lipid membranes (Tomity and Csillik, 1964), and a reduction of electrical conductance in artificial lipid membranes (Goudeau, 1968) have been described with cold.

With increasing cold, there is an arrest of axo-

with normally innervated skin. Muscle wasting in the feet only becomes evident as leg swelling diminishes.

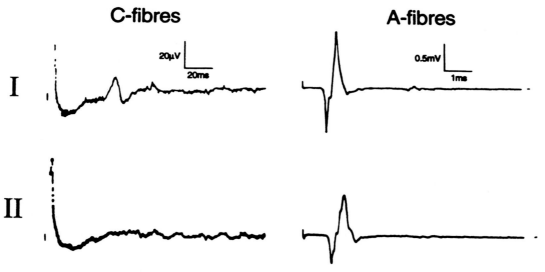

Fig. 3. Changes induced in compound action potentials by high grade nerve heating. The left and right columns show C- and A-fibre compound action potentials, respectively. I shows a control record. Note in II, the disappearance of the C-fibre compound action potential but persistence of the A-fibre compound action potential, immediately after thermal injury [from Xu and Pollock (1994) with kind permission of Oxford University Press].

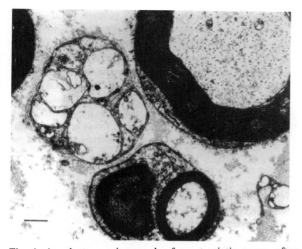

Fig. 4. An electron micrograph of a rat sciatic nerve, after high grade nerve heating, confirming extensive degeneration of unmyelinated fibres and of a small myelinated fibre, but preservation of the large myelinated fibre. Bar = 1 μm [from Xu and Pollock (1994), with kind permission of Oxford University Press].

plasmic transport (Figs. 6 and 7). Successive populations of peripheral nerve fibres subsequently undergo axonal degeneration. This begins with a low grade thermal loss of large myelinated axons, followed by small myelinated fibres. Finally in very severe cold lesions unmyelinated axons also degenerate (Basbaum, 1973; Nukada et al., 1981).

Pathogenic mechanisms in nerve thermal injury

The vasa nervorum are particularly sensitive to nerve thermal injury. Blood nerve barrier function is impaired after both hyper and hypothermic nerve injury (Basbaum, 1973; Nukada et al., 1981; Xu and Pollock, 1994) (Fig. 8). Histological analysis of thermally injured nerve typically shows thromboses in endoneurial, perineurial, and epineurial blood vessels (Denny-Brown et al., 1945; Lele, 1963; Xu and Pollock, 1994) (Fig. 9).

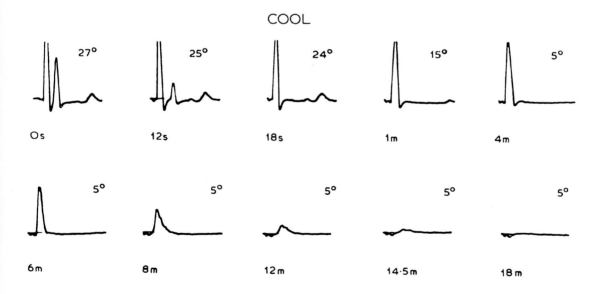

Fig. 5. Tracings demonstrate the effects of cooling on the compound action potential in cat sciatic nerve with a thermoelectric device applied to the nerve [from Basbaum (1973), with kind permission of the Editor and Publisher].

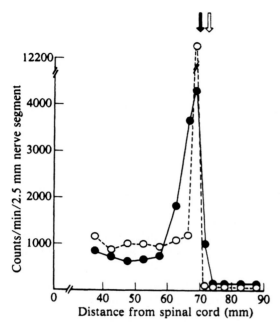

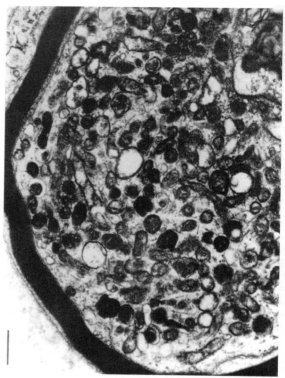

Fig. 6. Block of fast axoplasmic transport by cold. A typical example is shown (filled circles) in which cold (5°C) was applied for 2 h to the rat sciatic nerve (filled arrow: proximal end of cooled nerve segment). The contralateral sciatic nerve (open circles) was ligated just prior to cooling contralateral nerve (open arrow: point of ligation) [from Nukada et al. (1981), with kind permission of Oxford University Press].

Fig. 7. Electron micrograph of transverse section from rat sciatic nerve 3 days after cold injury. The swollen axoplasm is filled with large membranous bodies suggesting arrest of axoplasmic flow. Bar = 0.5 μm [from Nukada et al. (1981), with kind permission of Oxford University Press].

Synthesis of proteins that mediate thrombosis and fibronolysis are an integral function of endothelial cells. These products include von Willebrand Factor (vWF), thrombospondin (TSP), Tissue Plasminogen Activator (tPA) and Plasminogen Activator Inhibitor-1 (PAI-1). In an *in vitro* human endothelial model, levels of tPA, vWF, TSP and PAI-1 were measured between 37–43°C (Strother et al., 1986). TSP and vWF levels increased after 3 h at 41–43°C. PAI-1 levels rose and tPA decreased with increasing temperature. Prolonged exposure to 43°C reduced levels of both PAI-1 and tPA. These changes result in a prothrombotic tendency with heat injury. Clinical correlation of these observations was reported by Mustafa et al. (1985) in patients with heat stroke. In these patients activation of the coagulation system was evident as a disseminated intravascular coagulation syndrome.

Endothelial integrity fails with heat injury (Ang and Dawes, 1994). This was illustrated using permeability to albumin and low density lipoprotein in an human endothelial model. That endothelial cells are critical in tissue injury should not be surprising since endothelial structural and synthetic integrity are correlated with tissue graft survival and reperfusion tissue damage (Nanney et al., 1983; Gao et al., 1991).

Recent work in humans by Rydholm et al. (1995), concentrating on second messenger mechanisms for tPA and PAI-1 production in heat injury, suggests that catecholamines are not in-

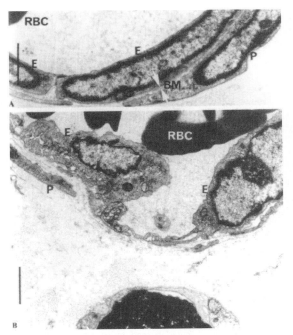

Fig. 8. Electron micrograph of transverse section through endoneural vessels of rat sciatic nerve. A, control. B, 7 days after cold injury. Note swelling of endothelial cell bodies, retraction of endothelial peripheral processes and lateral displacement of pericyte. Interstitial oedema separates a degenerating myelinated fibre from the endoneural capillary. Bars = 1.5 μm. BM = basement membrane. E = endothelial cell. P = pericyte. RBC = red blood cell [from Nukada et al. (1981), with kind permission of Oxford University Press].

volved in stimulation of these factors. However, thrombin has been shown to stimulate endothelial production of both tPA and PAI-1. This work suggests that physiological mechanisms explain thromboses and ischaemia in nerve thermal injury. Comparable studies with cold injury using this model have not been reported, although Ungley and Blackwood (1942) observed no difficulty in obtaining venous or arterial blood from hypothermic limbs.

Platelet abnormalities are well described in heat injury. In hyperthermic syndromes, thrombocytopenia may occur within 24 h and platelet microthrombi may be seen histologically in neural tissues (Stefanini, 1975; Chao et al., 1981). Early platelet changes are thought to be due to in-

travascular activation, and persistent changes to marrow injury and to the disseminated intravascular syndrome.

In hypothermia, platelet numbers are reduced, due to sequestration in splanchnic areas, such as spleen and liver. This appears to be largely reversible with rewarming (Villalobos et al., 1958). In addition, platelets progressively lose their ability to aggregate, with none evident between 2 and 4°C (Kattlove et al., 1970). This state is also reversible and is likely to be due to the temperature sensitivity of platelet microtubules (Behnke, 1967).

Thrombocytopenia may be found within an hour of birth in hypothermic neonates (< 34°C) (Chadd and Gray, 1972). A coagulopathy is also evident in these children who have a high risk of haemorrhage, particularly into lung or brain, with a mortality greater than 50%. Yoshihara et al. (1985) have demonstrated increased fibrinolytic activity in this setting. The coagulation cascade is strikingly inhibited below 35°C, with prothrombin time and activated partial thromboplastin time more sensitive than thrombin time below 33°C (Reed et al., 1990). Johnston et al. (1994) calculated that hypothermia around 29°C, is equivalent to a major clotting disorder. They suggested that enzyme failure accounts for the differential sensitivity of the activated partial thromboplastin time to cold in view of the greater number of enzymes involved.

Thermal injury may also alter the metabolic demand for oxygen. In heated tissue, metabolic rate increases proportionately (Goetz and Klawans, 1979; Simon, 1993) and this combined with the increased avidity of oxyhaemoglobin for oxygen may result in an hypoxic potential.

Chemical mediators of tissue damage in thermal injury have been extensively debated. It is likely that a range of chemical substances are involved (Boykin et al., 1980; Wahl et al., 1988; Sharma et al., 1994). Mediators in brain, skin, and spinal cord have been reported (Sharma et al., 1992, 1994). Histamine, 5-hydroxytryptamine (5 HT), and prostaglandins exacerbate clinical and

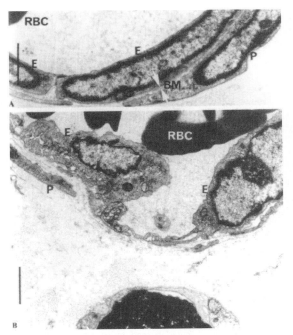

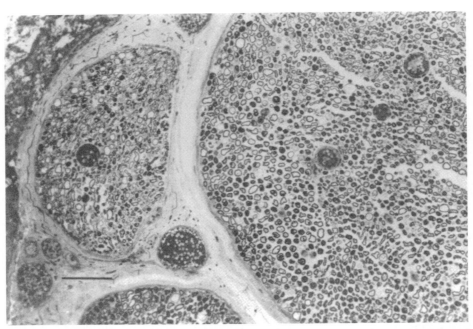

Fig. 9. A transverse section of rat sciatic nerve 2 days after low grade nerve heating showing widespread endoneural and epineural vascular thromboses. Bar = 800 μm [from Xu and Pollock (1994), with kind permission of Oxford University Press].

histological manifestations of heat injury in neural and vascular tissue. This appears to be via histamine-2 (H-2) and 5 HT-2 receptors. The clinical and histological effects of thermal injury are attenuated by prior administration of the specific inhibitors, cimetidine and ketaserine (Sharma et al., 1994).

Boykin et al. (1980) suggest histamine mediates the delayed distant effects of heat injury via H-2 receptors. They demonstrated that histamine depletion or cold, applied immediately to a heated area, have a similar effect, both locally and at a distance, to that of an H-2 antagonist.

Thus the above evidence suggests a variety of mediators are responsible for nerve thermal injury. Analysis of these principal chemical mediators is awaited in peripheral nerve, but there is considerable encouragement from work already accomplished in heat injured brain and spinal cord (Wahl et al., 1988; Sharma et al., 1992, 1993, 1994). Immediate effects pertain to conformational alterations of nerve structure. Later ischaemic changes are mediated by injured endothelium and the inflammatory cascade. In clinical cold injury, the temporal course of symptoms and histological change suggests a breakdown in the blood–nerve barrier and possibly re-perfusion injury. This response is seen in organ transplantation and tissue allografts where survival and successful function is closely correlated to endothelial integrity (Nanney et al., 1983; Gao et al., 1991). In contrast, activation of the coagulation-platelet-endothelial system is more likely in heat injury.

There is an underlying theme in the literature of thermal injury that despite a diversity of syndromes there is a single unifying pathological entity of nerve ischaemia. This is the result of the exquisite sensitivity of the vasa nervorum to variations in temperature. Future research into nerve thermal injuries should therefore be directed at strategies which protect endothelial cells or reverse intimal damage. If successful, such strategies are likely to greatly advance treatment options for these disabling disorders.

References

Adam, A.M., Hughes, R.A.C., Payan, J. and McColl, I. (1987) Letter: Peripheral neuropathy and hyperthermia. *Lancet*, 1: 1270–1271.

Ang, C. and Dawes, J. (1994) The effects of hyperthermia on human endothelial monolayers: modulation of thrombotic potential and permeability. *Blood Coagul. Fibrinolysis*, 5: 193–199.

Basbaum, C.B. (1973) Induced hypothermia in peripheral nerve: electron microscopic and electrophysiological observations. *J. Neurocytol.*, 2: 171–187.

Bassett, F.H., Kirkpatrick, J.S., Engelhardt, D.L. and Malone, T.R. (1992) Cryotherapy-induced nerve injury. *Am. J. Sports Med.*, 20: 516–518.

Behnke, O. (1967) Incomplete microtubules observed in mammalian blood platelets during microtubule polymerization. *J. Cell Biol.*, 34: 697–701.

Blatteis, C.M. (1992) Role of the OVLT in the febrile response to circulating pyrogens. *Prog. Brain Res.*, 91: 409–412.

Bouges, F., Vijayan, G. and Janfeerally, F. (1987) Peripheral neuropathy after heat stroke (letter). *Lancet*, 1: 224.

Boykin, J.V., Eriksson, E., Sholley, M.M. and Pittman, R.N. (1980) Histamine-mediated delayed permeability response after scald burn inhibited by cimetidine or cold-water treatment. *Science*, 209: 815–817.

Bull, J., Lees, D., Schuette, W., Whang-Peng, J., Smith, R., Bynum, G., Atkinson, E.R., Gottdiener, J.S., Gralnick, H.R., Shawker, T.H. and Devita, V.T. (1979) Whole body hyperthermia: A phase 1 trial of a potential adjuvant to chemotherapy. *Ann. Intern. Med.*, 90: 317–323.

Carter, J.L., Shefner, J.M. and Krarup, C. (1988) Cold-induced peripheral nerve damage: involvement of touch receptors of the foot. *Muscle Nerve*, 11: 1065–1069.

Chadd, M.A. and Gray, O.P. (1972) Hypothermia and coagulation defects in the newborn. *Arch. Dis. Child.*, 47(255): 819–821.

Chao, T.C., Sinniah, R. and Pakiam, J.E. (1981) Acute heat stroke deaths. *Pathology*, 13: 145–156.

Dahlin, L.B., Shyu, B.C., Danielsen, N. and Andersson, S.A. (1989) Effects of nerve compression or ischaemia on conduction properties of myelinated and non-myelinated nerve fibres. An experimental study in the rabbit common peroneal nerve. *Acta Physiol. Scand.*, 136: 97–105.

Denny-Brown, D., Adams, R.D. and Brenner, C. (1945) The pathology of injury to nerve induced by cold. *J. Neuropathol. Exp. Neurol.*, 4(4): 305–317.

Dhopesh, V.P. and Burns, R.A. (1976) Letter: Loss of nerve conduction in heat stroke. *New Engl. J. Med.*, 294: 557–558.

Efthimiou, J., Butler, J., Woodham, C., Benson, M.K. and Westaby, S. (1991) Diaphragm paralysis following cardiac surgery: role of phrenic nerve cold injury. *Ann. Thorac. Surg.*, 53: 1005–1008.

Emami, B., Myerson, R.J., Scott, C., Gibbs, F., Lee, C. and Perez, C.A. (1991) Phase I/II study. Combination of radiotherapy and hyperthermia in patients with deep-seated malignant tumours: a report of a pilot study by the Radiation Therapy Oncology Group. *Int. J. Radiat. Oncol. Biol. Phys.*, 20: 73–79.

Fujimura, H., Lacroix, C. and Said, G. (1991) Vulnerability of nerve fibres to ischaemia. A quantitative light and electron microscope study. *Brain*, 114: 1929–1942.

Gao, W., Takei, Y., Marzi, I., Lindert, K.A., Caldwell-Kenkel, J.C., Currin, R.T., Tanaka, Y., Lemasters, J.J. and Thurman, R.G. (1991) Carolina rinse solution — A new strategy to increase survival time after orthotopic liver transplantation in the rat. *Transplantation*, 52(3): 417–424.

Garvey, P.H., Jones, J. and Warren, S.L. (1940) Polyradiculoneuritis (Guillain-Barre syndrome) following the use of sulfanilamide and fever therapy. *J. Am. Med. Assoc.*, 115: 1955–1962.

Gerad, H., Van Echom, D.A. and Whitacre, M. et al. (1984) Doxorubicin, cyclophosphamide and whole body hyperthermia for treatment of advanced soft tissue sarcoma. *Cancer*, 53: 2585–2591.

Goetz, C.G. and Klawans, H.L. (1979) Heat stroke and malignant hyperthermia. In: P.J. Vinkin and G.W. Bruyn (Eds.), *Handbook of Clinical Neurology*, Vol. 38, Elsevier, New York, pp. 543–561.

Goudeau, J. (1968) Influence de la temperature sur la permeabilité, des membranes artificielles lipidiques aux cations inorganoqies et organique. *J. Physiol.* (60 Suppl.) 2: 450–451.

Helm, P.A., Johnson, E.R. and Carlton, A.M. (1977) Peripheral neurological problems in the acute burn patient. *Burns*, 3: 123–125.

Helm, P.A., Pandian, G. and Heck, E. (1985) Neuromuscular problems in the burn patient: cause and prevention. *Arch. Phys. Med. Rehabil.*, 66: 451–453.

Henderson, B., Koepke, G.H. and Feller, I. (1971) Peripheral polyneuropathy amongst patients with burns. *Arch. Phys. Med. Rehabil.*, 52: 149–151.

Johnston, T.D., Ying Chen, M.S. and Reed, R.L. (1994) Functional equivalence of hypothermia to specific clotting factor deficiencies. *J. Trauma*, 37(3): 413–417.

Kao, T.Y., Chio, C.C. and Lin, M.T. (1994) Hypothalamic dopamine release and local cerebral blood flow during onset of heat stroke in rats. *Stroke*, 25: 2483–2487.

Kattlove, H. and Alexander, B. (1970) Effect of cold on bleeding (letter). *Lancet*, 2: 1359.

King, K., Negus, K. and Vance, J.C. (1981) Heat stress in motor vehicles: a problem in infancy. *Pediatrics*, 68: 579–582.

Klumpp, D. and Zimmermann, M. (1980) Irreversible differential block of A- and C-fibres following local nerve heating in the cat. *J. Physiol. (Lond.)*, 298: 471–482.

Lele, P.P. (1963) Effects of focussed ultrasonic radiation on peripheral nerve with observations on local heating. *Exp. Neurol.*, 8: 47–83.

Lin, M.T., Kao, T.Y. and Chen, C.F. (1995) Interleukin-1 receptor antagonist attenuates the heat stroke induced neuronal damage by reducing the cerebral ischaemia in rats. *Brain Res. Bull.*, 37: 595–598.

Malamud, N., Haymaker, W. and Custer, R.P. (1946) Heat stroke: a clinicopathologic study of 125 fatal cases. *Milit. Surg.*, 99: 397–449.

Marquez, S., Turley, J.E. and Peters, W.J. (1993) Neuropathy in burn patients. *Brain*, 116: 471–483.

Mehta, A.C. and Baker, R.N. (1970) Persistent neurological deficits in heat stroke. *Neurology*, 20: 336–340.

Mueller, A.R., Nalesnik, M.A., Langrehr, J.M., Rao, P.N., Snyder, J.T., Hoffman, R.A. and Schraut, W.H. (1993) Evidence that small bowel preservation causes primarily basement membrane and endothelial rather than epithelial cell injury. *Transplantation*, 56(6): 1499–1504.

Mustafa, K.Y., Omer, O. and Khogali, M. et al. (1985) Blood coagulation and fibrinolysis in heat stroke. *Br. J. Haematol.*, 61: 517–523.

Nanney, L.B., Newton, E.D., Franklin, J.D., Rees, R.S. and Lynch, J.B. (1983) Venous endothelial changes after experimental cooling of free flaps. *J. Surg. Res.*, 34: 271–278.

Nukada, H., Pollock, M. and Allpress, S. (1981) Experimental cold injury to peripheral nerve. *Brain*, 104: 779–811.

Oshima, T., Maeda, H., Takayasu, T., Fujioka, Y. and Nakaya, T. (1992) An autopsy case of infant death due to heat stroke. *Am. J. Forensic Med. Pathol.*, 13: 217–221.

Parada, M.A., Puig de Parada, M., Rada, P. and Hernandez, L. (1995) Sulpiride increase and dopamine decreases intracranial temperature in rats when injected in the lateral hypothalamus: an animal model for the neuroleptic malignant syndrome. *Brain Res.*, 674: 117–121.

Reed, R.L., Bracey, A.W., Hudson, J.D., Miller, T.A. and Fischer, R.P. (1990) Hypothermia and blood coagulation: Dissociation between enzyme activity and clotting factor levels. *Circ. Shock*, 32: 141–152.

Rydholm, H., Bostrom, S., Eriksson, E. and Risberg, B. (1995) Complex intracellular signal transduction regulates tissue plasminogen activator (tPA) and plasminogen activator inhibitor type 1 (PAI-1) synthesis in cultured human umbilical vein endothelium. *Scand. J. Clin. Lab. Invest.*, 55: 323–330.

Semsarian, C. (1994) Cold exposure, frost-bite and acute cerebral infarction. *Aust. New Zealand J. Med.*, 24: 217.

Sepulchre, C., Moati, F., Miskulin, M., Huisman, O., Moczar, E. and Robert, A.M. et al. (1979) Biochemical and pharmacological properties of a neurotoxic protein isolated from the blood serum of heavily burned patients. *J. Pathol.*, 127: 137–145.

Sharma, H.S., Nyberg, F., Cervos-Navarro, J. and Dey, P.K. (1992) Histamine modulates heat stress-induced changes in blood–brain barrier permeability, cerebral blood flow, brain oedema and serotonin levels: An experimental study in conscious young rats. *Neuroscience*, 50(2): 445–454.

Sharma, H.S., Olsson, Y. and Cervos-Navarro, J. (1993) Early perifocal cell changes and oedema in traumatic injury of the spinal cord are reduced by indomethacin, an inhibitor of prostaglandin synthesis. *Acta Neuropathol. (Berlin)*, 85: 145–153.

Sharma, H.S., Westman, J., Nyberg, F., Cervos-Navarro, J. and Dey, P.K. (1994) Role of serotonin and prostaglandins in brain oedema induced by heat stress. An experimental study in the young rat. *Acta Neurochir. (suppl.)* 60: 65–70.

Simon, H.B. (1993) Hyperthermia. *New Engl. J. Med.*, 329: 484–487.

Smith, J.L., Ritchie, J. and Dawson, J. (1915) Clinical and experimental observations on the pathology of trench frost-bite. *J. Pathol. Bacteriol.*, 20: 159–190.

Stefanini, M. (1975) Heat stroke. In: P.J. Vinkin and G.W. Bruyn (Eds.), *Handbook of Clinical Neurology*, Vol. 23, Elsevier, New York, pp. 669–682.

Strother, S.V., Bull, J.M.C. and Branham, S.A. (1986) Activation of coagulation during therapeutic whole body hyperthermia. *Thromb. Res.*, 43: 353–360.

Tomity, I. and Csillik, B. (1964) Submicroscopic alterations of myelin sheath ultrastructure due to low temperature. *Acta Morphol. Acad. Sci. Hungaricae*, 12: 387–394.

Ungley, C.C. and Blackwood, W. (1942) Peripheral vasoneuropathy after chilling 'Immersion foot and immersion hand'. *Lancet*, 2: 447–451.

Ungley, C.C., Channell, G.D. and Richards, R.L. (1943) The immersion foot syndrome. *Br. J. Surg.*, 33: 17–31.

Villalobos, T.J., Adelson, E., Riley, P.A. and Crosby, W.H. (1958) A cause of the thrombocytopenia and leucopenia that occur in dogs during deep hypothermia. *J. Clin. Invest.*, 37: 1–7.

Wahl, M., Unterberg, A., Baethmann, A. and Schilling, L. (1988) Mediators of blood–brain barrier dysfunction and formation of vasogenic brain oedema. *J. Cereb. Blood Flow Metab.*, 8: 621–634.

Wijesundene, A. (1992) Guillain-Barre syndrome in plasmodium falciparum malaria. *Postgrad. Med. J.*, 68: 376–377.

Xu, D. and Pollock, M. (1994) Experimental nerve thermal injury. *Brain*, 117: 375–384.

Yaqub, B.A. (1987) Neurologic manifestations of heat stroke at the Mecca pilgrimage. *Neurology*, 37: 1004–1006.

Yaqub, B.A., Al-Harthi, S.S., Al Orainey, I.O., Laajam, M.A. and Obeid, M.T. (1986) Heat stroke at the Mekkah Pilgrimage: clinical characteristics and course of 30 patients. *Q. J. Med.*, 59: 523–530.

Yoshihara, H., Yamamoto, T. and Mihara, H. (1985) Changes in coagulation and fibrinolysis in dogs during hypothermia. *Thromb. Res.*, 37: 503–512.

Zeisberger, E. and Merker, G. (1992) The role of the OVLT in fever and antipyresis. *Prog. Brain Res.*, 91: 403–408.

Zhi-Cheng, M. and Yi-Tang, W. (1991) Analysis of 411 cases of severe heat stroke in Nanjing. *Chin. Med. J.*, 104: 256–258.

SECTION V

Clinical aspects

H.S. Sharma and J. Westman (Eds.)
Progress in Brain Research, Vol 115

CHAPTER 22

Fever and antipyresis

Matthew J. Kluger*, Wieslaw Kozak, Lisa R. Leon, Dariusz Soszynski and
Carole A. Conn

*Lovelace Respiratory Research Institute, P.O. Box 5890, Albuquerque,
New Mexico 89185, USA*

Fever defined

As discussed in other chapters in this text, fever is
a regulated rise in body temperature. As such,
fever can be distinguished from 'hyperthermia',
which is the condition where body temperature is
passively elevated above the thermoregulatory
set-point (e.g. sitting in a sauna). Fever is one of
the most common acute phase responses to infection, trauma or injury.

Fevers are triggered by the release of 'endogenous pyrogens' from a large number of different
types of macrophage-like cells. These endogenous
pyrogens include the cytokines interleukin-1 (IL-
1), IL-6, and others. They act at the level of the
anterior hypothalamus to raise the thermoregulatory set-point, thus initiating a large number of
physiological and behavioural responses, which
result in the elevation of body temperature. There
are considerable data indicating that many of
these cytokines induce the production of
prostaglandin E_2 (PGE_2) within the anterior hypothalamus and that it is PGE_2 that is the proximal mediator that raises the thermoregulatory
set-point (see Chapter 8).

In addition to the release of endogenous pyrogens, there are also endogenous antipyretics or

cryogens, which act to modulate the febrile rise in
body temperature, thus generally preventing body
temperature from rising to dangerous levels. Over
the past ten years, investigators have shown that
arginine vasopressin, α-melanocyte stimulating
hormone, glucocorticoids, and, in some cases,
TNFα may act as endogenous antipyretics. This
highly regulated nature of fever, containing factors that raise body temperature and others that
prevent this rise in body temperature from becoming too high, supports the hypothesis that
fever has evolved as a beneficial host defence
response (see Kluger et al., 1996 for details).

Below we briefly review the role of endogenous
pyrogens and endogenous cryogens in the regulation of body temperature during fever.

The role of endogenous pyrogens and cryogens in fever

Although most reviews on cytokines identify IL-1,
TNF and other cytokines as being responsible for
the fever that accompanies infection or cancer,
this conclusion is based largely on studies demonstrating that injection of these cytokines produces
this acute phase response (APR). However, it is
not known whether these injections simulate the
plasma or central nervous system concentrations
of cytokines that occur during diseases known to
produce fever. Could these simply be pharmacological effects? For example, Shapiro et al. (1993)

---

*Corresponding author. Tel: +1 505 845-1169; fax: +1 505
845-1193; e-mail: mkluger@lrri.org

reported that ciliary neurotrophic factor (CNTF) is an endogenous pyrogen. In this well-designed and executed study, it was shown that i.v. injection of CNTF into rabbits produced a dose-dependent rapid-onset fever. These fevers were blocked by pretreatment of the rabbits with indomethacin, a potent antipyretic drug. But is CNTF an *endogenous* pyrogen or is it simply a pyrogen, which when injected at *pharmacologic* doses causes fever? Simply demonstrating that injection of a cytokine results in a specific APR does not prove that the cytokine is involved in that APR during disease. It was argued that before any factor can be established to have a physiologic role (i.e. truly be an *endogenous* mediator of fever) several criteria must be fulfiled (Kluger, 1991). These criteria, plus some supporting data are presented below.

Criterion No. 1. Application of the putative endogenous mediator (e.g. pyrogen) at the hypothetical site of action results in the response observed during infection (e.g. a rise in body temperature)

For example, if the anterior hypothalamus is the theoretical site of action of an endogenous pyrogen, then injection of the putative endogenous pyrogen at this locus should induce fever. As an aside, for many years it was assumed that there must be a circulating mediator of fever. This hypothesis was based on elegant studies done by many labouratories showing that during certain types of fevers, a pyrogen could be transferred from one animal to another from the blood. When investigators tried to isolate these putative pyrogens (e.g. IL-1) from the blood, there were mixed results. Most studies have failed to show a strong correlation between circulating putative pyrogens and fever, perhaps with the exception of IL-6. We now know that the brain is capable of producing virtually all of the putative endogenous pyrogens (see, for example, chapters in De Souza, 1993, parts A and B, or Fabry et al., 1994). Thus, during some fevers it is possible that there is no need for a *circulating* trigger for fever.

Criterion No. 2. When an exogenous factor (e.g. bacteria) induces fever (A) the released putative endogenous mediator has some quantitative relationship to the response (e.g. rise in temperature), and (B) the putative mediator is released in amounts similar to those that cause an equivalent response (e.g. rise in temperature) when the putative endogenous mediator is given at the hypothetical site of action

Fevers vary in magnitude and duration. Suppose a putative mediator is hypothesized as being secreted from fixed macrophages in the liver into the circulation. Then, when an animal is injected with a pathogen, the mediator should be released from the liver into the circulation roughly in proportion to the resultant fever. Furthermore, when a putative mediator is infused into an experimental animal to achieve the plasma concentration observed during infection, the rise in body temperature should be virtually indistinguishable from that following injection of the pathogen.

Criterion No. 2, however, is not essential because it assumes that the administration of an exogenous pyrogen does not influence (e.g. upregulate) the receptor for a putative endogenous mediator of fever. For example, were LPS to either directly or indirectly increase the number of receptors for some endogenous pyrogen, then the plasma concentration of that endogenous pyrogen might vary in an 'all-or-none' mode, rather than in proportion to the fever. Furthermore, this criterion assumes that during the course of the fever other factors (e.g. endogenous cryogens) are not influencing the fever. Nevertheless, it is probable that whatever turns out to be the 'circulating' mediator of fever (or other APR) will fulfil, to some extent, this criterion.

Criterion No. 3. Substances that prevent the production of the putative endogenous mediator should block the response (e.g. rise in body temperature)

If drug X blocks the *production* of a putative endogenous mediator of fever, this should result in the complete blockade of the rise in body temperature. If drug X does block the production of a putative endogenous mediator, but does not block fever, or only attenuates it, then clearly other mediators are also involved in fever.

Criterion No. 4. Substances that prevent the action of the putative endogenous mediator should block the response (e.g. rise in body temperature)

As for criterion No. 3, if drug X blocks the *action* of a putative endogenous mediator of fever, this should result in the complete blockade of the rise in body temperature. If drug X does block the action of a putative EP, but does not block fever, or only attenuates it, then clearly other mediators are also involved in the response.

Until a few years ago only criterion 1 listed above had been fulfilled for most cytokines implicated in fever. However, within the past few years there have been numerous studies assessing the roles of cytokines in fever using criteria 2, 3 and 4. These are described below.

Data relevant to criterion No. 2

Michie et al. (1988) found that intravenous injection of LPS to human patients resulted in fever and an increase in plasma concentration of TNF. They then infused these patients with TNF at a dose that attempted to simulate the plasma concentrations measured following injection of LPS, and this resulted in fever. These findings support the hypothesis that TNF is a pyrogen in human subjects. Although their results are impressive, two aspects of their study are difficult to interpret. One is that despite continuous infusion of TNF, the plasma concentration of TNF (as determined by ELISA) fell to non-detectable levels after 12 h. Perhaps the presence of high levels of TNF induces its rapid clearance? Since there are reports of discrepancies between immunoassays and bioassays for measurement of TNF (Duncombe and Brenner, 1988; Fomsgaard et al., 1988; Petersen and Moller, 1988), it is also possible that the measurements of TNF in the study by Michie et al. (1988) did not accurately reflect the biologically active TNF. A second unresolved aspect of the study by Michie et al. is that the patients developed fevers despite pre-treatment with indomethacin, a nonsteroidal anti-inflammatory drug that has potent antipyretic properties.

In studies from our laboratory, Klir et al. (1993) measured the concentrations of IL-1, TNF and IL-6 in the anterior hypothalamus (using push–pull perfusion) of rats injected intraperitoneally (i.p.) with LPS. The hypothalamic concentrations of TNF and IL-6 rose. There was no detectable increase in IL-1. When we simulated these hypothalamic concentrations of cytokines by slowly infusing either TNF or IL-6 intrahypothalamically, the infusion of TNF had no effect on body temperature. The infusion of IL-6 caused a large fever, thus supporting the hypothesis that IL-6, acting at the hypothalamus, is an endogenous pyrogen.

Data relevant to criterion No. 3

Injection of LPS (2.5 mg/kg, i.p.) into IL-1β knock-out mice (mice lacking a functional gene for synthesis of IL-1β) resulted in attenuated fever (Kozak et al., 1995). With subcutaneous (s.c.) injection of turpentine, control mice developed large fevers whereas IL-1β knock-out mice developed no fever (Fig. 1) (Zheng et al., 1995). These data support the hypotheses that induction of a localized inflammation (i.e. s.c. injection of turpentine) causes fever (and a reduction in activity) exclusively via IL-1β, whereas the induction of systemic inflammation (i.e. i.p. injection of LPS) exerts its actions only partially via IL-1β.

In ongoing studies, Lisa Leon and others within our group are studying the febrile responses of mice that lack the gene for IL-1 type I receptors. These mice develop normal fevers after i.p. injection of a high (2.5 mg/kg) and low (50 μg/kg) dose of LPS, but fail to develop any fever in response to s.c. injection of turpentine. These data indicate that a localized inflammation causes fever exclusively via the IL-1 type I receptor,

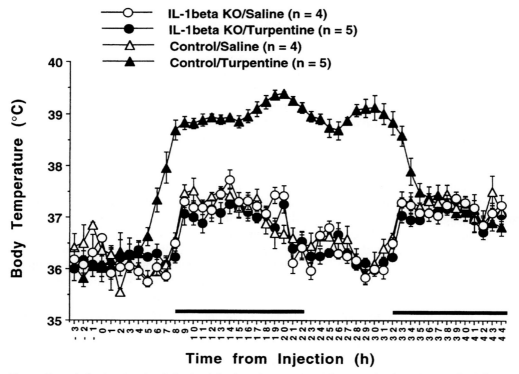

Fig. 1. Fever induction in mice following injection of turpentine. Mice were implanted with Mini-Mitter transmitters to monitor body temperature. One group lacked the gene for IL-1β (IL-1β knock-outs); the other group of mice were wild-type controls. They were then injected s.c. with 100 μl of turpentine or saline. Note that the wild-type controls injected with turpentine developed large fevers whereas the knock-out mice did not develop any fever (based on Zheng et al., 1995).

whereas the induction of systemic inflammation (i.e. i.p. injection of LPS) does not occur via the IL-1 type I receptor in mice. Perhaps these IL-1 type I receptor knock-out mice develop fevers in response to LPS as a result of the induction of another cytokine (e.g. MIP-1 or IL-6) or increased sensitivity to other pyrogens.

Chai et al. (1994) found that IL-6 deficient mice (lacking the gene for IL-6) fail to develop fevers in response to i.p. injection of LPS (50 μg/kg) and to recombinant mouse IL-1β (10 μg/kg). Results from our laboratory indicate that these knock-out mice develop normal fevers to the i.p. injection of 2.5 mg/kg LPS (Kozak et al., 1997). Thus, whereas IL-6 is critically important for fevers to low doses of LPS, high doses of LPS induce fever in mice via an IL-6-independent

pathway. Interestingly, as in IL-1β knock-out mice, injection of turpentine in IL-6 knock-out mice does not lead to fever (Kozak et al., 1997).

In interpreting data from experiments using transgenic mice, it is important to be cognizant of the tremendous redundancy in cytokine action. Animals that have never 'seen' IL-1β, IL-6, or other putative mediators of fever/inflammation may have developed compensatory mechanisms. Nevertheless, as shown above, much of the data obtained from cytokine knock-out mice are compatible with data obtained the old-fashioned way — i.e. using neutralizing antibodies and receptor blockers (see studies described below under 'Criterion 4').

Zabel et al. (1993) have shown that the drug pentoxifylline totally abolished the rise in plasma

TNF concentration in human volunteers given LPS intravenously without influencing the course of their fever, their 'flu-like symptoms' and leukocytosis. We found similar results in our experiments in LPS-injected rats that were pretreated with varying doses of pentoxifylline (LeMay et al., 1990). At moderate doses, this drug did not influence fever, but did significantly reduce the plasma concentration of TNF in LPS-injected rats. Taken together, these data support the hypothesis that TNF is not essential for the development of LPS-induced fever.

Data relevant to criterion No. 4

Work from our laboratory has shown that i.v. administration of antiserum to recombinant murine IL-1α had no effect on LPS-fever in the rat (Long et al., 1989). This latter finding might not be surprising since IL-1α is thought to be primarily cell-associated. IL-1β may be the secreted form of IL-1. We have found that antiserum to IL-1β did lead to a 57% attenuation in the magnitude of LPS-induced fever in rats (Long et al., 1990a). Rothwell et al. (1989) reported similar findings. Klir et al. (1994) have found that microinjection of neutralizing antibody to IL-1β into the anterior hypothalamus attenuates fever caused by i.p. injection of LPS, and also blocks the increase in hypothalamic IL-6. These data support the hypothesis that LPS-induced fever is triggered by IL-1β, and that this cytokine then causes fever via the hypothalamic release of IL-6. As noted above, we were unable to measure IL-1β in the push–pull perfusate bathing the anterior hypothalamus. A key question is why we were unable to measure IL-1β in the hypothalamic fluid? Stitt (1993) has argued that IL-1β might act outside the brain proper, perhaps in the organum vasculosum of the lamina terminalis (OVLT), to initiate fever. It is possible that our injection of antibody to IL-1β resulted in the antibody diffusing the short distance to the OVLT, inhibiting IL-1β in this region, thus blocking the IL-1β-induced rise in hypothalamic IL-6.

Nagai et al. (1988) and Kawasaki et al. (1989) found that administration of antibody to TNF resulted in a significant attenuation of LPS-fever in the rabbit. In these studies, rabbits that were injected with LPS and antibody to TNF developed fevers similar to rabbits that received only LPS during the first 2 h, but there was a significant reduction in the fever of the animals receiving antibody during hours two to four. Different results were obtained when we pretreated rats with antiserum to TNF in amounts that completely blocked any rise in plasma TNF, as determined by our sensitive WEHI assay (Long et al., 1990a,b). When rats injected with antiserum either i.p. or i.v. were then injected with LPS i.p., the resultant fevers were significantly enhanced, rather than suppressed. Our data are consistent with the hypothesis that in the rat TNF may be an endogenous antipyretic that limits the magnitude of fever. Similar findings were found by Smith and Kluger (1993), in rats inoculated with an MCA sarcoma. Antiserum to TNF prevented the tumor-induced fall in body temperature. Derijk and Berkenbosch (1994) found a similar attenuation in the fall in body temperature in rats injected with antiserum to TNF followed by injection of a high dose of LPS (500 μg/kg). In a more recent study, Klir et al. (1995) showed that injection of small, non-pyrogenic, doses of TNF i.p. into rats blocked LPS-induced fevers, confirming earlier findings by Long et al. (1992). In addition, Klir et al. (1995) found that i.p. injection of the TNF soluble receptor (TNF:Fc, Immunex) into rats, which at the dose injected prevents the biological activity of TNF, led to larger LPS-induced fevers, results that were then confirmed in a mouse model of fever by Kozak et al. (1995). Based on injections of TNF into various brain sites, our data support the hypothesis that the antipyretic actions of TNF reside at some location outside the central nervous system (CNS) (Klir et al., 1995).

How can we explain the differences between our experiments in rats and mice and those of Nagai et al. (1988) and Kawasaki et al. (1989) in rabbits? In the studies involving injection of monoclonal antibody to TNF in rabbits no data were presented demonstrating that their antibody neutralized TNF bioactivity in vivo. It is possible that injection of this antibody might have increased levels of TNF, producing greater antipyresis — thus, resulting in smaller fevers. In fact, in a study described below, injection of monoclonal antibody to TNF did indeed raise plasma levels of TNF in human subjects (Kwiatkowski et al., 1993).

In the study by Kwiatkowski et al. (1993) a single i.v. injection of a murine monoclonal antibody to TNF led to *smaller* fevers in children receiving otherwise conventional therapy for cerebral malaria. However, no evidence was presented indicating that the TNF was neutralized. In fact it was reported in this study that the circulating levels of TNF were actually significantly *higher* in those patients given the antibody. These investigators concluded that the presence of higher TNF in the circulation meant that less TNF could get to the CNS, and thus the fever was reduced. An alternative explanation, based on the data described above showing that injections of non-pyrogenic doses of TNF results in antipyresis, is that TNF is an endogenous cryogen, acting at a level outside the CNS — the higher levels of TNF led to a greater signal to reduce body temperature.

Further support for TNF playing a role as an endogenous cryogen or antipyretic comes from studies in our laboratory (Leon et al., 1997) using transgenic mice lacking both the p55 (type I) and p75 (type II) TNF receptors (TNFR double knock-out mice). The peripheral injection of a high dose of LPS (2.5 mg/kg, i.p.) resulted in an exacerbation of the early phase of fever (2–15 h) compared to LPS-injected TNFR wild-type mice. The late phase of fever (15–24 h) was virtually identical in both groups of mice. These results suggest that endogenous TNFα is involved in the early modulation or attenuation of fever to a high dose of LPS. We have not yet determined which type of TNF receptor is responsible for this modulation of fever.

The mechanism of this TNF antipyresis is unknown. Our data support the hypothesis that the antipyretic actions of TNF reside outside the CNS (Klir et al., 1995). TNF might be inducing the production and release of some antipyretic cytokine or other substance from sites outside the CNS, which then cross from the circulation to the CNS. As mentioned above, we (and others) have not been able to demonstrate any direct CNS fever-modulation when small physiologically relevant doses of TNF, or antibody to TNF, are injected intracerebroventricularly or directly into the anterior hypothalamus. Ebisui et al. (1994) have shown that injection of antiserum to TNF led to a marked attenuation of the rise of corticosterone induced by injection of LPS in the rat. Since we have recently shown that the LPS-induced rise in corticosterone results in attenuation of fever (Morrow et al., 1993), it is possible that TNF's antipyretic action is via the release of glucocorticoids. In a more recent study we have shown that the site of glucocorticoid suppression of fever is in the anterior hypothalamus (McClellan et al., 1994).

Macrophage inflammatory protein-1 (MIP-1) is another putative endogenous pyrogen. Davatelis et al. (1989) showed that a crude preparation MIP-1 led to prostaglandin-independent fevers. Miñano et al. (1990) then showed that MIP-1 led to fevers when injected intrahypothalamically into rats. Pretreatment of the injection site with indomethacin failed to prevent the development of fever. MIP-1 consists of two peptides, each about 8 kDa in size. Myers et al. (1993) showed that injection of both MIP-1α and MIP-1β caused fevers in rats. These data indicate that MIP-1 is capable of inducing fever when injected into rats, and that these fevers are not dependent on prostaglandins. But is MIP-1 actually in the fever pathway? Miñano et al. (1996) recently showed that microinjection of goat anti-mouse MIP-1β antibody into the preoptic anterior hypothalamus of rats markedly suppressed fever in response to an i.p. injection of LPS. The attenuation of fever occurred when the antibody was injected at the time of injection of LPS or even 3 h after the injection of LPS when fever was close to its maximum.

These data lead to a paradox. Antibody to MIP-1β blocks fevers caused by peripheral injection of LPS. It is well known that cyclooxygenase inhibitors block LPS-induced fevers. Yet MIP-1 fevers are presumably not mediated by prostaglandins. However, as described earlier in this review, studies using antibodies to IL-1β (or using IL-1β knock-out mice) indicate that this leads to the attenuation of LPS-induced fevers. Furthermore, IL-1β fevers are blocked by cyclooxygenase inhibitors. It is possible that injection of LPS or other inflammatory mediators induce the production of several cytokines necessary for the generation of full-blown fever. Neutralization of, for example, either IL-1β or MIP-1β leads to marked attenuation of fever (even though one presumably works via prostaglandins and the other via a prostaglandin-independent pathway).

Summary of the role of cytokines in fever

There are considerable data supporting the hypothesis that cytokines are responsible for the fever associated with infection and cancer. Although initially most of these data were obtained by injection of cytokines (Criterion 1), within the past 5 years considerable data have been published regarding the roles of cytokines in LPS-induced fever (primarily for IL-1β, MIP-1, TNF, and IL-6) based on criteria 2, 3, and 4.

The role of prostaglandins in fever

There is an enormous body of data supporting the hypothesis that PGE$_2$ is involved in most fevers (see Chapter 8). Milton and Wendlandt (1971) first showed that prostaglandins of the E (PGE) series will produce fever when injected into the cerebral ventricles of cats and rabbits. Studies by Feldberg and Saxena (1971), and Stitt (1973) showed that microinjections of prostaglandins into the preoptic/anterior hypothalamus produced fever in cats and rabbits; microinjections into

other areas of the brain (posterior hypothalamus and midbrain reticular formation) failed to produce a fever. Milton and Wendlandt (1971) were probably the first to propose that pyrogens might induce a fever through the production of specific prostaglandins, and that antipyretic drugs reduce fever by blocking its synthesis. Dozens of publications over the past 25 years have supported a role of prostaglandins in most fevers. It is probable that most (but not all — e.g., for MIP-1) fever-inducing actions of cytokines are mediated by prostaglandins.

Endogenous antipyretic hormones

Many hormones, such as glucocorticoids, arginine vasopressin, and α-melanocyte stimulating hormone modulate this febrile rise in body temperature. The roles of these hormones in modulation of fever are briefly described below.

Glucocorticoids

Virtually all stresses activate the hypothalamic-pituitary-adrenal (HPA) axis resulting in an elevation of circulating glucocorticoids. The ability of cytokines (e.g. IL-1, IL-6) to activate the HPA axis is well documented. Work from our laboratory on adrenalectomized rats supports the hypothesis that glucocorticoids suppress the production/release of IL-6 and attenuate fever (Morrow et al., 1993). In our studies, adrenalectomized rats injected with LPS developed both higher fevers and significantly higher plasma concentrations of IL-6 (vs. controls). This effect was abolished by replacement glucocorticoid treatment. Treatment of intact (non-adrenalectomized) rats with RU38486 (a glucocorticoid type II receptor antagonist) resulted in animals that were 'functionally' adrenalectomized. These animals also developed larger LPS-induced fevers, supporting the hypothesis that glucocorticoid effects are receptor-mediated. Support for the hypothesis that glucocorticoids limit the production of inflammatory mediators has also been provided by data showing that carrageenan-induced inflammation is more intense and lasts longer in hypophysectomized rats (Stenberg et al., 1990) and that the glucocorticoid receptor antagonist, RU38486, permits the development of severe inflammatory disease in response to streptococcal cell wall peptidoglycan polysaccharide (Sternberg et al., 1989).

Arginine vasopressin

Arginine vasopressin (AVP) fulfils many of the criteria of an endogenous cryogen or antipyretic (Kasting, 1989; Kluger, 1991). Exogenous administration of AVP in central temperature regulatory sites of a variety of species results in an attenuation of fever without having an effect on afebrile body temperature (Naylor et al., 1985; Wilkinson and Kasting, 1990; Fyda et al., 1990; Federico et al., 1992). These effects can be reversed with the administration of the AVP V_1 (vasopressor)-type receptor antagonist $d(CH_2)_5Tyr(Me)AVP$ (Kovacs et al., 1992). The sensitive central sites of AVP's exogenous actions include the ventral septal area (VSA) and medial amygdaloid nucleus (Naylor et al., 1985; Federico et al., 1992). Receptor localization studies demonstrated the presence of the V_1-type receptor in these areas (Poulin et al., 1988; Willcox et al., 1992). Centrally administered AVP V_1-type receptor antagonist or AVP antiserum have resulted in prolonged and exacerbated fevers (Malkinson et al., 1987; Landgraf et al., 1990; Cridland and Kasting, 1992).

There are some data supporting the hypothesis that salicylates (and other antipyretic drugs) may be blocking fever in part by inducing the production of AVP (e.g. Alexander et al., 1989). Thus, it is possible that prostaglandins exert a negative feedback on AVP release.

α-Melanocyte stimulating hormone

The discovery that central or peripheral administration of α MSH attenuates fever in rats (Bull et al., 1990; Martin et al., 1990), as well as several other species (e.g. Glyn and Lipton, 1981; Murphy et al., 1983; Deeter et al., 1989; Goelst et al., 1991; Martin et al., 1991; Davidson et al., 1992)

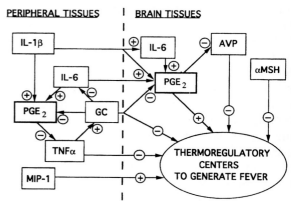

Fig. 2. Model of fever based on recent data. (+) = stimulatory action; (−) = inhibitory action. Injection of LPS or other inflammatory stimuli induces the production of the cytokines IL-1, IL-6, MIP-1 and others from various organs in the viscera and brain. Some of these cytokines exert their fever-inducing activity via prostaglandins (e.g. IL-1, IL-6) and others (e.g. MIP-1) appear to act independently of prostaglandins. Hormones such as arginine vasopressin (AVP), α melanocyte stimulating hormone (α MSH), and glucocorticoids exert antipyretic action perhaps via suppression of production of cytokines or via some direct action on the thermoregulatory centres involved in the development of fever. TNF may be exerting its antipyretic properties via either an elevation in glucocorticoids or some other pathway.

has raised the question as to the role of these endogenous peptides in the regulation of febrile and normal body temperature. Shih et al. (1986) have provided direct evidence as to the role of endogenous α MSH in the febrile response to IL-1 by intracerebroventricularly administering an antiserum to the peptide. The effective elimination of endogenously produced α MSH within the CNS caused a prolongation and enhancement of the febrile response to endogenous pyrogen for up to 9 h post-injection, suggesting that release of the peptide following pyrogen exposure normally limits the febrile response.

Plasma concentrations of α MSH increase following LPS injection (Martin and Lipton, 1990) as well as other stresses. Intravenous administration of α MSH reduced fever following LPS and IL-1β in rabbits (Davidson et al., 1992). It is postulated that α MSH elicits its antipyretic properties by antagonizing the actions of endogenous pyrogens such as interleukin-1. This hypothesis has not been extensively explored.

Summary of the roles of glucocorticoids, AVP and αMSH in modulation of fever

All three of these hormones have been shown to attenuate fever. Any or all of these hormones may play a physiologic role in attenuating fever.

The overall model of fever induced by LPS is shown in Fig. 2.

References

Alexander, S.J., Cooper, K.E. and Veale, W.L. (1989) Sodium salicylate: alternate mechanism of central antipyretic action in the rat. *Pflug. Arch.*, 413: 451–455.

Bull, D.F., King, M.G., Pfister, H.P. and Singer, G. (1990) α-Melanocyte-stimulating hormone conditioned suppression of a lipopolysaccharide induced fever. *Peptides*, 11(5): 1027–1030.

Chai, Z., Gatti, S., Poli, V. and Bartfai, T. (1994) IL-6 gene expression is necessary for fever induction in response to LPS in mice: a study on IL-6 deficient mice. In: G. Silvia, Ph.D. thesis. Interleukin 1, tumor necrosis factor α and interleukin 6 in the rat central nervous system: production and effects with particular attention to the fever response, Stockholm University.

Cridland, R.A. and Kasting, N.W. (1992) A critical role for central vasopressin in regulation of fever during bacterial infection. *Am. J. Physiol.*, 263: R1235–R1240.

Davatelis, G., Wolpe, S.D., Sherry, B., Dayer, J-M., Chicheportiche, R. and Cerami, A. (1989) Macrophage inflammatory protein-1: a prostaglandin-independent endogenous pyrogen. *Science*, 243: 1066–1068.

Davidson, J., Milton, A.S. and Rotondo, D. (1992) α-Melanocyte-stimulating hormone suppresses fever and increases in plasma levels of prostaglandin, E_2 in the rabbit. *J. Physiol.*, 451: 491–502.

Deeter, L.B., Martin, L.W. and Lipton, J.M. (1989) Antipyretic properties of centrally administered α-MSH fragments in the rabbit. *Peptides,*, 9: 1285–1288.

Derijk, R.H. and Berkenbosch, F. (1994) Hypothermia to endotoxin involves the cytokine tumor necrosis factor and the neuropeptide vasopressin in rats. *Am. J. Physiol.*, 266: R9–R14.

De Souza, E.B. (1993) *Neurobiology of Cytokines, Parts A and B.* Methods in Neurosciences, Academic Press, San Diego.

Duncombe, A.S. and Brenner, M.K. (1988) Is circulating tumor necrosis factor bioactive? *New Engl. J. Med.*, 319: 1227.

Ebisui, O., Fukata, J., Murakami, N., Kobayashi, H., Segawa, H., Muro, S., Hanaoka, I., Naito, Y., Masui, Y., Ohoto, Y., Imura, H. and Nakao, K. (1994) Effect of IL-1 receptor antagonist and antiserum to TNF-α on LPS-induced plasma ACTH and corticosterone rise in rats. *Am. J. Physiol.*, 266: E986–E992.

Fabry, Z., Raine, C.S. and Hart, M.N. (1994) Nervous tissue as an immune compartment: the dialect of the immune response in the CNS. *Immunol. Today*, 218: 218–224.

Federico, P., Veale, W.L. and Pittman, Q.J. (1992) Vasopressin-induced antipyresis in the medial amygdaloid nucleus of conscious rats. *Am. J. Physiol.*, 262: R901–R908.

Feldberg, W. and Saxena, P.N. (1971) Further studies on prostaglandin, E_1 fever in cats. *J. Physiol. (Lond.)*, 219: 739–745.

Fomsgaard, A., Worsaae, H. and Bendtzen, K. (1988) Detection of tumor necrosis factor from lipopolysaccharide-stimulated human mononuclear cells by enzyme-linked immunosorbent assay and cytotoxicity bioassay. *Scand. J. Immunol.*, 27: 143–147.

Fyda, D.M., Mathieson, W.B., Cooper, K.E. and Veale, W.L.(1990) The effectiveness of arginine vasopressin and sodium salicylate as antipyretics in the Brattleboro rat. *Brain Res.*, 512: 243–247.

Glyn, J.R. and Lipton, J.M. (1981) Hypothermic and antipyretic effects of centrally administered, ACTH (1-24) and α-melanotropin. *Peptides*, 2(2): 177–187.

Goelst, K., Mitchell, D. and Laburn, H. (1991) Effects of α-melanocyte stimulating hormone on fever caused by endotoxin in rabbits. *J. Physiol.*, 441: 469–476.

Kasting, N.W. (1989) Criteria for establishing a physiological role for brain peptides. A case in point: the role of vasopressin in thermoregulation during fever and antipyresis. *Brain Res. Rev.*, 14: 143–153.

Kawasaki, H., Moriyama, M., Ohtani, Y., Naitoh, M., Tanaka, A., and Nariuchi, H. (1989) Analysis of endotoxin fever in rabbits by using a monoclonal antibody to tumor necrosis factor (cachectin). *Infect. Immun.*, 57: 3131–3135.

Klir, J.J., Roth, J., Szelenyi, Z., McClellan, J.L. and Kluger, M.J. (1993) Role of hypothalamic interleukin-6 and tumor necrosis factor α in LPS-fever in rat. *Am. J. Physiol.*, 265: R512–R517.

Klir, J.J., McClellan, J.L. and Kluger, M.J. (1994)Interleukin-1β causes the increase in anterior hypothalamic interleukin-6 during LPS-induced fever in rats. *Am. J. Physiol.*, 266: R1845–R1848.

Klir, J.J., McClellan, J.L., Kozak, W., Szelenyi, Z., Wong, G.H.W. and Kluger, M.J. (1995) Systemic but not central administration of tumor necrosis factor α attenuates LPS-induced fever in rats. *Am. J. Physiol.*, 268: R480–R486.

Kluger, M.J. (1991) Fever: role of endogenous pyrogens and cryogens. *Physiol. Rev.*, 71: 93–127.

Kluger, M.J., Kozak, W., Conn, C., Leon, L. and Soszynski, D. (1996) The adaptive value of fever. In: B.A. Cunha (Ed.),

474

Fever. Infectious Disease Clinic of North America, W.B. Saunders, Philadelphia, pp. 1–20.

Kovacs, G.L., Baars, A.M. and Wied, D.D. (1992) Antipyretic effect of central arginine[8]-vasopressin treatment: V1 receptors specifically involved? *Life Sci.*, 50: 1625–1630.

Kozak, W., Conn, C.A., Klir, J.J. and Kluger, M.J. (1995) Tumor necrosis factor soluble receptor and antiserum against tumor necrosis factor enhance lipopolysaccharide fever in mice. *Am. J. Physiol.*, 269: R23–R29.

Kozak, W., Zheng, H., Conn, C.A., Soszynski, D., Van der Ploeg, L. and Kluger, M.J. (1995) Thermal and behavioural effects of lipopolysaccharide and influenza in interleukin-1 β deficient mice. *Am. J. Physiol.*, 269: R969–R977.

Kozak, W., Poli, V., Soszynski, D., Conn, C.A., Leon, L.R. and Kluger, M.J. (1997) Sickness behavior in mice deficient in interleukin-6 during turpentine abscess and influenza pneumonitis. *Am. J. Physiol.*, 272: R621–R630.

Kwiatkowski, D., Molyneux, M.E., Stephens, S., Curtis, N., Klein, N., Pointaire, P., Smit, M., Allan, R., Brewster, D.R., Grau, G.E. and Greenwood, B.M. (1993) Anti-TNF therapy inhibits fever in cerebral malaria. *Q. J. Med.*, 86: 91–98.

Landgraf, R., Malkinson, T.J., Veale, W.L., Lederis, K. and Pittman, Q.J. (1990) Vasopressin and oxytocin in rat brain in response to prostaglandin fever. *Am. J. Physiol.*, 259: R1056–R1062.

LeMay, L.G., Vander, A.J. and Kluger, M.J. (1990) The effects of pentoxifylline on lipopolysaccharide (LPS) fever and plasma interleukin-6 (IL-6) and tumor necrosis factor (TNF) in the rat. *Cytokine*, 2: 300–306.

Leon, L.R., Kozak, W., Peschon, J. and Kluger, M.J. (1997) Exacerbated febrile responses to LPS, but not turpentine, in TNF double receptor knock-out mice. *Am. J. Physiol.*, 272: R563–R569.

Long, N.C., Kluger, M.J. and Vander, A.J. (1989) Antiserum against mouse IL-1 alpha does not block stress hyperthermia or LPS fever in the rat. In: Lomax and Schonbaum (Eds.), *Thermoregulation: Research and Clinical Applications*, 7th International Symposium on Pharmacology of Thermoregulation, Odense, Denmark, 1988, Karger, Basel, pp. 78–84.

Long, N.C., Otterness, I., Kunkel, S.L., Vander, A.J. and Kluger, M.J. (1990a) The roles of interleukin-1 β and tumor necrosis factor in lipopolysaccharide-fever in rats. *Am. J. Physiol.*, 259: R724–R728.

Long, N.C., Kunkel, S.L., Vander, A.J. and Kluger, M.J. (1990b) Antiserum against TNF enhances LPS fever in the rat. *Am. J. Physiol.*, 258: R332–R337.

Long, N.C., Morimoto, A., Nakamori, T. and Murakami, N. (1992) Systemic injection of TNF-α attenuates fever due to IL-1 β and LPS in rats. *Am. J. Physiol.*, 263: R987–R991.

Malkinson, T.J., Bridges, T.E., Lederis, K. and Veale, W.J.(1987) Perfusion of the septum of the rabbit with vasopressinantiserum enhances endotoxin fever. *Peptides*, 8: 385–389.

Martin, L.W. and Lipton, J.M. (1990) Acute phase response

toendotoxin: rise in plasma α-MSH and effects of α-MSH injection. *Am. J. Physiol.*, 259: R768–R772.

Martin, S.M., Malkinson, T.J., Veale, W.L. and Pittman, Q.J. (1990) Depletion of brain α-MSH alters prostaglandin and interleukin fever in rats. *Brain Res.*, 526: 351–354.

Martin, L.W., Catania, A., Hiltz, M.E. and Lipton, J.M. (1991) Neuropeptide α-MSH antagonizes, IL-1- and TNF-induced fever. *Peptides*, 12: 297–299.

McClellan, J.L., Klir, J.J., Morrow, L.E. and Kluger, M.J. (1994) The central effects of glucocorticoid receptor antagonist, RU38486 on lipopolysaccharide and stress-induced fever. *Am. J. Physiol.*, 267: R705–R711.

Michie, H.R., Spriggs, D.R., Manogue, K.R., Sherman, M.L., Revhaug, A., O'Dwyer, S.T., Arthur, K., Dinarello, C.A., Cerami, A., Wolff, S.M., Kufe, D.W. and Wilmore, D.W. (1988) Tumor necrosis factor and endotoxin induce similar metabolic responses in human beings. *Surgery*, 104: 280–286.

Milton, A.S. and Wendlandt, S. (1971) Effects on body temperature of prostaglandins of the A, E and F series on injection into the third ventricle of unanesthetized cats and rabbits. *J. Physiol. (Lond.)*, 218: 325–336.

Miñano, F.J., Sancibrian, M., Vizcaino, M., Paez, X., Davatelis, G., Fahey, T., Sherry, B., Cerami, A. and Myers, R.D. (1990) Macrophage inflammatory protein-1: unique action on the hypothalamus to evoke fever. *Brain Res. Bull.*, 24: 849–852.

Miñano, F.J., Fernandez-Alonso A., Benamar, K., Myers, R.D., Sancibri n, M., Ruiz, R.M. and Armengol, J.A. (1996) Macrophage inflammatory protein-1 β (MIP-1 β) produced endogenously in brain during *E. coli* fever in rats. *Eur. J. Neurosci.*, 8: 424–428.

Morrow, L.E., McClellan, J.L., Conn, C.A. and Kluger, M.J. (1993) Glucocorticoids alter fever and IL-6 responses to psychological stress and to lipopolysaccharide. *Am. J. Physiol.*, 264: R1010–1016.

Murphy, M.T., Richards, D.B. and Lipton, J.M. (1983) Antipyretic potency of centrally administered α-melanocyte stimulating hormone. *Science*, 221: 192–193.

Myers, R.D., Paex, X., Roscoe, A.K., Sherry, B. and Cerami, A. (1993) Fever and feeding: differential actions of macrophage inflammatory protein-1 (MIP-1), MIP-1 α and MIP-1 β on rat hypothalamus. *Neurochem. Res.*, 18: 667–673.

Nagai, M., Saigusa, T., Shimada, Y., Inagawa, H., Oshima, H., and Iriki, M. (1988) Antibody to tumor necrosis factor (TNF) reduces endotoxin fever. *Experientia*, 44: 606–607.

Naylor, A.M., Ruwe, W.D., Kohut, A.F. and Veale, W.L. (1985) Perfusion of vasopressin within the ventral septum of the rabbit suppresses endotoxin fever. *Brain Res. Bull.*, 15: 209–213.

Petersen, C.M. and Moller, B.K. (1988) Immunological reactivity and bioactivity of tumour necrosis factor. *Lancet*, April 23, 934–935.

Poulin, P., Lederis, K. and Pittman, Q.J. (1988) Subcellular localization and characterization of vasopressin binding sites in the ventral septal area, lateral septum, and hippocampus of the rat brain. *J. Neurochem.*, 50: 889–898.

Rothwell, N.J., Busbridge, N.J., Humphray, H. and Hissey, P. (1989) Central actions of interleukin-1β on fever and thermogenesis. *Cytokine*, 1: 153.

Shapiro, L., Zhang, X.-X., Rupp, R.G., Wolff, S.M. and Dinarello, C.A. (1993) Ciliary neurotrophic factor is an endogenous pyrogen. *Proc. Natl. Acad. Sci. USA*, 90: 8614–8618.

Shih, S.T., Khorram, O., Lipton, J.M. and McCann, S.M. (1986) Central administration of α-MSH antiserum augments fever in the rabbit. *Am. J. Physiol.*, 250: R803–R806.

Smith, B.K. and Kluger, M.J. (1993) Anti-TNF-α antibodies normalized body temperature and enhanced food intake in tumor-bearing rats. *Am. J. Physiol.*, 265: R615–R619.

Stenberg, V.I., Bouley, M.G., Katz, B.M., Lee, K.J. and Parmar, S.S. (1990) Negative endocrine control system for inflammation in rats. *Agents Actions*, 29: 189–195.

Sternberg, E.M., Hill, J.M., Chouras, G.P., Kamilaris, T., Kistwak, S.J., Gold, P.W. and Wilder, R.L. (1989) Inflammatory mediator-induced hypothalamic-pituitary-adrenal axis activation is defective in streptococcal cell wall arthritis-susceptible Lewis rats. *Proc. Natl. Acad. Sci.*, 86: 2374–2378.

Stitt, J.T. (1973) Prostaglandin E$_1$ fever induced in rabbits. *J. Physiol.*, 232: 163–179.

Stitt, J.T. (1993) Central regulation of body temperature. In: *Exercise, Heat and Thermoregulation, Perspectives in Exercise Science and Sports Medicine*, Vol. 6, Brown and Benchmark, pp. 1–39.

Wilkinson, M.F. and Kasting, N.W. (1990) Centrally acting vasopressin contributes to endotoxin tolerance. *Am. J. Physiol.*, 258: R443–R449.

Willcox, B.J., Poulin, P., Veale, W.L. and Pittman, Q.J. (1992) Vasopressin-induced motor effects: localization of a sensitive site in the amygdala. *Brain Res.*, 596: 58–64.

Zabel, P., Schade, F.U. and Schlaak, M. (1993) Inhibition of endogenous TNF formation by pentoxifylline. *Immunobiology*, 187: 447–463.

Zheng, H., Fletcher, D., Kozak, W., Jiang, M., Hofmann, K, Conn, C.A., Soszynski, D., Grabiec, C., Trumbauer, M.E., Shaw, A., Kostura, M.J., Stevens, K., Rosen, H., North, R.J., Chen, H.Y., Tocci, M.J., Kluger, M.J. and Van der Ploeg, L.H.T. (1995) Resistance to fever induction and impaired acute-phase response in interleukin-1β deficient mice. *Immunity*, 3: 9–19.

H.S. Sharma and J. Westman (Eds.)
Progress in Brain Research, Vol 115

CHAPTER 23

Regional differentiation of sympathetic efferents during fever

Masami Iriki[1,*] and Takeshi Saigusa[2]

[1]*Yamanashi Institute of Environmental Sciences, Fujiyoshida, Yamanashi 403, Japan*
[2]*Yamanashi Medical University, Tamaho, Nakakoma, Yamanashi 409-38, Japan*

Introduction

Fever and hyperthermia are two different conditions in which body temperature is elevated above its normal level. These two states are defined in the *Glossary of Terms for Thermal Physiology* (Anonymous, 1987) as follows:

Fever: A state of elevated core temperature which is often, but not necessarily, part of the defensive responses of multicellular organisms (host) to the invasion of live (microorganisms) or inanimate matter recognized as pathogenic or alien by the host. The rise in core temperature is usually designated as due to an elevation of the set-point of body temperature, according to which the higher temperature is actively established by the operation of thermoeffectors.

Hyperthermia: The condition of a temperature regulator when core temperature is above its set-range specified for the normal active state of the species. Note: When temperature regulation against overheating is active, hyperthermia is the consequence of the temporary or permanent imbalance between heat load and the capability to dissipate heat. Impairment of temperature regulation may contribute to the development of hyperthermia.

From the viewpoint of temperature regulation, hyperthermia is a condition in which heat defence responses, such as skin vasodilatation, sweating or thermal panting are induced. Conversely, fever, at least in the phase of rising core temperature, is a condition in which the pathologically elevated set temperature is higher than the actual core temperature, causing activation of cold defence responses like skin vasoconstriction and generation of metabolic heat by shivering.

Fever, however, is not only a state of altered temperature regulation but includes various humoral and cellular defence responses. Accordingly, the term 'fever syndrome' was advocated to account for the complexity of fever as a generalized host defence response (Iriki, 1988).

The analysis of the involvement of the efferent sympathetic system in the control of thermally induced and febrile thermoregulatory adjustments has to consider its property to produce regionally non-uniform changes of activity which has been termed 'regional sympathetic differentiation' (Iriki and Simon, 1978). Depending on the kind of stimulation, different patterns of regional differentiation may be elicited. In this chapter the patterns displayed in the state of fever will be addressed to elucidate the contribution of this response type of sympathetic innervation to the thermoregulatory vasomotor adjustments, as well as to non-thermal factors in the general defence response of the 'fever syndrome'.

---

*Corresponding author.

478

Sympathetic response during fever in anesthetized rabbits

The chain of events leading from the impact of a pyrogenic substance like a bacterial endotoxin or lipopolysaccharide (LPS) to the generation of fever is schematically indicated in Fig. 1. The exogenous pyrogen stimulates immuno-active cells, for instance macrophages, to induce a sequence of effects leading to the production of cytokines, like interleukin 1 (IL-1), interleukin 6 (IL-6), tumor necrosis factor (TNF), interferons (IFN), macrophage inflammatory protein 1 (MIP-1), which act as endogenous pyrogens (EP). Since the febrile response to EP is prevented by prior administration of cyclooxygenase inhibitors, for instance, indomethacin, it is assumed that generation of fever requires the release of prostanoids such as prostaglandin E_2 (PGE_2) as a central mediator (Hashimoto et al., 1988; Rothwell, 1992), although there are still controversies about this point (Simpson et al., 1994). On the other hand, stimulation of fever by hypothalamic application of PGE_2 corresponds to the view that this mediator directly modifies the activity of neurons in the thermoregulatory centre to induce the cold defence activities necessary to generate the febrile rise in body temperature (Iriki, 1988).

When fever is induced experimentally, LPS as the effective component of bacterial endotoxin is frequently used as exogenous pyrogen. This applies also to the following series of experiments in which the fever-induced pattern of sympathetic differentiation was analyzed. The responses of body temperature, general circulation and regional sympathetic efferents to the intravenous (i.v.) LPS administration were studied in urethane-anesthetized rabbits (1.5 g/kg intraperitoneally) and are presented in Figs. 2A,B (Saigusa, 1989; Saigusa et al., 1989). Core (rectal, T_{re}) and ear skin (T_{ear}) temperatures were measured with thermistors. Blood pressure was recorded with a transducer connected to a femoral artery catheter to determine mean arterial pressure (MAP), and heart rate (HR) was derived from the pressure pulses. Electrical activity was recorded from renal

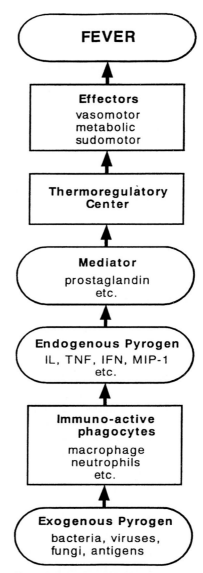

Fig. 1. Mechanism by which fever is induced by an exogenous pyrogen.

and splanchnic sympathetic nerve fibers by means of bipolar electrodes which consisted of fine multistrand silver wire and were kept in position by molding with self-curing silicone gel. The amplified electrical activity recorded from the sympathetic branch was fed into an integrating circuit, the integrator was reset at intervals of 5 s and the

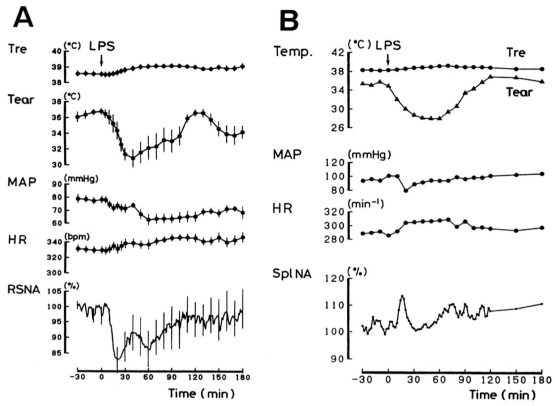

Fig. 2. Time courses of rectal temperature (T_{re}), ear skin temperature (T_{ear}), mean arterial pressure (MAP), heart rate (HR), and renal sympathetic nerve activity (RSNA) (A) or splanchnic nerve activity (SplNA) (B) from 30 min before to 180 min after i.v. injection of lipopolysaccharide (LPS). A: $n = 7$, LPS 1 μg/kg, means with standard errors, B: single experiment, LPS 100 ng/kg (A: Saigusa, 1989; B: Saigusa et al., 1989).

amplitudes were taken as the indicator for sympathetic nerve activity.

Within 10–20 min after i.v. administration of LPS (1 μg/kg), T_{re} started to rise. During the phase of rising temperature T_{ear} decreased, indicating enhanced vasoconstriction due to increased activity in sympathetic nerve fibers innervating skin vessels (SkSNA). The diagram of Fig. 2A shows that directly recorded renal sympathetic nerve activity (RSNA) was reduced. Since MAP decreased, this inhibition was not reflexly induced. On the other hand, the data of Fig. 2B show that, at the same time, splanchnic sympathetic activity (SplNA) was augmented rather than inhibited. Since this response was apparent be-

fore MAP decreased, it was not generated reflexly, although it may have been modified by the change in baroreceptor input.

As examples for the effects of EP, Figs. 3A,B shows the time courses of monophasic fever responses induced by i.v. administration of 1 μg/kg IL-1 (Fig. 3A) and of 10 μg/kg TNF-α (Fig. 3B) in rabbits anesthetized with urethane. The rise in SkSNA (inferred from the decrease of T_{ear}) was associated with the decrease in directly recorded RSNA and, thus, revealed a pattern of regional differentiation which corresponded to that induced by LPS.

The specificity of the presumed mediator function of PGE_2 in the generation of fever is docu-

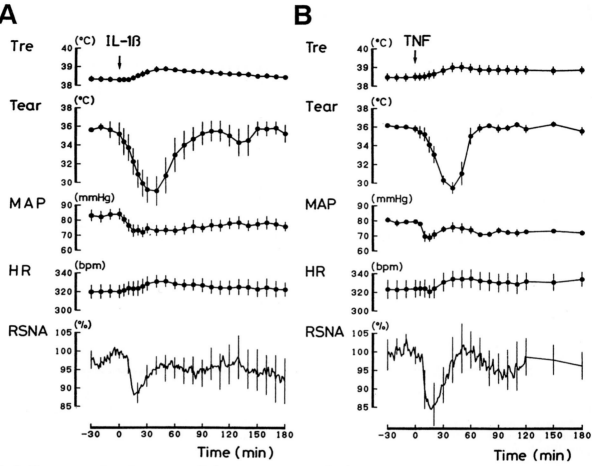

Fig. 3. Time courses of rectal temperature (T_{re}), ear skin temperature (T_{ear}), mean arterial pressure (MAP), heart rate (HR), and renal sympathetic nerve activity (RSNA) from 30 min before to 180 min after i.v. injection of interleukin 1β (A) and of tumor necrosis factor α (B). $n = 7$, means with standard errors (Saigusa, 1989).

mented by the single experiment in urethane-anesthetized rabbits shown in Figs. 4A,B. The rise in T_{re} induced by intracerebroventricular (i.c.v.) application of 8 μg/kg PGE_2 was associated with a decrease in T_{ear} indicating enhanced SkSNA and, as demonstrated directly, by a decrease in RSNA and an opposing rise in SplNA. This response pattern was identical with that during fevers induced by LPS and EP.

Table 1 summarizes in its lower part the rises in core temperature and the qualitatively identical response patterns of regional sympathetic

nerve activity during the fevers elicited in ure-thane-anesthetized rabbits by LPS, IL-1, TNF and PGE_2. In order to generate the febrile rise of T_{re} as the consequence of the presumed rise of the temperature set-point, not only skin vasoconstriction may be induced but, depending on the thermal conditions, heat production by shivering or non-shivering thermogenesis may be activated or heat loss by panting and sweating may be inhibited. Thus, the entire scope of thermoregulatory activities is available when a febrile rise of body temperature has to be produced. Therefore, as a

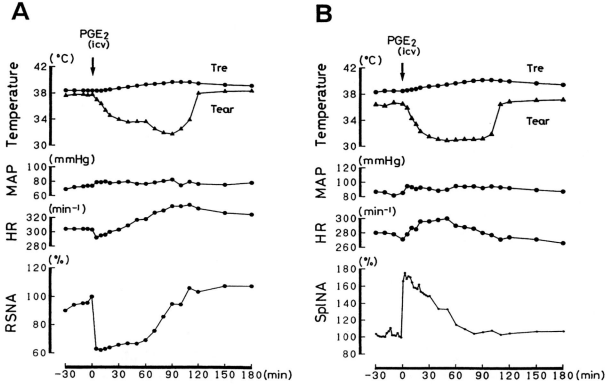

Fig. 4. Time courses of rectal temperature (T_{re}), ear skin temperature (T_{ear}), mean arterial pressure (MAP), heart rate (HR), and renal sympathetic nerve activity (RSNA) (A) and splanchnic nerve activity (SplNA) (B) during fever induced by PGE_2 8 μg/kg i.c.v. injection in one experiment (Saigusa et al., 1989).

TABLE 1

Comparison of changes in regional differentiation of sympathetic efferents during spinal cooling and fever induced by administration of lipopolysaccharide (LPS), interleukin 1 (IL1), tumor necrosis factor (TNF) and prostaglandin E_2 (PGE_2) in anesthetized rabbits

	Temperature response	Sympathetic efferents		
		Cutaneous ear	Renal	Splanchnic
Spinal cooling	ϕ	+	−	−
LPS (i.v.)	↑	+	−	+
IL1 (i.v.)	↑	+	−	
TNF (i.v.)	↑	+	−	
PGE_2 (i.c.v.)	↑	+	−	+

↑ = fever; + = Activation; − = Inhibition; ϕ = no change; i.v. = intravenous; i.c.v. = intracerebroventricular.

482

first guess, the pattern of regional sympathetic differentiation during the febrile rise in core temperature should correspond to that observed during cold exposure.

However, the single experiment of Fig. 5 shows that, unlike the febrile response, SplNA decreased rather than increased in an urethane-anesthetized rabbit, when a cold defence response was induced by cooling the thermosensors of the spinal cord. For the same cold stimulus previous studies had demonstrated that RSNA decreased as well (Iriki and Simon, 1978). Thus, the pattern of regional sympathetic differentiations during fever differs from that during cold exposure in the rise of SplNA in the former and the decrease of SplNA in the latter condition. For reasons of comparison the pattern induced by cold stimulation is included in Table 1 (upper line).

As a first conclusion to be derived from the comparison of the febrile response with the cold defence response it is stated that the patterns of cold-induced and fever-induced regional sympathetic differentiation are not identical, especially with respect to the course of SplNA. In addition, functional correlates exist which support this hypothesis. The decrease in SplNA during cold stimulation was reflected by an increase in blood flow in visceral organs innervated by the splanchnic nerve (Kullmann et al., 1970). In fever, the increase of SplNA was confirmed by recordings from functionally different portions of the splanchnic nerve among which the branches to the spleen and to the adrenals both increased their activities (Niijima et al., 1991). The response of the splenic branch would correspond to the observation of a fever-induced, adrenergic inhibition of splenic killer cell activity (Take et al., 1993), while the response of the adrenal branch would suggest enhanced catecholamine release in the state of fever.

As indicated by the term 'fever syndrome', the transient state of cold defence, due to an elevated set-point of body temperature, is only one out of a multitude of neuro-humoral processes in a complex host defence response. Fig. 6 summarizes, in

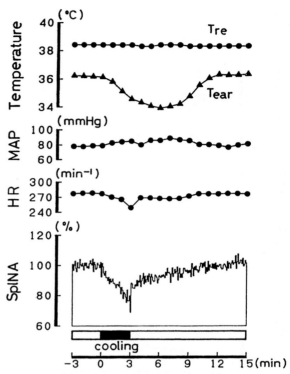

Fig. 5. Time course of rectal temperature (T_{re}), ear skin temperature (T_{ear}), mean arterial pressure (MAP), heart rate (HR) and splanchnic nerve activity (SplNA) during spinal cord cooling in one experiment (Saigusa et al., 1989).

its left part, the various cytokines identified as fever-inducing agents and, in its right part, the multifarious adjustments of endocrine systems, blood plasma composition and homeostatic regulatory functions, including the synthesis of prostaglandins among which PGE_2 functions centrally as the inducer of the febrile rise of body temperature. It is most likely that the multitude of response components leads to interferences which may also affect autonomic sympathetic control. Therefore, it is not surprising that fever-induced regional differentiation of regional sympathetic activity deviates from that observed as a component of the physiological cold defence response. It is necessary to study further, how and to what extent the sympathetic nervous system takes part in the control of host defence mecha-

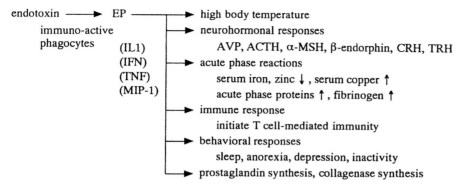

Fig. 6. Manifold responses evoked by endotoxins/EP — 'fever syndrome' (Iriki, 1988).

nisms within the scope of the 'fever syndrome', and to elucidate the functional changes induced in the various target organs.

Pattern generation in the sympathetic outflow as a physiological phenomenon

Before dealing with the most recent observations on fever-induced regional sympathetic differentiation, it seems necessary to review the scope of response patterns which were disclosed, so far, in connection with a variety of thermoregulatory as well as non-thermoregulatory activities. Originally, the concept of regional sympathetic differentiation was derived from studies on pentobarbital-anesthetized rabbits and cats in which antagonistic responses of sympathetic efferents innervating the skin and visceral organs were observed, when the spinal cord was thermally stimulated (Walther et al., 1970), and supported by the observation of corresponding antagonistic changes in regional blood flow when the same stimuli were applied to pentobarbital-anesthetized dogs (Kullmann et al., 1970). Fig. 7 presents the original data. This observation enforced a substantial correction of the hitherto favoured concept that the sympathetic nervous system rather produced 'mass actions' to the effect that recording from one sympathetic branch reflected the general state of sympathetic activity with, at most, quantitative differences in its regional expression. The same response pattern was subsequently shown to be induced by thermal stimuli of the hypothalamus and the skin (Iriki et al., 1971; Riedel et al., 1972). The state of knowledge that had been attained at the time of a first review (Iriki and Simon, 1978) is summarized in Table 2 which presents regional changes of sympathetic activity in a variety of homeostatic and non-homeostatic conditions. In addition to thermal stimuli, regional differentiation of sympathetic efferents was reported to be induced by hypoxic and hypercapnic stimulation, coronary occlusion, cutaneous, non-noxious and noxious stimulation, visceral stimulation and mental arithmetic. Baroreceptor stimulation did not induce clear-cut antagonistic regional responses but nevertheless affected skin innervation differently from that of other organs. A recent example for a quantitatively non-uniform response of regional sympathetic activities is presented by the effects of i.c.v. applications of insulin on lumbar, renal and adrenal sympathetic activities (Muntzel et al., 1994).

Important additional information was provided by studies showing that non-uniformity of sympathetic responses could be displayed by different filaments of a sympathetic branch innervating a particular organ, as demonstrated for the cardiac (Simon and Riedel, 1975) and renal (Riedel and Peter, 1977) sympathetic innervation and especially by recording single fiber activity of efferents to the hindlimb skin of the cat (Gregor et al., 1976). These findings strongly suggested a highly differentiated sympathetic control of diverse

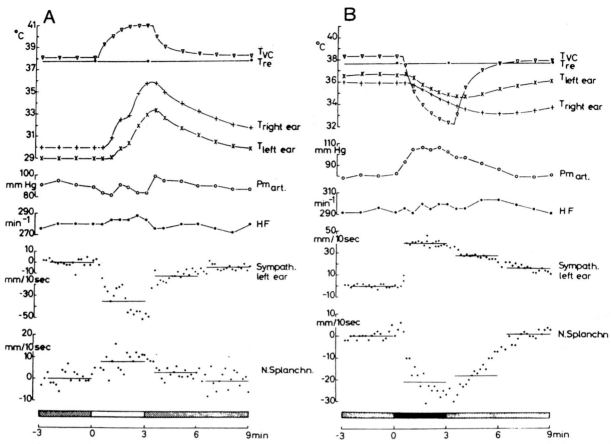

Fig. 7. Time courses of rectal temperature (T_{re}), vertebral canal temperature (T_{vc}), right and left ear temperatures ($T_{right\,ear}$, $T_{left\,ear}$), mean arterial pressure ($Pm_{art.}$), heart rate (HF), cutaneous sympathetic nerve activity (Sympath.$_{left\,ear}$), and splanchnic nerve activity (N.Splanchn.) during spinal cord warming (A white bar) and cooling (B black bar) in two (A and B) anesthetized, paralysed rabbits (Walther et al., 1970).

functions in a single organ. In the special case of skin innervation, these fibers could be identified, according to their discharge characteristics, as fibers mediating vasoconstriction or active vasodilatation. A similar observation was the reciprocal control of sudomotor and vasoconstrictor efferents in the hairless skin of the cat's paw (Jänig and Kümmel, 1981). The non-uniformity of activities in the sympathetic innervation according to their different functions as vasoconstrictor, vasodilator, sudomotor and pilomotor fibers was disclosed in detail by observing the responses to thermal, hypoxic, cutaneous noxious and non-noxious, and visceral stimuli (Jänig, 1985).

Taken together, the phenomenon of differential responses in sympathetic efferents is expressed at two levels. The first level is regional differentiation of responses in sympathetic nerve branches innervating different organs. The response patterns exhibit a high degree of variability, as shown in Table 2, and it may be expected that the variability of the patterns will become more obvious when sympathetic nerve branches to more organs will be included in the analysis. The second level of local differentiation is disclosed by recordings from different filaments, or nerve fibers, supplying a particular organ, such as the skin, and reflects selective control of different

TABLE 2

Summary of conditions in which regional differentiation of sympathetic efferents were observed, in direct recordings of nerve discharges (modified from Iriki and Simon, 1978)

Experimental conditions	Sympathetic efferents				
	Cutaneous	Splanchnic	Cardiac	Muscle	Renal
Cold stimulation (central and peripheral)	+	−	−		−
Warm stimulation (central and peripheral)	−	+	+		+
Fever	+				−
Hypoxic stimulation					
Primary tissue	−	+	+		
Mild arterial	−	+	−	+	+
Severe arterial	+	+	+	+	+
Hypercapnic stimulation	−	+	−		
Chemoreceptor stimulation	−			+	
Baroreceptor stimulation	ϕ	−	−	−	−
Atrial dilatation		ϕ	+	ϕ	−
Coronal occlusion	−	+			
Cutaneous stimulation					
Non-noxious	+(−)			−	
Noxious	−(+)			+	
Mental arithmetic	+			−	

+ = activation; − = inhibition; ϕ = no change.

organ functions. This high degree of diversity suggests that the mechanisms by which these patterns are generated may involve different levels of organization of central nervous sympathetic control.

Role of the baroreflex system

Although baroreceptor denervation was shown to modify some of the patterns of regional sympathetic innervation, others were found to remain unaffected and, thus, demonstrated that baroreflex control is not essential for the generation of sympathetic differentiation (Simon and Riedel, 1975). At least, its involvement cannot be simply concluded when a regional sympathetic response happens to change inversely to a change of arterial pressure (Grewe et al., 1995). However, the baroreceptor signals may contribute to the expression of the differential response, because they do not uniformly affect the sympathetic output. For instance, baroreflex inhibition is more pronounced in renal than splanchnic sympathetic efferents (Meckler and Weaver, 1988) or in mesenteric nerves (Stein and Weaver, 1988), whereas activity of sympathetic efferents to the skin is little affected by changes in blood pressure (Iriki et al., 1979). These results are consistent with a model of multiple routes over which baroreceptor influences are distributed to the central circuits controlling different sympathetic nerves (Gebber et al., 1994).

Alterations of the peripheral segmental input

Preliminary evidence exists that patterns observed in the sympathetic efferent innervation may be altered in chronic conditions of an altered peripheral input. For example, cats may exhibit reflex sympathetic dystrophy when a neurinoma develops after peripheral nerve dissection causing chronic pain, i.e. a chronically enhanced nociceptive input to the spinal cord. In this condition, the response patterns of functionally different nerve fibers in the efferent sympathetic innervation to the skin were altered in comparison to the intact state, when thermal and hypoxic or baroreflex stimuli were applied (Jänig, 1992). This observation indicates that the peripheral input contributes to the expression of a particular response pattern in the sympathetic efferent innervation.

Central organization of pattern generation in homeostatic regulatory activities

The involvement of different levels of central integration in pattern generation was investigated by studying anesthetized, decerebrated or spinalized rabbits (Walther et al., 1971; Iriki and Kozawa, 1976). The results are summarized in Table 3. The well-established thermally induced pattern, i.e. antagonistic changes between SkSNA on the one hand and cardiac sympathetic nerve activity (CSNA) and SplNA on the other hand, was preserved after midcollicular decerebration. For the spinalized rabbit, the thermally induced pattern shown in Table 3 was extrapolated from the experimental observation of an antagonism between SkSNA and SplNA in response to spinal cooling and the experimentally documented ability of spinalized animals to produce cold shivering as a thermoregulatory response (Kosaka et al., 1967). However, with respect to the regional sympathetic differentiation caused by chemoreceptor stimulation, the well established antagonism between reduced SkSNA and CSNA on the one hand and enhanced SplNA on the other, which was observed in intact animals as a response to arterial hypoxia, was replaced by general activation after decerebration. Not included in Table 3 are circumstantial observations in spinalized animals indicating a general rise in efferent sympathetic activity in response to mild arterial hypoxia. Thus, the hypoxia-induced sympathetic response pattern seems to require not only intact connections between the chemoreceptor input at the

medullary level and the spinal cord, but in addition also signal processing in the upper brain stem.

Spinal and medullary contributions to reflexly induced pattern generation

As a property of segmental or intersegmental reflex circuits in the control of efferent sympathetic activity, the concept of 'spinal sympathetic functional units' was proposed (Jänig, 1985). Indeed, the reflex patterns observed in chronically spinalized animals, in comparison to the patterns elicited in animals with an intact neuraxis, indicated the importance of intraspinal neuronal circuits by which these reflex patterns could be generated.

As far as the involvement of supraspinal reflex circuits is concerned, particular attention was drawn to the rostral ventrolateral medulla (RVLM). Using electrical stimuli, local chemical activation by microinjecting DL-homocysteic acid, or local chemical inhibition by microinjecting glycine, the role of the RVLM in regional sympathetic differentiation was studied. With this approach, differential actions on regional sympathetic efferents could be demonstrated for splenic and intestinal sympathetic activities (Hayes and Weaver, 1990), for splenic and mesenteric sympathetic activities (Yardley et al., 1989), for sympathetic innervation of the kidney and the vasculature of the skeletal muscle vasculature (Dean et al., 1992), and for the activities of sympathetic efferents to the kidney, muscle and visceral organs (McAllen and May, 1994). Since the sites from which the three different responses could be driven overlapped but showed clear differences, a topographical separation of the different populations of neurons was concluded (Dampney and McAllen, 1988; McAllen and May, 1994), whereas the quantitatively different responses of renal and splanchnic nerves did not indicate a viscerotopic organization at the medullary level (Beluli and Weaver, 1991). Interestingly, stimuli in the ventrolateral medulla provided evidence for a topographical organization of sites controlling skin

TABLE 3

The pattern of regional differentiation of sympathetic efferents induced by thermal and hypoxic stimuli in intact, decerebrated, and spinalized rabbits (Iriki and Nagai, 1981)

			Sympathetic efferents		
			Cutaneous ear	Cardiac	Splanchnic
Intact	Spinal cord	Warming	−	+	+
		Cooling	+	−	−
	Arterial	Hypoxia	−	−	+
Decereb.	Spinal cord	Warming	−	+	+
		Cooling	+	−	−
	Arterial	Hypoxia	+	+	+
Spinalized	Spinal cord	Warming	−[a]	+	+[a]
		Cooling	+[a]	−[a]	−[a]

+ = increase; − = decrease. [a] From indirect experiments.

vasoconstriction which might be relevant for regional vasomotor control of vascular beds in thermoregulation (Key and Wigfield, 1994).

Taken together, the analysis of spinal and medullary relay stations in central sympathetic control suggests the existence of control circuits by which certain patterns of regional differentiation of efferent activity may be generated. The degrees to which these networks contribute to the fully expressed sympathetic response patterns elicited by the various homeostatic or non-homeostatic control activities, remain to be elucidated.

Role of putative mediators in sympathetic differentiation during fever

Since body temperature is the resultant of a multitude of metabolic, vasomotor and behavioural states of activity, it is not surprising that it is affected by a host of putative transmitters and mediators injected either centrally or systemically. For various compounds with putative mediator functions, such as somatostatin, some of the endogenous opioids, bradykinin, and thyrotropin releasing hormone (TRH), hyperthermic effects of central applications have been documented.

However, as one consequence of the complexity of underlying mechanisms, these effects have never been fully consistent (Clark and Lipton, 1985). Our own current work to approach this problem with special respect to the generation of fever has, so far, considered the role of PGE_2 as the best documented central mediator of the febrile response and TRH as a genuine neuropeptide with a well-documented hyperthermic action in rabbits, when centrally applied.

For PGE_2, the available evidence suggests that it is not involved in the stimulation of various systemic humoral adjustments which constitute the 'fever syndrome', such as the increases in plasma concentration of Cu and of N-acetylneuraminic acid (NANA) which are typical for the 'acute phase reaction' induced, for instance, by LPS as an established exogenous pyrogen (Blatteis et al., 1984). However, this does not compromise the well-established role of PGE_2 as the central mediator of the thermal febrile response. While it is clear that PGE_2 also induced the differential sympathetic response by which the effects of established exogenous and endogenous pyrogens are characterized, some uncertainties exist about possible differences in the sites of action from where the hyperthermic and the sympathetic responses originate. This question was studied by applying intracephalic microinjections of 500 ng PGE_2 in anesthetized rabbits. T_{re} was recorded to determine the appearance of fever. The regional sympathetic responses were assessed indirectly for the skin by observing the course of T_{ear} and directly for RSNA by recording its electrical activity.

Fig. 8 shows the effects of an intracephalic PGE_2 injection applied at the site indicated by the inset figure. Rectal temperature increased significantly and the typical response of an increase in SkSNA and a decrease of RSNA was observed (Huang, 1993).

Microinjections of PGE_2 were performed at 50 sites in the ventral portions of the diencephalon. A febrile response was assumed when T_{re} rose by 0.3°C or more within 1 h after injection. By this criterion 13 out of 50 injections sites effectively mediated fever. Their location is shown in Fig. 9. The effective sites were located in the rostral hypothalamus and preoptic area. The same injections also elicited the typical regional sympathetic differentiation (Huang, 1993). Thus, the febrile rise of core temperature and the appearance of regional sympathetic differentiation following circumscribed intrahypothalamic applications of PGE_2 in the vicinity of the supraoptic nucleus exhibited a close spatial relationship which supports the view of PGE_2 as a physiological mediator for those fever response components which are associated with the rise in core temperature.

TRH was i.c.v. injected in anesthetized rabbits in a dose of 10 μg/kg in order to see which kind of regional sympathetic response was associated with its known hyperthermic effect (Huang et al., 1992). It is clear from Fig. 10 that central TRH application had the expected hyperthermic effect, causing a long-lasting rise of T_{re}. However, the course of T_{ear} indicated an only short-lasting rise in SkSNA which was accompanied by a short-lasting rise in RSNA. In addition, respiratory rate rose rather than fell, as it would be expected for a concerted cold defence response. Thus, typical sympathetic differentiation is missing in the hyperthermic action of TRH.

Taken together the analysis of two putative mediators confirmed the central nervous mediator function of PGE_2 for those aspects of the 'fever syndrome' which are associated with the rise in core temperature and the underlying thermoregulatory activities, including the control of regional sympathetic activity. For TRH, such a general central mediator function does not seem to exist. Nevertheless, this neuropeptide may function as a mediator controlling certain components of a cold defence or fever response, for instance, metabolic activation.

Role of anesthesia in the generation of differential sympathetic response patterns

Anesthesia is known to interfere with temperature regulation and, consequently, it may also affect the actions of pyrogens on the regulation of body temperature in general and the generation of regionally differentiated sympathetic response patterns in particular. However, regional sympathetic differentiation in the course of fever was studied mostly in anesthetized animals because of the difficulties associated with the recordings of regional sympathetic activity in conscious animals. This difficulty was overcome by preparing animals with a chronically implanted device to record RSNA. In studies on rabbits a bipolar stainless steel electrode was connected to the renal sympathetic nerve 5–10 days prior to the experiments. With T_{ear} as an indirect indicator for the degree of sympathetic vasoconstrictor activity in the skin, it was possible to study effects of pyrogens on regional sympathetic differentiation in the state of consciousness (Ohashi and Saigusa, 1997).

Fig. 11 summarizes the results of three series of experiments in which LPS, IL-1β and TNF-α were applied i.v. as pyrogens. According to the left-hand diagram, LPS at a dose of 1 μg/kg induced a long-lasting rise of T_{re} with a tendency for a biphasic fever response. The decrease of T_{ear} indicated an early phase of enhanced SkSNA. At the same time RSNA increased, unlike the response of anesthetized rabbits. Although MAP

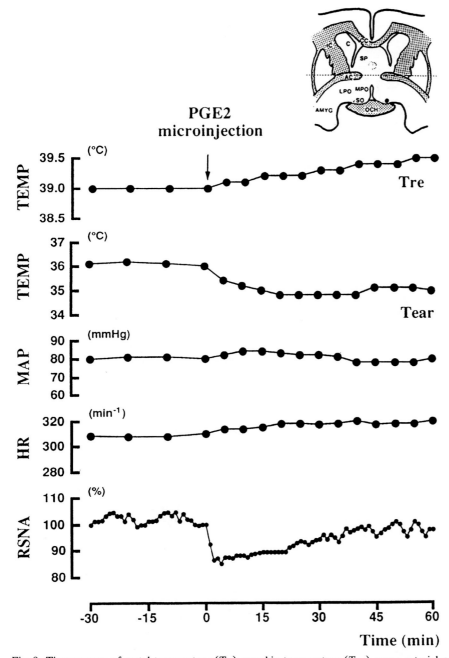

Fig. 8. Time courses of rectal temperature (T_{re}), ear skin temperature (T_{ear}), mean arterial pressure (MAP), heart rate (HR), and renal sympathetic nerve activity (RSNA) during fever induced by microinjection of PGE_2 500 ng (indicated by an arrow). The site of microinjection was histologically identified and is indicated as a small black dot on the right side immediately dorsal to the optic chiasma (OCH) (Huang, 1993).

490

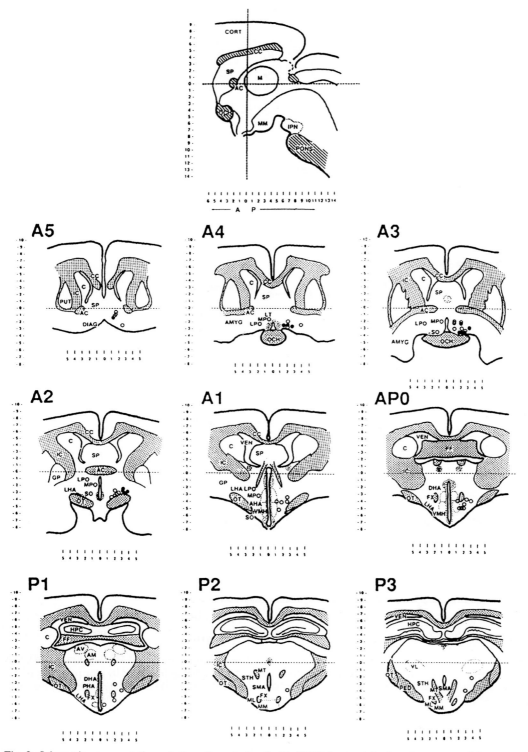

Fig. 9. Schematic representation of sites of prostaglandin E_2 (PGE_2)-microinjection shown on serial cross sections of the rabbit brain according to the stereotaxic coordinates by Sawyer et al. Closed circles (●) show the loci where PGE_2 caused an increase in body temperature of more than 0.3°C, and open circles (○) show the loci where PGE_2 was not effective. LHA, lateral hypothalamic area; LPO, lateral preoptic area; MPO, medial preoptic area; SO, supraoptic nucleus (Huang, 1993).

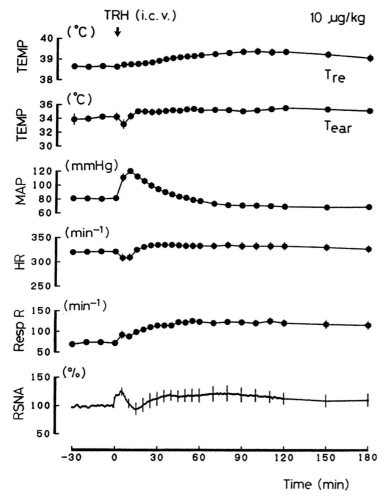

Fig. 10. Time courses of rectal temperature (T_{re}), ear skin temperature (T_{ear}), mean arterial pressure (MAP), heart rate (HR), respiratory rate (Resp R), and renal sympathetic nerve activity (RSNA) in urethane-anesthetized rabbits from 30 min before to 180 min after i.c.v. injection of TRH 10 μg/kg $n = 5$, means with standard errors (Huang et al., 1992).

decreased, the increase in RSNA could not be entirely explained by a baroreflex release, because RSNA began to rise before MAP started to decrease. The rise of RSNA was also observed in fever elicited by a lower dose of 500 ng/kg LPS which did not induce a decrease in MAP (Ohashi and Saigusa, 1997).

As shown by the middle diagram, a dose of 100 ng/kg IL-1β administered i.v. induced a fever very similar to that following LPS. The rise in SkSNA, as indicated by the decrease in T_{ear}, was accompanied by a rise in RSNA which was clearly

not attributable to a baroreflex release, because MAP rose rather than fell in this condition.

The right-hand diagram shows the response to 10 μg/kg TNF-α which displayed a rapid and early rise in T_{re} followed by partial defervescence and a sustained phase of moderately elevated T_{re}. The course of T_{ear} indicated an early activation of SkSNA which was concomitant with the early fever response and a rise in RSNA for which, again, the course of MAP excluded baroreflex release as a cause.

According to the three series of experiments in

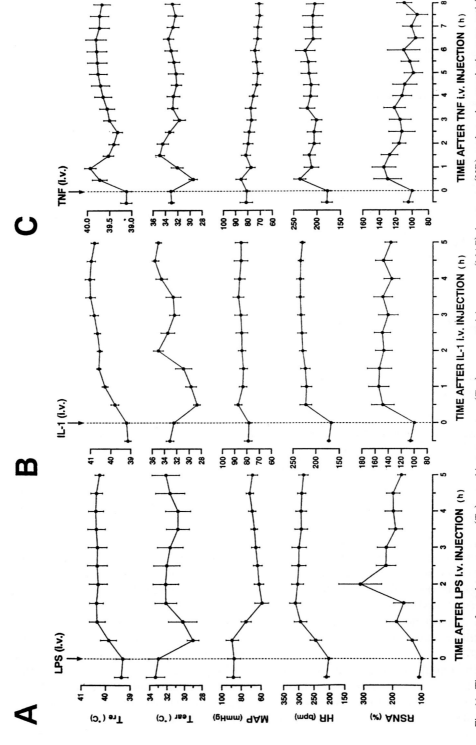

Fig. 11. Time courses of rectal temperature (T_{re}), ear skin temperature (T_{ear}), mean arterial pressure (MAP), heart rate (HR), and renal sympathetic nerve activity (RSNA) in conscious rabbits after i.v. injection of lipopolysaccharide (LPS) 1 μg/kg (A), interleukin 1β (IL-1β) 100 ng/kg (B), and tumor necrosis factor α (TNF-α) 10 μg/kg (C). n = 6, means with standard errors (modified from Ohashi and Saigusa, 1997).

Fig. 11, the antagonism in the reactions of SkSNA and RSNA observed at the start of the fever response in anesthetized rabbits was not found in the conscious animals. This finding differs, in part, from the results of an earlier study in conscious rabbits which received a dose of 4 μg/kg LPS. While in this study the onset of fever was accompanied by an initial decrease in RSNA, this response changed into a subsequent, long-lasting increase starting 60 min after the injection of LPS (Riedel et al., 1982). There are, however, differences in the experimental arrangements between this previous and the present study. The batch of LPS used in the recent studies (Ohashi and Saigusa, 1997) seemed more potent and may have displayed a different spectrum of thermal and non-thermal effects in the generation of the fever. Further, the recovery time after the implantation of the recording electrode was 3–5 days in the earlier experiments but 5–10 days in the recent studies which might imply an improved condition of the animals. On the other hand, the course of RSNA in the earlier study (Riedel et al., 1982) was ascertained by a corresponding course of renal blood flow which had been determined in parallel experiments by electromagnetic flowmetry. Further, Fig. 12 shows that peripheral cooling applied in this study elicited antagonistic changes of SkSNA and RSNA as they are typical for thermally induced responses. As an important factor modulating regional sympathetic responses, the ambient thermal condition has to be taken into consideration. The recent study (Ohashi and Saigusa, 1997) was carried out at a thermoneutral (25°C) ambient temperature. The previous analysis of sympathetic differentiation under the influence of LPS (Riedel et al., 1982) was carried out in warm ambient conditions (32°C) in which heat loss mechanisms were activated to some degree. Warm ambient conditions may have prevented shivering as a cold defence response in the early phase of fever. It was previously shown that the onset of shivering in response to cold stimulation and the resulting demand for an increase in muscle blood flow could overrule the original response pattern of the sympathetic nervous sys-

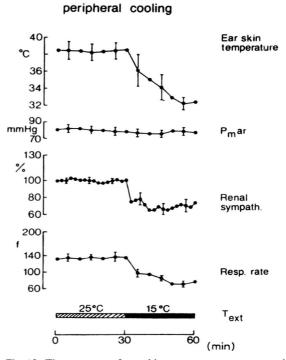

Fig. 12. Time courses of ear skin temperature, mean arterial pressure ($P_m$ar), renal sympathetic nerve activity (Renal sympath.) and respiratory rate (Resp. rate) before and after peripheral cooling (ambient temperature change from 25°C to 15°C) in conscious rabbits. $n = 11$, means with standard errors (Riedel et al., 1982).

tem (Kullmann et al., 1970). Taken together, apparent differences in the expression of fever-induced regional sympathetic responses under different experimental conditions, while not readily explainable, may be taken as evidence for the complexity of pattern generation in the sympathetic response to fever, or to other physiological and pathophysiological stimuli, as the consequence of interactions of a multitude of effector activities.

The involvement of PGE_2 as a key mediator in fever generation of conscious rabbits was investigated by blocking its synthesis with the cyclooxygenase inhibitor indomethacin, of which a dose of 20 mg/kg was administered subcutaneously (s.c.) 30 min before the i.v. injection of IL-1β at a dose

494

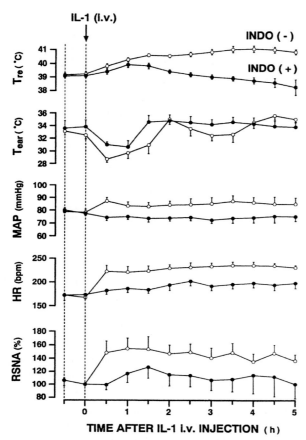

IL-1 (I.v.)

INDO (-)

INDO (+)

TIME AFTER IL-1 i.v. INJECTION (h)

Fig. 13. Effects of pretreatment with subcutaneous injection of indomethacin (INDO) 20 mg/kg on the changes of rectal temperature (T_{re}), ear skin temperature (T_{ear}), mean arterial pressure (MAP), heart rate (HR) and renal sympathetic nerve activity (RSNA) induced by i.v. administration of recombinant rabbit interleukin 1β (IL-1β) 100 ng/kg in conscious rabbits. INDO was injected 30 min before IL-1β injection (closed circles). The original responses induced by IL-1β without INDO-pretreatment (Fig. 11B) have been superimposed (open circles). $n = 6$, means with standard errors (modified from Ohashi and Saigusa, 1997).

of 100 ng/kg (Ohashi and Saigusa, 1997). As shown by Fig. 13, this sequence of treatments did not completely prevent the onset of the fever response, while its duration was clearly diminished. The partial fever suppression was in accordance with a previous study (Hashimoto et al., 1988) and with the general observation that the

degree of fever suppression depends on the dose and route of administration (Watanabe, 1992). However, Fig. 13 indicates that even partial suppression of fever by indomethacin, while still associated with an initial increase in SkSNA, prevented any significant change of RSNA during fever.

As a summary, Table 4 compares the data obtained from the studies in conscious rabbits, especially the effect of a cold stimulus with that of LPS, IL-1 and TNF on SkSNA and RSNA. While the antagonism between the activities of these two nerve branches was typical for the response to cold stimulation of conscious as well as anesthetized rabbits, the same antagonism was seen during fever in anesthetized rabbits but had disappeared in febrile, conscious rabbits.

Conclusions

In the assessment of the phenomenon of regional sympathetic differentiation, the use of anesthesia as an experimental tool is being replaced by procedures in which animals are equipped with chronically implanted recording electrodes. In this way it is attempted to sort out modulations of sympathetic activity by the anesthetics themselves. Reconfirmation or correction of data on sympathetic differentiation described previously, will require numerous future studies. However, some evidence is already available to discuss interactions of anesthetics with sympathetic control.

Sympathetic activity may be suppressed by some anesthetics, but their actions are not homogeneous in this respect. For example, pentobarbital or chloralose differentially affect sympathetic outflows to different organs such as the heart, kidney and adrenal gland (Matsukawa et al., 1993), CSNA was decreased by both anesthetics, while RSNA was decreased by pentobarbital but increased by chloralose. In studies on sympathetic activity, urethane or urethane-chloralose were frequently used under the premise that their influence was a minor one.

A number of studies exist on conscious cats

with chronically implanted recording electrodes in which the responses of regional sympathetic activity to various stimuli, such as blood pressure changes (Ninomiya et al., 1988), coronary occlusion (Ninomiya et al., 1986) and static exercise (Matsukawa et al., 1991) were analyzed. The data indicated for CSNA and RSNA that response generation involved descending inputs from higher brain centres rather than only simple feedback loops triggered by peripheral receptors. The degree of differentiation displayed by multiple, functionally different sympathetic efferents remains to be determined.

Thermoregulatory responses may also be depressed or distorted by anesthetics as the consequence of a decrease of threshold temperature for cold defence, an increase of threshold temperature for heat defence and generally reduced sensitivities of the effector responses. For humans, decreased threshold temperatures and sensitivities of cutaneous vasoconstriction, nonshivering thermogenesis and shivering were recently reported (Sessler, 1994), but these changes were only quantitative and not qualitative ones. Paradoxical effects of thermal stimuli on thermoregulatory effectors as a consequence of anesthesia, however, may also occur (Martin et al., 1977).

In the 'fever syndrome', as summarized in Fig. 6, the activation of cold defence activities at normal body temperature is only one out of many aspects of the general defence response in which the sympathetic nervous system plays various important roles. Therefore, the mechanisms to develop the pattern of responses of sympathetic efferents necessarily includes factors that are not relevant for thermoregulatory adjustments as such. With special respect to fever, the recently observed discrepancy between the results obtained with and without anesthesic indicates that there are at least two mechanisms contributing to the pyrogen-induced modulation of the sympathetic efferents which seem to be impaired by anesthesia to different degrees. Urethane is known to suppress preferentially the responses produced by polysynaptic, integrated neuronal networks, while autonomic reflex functions are much better preserved. Therefore, the presented results imply that the typical sympathetic response pattern to cold stimulation, which seems to be little affected by anesthesia, may be generated by a less complex neuronal network. Under this premise, visceral sympathetic activation, which is not seen in physiological cold defence responses, may require a more complex neuronal network, involving higher central nervous centres, because it is at least partially suppressed during fever of anesthetized animals. This working hypothesis has to be taken into consideration in the future work on the elucidation of regional sympathetic contributions to the generation of the 'fever syndrome'.

TABLE 4

Comparison of changes in regional differentiation of sympathetic efferents during spinal cooling and fever induced by administration of lipopolysaccharide (LPS), interleukin 1 (IL1), and tumor necrosis factor (TNF) in conscious rabbits

	Temperature response	Sympathetic efferents	
		Cutaneous ear	Renal
Spinal cooling	ϕ	+	−
LPS (i.v.)	↑	+	+
IL1 (i.v.)	↑	+	+
TNF (i.v.)	↑	+	+

↑ = fever; + = Activation; − = Inhibition; ϕ = no change; i.v. = intravenous.

496

Acknowledgement

We would like to express our gratitude to Professor E. Simon, Kerckhoff-Institut in Bad Nauheim, for his critical reading of the manuscript and valuable suggestions.

References

Anonymous (1987) Glossary of terms for thermal physiology — Second edition. *Pflüg. Arch.*, 410: 567–587.

Beluli, D.J. and Weaver, L.C. (1991) Differential control of renal and splenic nerves without medullary topography. *Am. J. Physiol.*, 260: H1072–H1079.

Blatteis, C.M., Hunter, W.S., Llanos-Q, J., Ahokas, R.A. and Mashburn, T.A. Jr. (1984) Activation of acute-phase responses by intrapreoptic injections of endogenous pyrogen in guinea pigs. *Brain Res. Bull.*, 12: 689–695.

Clark, W.G. and Lipton, J.M. (1985) Changes in body temperature after administration of amino acids, peptides, dopamine, neuroleptics and related agents: II. *Neurosci. Biobehav. Rev.*, 9: 299–371.

Dampney, R.A.L. and McAllen, R.M. (1988) Differential control of sympathetic fibres supplying hindlimb skin and muscle by subretrofacial neurones in the cat. *J. Physiol.*, 395: 41–56.

Dean, C., Seagard, J.L., Hopp, F.A. and Kampine, J.P. (1992) Differential control of sympathetic activity to kidney and skeletal muscle by ventral medullary neurons. *J. Auton. Nerv. Syst.*, 37: 1–10.

Gebber, G.L., Zhong, S., Barman, S.M. and Orer, H.S. (1994) Coordination of the cardiac-related discharges of sympathetic nerves with different targets. *Am. J. Physiol.*, 267: R400–R407.

Gregor, M., Jänig, W. and Riedel, W. (1976) Response pattern of cutaneous postganglionic neurones to the hindlimb on spinal cord heating and cooling in the cat. *Pflüg. Arch.*, 363: 135–140.

Grewe, W., Jänig, W. and Kümmel, H. (1995) Effects of hypothalamic thermal stimulations on sympathetic neurones innervating skin and skeletal muscle of the cat hindlimb. *J. Physiol., 488: 139–152.*

Hashimoto, M., Bando, T., Iriki, M. and Hashimoto, K. (1988) Effect of indomethacin on febrile response to recombinant human interleukin 1-α in rabbits. Am. J. Physiol., 255: R527–533.

Hayes, K. and Weaver, L.C. (1990) Selective control of sympathetic pathways to the kidney, spleen and intestine by the ventrolateral medulla in rats. *J. Physiol.*, 428: 371–385.

Huang, X.-C. (1993) Effects of hypothalamic microinjection of PGE_2 on body temperature and sympathetic nervous activities in the rabbit. *Int. J. Biometeorol.*, 37: 222–228.

Huang, X.-C., Saigusa, T. and Iriki, M. (1992) Comparison of TRH and its analog (NS-3) in thermoregulatory and cardiovascular effects. *Peptides*, 13: 305–311.

Iriki, M. (1988) Fever and fever syndrome — Current problems. *Jpn. J. Physiol.*, 38: 233–250.

Iriki, M. and Kozawa, E. (1976) Patterns of differentiation in various sympathetic efferents induced by hypoxic and by central thermal stimulation in decerebrated rabbits. *Pflüg. Arch.*, 362: 101–108.

Iriki, M., Kozawa, E., Korner, P.I. and Dorward, P.K. (1979) Arterial and cardiopulmonary baroreceptor and chemoreceptor influences and interactions on ear sympathetic nerve discharge in the rabbit. *Jpn. J. Physiol.*, 29: 551–558.

Iriki, M. and Nagai, M. (1981) Peripheral effector mechanism of temperature regulation — Regulation by vascular activities. In: Z. Szelényi and M. Székely (Eds.), *Advances in Physiological Sciences*, Vol. 32, Contributions to Thermal Physiology, Pergamon, Oxford, pp. 365–374.

Iriki, M., Riedel, W. and Simon, E. (1971) Regional differentiation of sympathetic activity during hypothalamic heating and cooling in anaesthetized rabbits. *Pflüg. Arch.*, 328: 320–331.

Iriki, M. and Simon, E. (1978) Regional differentiation of sympathetic efferents. In: M. Itoh (Ed.), *Integrative Control Functions of the Brain, I*, Kodansha, Tokyo, pp. 221–238.

Jänig, W. (1985) Organization of the lumbar sympathetic outflow to skeletal muscle and skin of the cat hindlimb and tail. *Rev. Physiol. Biochem. Pharmacol.*, 102: 119–213.

Jänig, W. (1992) Pathophysiological mechanisms operating in reflex sympathetic dystrophy. In: F. Sicuteri (Ed.), *Advances in Pain Research and Therapy*, Vol. 20, Raven Press, New York, pp. 111–127.

Jänig, W. and Kümmel, H. (1981) Organization of the sympathetic innervation supplying the hairless skin of the cat's paw. *J. Auton. Nerv. Syst.*, 3: 215–230.

Key, B.J. and Wigfield, C.C. (1994) The influence of the ventrolateral medulla on thermoregulatory circulations in the rat. *J. Auton. Nerv. Syst.*, 48: 79–89.

Kosaka, M., Simon, E. and Thauer, R. (1967) Shivering in intact and spinal rabbits during spinal cord cooling. *Experientia*, 23: 385–387.

Kullmann, R., Schönung, W. and Simon, E. (1970) Antagonistic changes of blood flow and sympathetic activity in different vascular beds following central thermal stimulation. I. Blood flow in skin, muscle and intestine during spinal cord heating and cooling in anesthetized dogs. *Pflüg. Arch.*, 319: 146–161.

Martin, H., Göbel, D. and Simon, E. (1977) Vasodilatator vs.. vasoconstrictor responses in the skin to cooling hypothalamus of anaesthetized dogs. *J. Therm. Biol.*, 2: 49–51.

Matsukawa, K., Ninomiya, I. and Nishiura, N. (1993) Effects of anesthesia on cardiac and renal sympathetic nerve activities and plasma catecholamines. *Am. J. Physiol.*, 265: R792–R797.

Matsukawa, K., Mitchell, J.H., Wall, P.T. and Wilson, L.B. (1991) The effect of static exercise on renal sympathetic nerve activity in conscious cats. *J. Physiol.*, 434: 453–467.

McAllen, R.M. and May, C.N. (1994) Differential drives from rostral ventrolateral medullary neurons to three identified sympathetic outflows. *Am. J. Physiol.*, 267: R935–R944.

Meckler, R.L. and Weaver, L.C. (1988) Characteristics of ongoing and reflex discharge of single splenic and renal sympathetic postganglionic fibres in cats. *J. Physiol.*, 396: 139–153.

Muntzel, M.S., Morgan, D.A., Mark, A.L. and Johnton, A.K. (1994) Intracerebroventricular insulin produces nonuniform regional increases in sympathetic nerve activity. *Am. J. Physiol.*, 267: R1350–R1355.

Niijima, A., Hori, T., Aou, S. and Oomura, Y. (1991) The effects of interleukin-1 β on the activity of adrenal, splenic and renal sympathetic nerves in the rat. *J. Auton. Nerv. Syst.*, 36: 183–192.

Ninomiya, I., Matsukawa, K., Honda, T., Nishiura, N. and Shirai, M. (1986) Cardiac sympathetic nerve activity and heart rate during coronary occlusion in awake cats. *Am. J. Physiol.*, 251: H528–H537.

Ninomiya, I., Matsukawa, K. and Nishiura, N. (1988) Central and baroreflex control of sympathetic nerve activity to the heart and kidney in a daily life of the cat. *Clin. Exp. Hypertens. Theory Pract.*, A10 (Suppl. 1): 19–31.

Ohashi, K. and Saigusa, T. (1997) Sympathetic nervous responses during cytokine-induced fever in conscious rabbits. *Pflüg. Arch.*, 433: 691–698.

Riedel, W., Iriki, M. and Simon, E. (1972) Regional differentiation of sympathetic activity during peripheral heating and cooling in anesthetized rabbits. *Pflüg. Arch.*, 332: 239–247.

Riedel, W., Kozawa, E. and Iriki, M. (1982) Renal and cutaneous vasomotor and respiratory rate adjustments to peripheral cold and warm stimulations and to bacterial endotoxin in conscious rabbits. *J. Auton. Nerv. Syst.*, 5: 177–194.

Riedel, W. and Peter, W. (1977) Non-uniformity of regional vasomotor activity indicating the existence of 2 different systems in the sympathetic cardiovascular outflow. *Experientia*, 33: 337–338.

Rothwell, N.J. (1992) Eicosanoids, thermogenesis and thermoregulation. *Prostaglandins Leukotrienes Essent. Fatty Acids*, 46: 1–7.

Saigusa, T. (1989) Participation of interleukin-1 and tumor necrosis factor in the responses of the sympathetic nervous system during lipopolysaccharide-induced fever. *Pflüg. Arch.*, 416: 225–229.

Saigusa, T., Huang, X.-C. and Iriki, M. (1989) Regional differentiation of sympathetic nerve activity during spinal cord cooling and fever caused by LPS and PGE$_2$. In: P. Lomax and E. Schönbaum (Eds.), *Thermoregulation: Research and Clinical Applications*, Karger, Basel, pp. 91–94.

Sessler, D.I. (1994) Thermoregulation and heat balance: General anesthesia. In: E. Zeisberger, E. Schönbaum and P. Lomax (Eds.), *Thermal Balance in Health and Disease*, Birkhäuser, Basel, pp. 251–265.

Simon, E. and Riedel, W. (1975) Diversity of regional sympathetic outflow in integrative cardiovascular control; Patterns and mechanisms. *Brain Res.*, 87: 323–333.

Simpson, C.W., Ruwe, W.D. and Myers, R.D. (1994) Prostaglandins and hypothalamic neurotransmitter receptors involved in hyperthermia; a critical evaluation. *Neurosci. Biobehav. Rev.*, 18: 1–20.

Stein, R.D. and Weaver, L.C. (1988) Multi- and single-fibre mesenteric and renal sympathetic responses to chemical stimulation of intestinal receptors in cats. *J. Physiol.*, 396: 155–172.

Take, S., Mori, T., Katafuchi, T. and Hori, T. (1993) Central interferon-α inhibits natural killer cytotoxicity through sympathetic innervation. *Am. J. Physiol.*, 265: R453–R459.

Walther, O.-E., Iriki, M. and Simon, E. (1970) Antagonistic changes of blood flow and sympathetic activity in different vascular beds following central thermal stimulation. II. Cutaneous and visceral sympathetic activity during spinal cord heating and cooling in anesthetized rabbits and cats. *Pflüg. Arch.*, 319: 162–184.

Walther, O.-E., Riedel, W., Iriki, M. and Simon, E. (1971) Differentiation of sympathetic activity at the spinal level in response to central cold stimulation. *Pflüg. Arch.*, 329: 220–230.

Watanabe, M. (1992) Characteristics of TNFα- and TNFβ-induced fever in the rabbit. *Jpn. J. Physiol.*, 42: 101–116.

Yardley, C.P., Stein, R.D. and Weaver, L.C. (1989) Tonic influences from the rostral medulla affect sympathetic nerves differentially. *Am. J. Physiol.*, 256: R323–R331.

H.S. Sharma and J. Westman (Eds.)
Progress in Brain Research, Vol 115

CHAPTER 24

Thermoregulation and body fluid in hot environment

Taketoshi Morimoto*, Toshiyuki Itoh and Akira Takamata

Department of Physiology, Kyoto Prefectural University of Medicine, Kamigyo-ku, Kyoto 602, Japan

Introduction

The physiological responses to a heat load in homeothermic animals include cutaneous vasodilation to transfer heat from the body core to the body surface by circulation and evaporative heat loss from the body surface. The redistribution of blood to the skin to dissipate body heat causes a lowering of central venous pressure, and evaporative heat loss leads to dehydration. Both of these thermoregulatory responses have important effects on cardiovascular function and body fluid homeostasis and, inversely, dehydration and heat-induced changes in circulatory function limit thermoregulatory responses.

Body fluid homeostasis has particular significance in mammals because water is the most abundant component in their body, comprising about 50–70% of body weight. The importance of water comes not only from its amount in the body but also from its physicochemical characteristics, which are very different from other solvents. Its high specific heat, high thermal conductivity, and high latent heat of evaporation are crucial to maintain body temperature homeostasis. In addition, its power as a solvent, its high dielectric constant and related ionizing potential, and its

high surface tension provide the constant internal environment necessary to maintain cellular function and cell integrity.

In this review we explore the effect of thermoregulatory responses on body fluid and circulation. Modifications of thermoregulatory control induced by dehydration are discussed in regard to the influence of hyperosmolality and hypovolemia. We also deal with the effect of hyperosmolality and hypovolemia on hypothalamic thermoregulatory mechanisms and the competition between body temperature, cardiovascular and body fluid homeostasis.

Effect of heat load on body fluid

The total body water (TBW) is divided by cell membrane into intracellular fluid (ICF) and extracellular fluid (ECF) compartments. ICF ($\sim$ 45% of body weight) sustains cell integrity and cell function, and ECF ($\sim$ 20% of body weight) provides the constant internal environment necessary to support cell function. ECF is further subdivided into interstitial fluid (ISF, $\sim$ 15% of body weight) and plasma (PV, $\sim$ 5% of body weight) by capillary endothelium. The circulation of plasma induces convective heat transfer within the body.

Because sweat is a hypotonic solution compared to plasma, thermal sweating causes elevation of body fluid osmolality, which in turn causes

---

*Corresponding author. Tel: +81 75 2515310; fax: +81 75 2510295; e-mail: morimoto@phys.kpu-m.ac.jp

a fluid shift between fluid compartments. Figure 1 shows the reduction in body fluid due to sweating and the distribution of these body fluid loss, measured in eight men after 2 h exercise in heat and after 3 h recovery without fluid replacement (Morimoto et al., 1981). With the 2 h exercise in hot environment, subjects lost about 27 ml/kg body weight, and 26% of this loss (7.1 ml/kg) came from plasma. There was further reduction in body weight during the 3 h of recovery period due to residual sweating and urine output. Although the subjects consumed no water, the reduction of PV recovered to 8% (2.7 ml/kg) after 3 h of recovery. However, loss of ICF volume increased from 20% to 44% (6.1 to 14.8 ml/kg), which indicates a mobilization of ICF into the compartments of ISF and plasma.

To further quantitate water loss from each body fluid compartment and to assess the difference in the buffering capacity of organs to thermal dehydration, dehydration amounting to about 10% of body weight was loaded to adult male rats by exposing them to a hot, dry environment (DBT 36°C, RH 20%) over 6–8 h (Nose et al., 1983). The TBW, ECF, and PV volumes were determined both for individual tissue and the whole

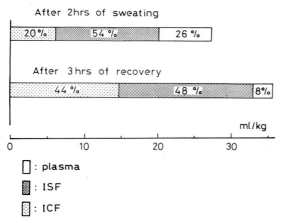

Fig. 1. Loss of body weight in eight subjects due to sweating, and reduction in body fluid compartments. Values were obtained after 2 h of sweating with exercise in hot environment, and after 3 h of recovery with no drinking. Based on data from Morimoto et al. (1981).

body by using the constant dry weight method as well as ^{51}Cr-EDTA and ^{125}I-RIHSA dilution methods, and ISF volume was calculated as the difference between TBW and ECF. As shown in Fig. 2, TBW decreased by 10%. This reduction largely came from ICF and ISF: 46% from ICF, 48% from ISF, and only 5% from PV. As for the water loss from organs, the major portion of the water loss during the thermal dehydration in rats occurred in muscle (40%) and skin (30%). In addition, the water content in brain tissue was maintained at a fairly constant level without significant change from the control value. These results indicate that, under heat-induced dehydration, both ECF and ICF of muscle and skin play an important role in compensating water loss and in maintaining brain circulation.

The mechanism of the fluid shift from ICF to ECF is accounted for by the elevated osmolality of ECF due to dehydration. However, the mechanism responsible for fluid shift from ISF to the intravascular spaces within ECF has not yet been clarified. Fluid movement across the capillary endothelium is determined by the difference between hydrostatic and colloid osmotic pressures in the capillary and ISF spaces (the so-called Starling force). Senay (1970) measured changes in blood osmolality, plasma protein, and hematocrit in heat-exposed humans and, as a mechanism for the maintenance of blood volume under heat stress, he postulated an inflow of extravascular protein from the cutaneous tissue space into the vascular space with an increase of lymph flow, based on an observed increase in plasma protein content.

In his experiment, however, heat loading was induced by exercise in hot environment. The effects of exercise and heat stress to the increase of plasma protein content were differentiated by us (Morimoto et al., 1979), and our data indicated that the rate of transfer of subcutaneous protein into the vascular space was increased by exercise rather than by heat per se. In addition, we have recently observed that mRNA for albumin synthesis in rats increases in response to hyperos-

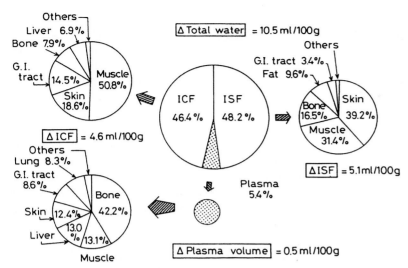

Fig. 2. Water losses from ISF, ICF and plasma compartments and their distribution in various organs of thermally dehydrated rat. Values are mean of seven rats. Based on data from Nose et al. (1983).

molality induced by thermal dehydration (unpublished observation). We have also found that plasma Na^+ concentration increases proportionately with the increase in plasma lactate concentration during exercise of intensities higher than 70% of the maximum aerobic power (Nose et al., 1991). These results suggest that both colloidal and ionic osmotic pressures are involved in the fluid shift from ISF to PV space. In addition, upon isotonic volume loading with physiological saline solution, a greater fraction of the infused saline was retained in the vascular space in hyperthermic than in normothermic dog (Miki et al., 1983a), which suggests that the increase in the vascular bed induced by heat stress is also involved in the retention of plasma fluid in vascular space, as previously reviewed in detail (Morimoto, 1990).

Effects of dehydration on thermoregulation

Adolph et al. (1947) showed a close relationship between water debt and the rise in rectal temperature during desert walking with and without water intake. Their data suggest that dehydration by about 1% of the body weight causes a rise in rectal temperature of about 0.3°C. This rate of increase in rectal temperature associated with dehydration has been confirmed repeatedly by other investigators (Sawka, 1992; Yorimoto et al., 1995). Thermal dehydration causes both osmolality elevation and volume reduction in body fluid. Thus, to study the mechanism responsible for the increase in body temperature in a dehydrated state, the effect of hyperosmolality and hypovolemia should be differentiated.

Hyperosmolality and thermoregulation

It is well recognized that the central nervous system (CNS) plays an important role in thermoregulation (Boulant, 1996). As shown below, results from *in vivo* and *in vitro* experiments have suggested that osmotic factor modulates neural mechanisms for body temperature regulation.

In order to study the relationship between normovolemic hyperosmolality and thermoregulation in human, Fortney et al. (1984) infused 3% saline to dehydrated subjects and induced normovolemic hyperosmolality. An increase in plasma osmolality by about 12 mOsm/kg H_2O induced increases in esophageal temperature threshold for cutaneous vasodilation and sweating, a reduction in the slope of the linear relationship between forearm blood flow and esophageal temperature, and a decrease in maximal exercise blood flow. Recently, this effect of hyperosmolality on thermoregulatory responses was further studied quantitatively (Takamata et al., unpublished data). They modified plasma osmolality by the infusion of saline solutions of various concentrations at different rates, while maintaining a constant blood volume. The increase in plasma osmolality caused a linear increase in the esophageal temperature threshold for cutaneous vasodilation and sweating. The reduction in the maximal level of forearm blood flow also showed a linear reduction as plasma osmolality increased. In addition, water intake in dehydrated human subject eliminated osmotic inhibition of thermal sweating associated with a rapid reduction in plasma vasopressin and thirst before any change in plasma osmolality was observed. This finding suggests that the osmoreceptor which induces thirst and vasopressin secretion is involved in the osmotic inhibition of sweating (Takamata et al., 1995).

Baker and Doris (1982a) showed that in dehydrated cats with hypothalamic thermodes, the rate of evaporation in response to hypothalamic heating was reduced. They also infused hypertonic NaCl solution intravenously and showed lower rates of evaporative heat loss during hypothalamic heating (Baker and Doris, 1982b). In heat-stressed monkeys, a decrease in sweating rate and an increase in rectal temperature have been observed to occur subsequent to infusion of hypertonic artificial cerebrospinal fluid into the third ventricle (Owen et al., 1989).

The above results clearly indicate the osmoregulatory modulation of thermoregulatory responses in hyperthermia (Baker, 1989). In relation to the involvement of osmotic factor in thermoregulation, it may be of interest to note here the reduction in evaporative cooling upon dehydration and resulting elevation in body temperature. This phenomenon, first found in camels by Schmidt-Nielsen et al. (1967), has been reported in ungulates (Taylor, 1970), goats (Dmi'el and

Robertshaw, 1983), and dogs (Baker et al., 1983; Horowitz and Nadel, 1984). Schmidt-Nielsen et al. (1967) pointed out that the body temperature elevation upon dehydration is advantageous in camels, because such a response conserves water during the period of heat storage and reduces heat gain in hot and dry desert condition. In a temperate environment, the elevation of body temperature should be advantageous for heat loss from the body due to the increased temperature gradient between the body and the environment, working in favour of the lower requirement for evaporative heat loss. In addition, it is possible to hypothesize that the reduced evaporation leads to relative lowering of body fluid osmolality and hence decreases the above mentioned hypothalamic responsiveness to elevated body temperature.

The effects of osmotic changes on the activity of preoptic thermosensitive neurons have also been reported. The majority of the response pattern observed is a decreased firing rate of warm-sensitive neurons following hyperosmotic stimuli, applied either locally (Silva and Boulant, 1984; Nakashima et al., 1985) or peripherally (Koga et al., 1987). Hori et al. (1988) and Hori (1991) suggested that hyperosmolality reduces the activity in about half of warm-sensitive neurons and in three quarters of cold-sensitive neurons and that both central and hepatoportal osmoreceptors are involved in their response. In addition, it has been shown that these thermosensitive neurons also respond to changes in blood pressure (Koga et al., 1987). The major pattern of response observed is the excitation of warm-sensitive neurons and the inhibition of cold-sensitive neurons during a fall in blood pressure, causing a lowering of body temperature by increasing heat loss and decreasing heat gain. Hori (1991) suggested that the response of thermosensitive neurons to acute reduction in blood pressure has a critical significance for survival, adapting the organism to impaired blood supply by lowering tissue metabolism via systemic hypothermia.

The finding that thermosensitive neurons respond to both osmotic and blood pressure stimuli suggests a possible interaction between the control mechanisms of body fluid volume and osmolality. Our results on the regulation of drinking behaviour in response to thermal dehydration indicated that osmoregulation precedes the regulation of blood volume (Morimoto et al., 1993; Greenleaf and Morimoto, 1996). The precedence of osmoregulation to volume regulation might be explained by changes in plasma osmolality stimulating the osmoreceptor mechanism directly. On the other hand, hyperosmolality induces a fluid shift from ICF to ECF and compensates for hypovolemia. In addition, cardiovascular responses maintain both arterial and central venous pressures.

Hypovolemia and thermoregulation

In human subjects, during exercise in a hot environment, skin blood flow increases in proportion to the increase in esophageal temperature. The esophageal temperature threshold for cutaneous vasodilation and the attainable maximal skin blood flow are modified by various factors.

Isotonic hypovolemia causes an upward shift of the esophageal temperature threshold for cutaneous vasodilation under the combined stresses of heat and exercise, while isotonic hypervolemia does not influence this threshold. The increase in skin blood flow per unit increase in esophageal temperature is not altered by the reduction in blood volume but the maximal level of attainable forearm blood flow was reduced (Nadel et al., 1980). Mack et al. (1988) applied negative pressure to the lower body of exercising subjects and found reductions of forearm blood flow in proportion to the pressure applied to the lower body and the reduction induced an increase in body temperature. Thermal sweating response to increased body core temperature during exercise was also inhibited by baroreceptor unloading with lower body negative pressure (Mack et al., 1995).

The relationship between esophageal temperature and skin blood flow is affected by other factors, which include posture (Johnson et al., 1974), water immersion (Nielsen et al., 1984),

saline infusion (Nose et al., 1990), and fluid ingestion (Montain and Coyle, 1992). All of these factors cause changes in central venous pressure, and these findings support the involvement of unloading of cardiopulmonary baroreceptors in the vasoconstriction in the forearm observed during exercise in heat (Rowell, 1983). It is of interest that the vasoconstriction in the forearm is observed at around 38°C during exercise in hot environment in humans, much lower than the 40°C observed in anesthetized rats, which might be explained by the increased demand for blood flow to muscle.

Integrated thermoregulation and cardiovascular adjustments

Cardiovascular response to heat load is to maintain cardiac output in response to the increased demand for skin blood flow. However, because thermal dehydration modifies blood volume and its distribution, there is a complicated interaction among body temperature regulation, cardiovascular function, and body fluid homeostasis.

Miki et al. (1983b) elevated body temperature of dogs gradually up to ~ 42°C, and continuously measured cardiovascular responses and changes in blood volume distribution within the body. During moderate hyperthermia up to ~ 40°C, the mean systemic arterial pressure (MAP) was maintained with an increase in cardiac output of about 20%, and this increase was caused by both heart rate and stroke volume. The total peripheral vascular resistance (TPR) decreased linearly with the rise in core temperature, and central venous pressure (CVP) was maintained. When body temperature was further elevated up to ~ 42°C (severe hyperthermia, Fig. 3), CVP showed a gradual fall with the reduction of stroke volume. Although the heart rate was significantly increased by ~ 47 beats/min, cardiac output and TPR were reduced and an abrupt fall in MAP was observed when CVP was lowed by ~ 3 mmHg. The total blood volume determined by ^{51}Cr-RBC dilution method did not change during moderate and severe hyperthermia. The central

504

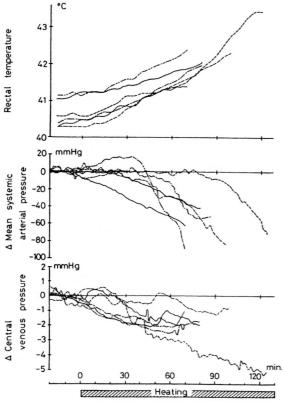

Fig. 3. The time course of rectal temperature, mean systemic arterial and central venous pressures during induced severe hyperthermia in dogs. The values are presented as the differences from the values under moderate hyperthermia. From Miki et al. (1983b).

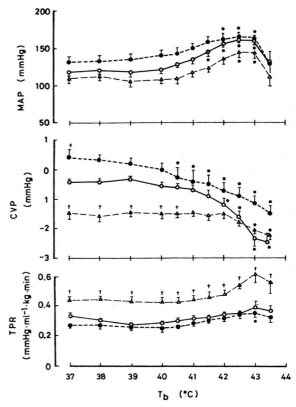

Fig. 4. Mean arterial pressure (MAP), central venous pressure (CVP) and total peripheral resistance (TPR) in response to elevation of body temperature (T_b) in hypervolemia (●), normovolemia (○), and hypovolemia (△). Values are mean and S.E. of six rats. *$P < 0.05$ from value at T_b = 37°C. †$P < 0.05$ from normovolemia. Based on data from Takamata et al. (1990).

blood volume, determined by the indicator mean transit time method, did not change during moderate hyperthermia, while a significant decrease compared with the control value was observed during severe hyperthermia. The systemic blood volume, calculated as the difference between the total blood volume and the central blood volume, increased significantly during severe hyperthermia. These results show that the shift of blood from central circulation to systemic circulation is responsible for the lowering of CVP, and causes the circulatory failure.

To analyze the effect of hydration state on cardiovascular responses to hyperthermia, circu-

latory responses to heat stress were measured in rats at three levels of blood volume: normovolemia (NBV), hypervolemia (HBV, +32% of the plasma volume induced by isotonic albumin solution infusion), and hypovolemia (LBV, −16% of the plasma volume induced by furosemide administration) during body heating at a rate of 0.1°C/min. As shown in Fig. 4, CVP was significantly higher in HBV and lower in LBV than in NBV. CVP started to decrease at ~ 40°C in HBV, ~ 41°C in NBV, and ~ 42°C in LBV, while the value at ~ 43.5°C in HBV was higher than the value of LBV at 37°C. The stroke volume closely correlated with the CVP. The heart rates of the three groups were almost all the same and they increased with the increase in body temperature. MAP showed no significant difference between the groups and was maintained at the preheating level up to ~ 40°C. Above this temperature, MAP increased by 30–40 mmHg up to ~ 43°C in each group. TPR increased at body temperatures higher than 40°C, and was inversely correlated with CVP. The slope of the linear relationship between TPR and CVP in the LBV group was three- to fourfold steeper than those in the NBV and HBV groups (Takamata et al., 1990).

To elucidate the involvement of cardiopulmonary baroreflexes to the regulation of TPR, a similar experiment was performed on vagotomized rats, and the changes in TPR were compared with those in the control rats without vagotomy. Circulatory responses in the group with intact vagus were similar to those in the previous experiment, whereas the responses to the hyperthermia and hypovolemia were reduced in the vagotomized group. The slope of TPR vs. CVP was reduced by about 40% in the vagotomized group compared with that in the control rats (Takamata, 1992).

These results suggest that the control of TPR during hyperthermia is influenced by a fall in CVP, while the heart rate is controlled by heat per se. A similar result has been reported by Kregel et al. (1988), who measured the TPR of the caudal artery of heat-exposed rats, and found that the blood flow, which has important implications for heat dissipation in rats, was increased as the body temperature was increased to 40°C, while it decreased at body temperatures higher than 40°C.

These findings, in combination with various results introduced in the previous section, indicate that, at extremely high body temperatures, excess cutaneous vasodilation is inhibited to maintain CVP and cardiac output, and suggests a possible role of the CVP in the control of TPR. To obtain more direct evidence to support such a role of

cardiopulmonary baroreflex in human subject, we directly measured right atrial pressure (RAP) using a Swan-Ganz catheter during exercise in a hot environment together with forearm blood flow (FBF), and determined the RAP at which FBF leveled off (Nose et al., 1994). Arterial blood temperature (T_b) rose rapidly to 37.7 ± 0.1°C in the first 10 min and then increased gradually to reach 38.6 ± 0.2°C at 50 min of exercise. FBF increased steadily to 10.8 ± 1.7 ml/min in the first 25 min, but thereafter reached a plateau. RAP increased sharply from 4.3 ± 0.8 mmHg to 7.6 ± 1.2 mmHg in the first 5 min but then declined significantly to 6.3 ± 1.0 mmHg at 20 min and subsequently continued to decrease gradually to reach 5.7 ± 1.0 mmHg by the end of exercise. The upper panel of Fig. 5 shows the relationship between T_b and FBF during 50 min of exercise, and the mean values for the five subjects are shown at 5-min intervals during the exercise. The increase in FBF was significantly correlated with the rise in T_b for the first 20 min of exercise ($r = 0.999$, $P < 0.001$) and, above the T_b level of 38.0°C, the slope was reduced and reached a plateau. The lower panel of Fig. 5 shows the relationship between FBF and RAP, and the increase in FBF showed a significant correlation with the decrease in RAP for the first 20 min of exercise ($r = 0.998$, $P < 0.001$). Almost no additional increase in FBF was observed when RAP was lower than 6.3 mmHg. These results suggest an interaction between body temperature and RAP in the leveling-off of FBF. It is certain that changes in RAP are transmitted to CNS via vagal nerve to a considerable extent, as indicated by the analysis of TPR vs. CVP relationship on vagotomized rats (Takamata, 1992). However, further studies are required for identification of this efferent pathway because, in his study, vagotomy induced only a partial reduction (40%) in the TPR vs. CVP relationship.

The above mentioned control of cardiovascular function is also under the influence of osmolality in cerebrospinal fluid (CSF). Recently, we succeeded in measuring continuously the sodium concentration in CSF ($[Na]_{csf}$) by placing a newly

506

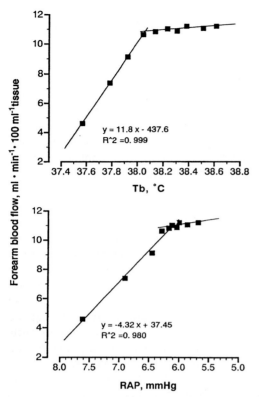

Fig. 5. The relationship between forearm blood flow and blood temperature (T_b) (upper panel) and right arterial pressure (RAP) (lower panel) during 50 min of exercise in a hot environment. Each point represents the mean value for five subjects obtained at 5-min intervals. Note that the forearm blood flow leveled off after 20 min of exercise when T_b reached 38.0°C, and RAP lowered to 6.3 mmHg. Based on data from Nose et al. (1994).

developed Na-sensitive electrode in the lateral ventricle (Nose et al., 1992). Chen (1996) applied this method to examine the effect of $[Na]_{csf}$ on cardiovascular adjustment in thermally dehydrated rats. After dehydration, MAP increased by 20 mmHg, mainly because of the increase in TPR despite a 9% decrease in blood volume, while $[Na]_{csf}$ increased by 13 mequiv./kg H_2O. After the infusion of hypotonic artificial CSF into the lateral ventricle, MAP and $[Na]_{csf}$ decreased and the changes in MAP and TPR were highly correlated with the change in $[Na]_{csf}$, which indicates

the involvement of $[Na]_{csf}$ in the maintenance of MAP during dehydration-induced hypovolemia.

Conclusion

Heat stress causes dehydration due to sweating, leading to hyperosmolality of body fluid and hypovolemia. Dehydration impairs thermoregulation, reducing both sweating and cutaneous vasodilation, while dehydration-induced hyperosmolality causes a shift of body fluid from ICF to ECF and also stimulates drinking behaviour, which counteracts the decrease in blood volume. The redistribution of blood flow for thermoregulation causes a lowering of CVP, which serves as an input signal for drinking behaviour and also for circulatory regulation including increases in total peripheral resistance and vascular compliance. During passive heating, these regulatory responses can maintain circulatory function up to about 40°C, while skin blood flow is restricted at body temperatures higher than 40°C. When increased blood circulation is required, upon exercise in heat for example, the equilibrium temperature is lowered to about 38°C, which causes an elevation of body temperature. These responses suggest a hierarchic structure for the homeostatic mechanism for thermoregulation, body fluid homeostasis, and circulation. Under dehydrated conditions, both hyperosmolality and hypovolemia reduce cutaneous evaporative heat loss and vasodilation. These responses serve to maintain cardiac output, in particular, the cerebral circulation, together with the body fluid shift from ICF and ISF to plasma. The central mechanism to control this subtle balance among body fluid, body temperature, and circulation is not well known.

Because we placed stress on the effect of hyperosmolality and hypovolemia on integrated thermoregulation in this review, other aspects of thermoregulatory mechanisms have not been treated in detail. Intensive reviews recently published should be referred to, for efferent control of cardiovascular adjustments (Johnson and Proppe, 1996), endocrinological responses (Francesconi, 1996), body fluid balance during heat stress (Mack and Nadel, 1996), and physiological responses to severe heat (Hales et al., 1996).

References

Adolph, E.F. et al. (1947) *Physiology of Man in the Desert*, Interscience, New York, pp. 172–196.

Baker, M.A. (1989) Thermoregulation in dehydrated vertebrates. In: M.K. Yousef (Ed.), *Progress in Biometeorology, Vol. 7, Milestones in Environmental Physiology*, SPB Academic Publishing, The Hague, pp. 101–107.

Baker, M.A. and Doris, P.A. (1982a) Effect of dehydration on hypothalamic control of evaporation in the cat. *J. Physiol. (Lond.)*, 322: 457–468.

Baker, M.A. and Doris, P.A. (1982b) Control of evaporative heat loss during changes in plasma osmolality. *J. Physiol. (Lond.)*, 328: 535–545.

Baker, M.A., Doris, P.A. and Hawkins, M.J. (1983) Effect of dehydration and hyperosmolality on thermoregulatory water losses in exercising dogs. *Am. J. Physiol.*, 244: R516–R521.

Boulant, J.A. (1996) Hypothalamic neurons regulating body temperature. In: M.J. Fregly and C.M. Blatteis (Eds.) *Handbook of Physiology, Section 4, Environmental Physiology, Vol. 1*, Oxford University Press, New York, pp. 105–126.

Chen, M. (1996) Na concentration of CSF and cardiovascular adjustment in thermally dehydrated rats. *Jpn. J. Physiol.*, 46: 75–81.

Dmi'el, R. and Robertshaw, D. (1983) The effect of dehydration on the control of panting and sweating in the black bedouin goat. *Physiol. Zool.*, 56: 412–418.

Fortney, S.M., Wenger, C.B., Bove, J.R. and Nadel, E.R. (1984) Effect of hyperosmolality on control of blood flow and sweating. *J. Appl. Physiol.*, 57: 1688–1695.

Francesconi, R.P. (1996) Endocrinological and metabolic responses to acute and chronic heat exposures. In: M.J. Fregly and C.M. Blatteis (Eds.) *Handbook of Physiology, Section 4, Environmental Physiology, Vol. 1*, Oxford University Press, New York, pp. 245–260.

Greenleaf, J.E. and Morimoto, T. (1996) Mechanisms controlling fluid ingestion: thirst and drinking. In: E.R. Buskirk and S.M. Puhl (Eds.), *Body Fluid Balance: Exercise and Sport*, CRC Press, Boca Raton, FL, pp. 3–17.

Hales, J.R.S., Hubbard, R.W. and Gaffin, S.L. (1996) Limitation of heat tolerance. In: M.J. Fregly and C.M. Blatteis (Eds.), *Handbook of Physiology, Section 4, Environmental*

Physiology, Vol. 1, Oxford University Press, New York, pp. 285–355.

Hori, T. (1991) An update on thermosensitive neurons in the brain: from cellular biology to thermal and non-thermal homeostatic functions. *Jpn. J. Physiol.*, 41: 1–22.

Hori, T., Nakashima, T., Koga, H., Kiyohara, T. and Inoue, T. (1988) Convergence of thermal, osmotic and cardiovascular signals on preoptic and anterior hypothalamic neurons in the rat. *Brain Res. Bull.*, 20: 879–885.

Horowitz, M. and Nadel, E.R. (1984) Effect of plasma volume on thermoregulation in the dog. *Pflügers Arch.*, 400: 211–213.

Johnson, J.M. and Proppe, D.W. (1996) Cardiovascular adjustments to heat stress. In: M.J. Fregly and C.M. Blatteis (Eds.), *Handbook of Physiology, Section 4, Environmental Physiology, Vol. 1*, Oxford University Press, New York, pp. 215–243.

Johnson, J.M., Rowell, L.B. and Brengelmann, G.L. (1974) Modification of the skin blood flow-body temperature relationship by upright exercise. *J. Appl. Physiol.*, 37: 880–886.

Koga, H., Hori, T., Inoue, T., Kiyohara, T. and Nakashima, T. (1987) Convergence of hepatoportal osmotic and cardiovascular signals on preoptic thermosensitive neurons. *Brain Res. Bull.*, 19: 109–113.

Kregel, K.C., Wall, P.T. and Gisolfi, C.V. (1988) Peripheral vascular responses to hyperthermia in the rat. *J. Appl. Physiol.*, 64: 2582–2588.

Mack, G.W. and Nadel, E.R. (1996) Body fluid balance during heat stress in humans. In: M.J. Fregly and C.M. Blatteis (Eds.) *Handbook of Physiology, Section 4, Environmental Physiology, Vol. 1*, Oxford University Press, New York, pp. 187–214.

Mack, G., Nose, H. and Nadel, E.R. (1988) Role of cardiopulmonary baroreflexes during dynamic exercise. *J. Appl. Physiol.*, 65: 1827–1832.

Mack, G., Nishiyasu, T. and Shi, X. (1995) Baroreceptor modulation of cutaneous vasodilator and sudomotor responses to thermal stress in humans. *J. Physiol. (Lond.)*, 483: 537–547.

Miki, K., Morimoto, T., Nose, H., Itoh, T. and Yamada, S. (1983a) Canine blood volume and cardiovascular function during hyperthermia. *J. Appl. Physiol.*, 55: 300–306.

Miki, K., Morimoto, T., Nose, H., Itoh, T. and Yamada, S. (1983b) Circulatory failure during severe hyperthermia in dog. *Jpn. J. Physiol.*, 33: 269–278.

Montain, S.J. and Coyle, E.F. (1992) Fluid ingestion during exercise increases skin blood flow independent of increases in blood volume. *J. Appl. Physiol.*, 73: 903–910.

Morimoto, T. (1990) Thermoregulation and body fluids: role of blood volume and central venous pressure. *Jpn. J. Physiol.*, 40: 165–179.

Morimoto, T., Shiraki, K., Miki, K. and Tanaka, Y. (1979)

Effect of exercise and thermal stress on subcutaneous protein transport. *Jpn. J. Physiol.*, 29: 559–567.

Morimoto, T., Miki, K., Nose, H., Yamada, S., Hirakawa, K. and Matsubara, C. (1981) Changes in body fluid volume and its composition during heavy sweating and the effect of fluid and electrolyte replacement. *Jpn. J. Biometeorol.*, 18: 31–39.

Morimoto, T., Nose, H., Sugimoto, E., Yawata, T. and Okuno, T. (1993) Role of sodium chloride in rehydration from thermal dehydration. In: H. Kakihana, H.R. Hardy, Jr., T. Hoshi and K. Toyokura (Eds.) *Seventh Symposium on Salt*, Vol. 2, Elsevier, Amsterdam, pp. 389–393.

Nadel, E.R., Fortney, S.M. and Wenger, C.B. (1980) Effect of hydration state on circulatory and thermal regulations. *J. Appl. Physiol.*, 49: 715–721.

Nakashima, T., Hori, T., Kiyohara, T. and Shibata, M. (1985) Osmosensitivity of preoptic thermosensitive neurons in hypothalamic slices *in vitro*. *Pflügers. Arch.*, 405: 112–117.

Nielsen, B., Rowell, L.B. and Bonde-Petersen, F. (1984) Cardiovascular responses to heat stress and blood volume displacements during exercise in man. *Eur. J. Appl. Physiol.*, 52: 370–374.

Nose, H., Morimoto, T. and Ogura, K. (1983) Distribution of water losses among fluid compartments of tissues under thermal dehydration in the rat. *Jpn. J. Physiol.*, 33: 1019–1029.

Nose, H., Mack, G.W., Shi, X., Morimoto, K. and Nadel, E.R. (1990) Effect of saline infusion during exercise on thermal and circulatory regulations. *J. Appl. Physiol.*, 69: 609–616.

Nose, H., Takamata, A., Mack, G.W., Oda, Y., Okuno, T., Kang, D. and Morimoto, T. (1991) Water and electrolyte balance in the vascular space during graded exercise in humans. *J. Appl. Physiol.*, 70: 2757–2762.

Nose, H., Doi, Y., Usui, S., Kubota, T., Fujimoto, M. and Morimoto, T. (1992) Continuous measurement of Na concentration in CSF during gastric water infusion in dehydrated rats. *J. Appl. Physiol.*, 73: 1419–1424.

Nose, H., Takamata, A., Mack, G.W., Oda, Y., Kawabata, T., Hashimoto, S., Hirose, M., Chihara, E. and Morimoto, T. (1994) Right atrial pressure and forearm blood flow during prolonged exercise in a hot environment. *Pflügers Arch.*, 426: 177–182.

Owen, M.D., Matthes, R.D. and Gisolfi, C.V. (1989) Effect of cerebrospinal fluid hyperosmolality on sweating in the heat-stressed patas monkey. *J. Appl. Physiol.*, 67: 128–133.

Rowell, L.B. (1983) Cardiovascular adjustments to thermal stress. In: J.T. Shepherd and F.M. Abboud (Eds.), *Handbook of Physiology, Section 2, The Cardiovascular System, Vol. 3, Peripheral Circulation and Organ Blood Flow, Part 2*, American Physiological Society, Bethesda, pp. 967–1023.

Sawka, M.N. (1992) Physiological consequences of hypohydration: exercise performance and thermoregulation. *Med. Sci. Sports Exerc.*, 24: 657–670.

Schmidt-Nielsen, K., Schmidt-Nielsen, B., Jarnum, S.A. and Houpt, T.R. (1967) Body temperature of the camel and its relation to water economy. *Am. J. Physiol.*, 188: 103–112.

Senay, L.C., Jr. (1970) Movement of water, protein and crystalloids between vascular and extravascular compartments in heat-exposed men during dehydration and following limited relief of dehydration. *J. Physiol. (Lond.)*, 210: 617–635.

Silva, N.L. and Boulant, J.A. (1984) Effects of osmotic pressure, glucose, and temperature on neurons in preoptic tissue slices. *Am. J. Physiol.*, 247: R335–R345.

Takamata, A. (1992) Effect of vagotomy on cardiovascular adjustment to hyperthermia in rats. *Jpn. J. Physiol.*, 42: 641–652.

Takamata, A., Nose, H., Mack, G.W. and Morimoto, T. (1990) Control of total peripheral resistance during hyperthermia in rats. *J. Appl. Physiol.*, 69: 1087–1092.

Takamata, A., Mack, G.W., Gillen, C.M., Jozsi, A.C. and Nadel, E.R. (1995) Osmoregulatory modulation of thermal sweating in humans: reflex effects of drinking. *Am. J. Physiol.*, 268: R414–R422.

Taylor, C.R. (1970) Dehydration and heat: effects on temperature regulation of East African ungulates. *Am. J. Physiol.*, 219: 1136–1139.

Yorimoto, A., Nakai, S., Yoshida, T. and Morimoto, T. (1995) Relationship between drinking behaviour and body temperature during exercise in heat. *Jpn. J. Phys. Fitness Sports Med.*, 44: 357–364.

Subject Index